Cardiac Arrhythmia: Contemporary Cardiology

Cardiac Arrhythmia: Contemporary Cardiology

Edited by Rowan Cook

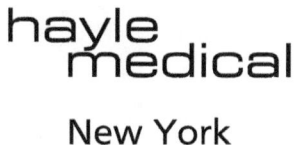

New York

Hayle Medical,
750 Third Avenue, 9th Floor,
New York, NY 10017, USA

Visit us on the World Wide Web at:
www.haylemedical.com

ISBN: 978-1-63241-922-4

Cataloging-in-publication Data

Cardiac arrhythmia : contemporary cardiology / edited by Rowan Cook.
    p. cm.
Includes bibliographical references and index.
ISBN 978-1-63241-922-4
1. Arrhythmia. 2. Heart--Diseases. 3. Heart beat. 4. Cardiology. I. Cook, Rowan.
RC685.A65 C37 2020
616.128--dc23

Table of Contents

Preface

Over the recent decade, advancements and applications have progressed exponentially. This has led to the increased interest in this field and projects are being conducted to enhance knowledge. The main objective of this book is to present some of the critical challenges and provide insights into possible solutions. This book will answer the varied questions that arise in the field and also provide an increased scope for furthering studies.

Cardiac arrhythmia or heart arrhythmia refers to a group of cardiac conditions, which is characterized by an irregular heartbeat. Arrhythmias can be of different types- supraventricular tachycardias, bradyarrhythmias, extra beats and ventricular arrhythmias. Arrhythmias are generally not considered serious but a person may become susceptible to complications such as heart failure or stroke, and cardiac arrest. Some common symptoms of arrhythmia are palpitations, which can be frequent, infrequent or continuous. If an arrhythmia causes a very fast, very slow or weak heartbeat, then lower blood pressure, light-headedness or dizziness are commonly experienced. Cardiac arrhythmias are generally detected during an auscultation of the heartbeat using a stethoscope, or by feeling peripheral pulses. The assessment of a cardiac abnormality using an electrocardiogram allows the diagnosis and evaluation of arrhythmia. Cardiac rhythm management can be achieved through medication, electro-cautery or cryo-cautery or by vagal maneuvres. Drugs such as anticoagulants and antiarrhythmics drugs may be prescribed. This book covers in detail the clinical perspectives in the development of cardiac arrhythmia. Different approaches, evaluations, methodologies and advanced studies on contemporary cardiology have been included herein. This is a collective contribution of a renowned group of international experts.

I hope that this book, with its visionary approach, will be a valuable addition and will promote interest among readers. Each of the authors has provided their extraordinary competence in their specific fields by providing different perspectives as they come from diverse nations and regions. I thank them for their contributions.

Editor

Increased expression of NF-AT3 and NF-AT4 in the atria correlates with procollagen I carboxyl terminal peptide and TGF-β1 levels in serum of patients with atrial fibrillation

Fei Zhao, ShiJiang Zhang, YiJiang Chen, WeiDong Gu, BuQing Ni, YongFeng Shao*, YanHu Wu and JianWei Qin

Abstract

Background: Atrial fibrillation (AF) is the most common cardiac arrhythmia in clinical practice. Unfortunately, the precise mechanisms and sensitive serum biomarkers of atrial remodeling in AF remain unclear. The aim of this study was to determine whether the expression of the transcription factors NF-AT3 and NF-AT4 correlate with atrial structural remodeling of atrial fibrillation and serum markers for collagen I and III synthesis.

Methods: Right and left atrial specimens were obtained from 90 patients undergoing valve replacement surgery. The patients were divided into sinus rhythm (n = 30), paroxysmal atrial fibrillation (n = 30), and persistent atrial fibrillation (n = 30) groups. NF-AT3, NF-AT4, and collagen I and III mRNA and protein expression in atria were measured. We also tested the levels of the carboxyl-terminal peptide from pro-collagen I, the N-terminal type I procollagen propeptides, the N-terminal type III procollagen propeptides, and TGF-β1 in serum using an enzyme immunosorbent assay.

Results: NF-AT3 and NF-AT4 mRNA and protein expression were increased in the AF groups, especially in the left atrium. NF-AT3 and NF-AT4 expression in the right atrium was increased in the persistent atrial fibrillation group compared the sinus rhythm group with similar valvular disease. In patients with AF, the expression levels of nuclear NF-AT3 and NF-AT4 correlated with those of collagens I and III in the atria and with PICP and TGF-β1 in blood.

Conclusions: These data support the hypothesis that nuclear NF-AT3 and NF-AT4 participates in atrial structural remodeling, and that PICP and TGF-β1 levels may be sensitive serum biomarkers to estimate atrial structural remodeling with atrial fibrillation.

Keywords: Atrial fibrillation, Atrial fibrosis, Transcription factor, NF-AT3, NF-AT4, Carboxyl terminal peptide from pro-collagen I, N-terminal type I procollagen propeptides, N-terminal type III procollagen propeptides

Background

Atrial fibrillation (AF) is the most common cardiac arrhythmia in clinical practice [1,2]. Valvular heart disease (VHD), which comprises pathological changes in the mitral or aortic valves, causes AF. Valvular surgery is an option to prevent heart failure in serious VHD patients [3,4]. AF is self-perpetuating because tachyarrhythmia causes electrophysiological and structural changes that exacerbate or maintain AF [5]. This structural remodeling can contribute to both the development and maintenance of AF [6,7]. Several factors associated with atrial structural remodeling have been identified [8], of which atrial fibrosis and myocyte hypertrophy are considered key [9].

Atrial fibrosis is a hallmark of arrhythmogenic structural remodeling [10,11]. Cardiac fibrosis is defined as a detrimental process causing imbalanced extracellular matrix deposition and heart degradation. Cardiac fibrosis causes excessive fibroblast proliferation and accumulation of extracellular matrix proteins in the cardiac

* Correspondence: shaoyongfeng6708@aliyun.com
Cardiothoracic Surgery Department, First Affiliated Hospital of Nanjing
Medical University, 300 Guangzhou RoadJiangsu Province, Nanjing 210029,
China

interstitial space [12]. Expansion of the extracellular matrix between cardiomyocytes may cause conduction delays and create alternate conduction pathways. These changes also result in ectopic foci and anisotropic conduction, creating nonuniform wave fronts that facilitate abnormal reentrant arrhythmias [13]. Unfortunately, the precise mechanisms of atrial remodeling in AF remain unclear.

Atrial structural remodeling consists primarily of collagens I and III, and the process of fibrosis is regulated by a cascade of fibro-proliferative signals, including TGF-β1 and angiotensin II [2,14]. Calcineurin is a Ca^{2+}-calmodulin-activated serine/threonine phosphatase that is ubiquitously expressed and plays an important role in transducing Ca^{2+}-dependent signals. Calcineurin is a heterodimer comprising a calmodulin binding catalytic subunit A and a Ca^{2+} binding regulatory subunit B. Calcineurin is required for activation of transcription and induction of cell hypertrophy in a number of cell types including cardiac myocytes [15,16]. Activation of calcineurin was reported to be increased in atrial tissues of patients with AF [17]. Calcineurin dephosphorylates NF-AT3 and NF-AT4, which induces their translocation from the cytosol to the nucleus where they activate the transcription of their target genes [17-19]. Transgenic mice that constitutively express calcineurin in cardiomyocytes can develop cardiac hypertrophy and a concomitant accumulation of collagen deposits surrounding the degenerating cardiomyocytes [19-21]. Calcineurin inhibitors such as cyclosporin A and FK506 can inhibit TGF-β1 expression to block increased extracellular matrix protein accumulation [22]. Furthermore, a constitutively active NF-AT 3 and NF-AT4 expressed in the hearts of transgenic mice produced cardiac wall fibrosis and cardiac myocyte enlargement, demonstrating the importance of a calcium-calcineurin-NF-AT3 pathway in cardiac fibrosis and hypertrophy [19].

The transcription factors NF-AT3 and NF-AT4 are the downstream effectors of calcineurin, and play an important role in the calcineurin-dependent pathway during cardiac hypertrophy [19,23]. Recent studies also directly and indirectly implicate the calcineurin-dependent pathway in the development of cardiac fibrosis [19,20,24,25]. In addition, the N-terminal propeptides of collagen types I or III (PINP and PIIINP, respectively) and the C-terminal propeptides (PICP) in the blood have been reported to be useful markers of collagen type I or III synthesis [26].

In the present study, we examined the correlation between nuclear NF-AT3 and NF-AT4 expression and distribution with collagens I and III expression levels in diseased atrial tissues of patients with AF. We also examined the correlations between serum levels of TGF-β1, PINP, PIIINP, and PICP with NF-AT3 and NF-AT4 expression in the nucleus and with collagen I and III expression in atrial tissues. In patients with AF, we found that the expression levels of nuclear NF-AT3 and NF-AT4 correlated with those of collagens I and III in the atria and with PICP and TGF-β1 in blood.

Methods
Patients
We recruited 90 VHD patients, comprising pathological changes in the mitral or aortic valves, or both, admitted to the First Affiliated Hospital of Nanjing Medical University for valve replacement surgery from January 2012 to January 2013. The patients were divided into three groups: sinus rhythm (SR; *n = 30*), persistent AF (PeAF; AF lasting >6 month, *n = 30*), and paroxysmal AF (PaAF; recurrent AF that terminated spontaneously in <7 days, *n = 30*). The control group (*n = 10*) comprised patients with congenital heart disease and SR who underwent heart surgery. We excluded four categories of patients from this study: (i) patients with renal dysfunction (serum creatinine >136 µmol/L) or Type II diabetes, (ii) patients whose coronary angiography and echocardiographic evaluation indicated coronary artery bypass grafting or associated procedures, (iii) patients >70 years, or those with a history of some diseases (e.g., hyperthyroidism) that influence AF risk, and (iv) patients with fibrosis disease that could affect serum fibrosis biomarkers. Preoperative medications, except warfarin and angiotensin-converting enzyme inhibitors, were continued until the morning of the surgery. Prior to surgery, an investigator assessed the preoperative clinical characteristics of the patients. Before discharge, another investigator recorded detailed operative data. The Ethics Committee of Nanjing Medical University approved the study protocol, and all patients provided written consent prior to enrollment. The investigation adhered to the principles outlined in the Declaration of Helsinki.

Human cardiac tissue collection and storage
The same cardiac anesthesiologist, perfusionist, and surgical team performed all surgeries. All patients underwent cardiopulmonary bypass with moderate hypothermia (33–34°C). Antegrade crystalloid cardioplegia was used to arrest the heart, and local hypothermia was maintained with ice slush. A cardioplegic solution was readministered every 20–30 min. Approximately 250 mg of right atrial appendage (RAA) tissue was collected from the cannulation site, and approximately 250 mg of left atrial appendage (LAA) tissue was collected in the PeAF and PaAF group before initiating extracorporeal circulation. In our department, LAA ligation and resection is a routine surgical maneuver in rheumatic valvular disease patients with AF. To minimize damage, we only collected LAA samples from the AF group; this surgical maneuver was not necessary in the SR group. The sample site was

similar because of similar surgical maneuvers. A 50 mg portion of RAA and LAA tissue was fixed in 4% paraformaldehyde for histology and immunohistochemistry. The remaining tissue was snap-frozen in liquid nitrogen for other analyses.

Reverse transcription-polymerase chain reaction (RT-PCR)

Total RNA was isolated from the atrial tissue samples and treated with RNase-free water according to the TRIzol® (Invitrogen, Carlsbad, CA, USA) method. Single-stranded cDNA was synthesized from the total RNA as follows. In brief, 2 μg RNA was preincubated with 1.5 μL oligo $(dT)_{18}$ primer (10 μmol/L; Genscript Technology Co., Nanjing, China), and diethylpyrocarbonate (DEPC)-treated water (0.1% DEPC; Keygen, China) in a total volume of 10 μL. This solution was incubated at 70°C for 10 min and then rapidly chilled on ice. The reaction was initiated by incubation at 42°C for 1 h in a Multigene™ Gradient TC9600-G-230 V thermal cycler (Labnet International Inc., Edison, NJ, USA) and was deactivated at 70°C for 15 min, followed by immersion in ice. The resultant cDNA was used as a template for subsequent PCR. Thirty cycles of PCR amplification were performed, with initial incubation at 94°C for 5 min and final extension at 72°C for 5 min. Each cycle comprised denaturation at 94°C for 30 s, annealing at 55°C for 30 s, and extension at 72°C for 30 s. The collagen I, collagen III, NF-AT3, and NF-AT4 genes were amplified using the following specific primers: *collagenI* (sense: 5′- TTCCTGC GCCTGATGTCC –3′, antisense: 5′- GGTTCAGTTTGG GTTGCTTGT –3′); *collagenIII* (sense: 5′- TCAACACC GATGAGATTATGAC –3′, antisense: 5′- CAAAGGATT GGCACTTATGC –3′); *NF-AT3* (sense: 5′- GGGACAAC AGAACCAGAGTAAC –3′, antisense: 5′- AAACAGAAT AGTCCACCTTGAGA –3′); *NF-AT4* (sense: 5′- TTGGA ACACCAGCCATCAGG –3′, antisense: 5′- GCTGCTC CTGTTCTTTTGCC –3′). The quantities of cDNA that produced an equal amount of GAPDH PCR product were used for PCR using the primers for *collagenI, collagenIII, NF-AT3,* and *NF-AT4*. PCR product levels were semiquantitatively determined using a digital camera and an image analysis system (Gel Doc™ XR; Bio-Rad, Hercules, CA, USA), followed by normalization against GAPDH expression.

Western blotting

In preparation of whole tissue extracts, atrial tissue samples were homogenized on ice in RIPA lysis buffer (Thermo Fisher Scientific Inc, Rockford, IL USA). Lysates were incubated on ice for 10 min at 4°C and subsequently centrifuged at $9300 \times g$ for 10 min. Supernatants were saved and stored at –70°C. Nuclear extracts were prepared as follows [17]. Approximately 250 mg of atrial tissue was washed with cold PBS, homogenized, and resuspended in 1 ml of hypotonic buffer. Homogenates were incubated for 10 min on ice and centrifuged (10 min, $800 \times g$ at 4°C). Pellets were resuspended in 0.15 ml of hypertonic buffer and incubated on ice for 20 min. Samples were centrifuged (10 min, $13\,000 \times g$ at 4°C), and supernatants (nuclear protein extract) were stored in aliquots at –80°C. Protein concentrations were determined using the Lowry method, and absorbance was measured spectrophotometrically (UV 2540; Shimadzu, Kyoto, Japan). Denatured samples were subjected to western blotting as follows. Samples containing 25 μg of protein were electrophoretically separated on a 10% SDS-polyacrylamide gel for 1.5 h at 120 V, and the proteins were transferred to nitrocellulose membranes (Pall Corporation, Ann Arbor, MI, USA). After blocking in 5% fat-free milk, the membranes were incubated overnight at 4°C with primary antibodies (dilution) against collagen I (1:200, Biosynthesis Biotechnology Company, Inc., Beijing, China), collagen III (1:200, Bioss), NF-AT3 [1:1000; Cell Signaling Technology Inc., USA], and NF-AT4 (1:1000; Cell Signaling Technology). Anti-GAPDH (1:1000; Cell Signaling Technology Inc.) and anti-lamin B (1:1000; Cell Signaling Technology Inc.) polyclonal antibodies were used as controls to normalize the data. The membranes were then incubated for 2 h at 37°C with secondary antibodies (goat anti-rabbit IgG diluted in PBS containing 5% fat-free milk and 0.1% Tween-20). The stained membranes were visualized using enhanced chemiluminescence with the ECL Plus reagent (GE Healthcare, Chalfont St. Giles, Buckinghamshire, UK). Western blotting was repeated at least thrice per sample with similar results.

Blood sampling and enzyme-linked-immunosorbent serologic assay (ELISA)

Venous blood samples were obtained in EDTA from every patient before surgery. Serum was separated by centrifugation ($1800 \times g$, 5 min, room temperature), and stored at –80°C until analysis. Serum PIIINP, PINP, TGF-β1, and PICP levels were determined by sensitive ELISA kits (Senxiong Biotechnology Industry Inc., Shanghai, China), according to the manufacturer's instructions. Assays were performed in duplicate in a single run and normalized to a standard curve.

Histology and immunohistochemistry

RAA and LAA samples were fixed with 4% paraformaldehyde in phosphate-buffered saline (pH 7.4) for 24 h. After alcohol dehydration, the tissues were embedded in paraffin and sectioned. The 2-μm-thick serial sections were then stained with Van Gieson's solution for microscopic examination. For NF-AT3 and NF-AT4 (Biosis) detection, immunoreactivity was performed on 4-μm-thick sections of the paraffin-embedded tissues. Brown staining in the cells or cell membranes was considered positive. Hypertrophic heart ventricle tissues were selected as a positive control, and negative controls were sections incubated with antibodies pre-absorbed with the NF-AT3 and NF-AT4 peptide (Abcam). The entire sections were scanned at low magnification (×100) initially to select regions, and then high magnification (×400) was used for focused investigation.

Statistical analyses

Values are expressed as the mean ± standard deviation. Differences among three or more groups were analyzed using the Kruskal–Wallis test. Differences between any two groups were analyzed using the Mann–Whitney U test. Chi-square and Fisher's exact tests were used to determine the differences between the groups. Univariate regression tests were used to assess the associations

Table 1 Analysis of clinical data

	SR + CHD	SR + VHD	PaAF + VHD	PeAF + VHD
Patient number	10	30	30	30
Sex, M/F (n)	4/6	16/14	13/17	12/18
Age (years)	16.20 ± 3.31	54.75 ± 3.68	55.61 ± 6.83	53.58 ± 4.63
Preoperative data				
Heart rate (beats/min)	102.4 ± 4.51	79 ± 6.00	81 ± 7.00	83 ± 9.20
NYHA class I/II/III/IV	2/7/1/0	0/12/10/8	0/7/13/10	0/5/12/13
Echocardiographic parameters				
LVDd	34 ± 2.30	53.55 ± 8.70	55.66 ± 14.13	54.97 ± 12.36
LVDs	24 ± 3.11	36.38 ± 1.26	39 ± 10.22	34.13 ± 11.03
EF (%)	64 ± 4.12	55.01 ± 4.80	53.08 ± 5.32	52.21 ± 5.21
LAD (mm)	23 ± 6.73	47.25 ± 5.19[c]	55.43 ± 6.80[a,c]	59.23 ± 5.92[b,c]
RAD (mm)	27 ± 8.71	38.40 ± 5.20	38.10 ± 4.64	38.20 ± 5.00
Preoperative length of stay	10.00 ± 9.36	15.00 ± 1.80	16.00 ± 11.53	16.00 ± 13.40
Valve disease				
Pure MVD	0	12	15	12
Mitral stenosis		4	5	6
Mitral regurgitation		5	6	2
Mitral stenoregurgitation		3	4	4
Pure AVD	0	10	6	5
Aortic valve stenosis		6	3	1
Aortic valve regurgitation		4	3	4
DVD	0	8	9	13
Preoperative drug				
Digitalis	0	18	28	30
Diuretic	4	22	24	28
Nitrate drug	0	26	23	27
Calcium channel blocker	0	10	12	11
β-blocker	3	10	22	30
ACEI	0	19	21	18
Operative data				
Surgical procedure				
MVR/AVR/DVR	0/0/0	12/10/8	15/6/9	12/5/13
CPB duration	78 ± 11.44	130 ± 12.42	141 ± 23.44	145 ± 13.23
Aortic clamp time	45.32 ± 33.32	79 ± 34.43	82 ± 35.26	90 ± 42.13

Data are presented as n or mean ± standard deviation.
AVD, aortic valve disease; CHD, Congenital heart disease; DVD, Double valvular disease (mitral and aortic valves); MVD, Mitral valvular disease; PaAF, Paroxysmal atrial fibrillation; PeAF, Persistent atrial fibrillation; SR, Sinus rhythm; VHD, Valvular heart disease.
[a]PaAF + VHD vs. SR + VHD; $P < 0.01$. [b]PeAF + VHD vs. SR + VHD; $P < 0.01$. [c]LAD vs. RAD; $P < 0.01$.

Table 2 PIIINP, PINP, PICP, and TGF-β1 blood levels

	PeAF + VHD (n = 30)	PaAF + VHD (n = 30)	SR + VHD (n = 30)	SR + CHD (n = 10)
PIIINP (ng/ml)	88.03 ± 46.08[b,c]	72.96 ± 43.30[d]	52.50 ± 29.32[e]	14.09 ± 2.732
PINP (ng/ml)	45.41 ± 42.17[c]	34.82 ± 28.60	18.95 ± 17.34	6.940 ± 3.007
TGF-β1 (pg/ml)	49.01 ± 28.67[a,b,c]	27.96 ± 13.16[d]	24.09 ± 14.10	11.43 ± 2.695
PICP (ng/ml)	43.42 ± 3.699[a,b,c]	36.06 ± 7.710[d]	29.75 ± 9.241[e]	12.52 ± 3.033

Data are presented as n or mean ± standard deviation.
CHD, Congenital heart disease; PaAF, Paroxysmal atrial fibrillation; PeAF, Persistent atrial fibrillation; PICP, carboxyl-terminal peptide from pro-collagen I; PINP,
N-terminal type I procollagen propeptides; PIIINP, N-terminal type III procollagen propeptides; SR, Sinus rhythm; VHD, Valvular heart disease.
[a]PeAF + VHD vs. PaAF + VHD; P < 0.05. [b]PeAF + VHD vs. SR + VHD; P < 0.05. [c]PeAF + VHD vs. SR + CHD; P < 0.05. [d]PaAF + VHD vs. SR + CHD; P < 0.05. [e]SR + VHD vs. SR + CHD; P < 0.05.

among the expression of NF-AT3 and NF-AT4 in the nucleus, collagens I and III in atrial tissue, and PINP, PIIINP, PICP, and TGF-β1 in the blood. Differences yielding p <0.05 were considered significant. Data were analyzed using GraphPad Prism version 5.01 and STATA version 10.0.530.0.

Results
Clinical characteristics and hemodynamic data
Preoperative hemodynamic and echocardiographic data are shown in Table 1. Statistical analysis showed that left atrial diameter, measured by echocardiography, was significantly larger in the PeAF group than in the SR group. Furthermore, the left atrial diameter was significantly larger than the right atrial diameter in all groups, except for the control group. Right atrial diameters, left ventricular end systolic dimensions (LVDs), and left ventricular end diastolic dimensions were not significantly different among the three VHD groups. The constituent ratios of patients with different heart functions were not significantly different among the three VHD groups.

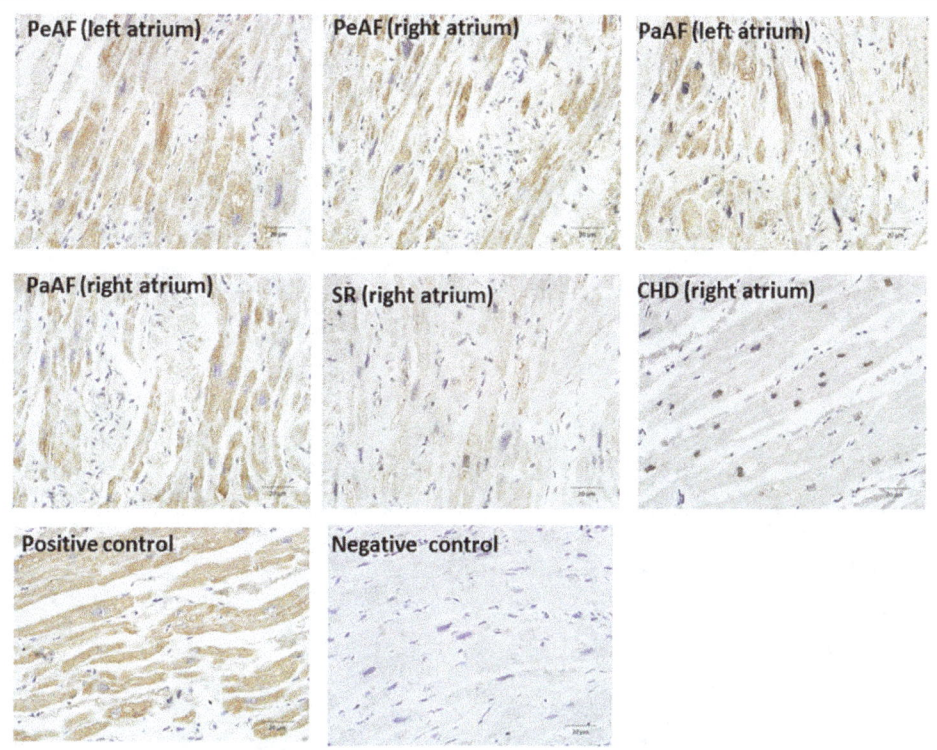

Figure 1 Immunohistochemistry for NF-AT3 (stained brown) in sections obtained from the CHD (right atrium), SR (right atrium), PaAF (right atrium), PaAF (left atrium), PeAF (right atrium), and PeAF (left atrium) groups. Nuclei are in blue. Elevated levels of NF-AT3 in the right and left atrial tissues were identified in the PeAF groups compared with the SR and CHD groups. Hypertrophic heart ventricle tissues were selected as a positive control, and negative controls were sections incubated with antibodies pre-absorbed with the NF-AT3 and NF-AT4 peptide. Magnification (×400). CHD, Congenital heart disease; SR, Sinus rhythm; PaAF, Paroxysmal atrial fibrillation; PeAF, Persistent atrial fibrillation; NF-AT3, Nuclear factor of activated T cells 3; NF-AT4, Nuclear factor of activated T cells 4.

Serum PINP, PIIINP, PICP, and TGF-β1 levels were increased in the AF groups

The levels of PICP and TGF-β1 were significantly increased in the PeAF group compared with the PaAF and SR groups. However, there were no differences in PIIINP levels between the PeAF and PaAF groups, while PIIINP levels in the PeAF group were only significantly higher than those in the SR group. Levels of PINP in the PeAF group were significantly greater than those in the control group, while there were no differences in PINP levels between the PeAF and the other groups (Table 2).

Expression of collagen I, collagen III, NF-AT3, and NF-AT4 mRNA and protein were increased in the AF groups

Immunohistochemistry showed that total NF-AT3 (Figure 1) and NF-AT4 (Figure 2) expression were upregulated in the AF groups compared with the SR and control groups. We also demonstrated that collagen I, collagen III, total NF-AT3, and NF-AT4 expression were upregulated in the AF groups using RT-PCR and western blotting (Figure 3A,B; Figure 4A,B). We also demonstrated that nuclear NF-AT3 and NFAT4 expression was upregulated in the AF group compared with the SR group (Figure 5A,B).

Analysis of the expression of NF-AT3 and NF-AT4 and collagens I and III in the right and left atria of patients with AF

In the left atrium of patients with AF, collagen I mRNA expression was not correlated with NF-AT3 and NF-AT4 mRNA expression. Collagen I protein expression was positively correlated with nuclear NF-AT3 expression (p <0.01), but not with nuclear NF-AT4 expression. Levels of collagen III mRNA expression were positively correlated with NF-AT4 mRNA expression (p < 0.01), but not with NF-AT3 expression. Collagen III protein expression was positively correlated with nuclear NF-AT3 (p <0.01) and nuclear NF-AT4 expression (p <0.01).

In the right atrium of patients with AF, collagen I mRNA expression was correlated with NF-AT3 (p <0.01) and NF-AT4 mRNA expression (p <0.01). Collagen I expression was correlated with nuclear NF-AT3 expression (p <0.01), but not with nuclear NF-AT4 expression. Collagen III mRNA expression was correlated with NF-AT3 (p <0.01) and NF-AT4 mRNA expression (p <0.01).

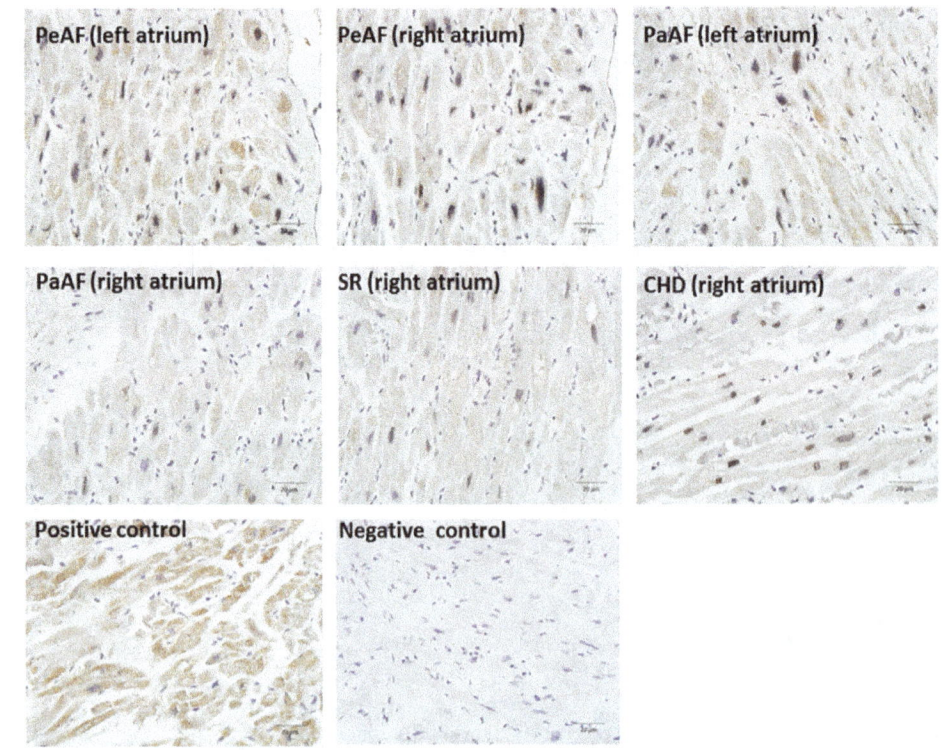

Figure 2 Immunohistochemistry for NF-AT4 (stained brown) in sections obtained from the CHD (right atrium), SR (right atrium), PaAF (right atrium), PaAF (left atrium), PeAF (right atrium), and PeAF (left atrium) groups. Nuclei are in blue. Elevated levels of NF-AT3 in the right and left atrial tissues were identified in the PeAF groups compared with the SR and CHD groups. Hypertrophic heart ventricle tissues were selected as a positive control, and negative controls were sections incubated with antibodies pre-absorbed with the NF-AT3 and NF-AT4 peptide. Magnification (×400). CHD, Congenital heart disease; NF-AT3, Nuclear factor of activated T cells 3; NF-AT4, Nuclear factor of activated T cells 4; PaAF, Paroxysmal atrial fibrillation; PeAF, Persistent atrial fibrillation; SR, Sinus rhythm.

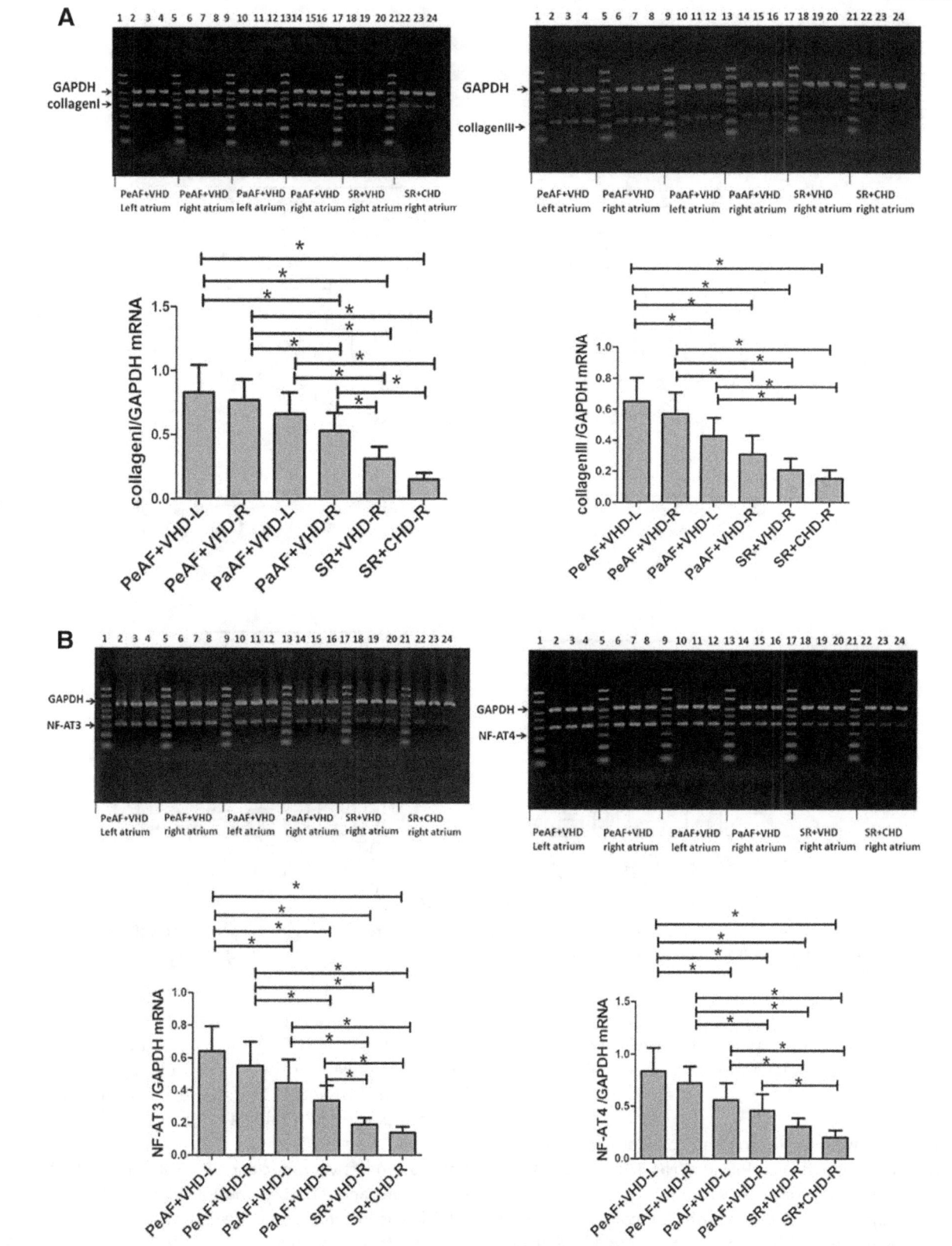

Figure 3 Collagen I,collagen III,NF-AT3 and NF-AT4 mRNA expression in the different groups (A) Collagen I and collagen III mRNA expression in the different groups. *P < 0.05. **(B)** NF-AT3 and NF-AT4 mRNA expression in the different groups. *P < 0.05. GAPDH indicates a representative blot. NF-AT3, Nuclear factor of activated T cells 3; NF-AT4, Nuclear factor of activated T cells 4.

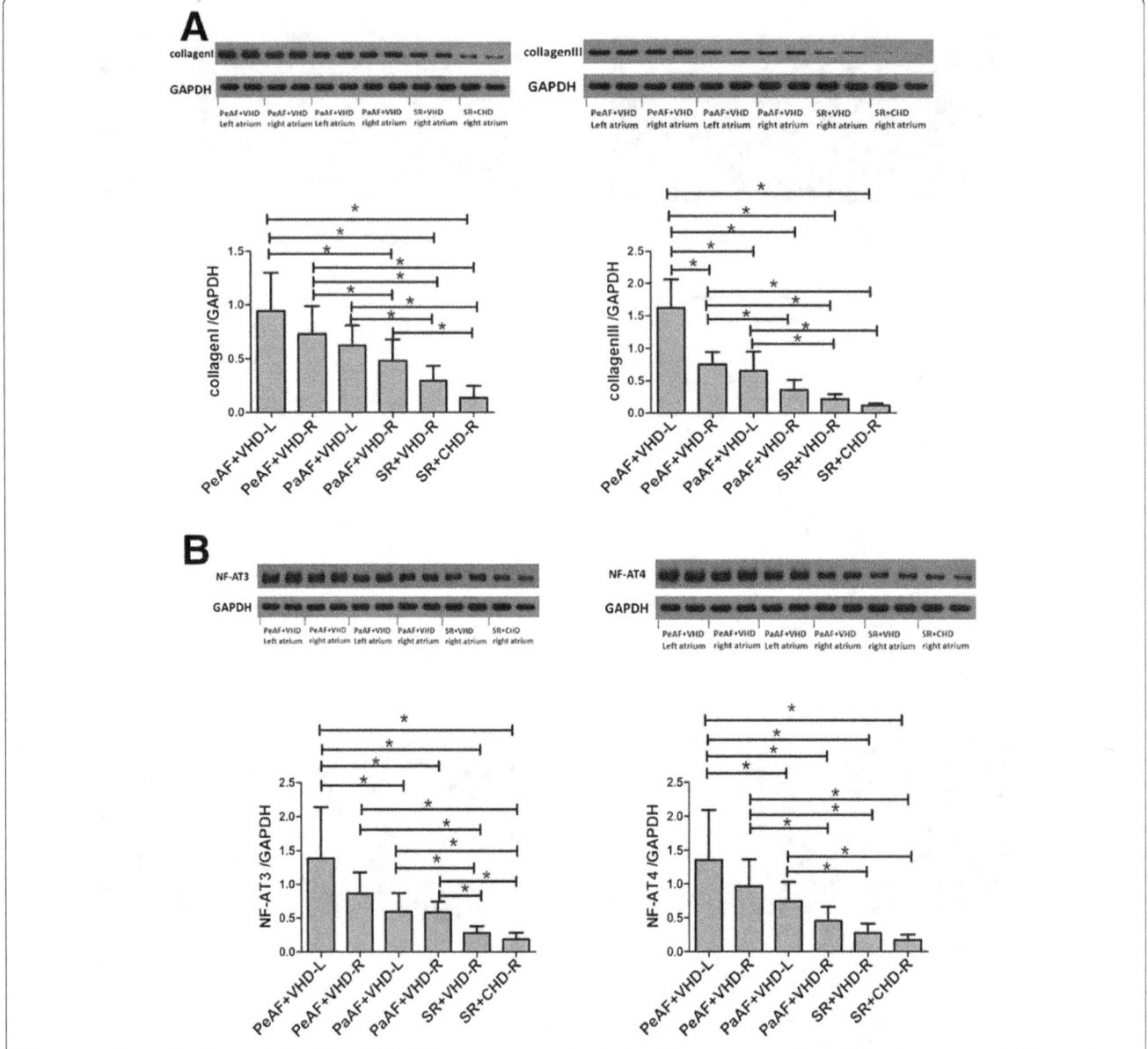

Figure 4 Collagen I,collagen III,NF-AT3 and NF-AT4 protein expression in the different groups (A) Collagen I and collagen III protein expression in the different groups. P < 0.05. **(B)** NF-AT3 and NF-AT4 protein expression in the different groups. *P < 0.05. GAPDH indicates a representative blot. NF-AT3, Nuclear factor of activated T cells 3; NF-AT4, Nuclear factor of activated T cells 4.

Collagen III expression was correlated with nuclear NF-AT3 expression (p <0.01) and nuclear NF-AT4 (p <0.01) (Table 3).

Correlation between collagen I and collagen III levels in the right and left atria with PIIINP, PINP, TGF-β1, and PICP levels in the blood of patients with AF

In the left atrium of patients with AF, collagen I levels were correlated with PICP (p = 0.001) and PINP levels (p = 0.003), but not with TGF-β1 levels. The level of collagen III was correlated with PIIINP (p <0.001) and TGF-β1 levels (p = 0.0042). Collagen I levels were

correlated with PICP (p = 0.019) and TGF-β1 levels (p <0.05), while there was no correlation of collagen III levels with PIIINP and TGF-β1 levels in the right atrium of patients with AF (Table 4).

Correlation between nuclear NF-AT 3 and NF-AT 4 levels in the right and left atria and PIIINP, PINP, TGF-β1, and PICP levels in the blood of patients with AF

In the left atrium of patients with AF, nuclear NF-AT3 levels were correlated with PICP (p <0.01) and TGF-β1 levels (p <0.01), while nuclear NF-AT4 levels correlated with PICP (p <0.01) and TGF-β1 levels (p <0.05). In the

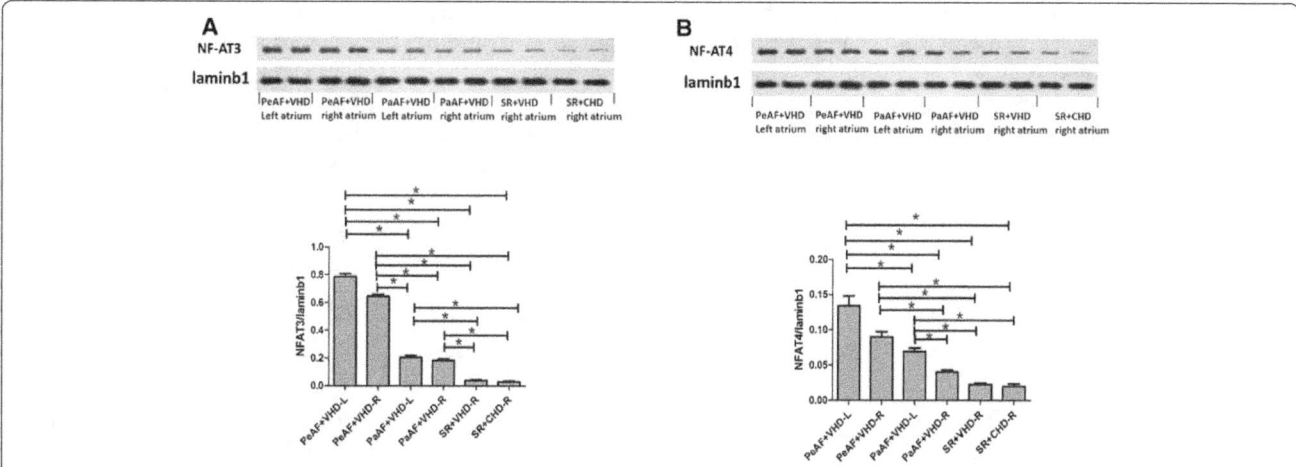

Figure 5 Nuclear NF-AT3 and Nuclear NF-AT4 protein expression in the different groups (A) Nuclear NF-AT3 protein expression in the **different groups.** *P < 0.05. **(B)** Nuclear NF-AT4 protein expression in the different groups. *P < 0.05. Laminb1 indicates a representative blot. NF-AT3, Nuclear factor of activated T cells 3; NF-AT4, Nuclear factor of activated T cells 4.

right atrium of patients with AF, nuclear NF-AT3 levels were correlated with PICP (p <0.01) and TGF-β1 levels (p <0.01), while nuclear NF-AT4 levels correlated with PINP (p <0.01) and PICP levels (p <0.05 (Table 5).

Analysis of NF-AT3 and NF-AT4 protein expression in the right atria of patients with different valvular disease
In the right atrium, the total NF-AT3 expression in patients in the AF group was higher than that in patients

Table 3 Correlation between expression of collagens and nuclear NF-AT3 and NF-AT4 in the left and right atria of patients with atrial fibrillation mRNA

		NF-AT3	NF-AT4
Collagen I mRNA	Left atrium	NF-AT3 mRNA	NF-AT4 mRNA
		Not significant	Not significant
	Right atrium	NF-AT3 mRNA	NF-AT4 mRNA
		r = 0.351, P < 0.01	r = 0.412, P < 0.01
Collagen III mRNA	Left atrium	NF-AT3 mRNA	NF-AT4 mRNA
		Not significant	r = 0.354, P < 0.01
	Right atrium	NF-AT3 mRNA	NF-AT4 mRNA
		r = 0.526, P < 0.01	r = 0.420, P < 0.01
		NF-AT3	**NF-AT4**
Collagen I protein	Left atrium	NF-AT3 protein	NF-AT4 protein
		r = 0.447, P < 0.01	No significant
	Right atrium	NF-AT3 protein	NF-AT4 protein
		r = 0.469, P < 0.01	Not significant
Collagen III protein	Left atrium	NF-AT3 protein	NF-AT4 protein
		r = 0.774, P < 0.01	r = 0.421, P < 0.01
	Right atrium	NF-AT3 protein	NF-AT4 protein
		r = 0.740, P < 0.01	r = 0.404, P < 0.01

NF-AT3, Nuclear factor of activated T cells 3; NF-AT4, Nuclear factor of activated T cells 4.

in the SR group with mitral valve disease (MVD). NF-AT3 expression in patients in the PeAF group was higher than that in patients in the PaAF and SR groups with double-valve disease (DVD) (p <0.05). The total NF-AT3 expression in patients in the AF group was higher than that in those in the SR group with aortic valve disease (AVD) (p <0.05). NF-AT3 expression in patients with MVD and DVD was higher than those with AVD in the PeAF group, while NF-AT3 expression in patients with MVD was higher than in those with DVD or AVD in the PaAF group (p <0.05). NF-AT3 expression in patients with MVD was higher than those with DVD or AVD in the SR group (p <0.05). NF-AT4 expression in patients in the PeAF group was higher than those in the PaAF and SR groups with MVD, while NF-AT4 expression in the PeAF group was higher than those in the PaAF and SR groups with DVD (p <0.05). NF-AT4 expression in patients in the PeAF group was higher than those in the SR group with AVD (p <0.05). NF-AT4 expression in patients with MVD and DVD was

Table 4 Correlation between serum fibrosis biomarkers and collagen levels in the right and left atria of patients with atrial fibrillation

		Fibrosis biomarker	
Collagen I	Left atrium	PICP	PINP
		r = 0.386, P = 0.001	r = 0.423, P = 0.003
	Right atrium	PICP	TGF-β1
		r = 0.336, P = 0.019	r = 0.258, P < 0.05
Collagen III	Left atrium	TGF-β1	PIIINP
		r = 0.469, P < 0.001	r = 0.291, P = 0.042
	Right atrium	Not significant	Not significant

PICP, carboxyl-terminal peptide from pro-collagen I; PINP, N-terminal type I procollagen propeptides; PIIINP, N-terminal type III procollagen propeptides.

Table 5 Correlation between markers of serum fibrosis and levels of nuclear NF-AT3 and NF-AT4 in the right and left atria of patients with atrial fibrillation

		Fibrosis biomarker	
Nuclear	Left atrium	PICP	TGF-β1
NF-AT3		r = 0.538, P < 0.01	r = 0.444, P < 0.01
	Right atrium	PICP	TGF-β1
		r = 0.538, P < 0.01	r = 0.387, P < 0.01
Nuclear	Left atrium	PICP	TGF-β1
NF-AT4		r = 0.282, P < 0.01	r = 0.324, P < 0.05
	Right atrium	PICP	PINP
		r = 0.264, P < 0.05	r = 0.316, P < 0.01

NF-AT3, Nuclear factor of activated T cells 3; NF-AT4, Nuclear factor of activated T cells 4; PICP, carboxyl-terminal peptide from pro-collagen I; PINP, N-terminal type I procollagen propeptides.

higher than those with AVD in the PeAF group, while NF-AT4 expression in patients with MVD was higher than those with AVD in the PaAF group (p <0.05). NF-AT4 expression in patients with MVD and DVD was higher than those with AVD in the SR group (p <0.05; Table 6).

Discussion

Atrial structural remodeling underlies AF development [8]. AF can cause structural remodeling that can exacerbate or maintain AF [5], while valvular disease also can induce atrial remodeling. However, the precise mechanisms of atrial remodeling in AF remain unclear. The development of sensitive serum biomarkers reflecting atrial remodeling may provide a simple method to determine the presence of atrial remodeling, allowing initiation of timely therapeutic interventions. In the present study, we determined that total NF-AT3 and NF-AT4 expression was increased in the PeAF group (particularly in the left atrium) and the AF group.

As dilated atria caused by valvular disease can affect atrial fibrosis and induce expression of related proteins, comparisons of left atria between the PeAF and SR groups may be confounded differences in left atrial sizes. By contrast, right atrial diameters were not significantly different between the three groups, and were thus considered suitable for studying the direct effects of AF on atrial remodeling. In the right atria, we found that NF-AT3 and NF-AT4 expression was increased in the PeAF group compared with that in the SR group with similar valvular disease. Moreover, NF-AT3 and NF-AT4 expression in patients with pure mitral valvular disease was increased compared with that in patients with pure aortic valvular disease in the PeAF, PaAF, and SR groups. These data suggest that expression of NF-AT3 and NF-AT4 are altered by atrial fibrillation and valvular disease (particularly MVD). Thus, atrial fibrillation may be an

Table 6 Protein expression of total NF-AT3 and NF-AT4 in right atria with different valvular disease in different group

NF-AT3

	PeAF group (n = 30)	PaAF group (n = 30)	SR group (n = 30)
MVD	0.990 ± 0.398[a,b,g] (n = 12)	0.695 ± 0.147[i,j] (n = 15)	0.313 ± 0.109[k,l] (n = 12)
DVD	0.880 ± 0.183[c,d,h] (n = 13)	0.516 ± 0.053 (n = 9)	0.331 ± 0.050 (n = 10)
AVD	0.522 ± 0.039[e,f] (n = 5)	0.396 ± 0.048 (n = 6)	0.170 ± 0.071 (n = 8)

NF-AT4

	PeAF group (n = 30)	PaAF group (n = 30)	SR group (n = 30)
MVD	1.109 ± 0.375[a,b,f] (n = 12)	0.559 ± 0.222[h] (n = 15)	0.332 ± 0.147[i] (n = 12)
DVD	1.010 ± 0.379[c,d,g] (n = 13)	0.415 ± 0.112 (n = 9)	0.331 ± 0.132[j] (n = 10)
AVD	0.492 ± 0.109[e] (n = 5)	0.244 ± 0.054 (n = 6)	0.158 ± 0.018 (n = 8)

Data are presented as n or mean ± standard deviation.
AVD, aortic valve disease; MVD, Mitral valvular disease; DVD, Double valvular disease (mitral and aortic valves); PaAF, Paroxysmal atrial fibrillation; PeAF, Persistent atrial fibrillation; SR, Sinus rhythm.
[a]MVD + PeAF group vs. MVD+ SR group; P < 0.05. [b]MVD + PaAF group vs. MVD + SR group; P < 0.05. [c]DVD + PeAF group vs. DVD + SR group; P < 0.05. [d]DVD + PeAF group vs. DVD + PaAF group; P < 0.05. [e]AVD + PeAF group vs. AVD + SR group; P < 0.05. [f]AVD + PaAF group vs. AVD + SR group P < 0.05. [g]MVD + PeAF group vs. AVD + PeAF group; P < 0.05. [h]DVD + PeAF group vs. AVD + PeAF group; P < 0.05. [i]MVD + PaAF group vs. AVD + PaAF group; P < 0.05. [j]MVD + PaAF group vs. DVD + PaAF group P < 0.05. [k]MVD + SR group vs. AVD + SR group; P < 0.05. [l]DVD + SR group vs. AVD + SR group; P < 0.05. DVD: Double valve disease; MVD: Mitral valve disease; AVD: Aortic valve disease.

important factor affecting NF-AT3/4 expression and atrial remodeling.

We also found a significant relationship between the expression of collagen and nuclear NF-AT3 and NF-AT4 (Table 6). Collagens I and III are secreted as pro-collagen precursors containing amino- and carboxyl-terminal propeptides, which are released into the serum by proteases after collagen deposition [27]. The N-terminal propeptides of collagen I or III (PINP and PIIINP, respectively) and the C-terminal propeptides (PICP) are used as markers of collagen type I or III synthesis [26]. We demonstrated that serum PINP, PIIINP, and PICP were increased in the PeAF group. Final analyses showed that PINP (PIN, r = 0.423 > PICP, r = 0.386) and TGF-β1 (TGF-β1, r = 0.469 > PIIINP, r = 0.291) were sensitive fibrosis biomarkers for the left atria of AF patients, while PICP (PICP, r = 0.336 > TGF-β1, r = 0.258) was a sensitive fibrosis biomarker for the right atria. To establish the extent of right and left atrial fibrosis, PICP and TGF-β1 are likely the most sensitive fibrosis biomarkers. We also found that serum PICP and TGF-β1 levels were the optimal biomarkers for indicating the effect of nuclear NF-AT3 and NF-AT4 on atrial fibrosis in patients with AF. Nuclear NF-AT3 expression in the right and left atria correlated significantly with PICP and TGF-β1 levels in the blood of patients with AF. Nuclear NF-AT4 levels in left atria correlated significantly with PICP and TGF-β1 levels, while those in the right atria correlated significantly with PICP and PINP levels in the blood of patients with AF. Therefore, we conclude that PICP and TGF-β1 may be useful serum fibrosis biomarkers to estimate the extent of atrial remodeling due to atrial fibrillation or other risk factors.

Conclusion

We demonstrate that NF-AT3 and NF-AT4 expression were increased in patients with atrial fibrillation. Furthermore, nuclear NF-AT3 and NF-AT4 expression were correlated significantly with levels of collagen I and III l in the atrium and with PICP and TGF-β1 levels in the blood. These data support the hypothesis that nuclear NF-AT3 and NF-AT4 participates in atrial structural remodeling, and that PICP and TGF-β1 levels may be sensitive serum biomarkers to estimate atrial structural remodeling. However, because there are many risk factors for AF, the mechanism of NF-AT3 and NF-AT4 expression in atrial structural remodeling requires further investigation.

Abbreviations
AF: Atrial fibrillation; AVD: Aortic valve disease; CHD: Congenital heart disease; DVD: Double valvular disease (mitral and aortic valves); MVD: Mitral valvular disease; NF-AT3: Nuclear factor of activated T cells 3; NF-AT4: Nuclear factor of activated T cells 4; PaAF: Paroxysmal atrial fibrillation; PeAF: Persistent atrial fibrillation; PICP: Carboxyl-terminal peptide from pro-collagen I; PIIINP: N-terminal type III procollagen propeptides; PINP: N-terminal type I procollagen propeptides; SR: Sinus rhythm; VHD: Valvular heart disease.

Competing interests
The authors declare that they have no competing interests.

Authors' contributions
ZF and SYF carried out the molecular genetic studies, participated in the sequence alignment and drafted the manuscript. NBQ and GWD carried out the immunoassays. ZSJ and CYJ participated in the design of the study and performed the statistical analysis. WY and QJW conceived of the study, and participated in its design and coordination and helped to draft the manuscript. All authors read and approved the final manuscript.

Acknowledgments
We thank Dr Jinhua Luo, Bin Zhang, Quan Zhu, and Sheng Zhao for their constructive suggestions and comments. We thank the members of the Keygen Biotechnology Institute for helpful comments. The authors thank Edanz for editorial assistance.

References
1. Wyse DG, Gersh BJ: Atrial fibrillation: a perspective: thinking inside and outside the box. *Circulation* 2004, **109**:3089–3095.
2. Burstein B, Nattel S: Atrial fibrosis: mechanisms and clinical relevance in atrial fibrillation. *J Am Coll Cardiol* 2008, **51**:802–809.
3. Ross J Jr: Left ventricular function and the timing of surgical treatment in valvular heart disease. *Ann Intern Med* 1981, **94**:498–504.
4. Otto CM: Valvular aortic stenosis: disease severity and timing of intervention. *J Am Coll Cardiol* 2006, **47**:2141–2151.
5. Wyse DG, Waldo AL, DiMarco JP, Domanski MJ, Rosenberg Y, Schron EB, Kellen JC, Greene HL, Mickel MC, Dalquist JE, Corley SD: A comparison of rate control and rhythm control in patients with atrial fibrillation. *N Engl J Med* 2002, **347**:1825–1833.
6. Lin CS, Pan CH: Regulatory mechanisms of atrial fibrotic remodeling in atrial fibrillation. *Cell Mol Life Sci* 2008, **65**:1489–1508.
7. Kostin S, Klein G, Szalay Z, Hein S, Bauer EP, Schaper J: Structural correlate of atrial fibrillation in human patients. *Cardiovasc Res* 2002, **54**:361–379.
8. Iwasaki YK, Nishida K, Kato T, Nattel S: Atrial fibrillation pathophysiology: implications for management. *Circulation* 2011, **124**:2264–2274.
9. Mazzini MJ, Monahan KM: Pharmacotherapy for atrial arrhythmias: present and future. *Heart Rhythm* 2008, **5**:S26–31.
10. Li D, Fareh S, Leung TK, Nattel S: Promotion of atrial fibrillation by heart failure in dogs: atrial remodeling of a different sort. *Circulation* 1999, **100**:87–95.
11. Allessie M, Ausma J, Schotten U: Electrical, contractile and structural remodeling during atrial fibrillation. *Cardiovasc Res* 2002, **54**:230–246.
12. Weber KT, Brilla CG: Pathological hypertrophy and cardiac interstitium. Fibrosis and renin-angiotensin-aldosterone system. *Circulation* 1991, **83**:1849–1865.
13. Eckstein J, Verheule S, de Groot NM, Allessie M, Schotten U: Mechanisms of perpetuation of atrial fibrillation in chronically dilated atria. *Prog Biophys Mol Biol* 2008, **97**:435–451.
14. Swartz MF, Fink GW, Sarwar MF, Hicks GL, Yu Y, Hu R, Lutz CJ, Taffet SM, Jalife J: Elevated pre-operative serum peptides for collagen I and III synthesis result in post-surgical atrial fibrillation. *J Am Coll Cardiol* 2012, **60**:1799–1806.
15. Palmer S, Groves N, Schindeler A, Yeoh T, Biben C, Wang CC, Sparrow DB, Barnett L, Jenkins NA, Copeland NG, Koentgen F, Mohun T, Harvey RP: The small muscle-specific protein Csl modifies cell shape and promotes myocyte fusion in an insulin-like growth factor 1-dependent manner. *J Cell Biol* 2001, **153**:985–998.
16. Miyashita T, Takeishi Y, Takahashi H, Kato S, Kubota I, Tomoike H: Role of calcineurin in insulin-like growth factor-1-induced hypertrophy of cultured adult rat ventricular myocytes. *Jpn Circ J* 2001, **65**:815–819.
17. Bukowska A, Lendeckel U, Hirte D, Wolke C, Striggow F, Rohnert P, Huth C, Klein HU, Goette A: Activation of the calcineurin signaling pathway induces atrial hypertrophy during atrial fibrillation. *Cell Mol Life Sci* 2006, **63**:333–342.
18. Diedrichs H, Hagemeister J, Chi M, Boelck B, Muller-Ehmsen J, Schneider CA: Activation of the calcineurin/NFAT signalling cascade starts early in human hypertrophic myocardium. *J Int Med Res* 2007, **35**:803–818.
19. Molkentin JD, Lu JR, Antos CL, Markham B, Richardson J, Robbins J, Grant SR, Olson EN: A calcineurin-dependent transcriptional pathway for cardiac hypertrophy. *Cell* 1998, **93**:215–228.
20. Berry JM, Le V, Rotter D, Battiprolu PK, Grinsfelder B, Tannous P, Burchfield JS, Czubryt M, Backs J, Olson EN, Rothermel BA, Hill JA: Reversibility of adverse, calcineurin-dependent cardiac remodeling. *Circ Res* 2011, **109**:407–417.
21. Dickhout JG, Carlisle RE, Austin RC: Interrelationship between cardiac hypertrophy, heart failure, and chronic kidney disease: endoplasmic reticulum stress as a mediator of pathogenesis. *Circ Res* 2011, **108**:629–642.
22. Islam M, Burke JF Jr, McGowan TA, Zhu Y, Dunn SR, McCue P, Kanalas J, Sharma K: Effect of anti-transforming growth factor-beta antibodies in cyclosporine-induced renal dysfunction. *Kidney Int* 2001, **59**:498–506.
23. Shibasaki F, Price ER, Milan D, McKeon F: Role of kinases and the phosphatase calcineurin in the nuclear shuttling of transcription factor NF-AT4. *Nature* 1996, **382**:370–373.
24. Shimoyama M, Hayashi D, Takimoto E, Zou Y, Oka T, Uozumi H, Kudoh S, Shibasaki F, Yazaki Y, Nagai R, Komuro I: Calcineurin plays a critical role in pressure overload-induced cardiac hypertrophy. *Circulation* 1999, **100**:2449–2454.
25. Herum KM, Lunde IG, Skrbic B, Florholmen G, Behmen D, Sjaastad I, Carlson CR, Gomez MF, Christensen G: Syndecan-4 signaling via NFAT regulates extracellular matrix production and cardiac myofibroblast differentiation in response to mechanical stress. *J Mol Cell Cardiol* 2013, **54**:73–81.

2

Very early recurrence predicts long-term outcome in patients after atrial fibrillation catheter ablation

Yangjing Xue[1†], Xiaoning Wang[3†], Saroj Thapa[1], Luping Wang[4], Jiaoni Wang[1], Zhiqiang Xu[1], Shaoze Wu[1], Luyuan Tao[1], Guoqiang Wang[1], Lu Qian[1], Lianming Liao[5], Baohua Liu[2*] and Kangting Ji[1*]

Abstract

Background: Long-term recurrence (LR) is a tendency that re-occurs within 3 months after catheter ablation for atrial fibrillation (AF). Whether very early recurrence (VER) within 7 days of post ablation is a prognostic factor of LR or not is unclear. For this reason, present study sought to examine the relationship between VER and LR.

Methods: In this prospective analysis 378 consecutive patients underwent an initial catheter ablation for paroxysmal or persistent AF. The association between VER and LR was analyzed by univariate and multivariate Cox regression, as well as time-dependent receiver operator characteristic (ROC) analysis.

Results: After a mean follow-up of 14.71 ± 8.58 months, 81 (65.90%) patients with VER experienced LR and were associated with lower event of free survival from LR (Log rank test, $P < 0.001$). Multivariate Cox regression analysis revealed that VER (HR = 7.02, 95% CI = 4.78–10.31; $P < 0.001$), left atrial enlargement (HR = 2.92, 95% CI = 1.88–4.54; $P < 0.001$), tendency in advanced age (HR = 1.50, 95% CI = 0.99–2.28; $P = 0.054$), and tendency in male (HR = 0.71, 95% CI = 0.50–1.01; $P = 0.060$) were independent predictors of LR. According to time-dependent ROC analysis, it was found that VER was more sensitive than common risk factors in predicting LR (0.74 vs 0.66, $P < 0.001$) and combination model further improved the C statistic for predicting LR (0.82 vs 0.66, $P < 0.001$).

Conclusions: After a single procedure of catheter ablation, patients with VER were strongly associated with LR and combination of VER and common risk factors could further improve prediction of patients who were at high risk for LR.

Keywords: Atrial fibrillation, Catheter ablation, Very early recurrence, Long-term recurrence

Background

Catheter ablation is the mainstay therapy for atrial fibrillation (AF), but the high rate of long-term recurrence (LR) is a limitation of the procedure. Non-paroxysmal AF, sleep apnea, obesity, left atrial enlargement, advanced age, hypertension, left atrial fibrosis and recurrence of AF within the first 3 months after catheter ablation have been identified to be the LR predictors [1–14]. Among them, recurrence of AF within the first 3 months is considered to be the most important predictor of long-term treatment failure [5–14]. Based on these studies, a so-called blanking period, the duration ranging from the first 7 days to 3 months post ablation, is proposed [5–15].

In the clinical practice, it has been found that lots of patients had episodes of AF as early as 7 days of post ablation. In the present study, it was aimed to examine the relationship of recurrence within 7 days, which we defined as very early recurrence (VER), and LR after 3 months. We hypothesized that VER was a prognostic factor of LR after 3 months.

* Correspondence: bhbh3699999@163.com; jikt@wzmc.edu.cn
†Equal contributors
²Department of Rehabilitation, the Second Affiliated Hospital and Yuying Children's Hospital of Wenzhou Medical University, Xueyuanxi Road, No 109, Wenzhou, Zhejiang 325000, China
¹Department of Cardiology, the Second Affiliated Hospital and Yuying Children's Hospital of Wenzhou Medical University, Xueyuanxi Road, No 109, Wenzhou, Zhejiang 325000, China
Full list of author information is available at the end of the article

Methods

This prospective study included 378 consecutive patients with paroxysmal (n = 168) or persistent (n = 210) AF who underwent an initial ablation at the Second Affiliated hospital and Yuying Children's Hospital of Wenzhou Medical University, from January 2013 and December 2014.

Paroxysmal AF is defined as AF that terminates spontaneously or under anti-arrhythmic drugs (AADs) within 7 days of onset. Persistent AF is defined as continuous AF sustaining for more than 7 days. Patients were excluded if they aged <20, had pregnancy, prior cardiac surgery, implanted pacemaker, chronic renal

Table 1 Baseline characteristics of the Patients[a]

Variables	Total	Long-term recurrence		P-value
	N = 378	Without N = 255	With N = 123	
Age, years	65.37 ± 10.44	63.69 ± 10.40	68.85 ± 9.68	<0.001
Age ≥ 65 years, n (%)	222 (58.70%)	131 (51.40%)	91 (74.00%)	<0.001
Male, n (%)	215 (56.90%)	156 (61.20%)	59 (48.00%)	0.015
BMI, kg/m^2	24.43 ± 3.08	24.07 ± 3.00	25.17 ± 3.15	0.001
Type of AF				
Paroxysmal, n (%)	168 (44.40%)	128 (50.20%)	40 (32.50%)	0.001
Persistent, n (%)	210 (55.60%)	127 (49.80%)	87 (67.50%)	0.001
Duration of AF, months	32.11 ± 44.82	33.44 ± 48.54	29.37 ± 35.91	0.409
Hypertension, n (%)	223 (59.00%)	141 (55.30%)	82 (66.70%)	0.035
Systolic BP, mmHg	135.17 ± 20.83	134.39 ± 21.27	136.80 ± 19.88	0.291
Diastolic BP, mmHg	82.94 ± 51.28	81.76 ± 42.34	85.39 ± 66.21	0.520
Diabetes, n (%)	56 (14.80%)	30 (11.80%)	26 (21.10%)	0.016
FBG, mmol/L	5.14 ± 1.15	5.09 ± 1.02	5.26 ± 1.39	0.117
History of HF, n (%)	46 (12.20%)	20 (7.80%)	26 (21.10%)	<0.001
Left ventricular EF, %	63.48 ± 7.52	63.82 ± 7.35	62.78 ± 7.85	0.211
Left atrial dimension, mm	40.82 ± 6.41	39.50 ± 5.72	43.56 ± 6.91	<0.001
Left atrial ≥50 mm, n (%)	39 (10.30%)	13 (5.10%)	26 (21.10%)	<0.001
Moderate valvular heart disease, n (%)	6 (1.60%)	3 (1.20%)	3 (2.40%)	0.357
CAD, n (%)	26 (6.90%)	12 (4.70%)	14 (11.40%)	0.016
Prior Stroke/TIA, n (%)	49 (13.00%)	31 (12.20%)	18 (14.60%)	0.502
CHADS2 Score	1.34 ± 1.19	1.17 ± 1.10	1.71 ± 1.30	<0.001
CHA2DS2-VASc Score	2.81 ± 1.81	2.49 ± 1.70	3.48 ± 1.83	<0.001
HAS-BLED Score	2.47 ± 1.06	2.32 ± 1.02	2.79 ± 1.07	<0.001
CRP within 24 h post-procedure, mg/dL	6.36 ± 10.27	6.38 ± 10.87	6.32 ± 8.94	0.954
Medication at hospital discharge				
Oral anticoagulant				
Warfarin, n (%)	297 (78.57%)	194 (76.10%)	103 (83.70%)	0.089
Dabigatran, n (%)	73 (19.31%)	54 (21.20%)	19 (15.40%)	0.186
Xa inhibitor, n (%)	8 (2.12%)	7 (2.70%)	1 (0.80%)	0.221
Statins, n (%)	269 (71.20%)	174 (68.20%)	95 (77.20%)	0.070
ACEI/ARB, n (%)	169 (44.70%)	103 (40.40%)	66 (53.70%)	0.015
Beta-blockers, n (%)	111 (29.40%)	70 (27.50%)	41 (33.30%)	0.239
Vaughan Williams class I or III AAD, n (%)	342 (90.50%)	235 (92.20%)	107 (87.00%)	0.109
Amiodarone, n (%)	328 (86.80%)	228 (89.40%)	100 (81.30%)	0.029
Propafenon, n (%)	14 (3.70%)	7 (2.70%)	7 (5.70%)	0.155

BMI body mass index, *AF* atrial fibrillation, *FBG* fasting blood glucose, *HF* heart failure, *EF* ejection fraction, *CAD* coronary artery disease, *TIA* transient ischemic attack, *CRP* C-reactive protein, *AAD* anti-arrhythmia drug

[a]Plus-minus values are means ± SD. Percentages do not sum to 100 because of rounding

failure requiring hemodialysis, and severe mitral valve disease. All patients gave written informed consent and the study protocol was approved by our institutional review board.

For every patient, step-wise ablation strategy was performed, including circumferential pulmonary vein isolation (PVI), complex fractionated atrial electrograms, and linear ablation. The electrophysiological evaluation of PVI was bi-directional conduction block between left atria (LA) and pulmonary veins (PVs). Whether to perform additional ablation including tricuspid valve isthmus ablation, continuous fractionated atrial electrogram ablation, and LA linear ablation was decided by the operator and/or the attending physician. The ablation procedure followed the method described by Liu X et al. [16, 17].

After the ablation procedure, patients remained hospitalized under continuous electrocardiography monitoring for at least 7 days. Patients received 24 h Holter monitoring at 3, 6 and 12 months follow-ups after procedure and every 12 months thereafter. Among follow-ups, all patients were encouraged to visit doctors for ECGs or Holter monitoring for any symptoms suggestive of AT onset.

AADs continued for 1–3 months after the ablation procedure. LR was defined as any asymptomatic or symptomatic atrial tachyarrhythmia (AT) lasting >30s off AADs after the initial 3-month blanking period. VER was defined as sustained AT (lasting >30s) on or off AADs recurred within 7 days post ablation.

Statistical analysis

Depending on the distribution, the continuous data were presented as median (25th–75th percentiles) or as mean ± SD. Categorical data were presented as counts or proportions. The differences between groups were assessed with the χ^2 test or Fisher's exact test for categorical data and the nonparametric Wilcoxon rank-sum test or Student test for continuous data.

Factors associated with recurrence arrhythmia during follow-ups were assessed in univariate and multivariable Cox proportional hazard models. Factors with P values <0.1 in univariate analyses were included in stepwise multivariate Cox regression models. Time-dependent receiver operator characteristic (ROC) curve analysis was generated to test the predictive discrimination of patients with or without LR. A two-tailed value of $P < 0.05$ was considered to indicate the statistical significance.

Results

Baseline characteristics of patients are summarized in Table 1. AF was paroxysmal in 168 (44.44%) patients and persistent in 210 (55.56%). Only 6 patients had moderate valvular heart disease. Risk of thromboembolic (CHADS2 and CHADS-VASc Score) and bleeding (HAS-BLED Score) complications were both significantly high in patients with LR. Warfarin usage at hospital discharge tended to be more frequent in patients with LR ($P = 0.089$). Advanced age (age ≥ 65 years), female gender, increased BMI, persistent AF, hypertension, diabetes, history of heart failure (HF), decreased left ventricular ejection fraction (EF), left atrial enlargement (left atrial ≥50 mm), statins usage, and ACEI/ARB usage were significantly more frequent in patients with LR.

After a single ablation procedure, 112 patients (29.63%) experienced VER within the first 7 days post ablation while LR cumulatively occurred in 123 (32.54%) patients after the initial 3-month blanking period.

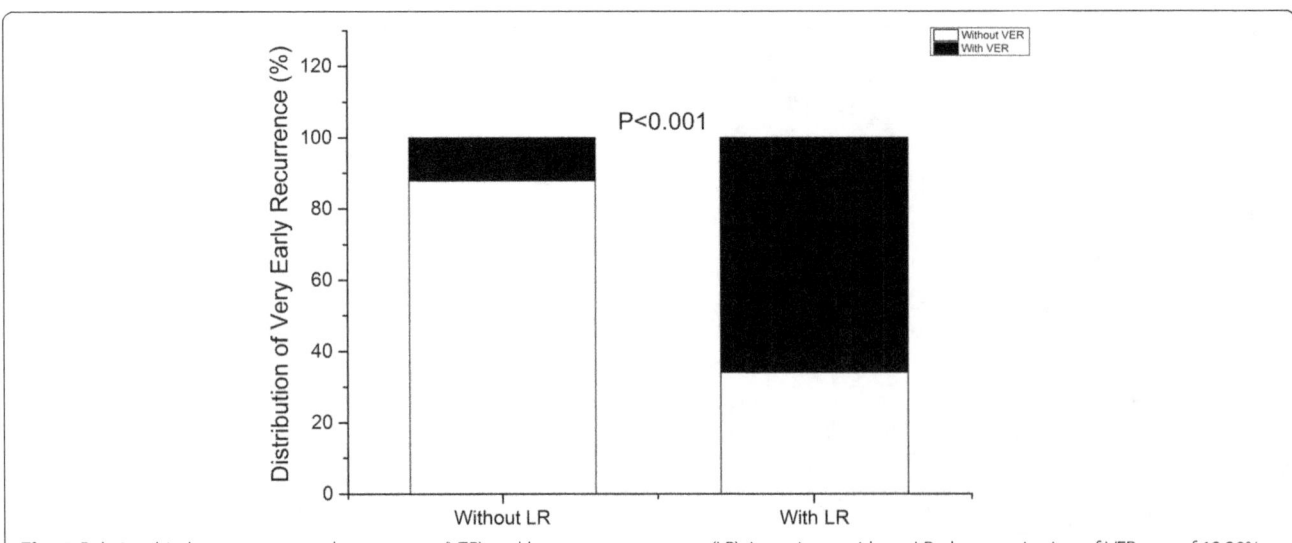

Fig. 1 Relationship between very early recurrence (VER) and long-term recurrence (LR). In patients without LR, the constitution of VER was of 12.20%; In patients with LR, the constitution of VER was of 65.90%

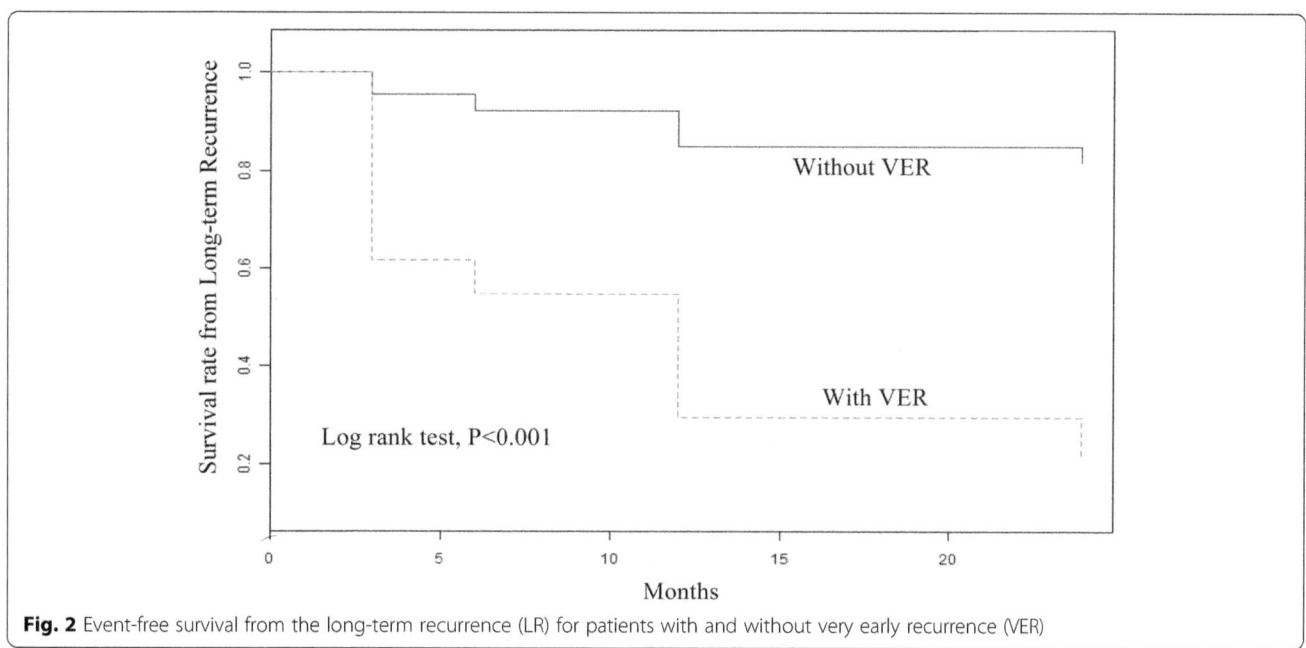

Fig. 2 Event-free survival from the long-term recurrence (LR) for patients with and without very early recurrence (VER)

Among these 112 patients with VER, 81 (65.90%) patients experienced LR (Fig. 1).

Figure 2 shows the event-free survival from the LR for patients with and without VER within 7 days. After a mean follow-up of 14.71 ± 8.58 months, patients with VER were associated with LR (Log rank test, $P < 0.001$).

Univariate Cox analysis was performed and identified that VER was associated with LR ($P < 0.10$), and similarly to the factors including advanced age (age ≥ 65 years), BMI, persistent AF, duration of AF, hypertension, diabetes, history of heart failure, left ventricular EF, left atrial enlargement, ACEI/ARB usage. In multivariable Cox regression analysis, independent predictors of LR in this study were VER (HR = 7.02, 95% CI = 4.78–10.31; $P < 0.001$), left atrial enlargement (HR = 2.92, 95% CI = 1.88–4.54; $P < 0.001$), tendency in advanced age (age ≥ 65 years) (HR = 1.50, 95% CI = 0.99–2.28; $P = 0.054$), and tendency in male (HR = 0.71, 95% CI = 0.50–1.01; $P = 0.060$) (Table 2).

To further assess the potential prognostic value of VER in predicting cumulative LR, we performed time-dependent ROC analysis. C statistic for VER was significantly greater than model based on established common risk factors (left atrial enlargement, age ≥ 65, male) in

this study (0.74 vs 0.66, $P < 0.001$) (Fig. 3). When VER was combined with the established common risk factors, VER improved the C statistic (0.82 vs 0.66, $P < 0.001$), indicating that the combination of VER with common risk factors has a greater potential to predict LR (Fig. 4).

Discussion

The major findings of this study are as follows; after a single procedure of catheter ablation for paroxysmal or

Table 2 The results of the multivariable Cox regression analysis of the independent correlates for the LR

Parameters	OR	95% CI Low	95% CI Upp	P-value
VER	7.02	4.78	10.31	<0.001
Left atrial enlargement	2.92	1.88	4.54	<0.001
Advanced age	1.50	0.99	2.28	0.054
Male	0.71	0.50	1.01	0.060

LR Long-term recurrence, *VER* Very Early Recurrence

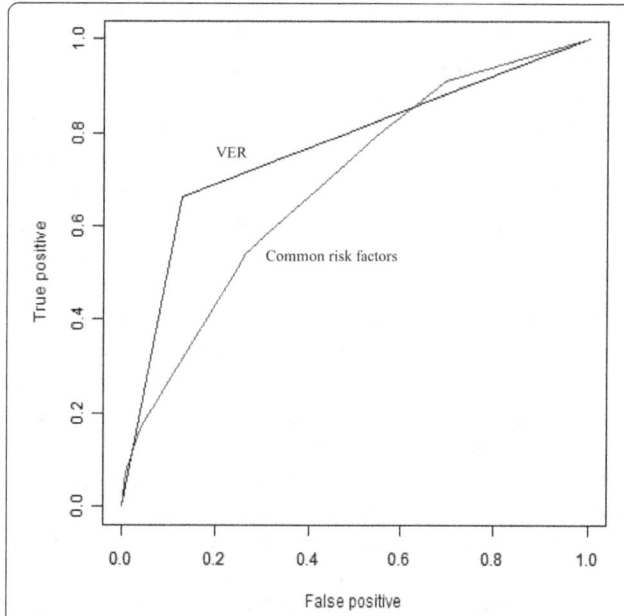

Fig. 3 Time-dependent ROC analysis based on very early recurrence (VER) and established common risk factors (0.74 vs 0.66, $P < 0.001$), respectively

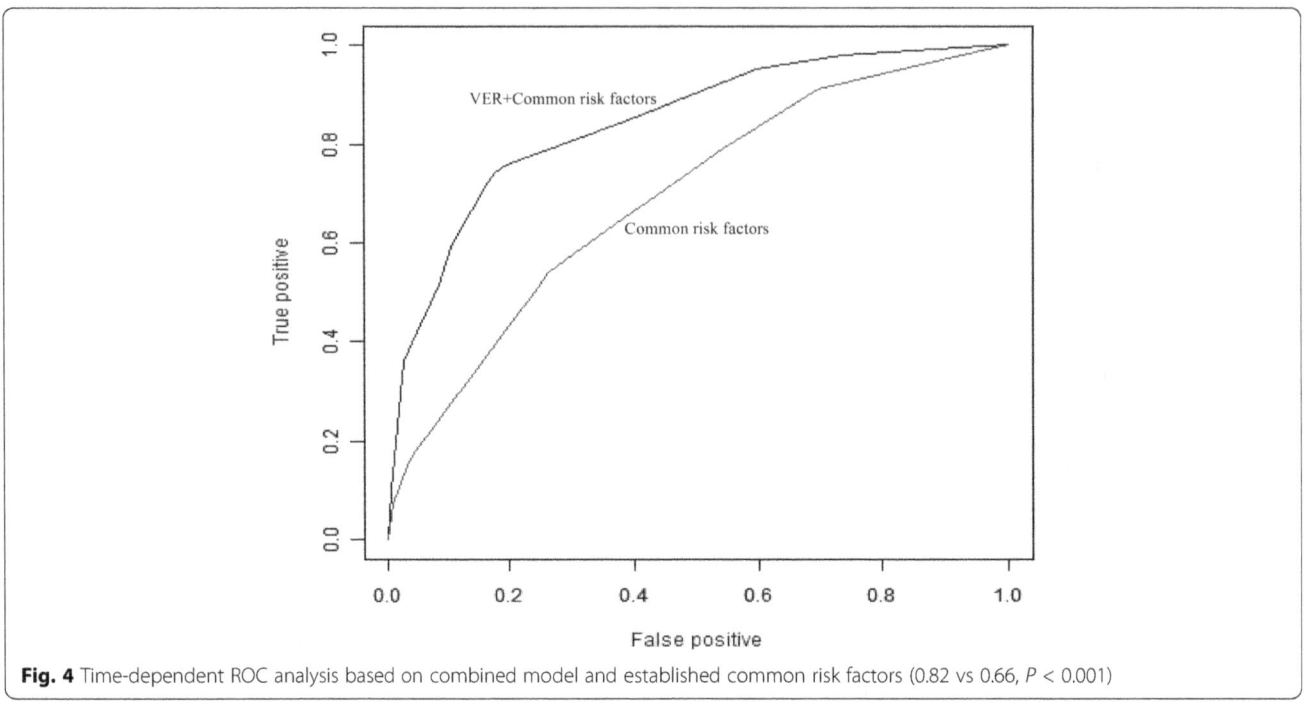

Fig. 4 Time-dependent ROC analysis based on combined model and established common risk factors (0.82 vs 0.66, $P < 0.001$)

persistent AF, (1) Above half of patients with VER (65.90%) experienced subsequent LR and were associated with lower event-free survival from LR, (2) VER was an independent predictor of LR after adjustment for common risk factors of AF, (3) VER was more sensitive than common risk factors in predicting LR and combination model was superior in predicting LR.

The purpose of catheter ablation is to eliminate underlying cardiac arrhythmia by destroying myocardial tissue through energy. However, due to the complexity of the underlying pathological mechanisms, AF recurs frequently after an initially successful ablation procedure. Reported frequency of LR ranges from 5 to 63%, depending on method and intensity of surveillance, technique used, patient characteristics, and definition of success, with a mean overall successful rate of approximately 70% [18]. In the present study, we found the cumulative LR was about 32.54% at a mean follow-up of 14.71 ± 8.58 months after a single procedure. Among most patients, AF recurred within 7 days.

Recurrence within 3 months following catheter ablation is relatively common regardless of catheter techniques used and is a predictor of LR [5–14]. However, definitions of recurrence time point within the blanking period vary in the reported studies. Arya et al. [9] defined early recurrence as a sustained episode of AF within 7 days immediately after the procedure, while others defined it by a sustained episode of AF within 2 weeks, [5] 1 month, [6, 7] 6 weeks, [8, 10] and 3 months [11–14] during the blanking period. The optimal time to define early recurrence remains to be

determined. In this study, we defined sustained AT episode within 7 days as VER since 112 patients (29.63%) experienced it. By using multivariate Cox analysis, VER independently predicted subsequent LR. Mechanisms of arrhythmia recurrence within 3 months of post ablation remain to be fully elucidated and may include reconnection of the PVs, [19] inflammatory response to thermal injury and/or pericarditis, [20, 21] imbalance of the autonomic nervous system, [22, 23] and a delayed effect of AF ablation [23, 24].

The use of 3-month blanking period has been proposed on the assumption that early recurrence will lead to delayed cure and should not prompt immediate re-ablation attempts [15, 25–27]. However, patients with early recurrence and delayed cure were of varied proportion [25–27] and the mechanisms and significance of early arrhythmia remains unclear [19–24]. Given the fact that early recurrence is a strong prognostic factor of LR, delayed re-intervention of tachyarrhythmia within blanking period may be a cause of failure to prevent LR. Indeed, Lellouche et al. [7] evaluated the use of early re-ablation on long-term outcome among patients with early recurrence. After a mean follow-up of 11 ± 11 months, patients with early re-ablation had a lower rate of clinical recurrences. Thus, detection of patients who are at high risk for LR and strategies of aggressive re-intervention may improve at long-term outcome. In our study, VER was more sensitive than common risk factors in prediction of LR. Moreover, when combining VER with common risk factors, it could further improve prediction of LR.

It must be noted that there are limitations in our study. Above all, it is a prospective cohort study and should be validated in large randomized controlled studies. Furthermore, monitoring of atrial tachyarrhythmia recurrence was based on the review of 12-lead electrocardiograms and Holter recordings at follow-up visits. It is likely that more invasive and detailed monitoring of atrial tachyarrhythmia should be offered. Finally, the precise mechanisms of VER and strategies to prevent VER were not investigated and required further research.

Conclusions

To sum up, the results of this study confirm that VER is observed frequently after a single procedure of catheter ablation and it was strongly associated with LR. Combination between VER and common risk factors could further improve prediction of patients who were at high risk for LR. Whether more aggressively invasive examinations and interventions are helpful for these patients, deserve further studies.

Abbreviations
AADs: Anti-arrhythmic drugs; AF: Atrial fibrillation; AT: Atrial tachyarrhythmia; LA: Left atria; LR: Long-term recurrence; PVI: Pulmonary vein isolation; PVs: Pulmonary veins; ROC: Receiver operator characteristic; VER: Very early recurrence

Acknowledgements
Not Applicable.

Funding
Not applicable.

Authors' contributions
KTJ and BHL analyzed and interpreted the patient data. YJX and XNW both were major contributors in writing the manuscript. YJX, XNW, ST, LPW, JNW, ZQX, SZW, LYT, GQW, LQ participated in data acquisition. YJX and LML performed statistical analysis. All authors read and approved the final manuscript.

Competing interests
The authors declare that they have no competing interests.

Author details
[1]Department of Cardiology, the Second Affiliated Hospital and Yuying Children's Hospital of Wenzhou Medical University, Xueyuanxi Road, No 109, Wenzhou, Zhejiang 325000, China. [2]Department of Rehabilitation, the Second Affiliated Hospital and Yuying Children's Hospital of Wenzhou Medical University, Xueyuanxi Road, No 109, Wenzhou, Zhejiang 325000, China. [3]Department of Intensive Care Unit, Zhengzhou Central Hospital Affiliated to Zhengzhou University, Tongbaibei Road, No 195, Zhengzhou, Henan 450000, China. [4]Department of Endocrinology, the Fourth Affiliated Hospital, Zhejiang University School of Medicine, Shangcheng Road, No N1, Yiwu, Zhejiang 322000, China. [5]Department of Oncology, Academy of Integrative Medicine, Fujian University of Traditional Chinese Medicine, Huatuo Road, No 1, Fuzhou, Fujian 350122, China.

References

1. Ouyang F, Tilz R, Chun J, Schmidt B, Wissner E, Zerm T, Neven K, Kokturk B, Konstantinidou M, Metzner A, et al. Long-term results of catheter ablation in paroxysmal atrial fibrillation: lessons from a 5-year follow-up. Circulation. 2010;122(23):2368–77.
2. Tzou WS, Marchlinski FE, Zado ES, Lin D, Dixit S, Callans DJ, Cooper JM, Bala R, Garcia F, Hutchinson MD, et al. Long-term outcome after successful catheter ablation of atrial fibrillation. Circ Arrhythm Electrophysiol. 2010;3(3):237–42.
3. Weerasooriya R, Khairy P, Litalien J, Macle L, Hocini M, Sacher F, Lellouche N, Knecht S, Wright M, Nault I, et al. Catheter ablation for atrial fibrillation: are results maintained at 5 years of follow-up? J Am Coll Cardiol. 2011;57(2):160–6.
4. Scherr D, Khairy P, Miyazaki S, Aurillac-Lavignolle V, Pascale P, Wilton SB, Ramoul K, Komatsu Y, Roten L, Jadidi A, et al. Five-year outcome of catheter ablation of persistent atrial fibrillation using termination of atrial fibrillation as a procedural endpoint. Circ Arrhythm Electrophysiol. 2015;8(1):18–24.
5. Oral H, Knight BP, Ozaydin M, Tada H, Chugh A, Hassan S, Scharf C, Lai SW, Greenstein R, Pelosi Jr F, et al. Clinical significance of early recurrences of atrial fibrillation after pulmonary vein isolation. J Am Coll Cardiol. 2002;40(1):100–4.
6. Lee SH, Tai CT, Hsieh MH, Tsai CF, Lin YK, Tsao HM, Yu WC, Huang JL, Ueng KC, Cheng JJ, et al. Predictors of early and late recurrence of atrial fibrillation after catheter ablation of paroxysmal atrial fibrillation. J Interv Card Electrophysiol. 2004;10(3):221–6.
7. Lellouche N, Jais P, Nault I, Wright M, Bevilacqua M, Knecht S, Matsuo S, Lim KT, Sacher F, Deplagne A, et al. Early recurrences after atrial fibrillation ablation: prognostic value and effect of early reablation. J Cardiovasc Electrophysiol. 2008;19(6):599–605.
8. Roux JF, Zado E, Callans DJ, Garcia F, Lin D, Marchlinski FE, Bala R, Dixit S, Riley M, Russo AM, et al. Antiarrhythmics after ablation of Atrial fibrillation (5A study). Circulation. 2009;120(12):1036–40.
9. Arya A, Hindricks G, Sommer P, Huo Y, Bollmann A, Gaspar T, Bode K, Husser D, Kottkamp H, Piorkowski C. Long-term results and the predictors of outcome of catheter ablation of atrial fibrillation using steerable sheath catheter navigation after single procedure in 674 patients. Europace. 2010;12(2):173–80.
10. Leong-Sit P, Roux JF, Zado E, Callans DJ, Garcia F, Lin D, Marchlinski FE, Bala R, Dixit S, Riley M, et al. Antiarrhythmics after ablation of atrial fibrillation (5A study): six-month follow-up study. Circ Arrhythm Electrophysiol. 2011;4(1):11–4.
11. Pokushalov E, Romanov A, Corbucci G, Bairamova S, Losik D, Turov A, Shirokova N, Karaskov A, Mittal S, Steinberg JS. Does atrial fibrillation burden measured by continuous monitoring during the blanking period predict the response to ablation at 12-month follow-up? Heart Rhythm. 2012;9(9):1375–9.
12. Kaitani K, Inoue K, Kobori A, Nakazawa Y, Ozawa T, Kurotobi T, Morishima I, Miura F, Watanabe T, Masuda M, et al. Efficacy of Antiarrhythmic drugs short-term use after catheter ablation for Atrial fibrillation (EAST-AF) trial. Eur Heart J. 2016;37(7):610–8.
13. Themistoclakis S, Schweikert RA, Saliba WI, Bonso A, Rossillo A, Bader G, Wazni O, Burkhardt DJ, Raviele A, Natale A. Clinical predictors and relationship between early and late atrial tachyarrhythmias after pulmonary vein antrum isolation. Heart Rhythm. 2008;5(5):679–85.
14. Koyama T, Sekiguchi Y, Tada H, Arimoto T, Yamasaki H, Kuroki K, Machino T, Tajiri K, Zhu XD, Kanemoto M, et al. Comparison of characteristics and significance of immediate versus early versus no recurrence of atrial fibrillation after catheter ablation. Am J Cardiol. 2009;103(9):1249–54.
15. Calkins H, Kuck KH, Cappato R, Brugada J, Camm AJ, Chen SA, Crijns HJ, Damiano Jr RJ, Davies DW, Di Marco J, et al. 2012 HRS/EHRA/ECAS expert consensus statement on catheter and surgical ablation of atrial fibrillation: recommendations for patient selection, procedural techniques, patient management and follow-up, definitions, endpoints, and research trial design: a report of the Heart Rhythm Society (HRS) task force on catheter and surgical ablation of Atrial fibrillation. Developed in partnership with the European heart rhythm association (EHRA), a registered branch of the European Society of Cardiology (ESC) and the European cardiac arrhythmia Society (ECAS); and in collaboration with the American College of Cardiology (ACC), American Heart Association (AHA), the Asia Pacific Heart Rhythm Society (APHRS), and the Society of Thoracic Surgeons (STS). Endorsed by the governing bodies of the American College of Cardiology Foundation, the American Heart Association, the European cardiac arrhythmia Society, the

European heart rhythm association, the Society of Thoracic Surgeons, the Asia Pacific Heart Rhythm Society, and the Heart Rhythm Society. Heart Rhythm. 2012;9(4):632–696 e621.

16. Liu X, Tan HW, Wang XH, Shi HF, Li YZ, Li F, Zhou L, Gu JN. Efficacy of catheter ablation and surgical CryoMaze procedure in patients with long-lasting persistent atrial fibrillation and rheumatic heart disease: a randomized trial. Eur Heart J. 2010;31(21):2633–41.

17. Zhang XD, Gu J, Jiang WF, Zhao L, Zhou L, Wang YL, Liu YG, Liu X. Optimal rhythm-control strategy for recurrent atrial tachycardia after catheter ablation of persistent atrial fibrillation: a randomized clinical trial. Eur Heart J. 2014;35(20):1327–34.

18. Marine JE. Catheter ablation therapy for supraventricular arrhythmias. JAMA. 2007;298(23):2768–78.

19. Lubitz SA, Fischer A, Fuster V. Catheter ablation for atrial fibrillation. BMJ. 2008;336(7648):819–26.

20. Grubman E, Pavri BB, Lyle S, Reynolds C, Denofrio D, Kocovic DZ. Histopathologic effects of radiofrequency catheter ablation in previously infarcted human myocardium. J Cardiovasc Electrophysiol. 1999;10(3):336–42.

21. Tanno K, Kobayashi Y, Kurano K, Kikushima S, Yazawa T, Baba T, Inoue S, Mukai H, Katagiri T. Histopathology of canine hearts subjected to catheter ablation using radiofrequency energy. Jpn Circ J. 1994;58(2):123–35.

22. Pappone C, Santinelli V, Manguso F, Vicedomini G, Gugliotta F, Augello G, Mazzone P, Tortoriello V, Landoni G, Zangrillo A, et al. Pulmonary vein denervation enhances long-term benefit after circumferential ablation for paroxysmal atrial fibrillation. Circulation. 2004;109(3):327–34.

23. Hsieh MH, Chiou CW, Wen ZC, Wu CH, Tai CT, Tsai CF, Ding YA, Chang MS, Chen SA. Alterations of heart rate variability after radiofrequency catheter ablation of focal atrial fibrillation originating from pulmonary veins. Circulation. 1999;100(22):2237–43.

24. Langberg JJ, Borganelli SM, Kalbfleisch SJ, Strickberger SA, Calkins H, Morady F. Delayed effects of radiofrequency energy on accessory atrioventricular connections. Pacing Clin Electrophysiol. 1993;16(5 Pt 1):1001–5.

25. O'Donnell D, Furniss SS, Dunuwille A, Bourke JP. Delayed cure despite early recurrence after pulmonary vein isolation for atrial fibrillation. Am J Cardiol. 2003;91(1):83–5.

26. Bertaglia E, Stabile G, Senatore G, Zoppo F, Turco P, Amellone C, De Simone A, Fazzari M, Pascotto P. Predictive value of early atrial tachyarrhythmias recurrence after circumferential anatomical pulmonary vein ablation. Pacing Clin Electrophysiol. 2005;28(5):366–71.

27. Jiang H, Lu Z, Lei H, Zhao D, Yang B, Huang C. Predictors of early recurrence and delayed cure after segmental pulmonary vein isolation for paroxysmal atrial fibrillation without structural heart disease. J Interv Card Electrophysiol. 2006;15(3):157–63.

3

Semaphorin 3A attenuates cardiac autonomic disorders and reduces inducible ventricular arrhythmias in rats with experimental myocardial infarction

Hesheng Hu[†], Yongli Xuan[†], Mei Xue, Wenjuan Cheng, Ye Wang, Xinran Li, Jie Yin, Xiaolu Li, Na Yang, Yugen Shi and Suhua Yan[*]

Abstract

Background: To investigate the effects of semaphorin 3A (sema 3A) on cardiac autonomic regulation and subsequent ventricular arrhythmias (VAs) in post-infarcted hearts.

Method and results: In order to explore the functions of sema 3A in post-infarcted hearts, lentivirus-Sema 3A-shRNA and negative control vectors were delivered to the peri-infarcted myocardium rats respectively. Meanwhile, recombinant sema 3A and control (0.9 % NaCl solution) were injected intravenously into infarcted rats to test the therapeutic potential of sema 3A. Results indicated that levels of sema 3A were higher in post-infarcted hearts compared with sham rats. However, sema 3A silencing leaded to sympathetic hyperinnervation, increased myocardial norepinephrine (NE) content and inducible VAs. Conversely, the intravenous administration of sema 3A to infarcted rats reduced sympathetic nerve sprouting, improved cardiac autonomic regulation, and decreased the incidence of inducible VAs. However, both infarct size and cardiac function were similar among infarcted hearts.

Conclusions: The upregulation and administration of sema 3A exerted beneficial effects on infarction-induced cardiac autonomic disorders by increasing cardiac electrical stability and reducing VAs. Sema 3A might be a potential therapeutic agent for cardiac autonomic abnormalities induced arrhythmias.

Keywords: Myocardial infarction, Semaphorin 3A, Cardiac autonomic nerve, Ventricular arrhythmia

Background

Despite advances in management strategies and patient education, ventricular arrhythmias (VAs) remain an unsolved problem, and the identification for patients at a high risk of sudden cardiac death due to myocardial infarction (MI) is still challenging [1, 2]. Increasing studies have identified that the neural mechanism is correlated with ventricular arrhythmogenesis [3–7]. Neural control of the heart is mediated through the parasympathetic and sympathetic branches of the autonomic nervous system, which jointly maintain the normal cardiac function and electrophysiological stability via innervation balance

and functional confrontation [8]. An imbalanced autonomic nervous system, especially the reduced parasympathetic and increased sympathetic tone, has been commonly found in post-infarcted patients [9]. MI complicated by sympathovagal imbalance occurs in some patients, despite of preserved ventricular function, sufficient exercises, and the use of beta-blockers [10]. All these findings suggest that cardiac autonomic disorders complicated MI is associated with an unfavorable prognosis, therefore, further studies should be performed.

Cardiac innervation is highly plastic and changed over time at different stages of cardiovascular disease [3]. MI induces nerve reinnervations including sympathetic nerve and cholinergic nerve fibers [11], and infarction-induced nerve sprouting is mainly sympathetic nerve

* Correspondence: yansuhua5537@163.com
[†]Equal contributors
Department of Cardiology, Shandong Provincial Qianfoshan Hospital, Shandong University, 250014 Jinan, China

fibers [3, 12]. The increasing sympathetic nerve density caused by autonomic imbalance is characterized by increased sympathetic and decreased parasympathetic activity [8]. Therefore, infarction-induced cardiac autonomic abnormalities might lead to sympathetic over-activation and subsequent VAs.

Cardiac innervation is sculpted by growth factors during infarction. Nerve growth factor (NGF), a chemoattractive factor, plays a key role in sympathetic nerve sprouting and hyperinnervation [13]. Our previous study demonstrated that NGF has pleiotropic effects on infarcted hearts, and downregulation of NGF does not improve prognosis [14]. However, cardiac reinnervation is also modulated by chemorepulsive factors such as sema-phoring 3A (sema 3A). Sema 3A is a secreted protein that regulates axon/dendrite growth and neuronal migration. It initiates growth cone collapse, inhibits axonal outgrowth, and plays crucial roles in neural, cardiac and peripheral vascular patterning [15]. Sema 3A-deficient mice exhibit sympathetic hyperinnervation, whereas sema 3A overexpressing mice lack sympathetic innervation in developing hearts [16]. Thus, sema 3A is an important regulatory factor that maintains the balance of cardiac autonomic nerve during heart development.

The changes in expression and function of semaphorins are correlated with the regenerative failure following nerve injury [15]. Sema 3A is upregulated during brain ischemia and spinal cord injury [17, 18]. Overexpression of sema 3A is also found in MI at the infarcted border [19]. Meanwhile, sema 3A-deficient mice were with high risk of sudden death and much more susceptible to VAs, which is characterized by a high level of sympathetic nerve density [16]. In addition, upregulating sema 3A by transfecting the sema 3A gene into the peri-infarcted zone could reduce sympathetic hyper-reinnervation and inducible VAs in post-infarcted hearts [19]. Moreover, variations in the sema 3A gene were identified in unexplained cardiac arrest patients with documented ventricular fibrillation [20]. Based on the above analyses, sema 3A expression plays an important role in cardiac innervation in heart development and diseased hearts. The importance of appropriate sema 3A expression in post-infarcted hearts is highlighted via downregulation or inhibition of myocardial sema 3A [19]. Therefore, sema 3A may be a potential therapeutic agent in sympathetic hyperinnervation and subsequent lethal VAs.

In the current study, the effects of sema 3A were investigated by regulating cardiac sema 3A expression via the local intramyocardial injection of lentiviral-mediated sema 3A shRNA and the intravenous injection of recombinant sema 3A. Our data revealed that silencing sema 3A augmented sympathetic hyperinnervation, increased myocardial NE content and inducible VAs. Conversely, the administration of exogenous sema 3A attenuated those abnormalities and protected infarcted hearts from inducible VAs.

Methods

Preparation of sema 3A shRNA lentiviral vector

RNA interference (RNAi) is a post-transcriptional process that is triggered by the introduction of double-stranded RNA (dsRNA), which leads to gene silencing in a sequence-specific manner. Lentiviral vectors provide a method of stably introducing exogenous DNA into cells that are difficult to transfect, allowing for the ectopic expression or silencing of genes for therapeutic or experimental purposes [21]. A small interference RNA (siRNA) design tool was used to design the RNA target sequences. Three selected siRNAs targeting different sites of the sema 3A gene were synthesized, and the corresponding DNA oligonucleotide (oligo) was cloned into a lentiviral expression vector. Then, the most effective short hairpin RNA (shRNA) target was determined by assessing the silencing efficacy in rat myocardial cells. The lentivirus expressing the optimal shRNA targeting sema 3A was then propagated and harvested using a virus packaging system (Telebio, Shanghai, China). Next, viral titers were determined using qPCR [22]. The shRNA construct (GFPi) targeting the reporter gene eGFP was included as a control. The lentivirus-sema 3A-shRNA titer was determined as 2.5×10^{12} vector genomes (vg)/ml, and the lentivirus-GFP titer was 1×10^{13} vg/ml.

MI model and sema 3A intervention in vivo

All animal experimental procedures were approved by the Ethics Committee for Animal Studies of Shandong University, China, and conformed to the Guide for the Care and Use of Laboratory Animals published by the United States National Institutes of Health (NIH publication No. 85–23, revised 1996).

Male Wistar rats (8 weeks old, 280–300 g) were obtained from animal center of Shandong University and housed under 12 h light/dark cycles in a temperature-controlled room with free access to food and water. The left anterior descending (LAD) coronary artery was ligated to induce MI, as described previously [14]. Briefly, rats were anesthetized with 30 mg/kg of 3 % sodium pentobarbital (intraperitoneal [ip]). The heart was then exposed using a fourth intracostal left lateral thoracotomy after mechanical ventilation. The LAD artery was ligated permanently at 2 mm from its origin. Coronary occlusion was confirmed by ST elevation on a surface electrocardiogram (ECG), as well as regional pallor and stiff movement of the left ventricle (LV). Meanwhile, Masson staining was conducted to determine the infarct size of rats on the day of sacrifice. With respect to clinical importance, only rats with moderate infarct size (30 to 50 %) were enrolled (data was not shown here).

In order to knockdown sema 3A expression, 80 μl virus solution including 1.09×10^9 TU/ml lentivirus-sema 3A-shRNA encoding green fluorescent protein(GFP) and containing sema 3A shRNA (MI-SiRNA group, $n = 17$) was injected intramyocardially at four sites in the peri-infarcted myocardium (~2 mm around the infarcted area), as reported previously [14]. The same amount of virus solution only encoding GFP (MI-GFP, $n = 16$) was injected to the rats in control groups. To investigate the potential therapeutic of sema 3A, the prepared recombinant sema 3A (Sino Biological Inc, China; MI-Sema group, $n = 11$; 1 mg/kg body weight) or PBS (MI-PBS group, $n = 9$) was injected intravenously weekly 3 days after coronary ligation for 4 weeks. An additional group of rats underwent only LAD ligation (MI-CON group, $n = 9$), and a group that underwent thoracotomy and pericardiotomy ($n = 15$) were used as the Sham group. After the incision was closed, the rats were allowed to recover from the anesthesia in a heated box, and were then returned to their individual cages.

Hemodynamic measurements and electrophysiological study

Five weeks after the operation, rats were tracheotomized, intubated, ventilated mechanically, and monitored after anesthesia. A pressure-volume catheter (SPR-869, Millar, Houston, TX, USA) was inserted into the right carotid artery of rats to measure the mean arterial blood pressure (MAP). Then, the transducer was advanced from the right carotid artery into the LV to get the pressure-volume (P-V) data. LabChart Pro software (AD Instruments, Sydney, Australia) was utilized to evaluate LV end-systolic pressure (LVESP), LV end-diastolic pressure (LVEDP), the maximal slope of LV systolic pressure increment (dP/dtmax), diastolic pressure decrement (dP/dtmin), end-diastolic volume (EDV), end-systolic volume (ESV) and LV ejection fraction (EF).

In addition, an electrophysiological study was performed to evaluate the susceptibility of rats in a stable condition to VAs. The protocol used for programmed electrical stimulation (PES) was performed as reported previously [4, 23]. After monitoring the surface ECG, a second thoracotomy was carried out. PES was performed via a specially modified electrode with a needle-point inserted into the epicardial surface of the infarcted border (2 mm deep). After measuring the pacing threshold, standard PES protocols were performed as follows: burst (cycle length 100 ms, S0), single (S1), double (S2), and triple (S3) extrastimuli. The coupling interval of the last extra stimulus was decreased from 80 ms to the value of ventricular effective refractory period with 2-ms steps. The experimental protocols were completed within 10 min. Ventricular tachyarrhythmias, including ventricular tachycardia and ventricular fibrillation, were considered non-sustained when they lasted < 15 beats and sustained when they lasted > 15 beats. Ventricular arrhythmia scores were determined by the inducibility quotient of ventricular tachyarrhythmias as follows: 0, non-inducible; 1, non-sustained tachyarrhythmias induced with three extrastimuli; 2, sustained tachyarrhythmias induced with three extrastimuli; 3, non-sustained tachyarrhythmias induced with two extrastimuli; 4, sustained tachyarrhythmias induced with two extrastimuli; 5, non-sustained tachyarrhythmias induced with one extrastimulus; 6, sustained tachyarrhythmias induced with one extrastimulus; 7, tachyarrhythmias induced during a train of eight stimuli ($8 \times S1$) at a basic cycle length of 100 ms; and 8, heart stopped before PES. The highest score was used when multiple forms of tachyarrhythmias occurred in one heart [23]. Finally, heart tissues were sampled according to corresponding experimental techniques.

Immunohistochemistry and Masson's trichrome staining
Immunohistochemistry and Masson's trichrome staining were performed as described previously [14]. Briefly, paraffin sections were deparaffinized, rehydrated, incubated and then treated with citric acid buffer. After incubated with serum-free protein blocking buffer (ZSGB-BIO, Beijing, China), sections were incubated with rabbit anti-TH (tyrosine hydroxylase, 1:100; Millipore, Billerica, MA, USA), rinsed and incubated in horseradish peroxidase-(HRP-) conjugated secondary antibodies, and then counterstained with hematoxylin. Finally, the sections were mounted and examined using a microscopy. The density is expressed as the ratio of labeled nerve fiber area to total area, while papillary muscles were excluded from the study because a variable sympathetic innervation has been reported [24].

In addition, samples from the apex, mid-LV, and base were paraffin-embedded, sectioned and stained with Masson's trichrome stain. The infarct size percentage was calculated as fibrosis area/total LV area × 100. All images were analyzed with ImageJ software ImagePro Plus 5.0 (Media Cybernetics, Bethesda, MD).

Western blotting
Proteins were extracted from cardiac issues prepared from the infarcted border using a Nuclear and Cytoplasmic Protein Extraction Kit (Beyotime, Haimen, China). Protein concentrations were quantified using a bicinchoninic acid (BCA) protein assay kit (Beyotime). From each extract, 40 μg proteins was separated using 10 % SDS-PAGE, and then transferred to polyvinylidene fluoride (PVDF) membranes (Bio-Rad, Hercules, CA, USA). Membranes were blocked in 5 % non-fat milk, followed by incubated with anti-TH (1:1000), anti-CHAT (choline acetyltransferase, 1:1500; Millipore, Billerica, MA, USA),

anti-NGF (1:1500, Epitomics, Burlingame, CA, USA), anti-sema 3A (1:1000, Abcam, Cambridge, England) or anti-GAPDH (glyceraldehyde-3-phosphate dehydrogenase, 1:3000; CoWin Bioscience, Beijing, China) antibodies. After washed with PBS, the membranes were incubated with the corresponding secondary antibodies, and images were developed using an enhanced chemiluminescence detection kit. Immunoreactive bands were visualized using a FluroChem E Imager (ProteinSimple, Santa Clara, CA, USA). The expression levels of the target proteins were measured and normalized to GAPDH.

Real-time quantitative PCR

Total RNA was isolated from samples at infarcted border zone (3 mm zone adjacent to the infarcted area), and the mRNA expression levels of TH, CHAT, NGF, and sema 3A were assessed by real-time quantitative RT-PCR using a PrimeScript RT reagent kit (TaKaRa, Dalian, China) in a Mastercycler EP realplex detection system (Roche, Indianapolis, IN, USA) as reported previously. For each sample, GAPDH and the target genes were amplified in duplicate in separate tubes. Each measurement was performed in triplicate. Gene expression was analyzed using the $2^{-\Delta\Delta CT}$ method described by Livak and Schmittgen [25]. The primers for each gene used in this study were as follows:

NGF forward 5'-TCGCTCACTCCACTATCCACTA-3', and reverse 5'-GACTCAACAGGGCAAGCATAC-3'; sema 3A forward 5'-GAGTGATGTAAGAAGGGTGTTCC-3', and reverse 5'-CAAGTTCCTGGTCGTGGATAAG-3'; TH forward 5'-GGCTTCTCTGACCAGGTGTATC-3', and reverse 5'-TAGCAATCTCTTCCGCTGTGTA-3'; CHAT forward 5'- AGCCCTCTGTATGAAGCAAT–3', and reverse GGACGCCATTTTGACTATCTTT-3'; GAPDH forward 5'-ACAGCAACAGGGTGGTGGAC-3', and reverse 5'-TTTGAGGGTGCAGCGAACTT-3'.

High performance liquid chromatography (HPLC)

According to previously reported studies [26, 27], we measured norepinephrine(NE) and acetylcholine (ACh) levels in heart tissue isolated from the infarcted border using HPLC with electrochemical detection. Briefly, fresh heart samples (50 mg) were transferred immediately into perchloric acid containing isopropylhomocholine as an internal control. They were then homogenized, centrifuged, and filtered to obtain an HPLC samples. HPLC was then used to quantify Ach and NE levels.

Statistical analyses

Data are presented as means ± standard deviations (SD). Independent t-tests were used to compare values between two groups. ANOVA followed by Tukey's test was used to compare differences between more than two groups. Analyses were performed using SPSS 17.0 software (SPSS Inc.,

Chicago, IL, USA). A value of $P < 0.05$ was considered statistically significant.

Results

Sema 3A knockdown using recombinant lentivirus vectors in vitro and in vivo

The mRNA and protein expression of sema 3A were assessed in a rat myocardial cell line to identify the knockdown efficacy of different siRNAs (Fig. 1). The results suggested that the sequence 5'-GGTGTTCCTTGGTCCA TATGC-3' resulted in the most effective knockdown of sema 3A in vitro. Therefore, this sequence was packaged and used for in vivo studies. Both mRNA and protein levels of sema 3A were higher in the MI-CON group than those in the Sham group at 1, 2, and 5 weeks after infarction ($P < 0.01$, Fig. 2). In addition, compared with the MI-GFP group, the expression of sema 3A was significantly lower in the MI-SiRNA group ($P < 0.01$, Fig. 2).

Effects of Sema 3A on inducible VAs, infarct size, and hemodynamics in post-infarcted hearts

There was no significant difference in the infarct size and hemodynamic data among the MI groups (Table 1). To assess the incidence of potential VAs, we designed an electrophysiological study to assess the cardiac electrical stability. Ventricular tachyarrhythmias were inducible by programmed stimulation in infarcted rats as showed in Fig. 3a–c. The percentage of inducible ventricular arrhythmia is negatively correlated with the expression level of sema 3A (Fig. 3d). The arrhythmia scores for sham rats were nearly 0 (Fig. 3e). Silencing sema 3A significantly increased the inducibility of ventricular tachyarrhythmia in infarcted rats compared with counterpart vehicle treatment; in contrast, sema 3A administration significantly decreased the inducibility of ventricular tachyarrhythmia (both $p < 0.05$) (Fig. 3e). Therefore, exogenous sema 3A could stabilize cardiac electrical activity and reduce the incidence of VAs.

Effects of silencing Sema 3A on sympathetic hyperinnervation, ratio of TH/CHAT and myocardial NE level

As shown in Figs. 4 and 5 and Table 2, MI caused nerve sprouting and sympathetic neural remodeling in the MI-CON and MI-GFP groups, and the TH-positive nerve densities were increased at the infarcted border. Meanwhile, the protein expression of TH and CHAT was higher in the MI-CON and MI-GFP groups. However, a higher TH-positive nerve density was detected in the MI-SiRNA group compared with the MI-GFP group (Fig. 4 and Table 2). Sema 3A silencing increased mRNA and protein levels of TH at the infarcted border (Table 2) but did not affected CHAT expression. Thus, the ratio of TH/CHAT protein was higher in MI-SiRNA

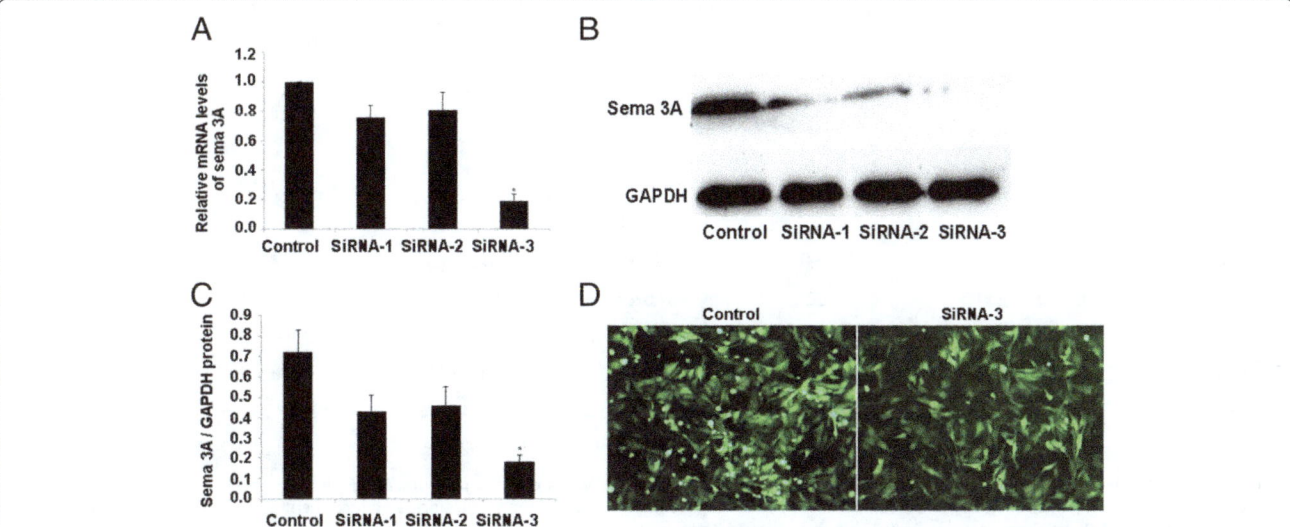

Fig. 1 The effectiveness of sema 3A-siRNA as determined by reduced protein and mRNA levels in vitro. **a** RT-PCR demonstrating sema 3A mRNA expression in rat myocardial cells transfected with sema 3A-shRNA 1 (*SiRNA-1*), 2 (*SiRNA-2*), and 3 (*SiRNA-3*), or PBS-control (*Control*) (*$P < 0.01$ vs. SiRNA-1). **b**, **c** Western blotting showing the expression of sema 3A in rat myocardial cells in various groups. (*$P < 0.01$ vs. SiRNA-1). **d** Image showing the effect of shRNA-3 in cultured rat myocardial cells using fluorescence microscopy

group compared with the MI-CON and MI-GFP groups (Table 2).

Myocardial NE and ACh were measured to evaluate autonomic nerve function. Both myocardial NE and ACh levels at the infarcted border were higher in the MI-CON and MI-GFP groups compared with the sham group. After sema 3A silencing, myocardial NE level was higher than that in the MI-GFP group. However, there were no significant differences of ACh levels between the MI-SiRNA and MI-GFP groups (Table 2).

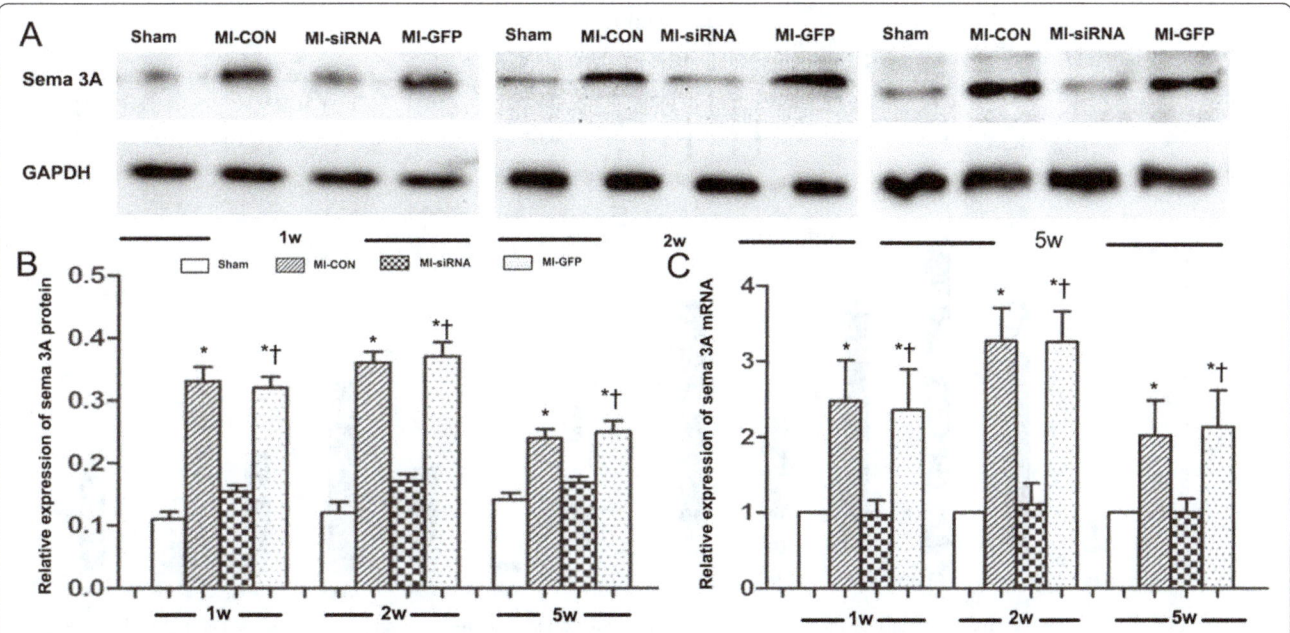

Fig. 2 The time-course expression of sema 3A in myocardial infarction (MI) models after lentivirus-sema 3A-shRNA treatment. **a**, **b** Western blotting was conducted to detect the effects of lentivirus-sema 3A-shRNA on the protein level of sema 3A (95 KDa) at various time points (1, 2, and 5 weeks). The relative expression of sema 3A was normalized to GAPDH (36 KDa). **c** Relative mRNA expression of *sema 3A* was detected using real-time quantitative RT-PCR. The relative gene expression of sema 3A was analyzed using the $2^{-\Delta\Delta CT}$ method. Data are presented as means ± SD. *$P < 0.05$ vs. sham group. †$P < 0.05$ vs. MI-siRNA group

Table 1 Hemodynamic data based on pressure-volume and infarct size 5 weeks after MI

	Sham	MI-CON	MI-GFP	MI-SiRNA	MI-Sema	MI-PBS
n	9	9	10	11	11	9
Infarct size (%)		42.7 ± 5.1	42.9 ± 4.7	44.3 ± 5.2	43.5 ± 4.2**	41.3 ± 4.9
HR (beats/min)	419.2 ± 19.1	424.5 ± 17.2*	421.4 ± 21.2	427.3 ± 19.2	419.2 ± 19.1**	420.1 ± 19.2
MAP (mmHg)	109.2 ± 3.7	92.4 ± 6.4*	93.2 ± 7.9	89.7 ± 8.1	92.7 ± 7.3**	93.7 ± 7.7
LVDSP (mmHg)	2.92 ± 0.97	6.3 ± 1.2*	5.8 ± 1.4	5.7 ± 1.6	6.1 ± 1.9**	5.9 ± 1.4
LVESP (mmHg)	119.3 ± 9.2	91.2 ± 5.9*	89.2 ± 6.1	90.2 ± 7.1**	88.3 ± 6.8**	91.4 ± 7.1
EDV (μl)	309.4 ± 21.3	483.2 ± 33.7*	467.6 ± 41.4	475.1 ± 48.1**	471.3 ± 47.4**	469.3 ± 45.3
ESV (μl)	106.1 ± 114	293.4 ± 19.4*	289.2 ± 23.1	291.2 ± 24.1**	289.4 ± 27.3**	285.7 ± 24.2**
EF (%)	61.2 ± 1.7	34.7 ± 0.7*	35.3 ± 06	34.9 ± 0.8	34.2 ± 0.9**	33.9 ± 1.0
dP/dtmax (mmHg/s)	5517.4 ± 129	3696.2 ± 90.2*	3712.7 ± 91.8	3637.4 ± 83.7	3707.2 ± 73.1**	3684.3 ± 80.5
dP/dtmin (mmHg/s)	−3989.1 ± 147	−2379.4 ± 77.5*	−2394.7 ± 90.3	−2427.4 ± 84.3	−2312.5 ± 74.9**	−2419.4 ± 94.2

Values are presented as means ± SD. HR, heart rate; *MAP* mean arterial pressure, *LVEDP* LV end-diastolic pressure, *LVESP* LV end-systolic pressure, *EDV* end-diastolic volume, *ESV* end-systolic volume, *EF* ejection fraction, *dP/dtmax and dP/dtmin* maximal slope of the systolic pressure increment and the diastolic pressure decrement, respectively. * $P < 0.05$ vs. sham group, ** $P > 0.05$ among various MI groups

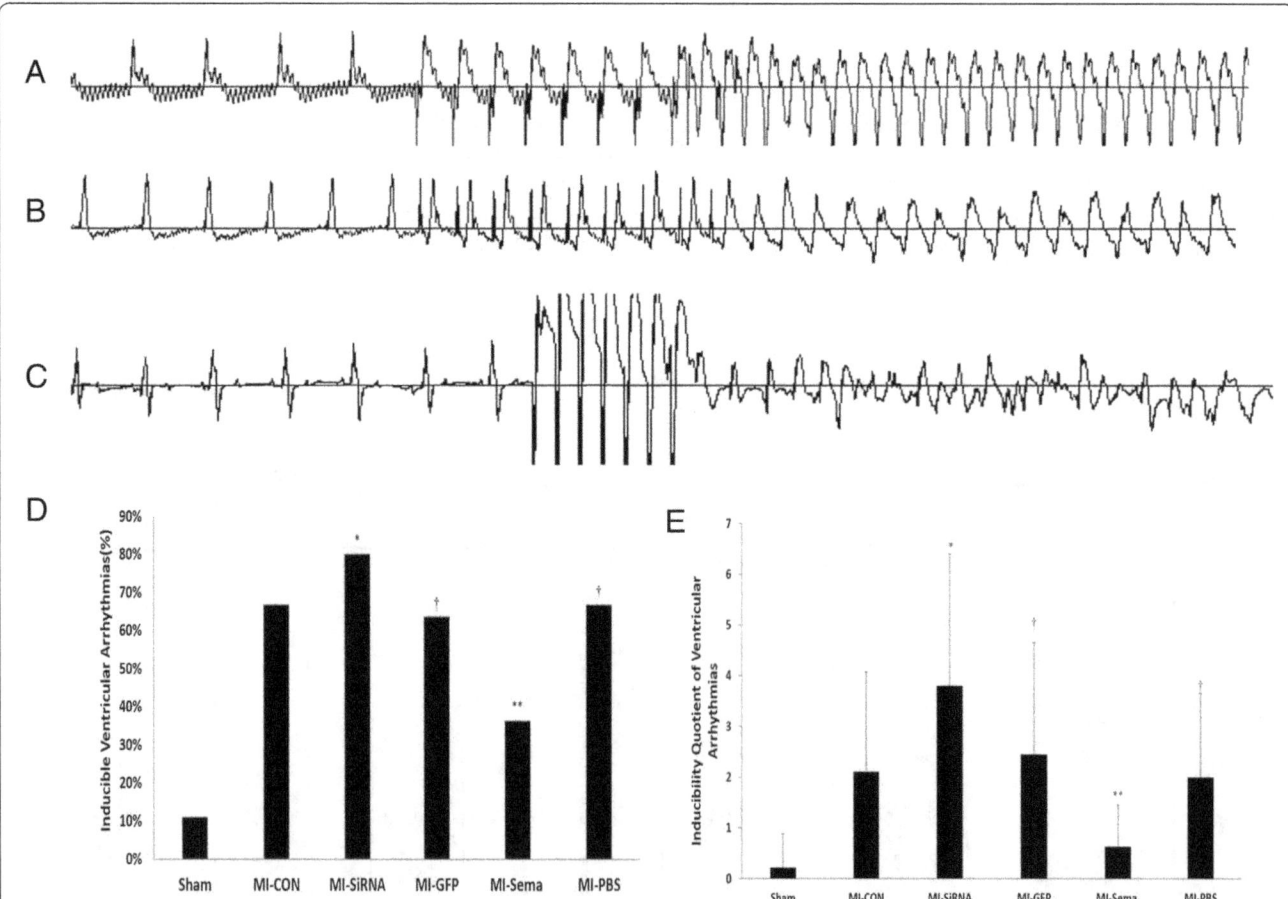

Fig. 3 Various ventricular arrhythmias induced by programmed electrical stimulation in infarcted rats. **a** Eight basic stimuli (S0) at cycle lengths of 100 ms and two extra stimuli (S1 and S2) induced monomorphic ventricular tachycardia (VT). **b** Eight basic stimuli (S0) and two extra stimuli (S1 and S2) induced polymorphic ventricular tachycardia. **c** Seven basic stimuli (S0) induced ventricular fibrillation (Vf). **d** The percentage of inducible total ventricular arrhythmias/ stimulation times.* $P < 0.05$ vs. MI GFP group; **$P < 0.01$ vs. MI-PBS group; †$P > 0.05$ vs. MI-CON group. **e** Inducibility quotient of induced ventricular arrhythmias 5 weeks after infarction. * $P < 0.01$ vs. MI GFP group; **$P < 0.01$ vs. MI-PBS group, †$P > 0.05$ vs. MI-CON group

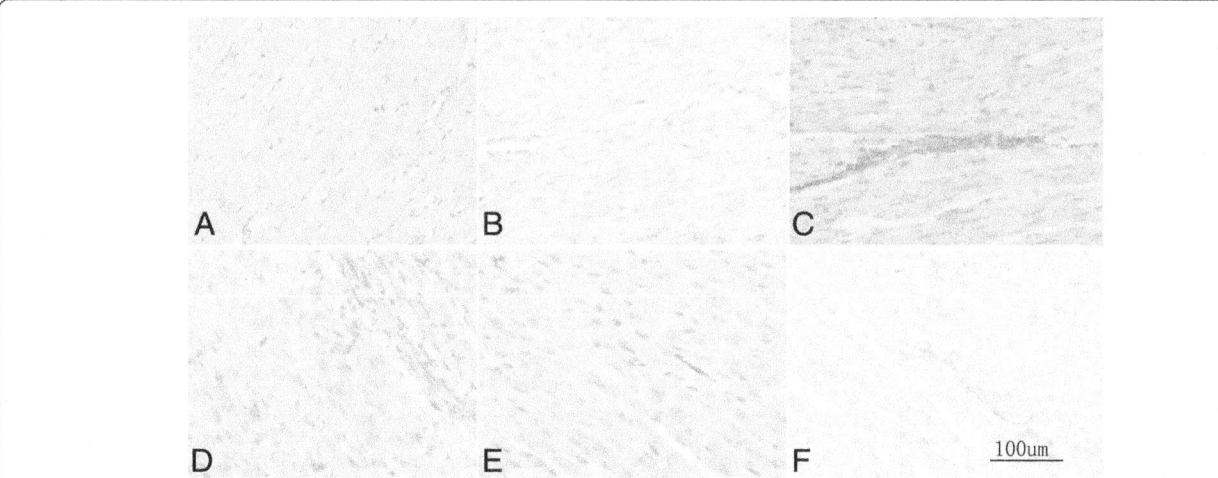

Fig. 4 Histological study of cardiac nerve fibers at the infarcted border zone in sham-operated and infarcted hearts. Immunohistochemistry staining for tyrosine hydroxylase (magnification × 200): (**a**), MI-CON (**b**), MI-SiRNA (**c**), MI-GFP (**d**), MI-PBS (**e**), and MI-Sema (**f**) groups

Sema 3A administration promoted cardiac innervation and function

To explore the potential therapeutic effects of sema 3A in infarcted hearts, recombinant sema 3A was injected as described previously [28]. Data revealed that intravenously administrated sema 3A dramatically decreased the sympathetic nerve density nerve fibers, accompanied by decreased protein and mRNA levels of TH and decreased TH/CHAT ratio (Fig. 3 and Table 2). In addition, as is shown in Fig. 5, knockdown or overexpression of sema 3A in infarcted rats did not seem to affect CHAT level, supported by the fact that neural remodeling post-infarction is mostly characterized by sympathetic hyperinnervation. Therefore, the alleviated TH/CHAT ratio by sema 3A is mainly through the downregulation of TH.

Myocardial NE levels were lower in the MI-Sema group compared with the MI-PBS group. However, there was no significant difference in myocardial ACh levels between the MI-PBS and MI-Sema groups (all $P > 0.05$). Moreover, both the mRNA and protein levels of NGF were comparable among the MI groups (Fig. 5), which suggested that sema 3A affected the post-infarcted cardiac autonomic nerve independent of NGF.

Discussion

Increased sympathetic tone and densities are important in the generation of VAs and subsequently sudden cardiac death. MI results in abnormal cardiac autonomic regulation in terms of both neural distribution and function. The MI-complicated abnormalities might cause unfavorable prognosis such as lethal VAs and sudden cardiac death [8, 29, 30]. The current study revealed that silencing sema 3A enhanced the abnormalities of cardiac autonomic regulation and increased the incidence of inducible VAs in post-infarcted hearts. Moreover, overexpression of sema 3A reduced sympathetic nerve sprouting, ameliorated cardiac autonomic imbalance, and decreased the incidence of inducible VAs. Infarct size and cardiac function were similar among the MI groups. Therefore, sema 3A has therapeutic potential for post-infarcted cardiac autonomic abnormalities.

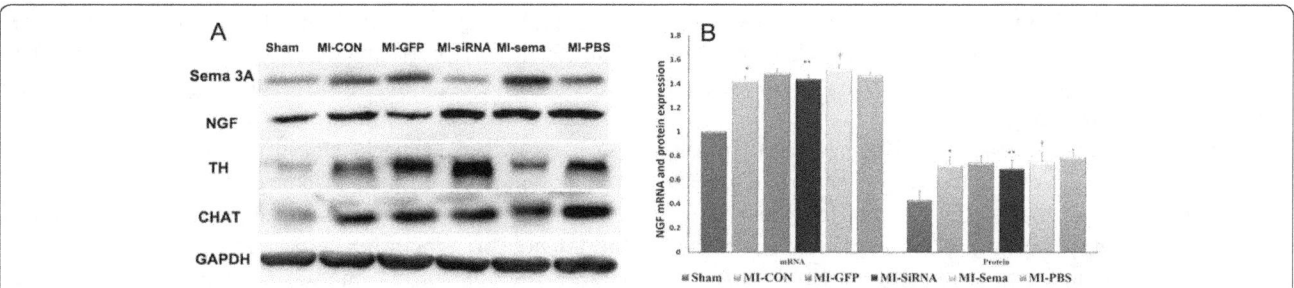

Fig. 5 The effects of sema 3A on the expression levels of NGF, TH and CHAT. **a** Representative western blots showing sema 3A (95 KDa), NGF (27 KDa), TH (58 KDa), CHAT (72KDa), and GAPDH (36 KDa) expression in various groups. **b** MI resulted in the increase of NGF mRNA and protein expression in the MI-CON group compared with the sham group (*$P < 0.05$). Both were similar in various MI groups. **$P > 0.05$ vs. MI-GFP group; †$P > 0.05$ vs. MI-PBS group

Table 2 Effects of sema 3A on autonomic abnormalities 5 weeks after infarction

		Sham	MI-CON	MI-GFP	MI-SiRNA	MI-Sema	MI-PBS
1-RT-PCR (target mRNA /GAPDH)	TH	1	2.93 ± 0.21	2.87 ± 0.18	3.82 ± 0.34*	1.84 ± 0.14**	3.12 ± 0.23***
	CHAT	1	1.66 ± 0.14	1.71 ± 0.17	1.67 ± 0.16	1.61 ± 0.14****	1.72 ± 0.17
2- IHC (um²/mm²)	TH-positive	1281 ± 75.1	3589 ± 278.1	3539 ± 176	4707 ± 193.2*	2330 ± 162.4**	3564 ± 118.9***
	Sema 3A protein	0.14 ± 0.02	0.35 ± 0.03	0.33 ± 0.025	0.167 ± 0.02*	0.44 ± 0.03**	0.31 ± 0.02***
3- WB (target protein/GAPDH)	TH protein	0.19 ± 0.03	0.45 ± 0.035	0.47 ± 0.029	0.67 ± 0.027*	0.35 ± 0.014**	0.48 ± 0.03***
	CHAT protein	0.085 ± 0.087	0.174 ± 0.013	0.174 ± 0.01	0.173 ± 0.011	0.167 ± 0.011**	0.179 ± 0.09
	TH/CHAT	2.18 ± 0.25	2.63 ± 0.26	2.67 ± 0.19	3.77 ± 0.20*	2.66 ± 0.18**	2.10 ± 0.10***
4- HPLC (pmol/mg)	NE	2.1 ± 0.12	4.3 ± 0.29	4.1 ± 0.31	5.1 ± 0.27*	2.9 ± 0.26**	3.9 ± 0.27***
	ACh	2.9 ± 0.26	3.9 ± 0.23	3.8 ± 0.27	3.5 ± 0.24	3.6 ± 0.28****	3.8 ± 0.27

(1) RT-PCR was used to assess the mRNA expression of TH, and CHAT in various groups. Sema 3A silencing increased the expression of GAP 43 and TH compared with the MI-GFP group ($P < 0.05$). However, the administration of sema 3A reduced the expression in TH compared with the MI-PBS group ($P < 0.05$). CHAT mRNA expression was comparable between various MI groups ($P > 0.05$). (2) Immunohistochemistry results revealed that the density of TH- and GAP 43- positive nerve fibers were higher in sema 3A-silenced infarcted-hearts compared with the MI-GFP group (both $P < 0.05$). Recombinant sema 3A reduced the number of TH- and GAP 43- positive nerve fibers compared with the MI-PBS group (both $P < 0.01$). There was no difference in the density of TH- nerve fibers among the MI-CON, MI-GFP, and MI-PBS groups (all $P > 0.05$). (3) Western blot (WB) showing increased protein expression of TH and CHAT in the MI-CON group compared with the sham group ($P < 0.05$). Sema 3A silencing increased the expression of TH protein, whereas sema 3A administration reduced TH protein expression. CHAT protein expression was comparable among the various MI groups. However, the ratio of TH/CHAT protein expression was increased in the MI-SiRNA group compared with the MI-GFP group ($P < 0.05$). The ratio was lower in the MI-Sema group compared with the MI-PBS group ($P = 0.021$), but there was no significant difference between the MI-Sema and sham groups ($P = 0.34$). (4) HPLC was used to assess local sympathetic and parasympathetic activity. MI resulted in increased myocardial NE and Ach levels in the MI-CON group compared with the sham group (both $P < 0.05$). NE content was increased in the MI-SiRNA group compared with the MI-GFP group ($P = 0.007$). In addition, NE content was reduced in the MI-Sema group compared with the MI-PBS group ($P = 0.024$). However, myocardial Ach levels were similar in the various infarcted groups ($P > 0.05$). * $P < 0.05$ vs. MI-GFP group, ** $P < 0.05$ vs. MI-SiRNA group, *** $P < 0.05$ vs. MI-sema group, **** $P > 0.05$ among various MI groups

Normal cardiac function and rhythm are maintained by balancing the actions of sympathetic and parasympathetic inputs to the heart [31]. The electrical and contractile activities of myocardium are modulated by the release of NE from sympathetic neurons and the secretion of ACh from parasympathetic neurons. However, the normal balance between cardiac autonomic neurons is disrupted by MI, which leads to increased sympathetic and decreased parasympathetic transmission in the heart [32]. Neurotrophins, such as sema 3A and NGF, regulate axonal growth, synaptic plasticity, survival, differentiation, myelination, and nerve patterning during both cardiac development and diseased pathologies [13, 16, 33–35].

Sema 3A is a neural chemorepellent as an axon guidance molecule that plays important roles in the development of the nervous system and axon growth [15]. Appropriate sema 3A expression in heart is required for sympathetic innervation patterning. Both sema 3A silencing and sema 3A overexpressing exhibited disrupted innervation patterning in mice [16]. In post-infarcted hearts, the lentivirus-mediated overexpression of sema 3A in the infarcted zone alleviated sympathetic hyper-reinnervation [19]. The increased expression of sema 3A in heart failure might partially account for the cardiac sympathetic denervation [36]. Consistent with the previous study [19], sema 3A expression was increased in the myocardium of MI rats. Besides, the mRNA and protein expression levels of TH were significantly higher in sema 3A-silenced rats compared with the MI-GFP and MI-CON groups. These results suggest that the upregulation

of sema 3A might partially suppress sympathetic nerve sprouting and subsequently decrease sympathetic nerve expression.

Previous studies revealed an increased expression of CHAT mRNA and protein in MI [11]. Nevertheless, in the current study, the ratio of TH/CHAT protein was higher in MI-SiRNA group than that in MI-CON and MI-GFP groups. Consistently, in the MI-SiRNA group, higher levels of NE were detected accompanied with a higher arrhythmic score and an increased incidence of inducible VAs. Previous studies revealed that sympathetic hyperinnervation and activation were correlated with a high incidence of lethal VAs and sudden cardiac death in post-infarcted hearts [5, 7, 8, 30]. In addition, pro-arrhythmia effects were reported in sema 3A-related neural remodeling animals [16, 19]. Recently, Nakano et al. demonstrated that a non-synonymous polymorphism in sema 3A was correlated with human unexplained cardiac arrest and ventricular fibrillation with inappropriate innervation patterning [20]. Taken together, these data suggest that sema 3A might play a critical role in maintaining cardiac electrical stability by preserving normal cardiac innervation in diseased hearts.

In damaged neural tissues, upregulated sema 3A could hinder neuroregeneration and remyelination [15]. Overexpression of sema 3A in the infarcted border via local myocardial gene transduction reduces sympathetic hyperinnervation and inducible VAs in post-infarcted hearts [19]. In our study, sema 3A expression was increased in vivo by intravenously injecting recombinant sema 3A. Five weeks after infarction, TH-positive nerve fibers, as well as its mRNA and protein levels, were all decreased in the MI-Sema group. However, there was no significant difference in the expression of CHAT and myocardial ACh levels between the MI-control and MI-Sema groups. The protein ratio of TH/CHAT was reduced to relatively normal levels, similar to that in the sham group ($P = 0.34$), via downregulating TH expression by sema 3A. The incidence of inducible VAs and myocardial NE levels were also lower in the MI-Sema group compared with the MI-CON and MI-PBS groups. Sympathetic overactivity complicated MI leads to an increase of NE concentration which encourages the early depolarization (EAD) and delayed afterdepolarization (DAD) by affecting influx and repolarization potassium current, and then trigger arrhythmia [37]. Moreover, NE may cause focal vasoconstriction and myocardial ischemia which facilitates- arrhythmogenesis [38]. Sema 3A suppresses the expressions and functions of myocardial transient outward current (Ito) and inward rectifier current (IK1) channels. Sema 3A ameliorates electrical remodeling in post-infarcted heart which is partly related with the inhibition of sympathetic nerve sprouting [39]. All these studies indicate that sympathetic innervation is also closely related to electrical homogeneity. Consistently, overexpression of sema 3A decreased sympathetic nerve sprouting activity and nerve density, improved TH/CHAT ratio and further reduced myocardial NE level according to our results. These effects may contribute to the increased cardiac electrical stability, resulting in reduced inducible VAs.

Infarct size and cardiac dysfunction are predictive factors of VAs in post-infarcted-hearts [40]. This current study revealed that these two factors were similar among MI groups, suggesting that sema 3A affected cardiac rhythm independent of infarct size and cardiac function in post-infarcted hearts. Sema 3A inhibits NGF-induced nociceptive afferent sprouting in spinal cords of adult rats [41]. However, both sema 3A silencing and overexpression did not alter the up-regulated NGF mRNA and protein in post-infarcted hearts. Cardiac innervation patterning is strictly controlled by the balance between NGF and sema 3A [16]. Treatment with exogenous sema 3A might alleviate the infarction-induced imbalance between NGF and sema 3A and suppress nerve sprouting, especially the sympathetic nerve. Furthermore, both sema 3A deficiency and supplementation did not alter the expression of CHAT protein and mRNA levels. Therefore, sema 3A treatment improved cardiac autonomic abnormalities mainly by affecting the sympathetic nerve.

Limitations

Coronary arteriosclerosis is the main cause of clinical MI in patients. In the current study, we ligated the left anterior descending coronary artery and created a MI model that was different from the clinical setting. Moreover, the different infarct sizes (small or large) and sites (anterior, inferior, or posterior wall) might partly affect the expression of neurotrophic factors and ventricular arrhythmogenesis. However, autonomic nerve function can be affected by animal emotions and surroundings. Clinically, heart rate variability (HBV), baroreflex sensitivity (BRS), and heart rate recovery (HRR) are used frequently to evaluate autonomic nerve function [42]. Myocaridial NE and ACh levels are also measured to assess nerve function. Nevertheless, additional studies are necessary to explore the mechanisms of effects of sema 3A on post-infarcted neural remodeling and its relationship with cardiac autonomic function. Such studies will provide further insights into sema 3A as a therapeutic target for autonomic abnormalities complicated cardiac electrical instability.

Conclusion

MI results in nerve injury and upregulation of the neuronal regulator sema 3A. Endogenous sema 3A partially inhibits nerve sprouting, whereas the downregulation of sema 3A aggravates the cardiac autonomic disorders and increases the potential of lethal VAs in post-infarcted hearts. Intravenous injection of sema 3A improves the autonomic abnormalities at the levels of both innervation and nerve function, mainly sympathetic nerve, and subsequently increases cardiac electrical stability and reduces inducible VAs. Therefore, sema 3A might be a therapeutic target for autonomic disorders induced VAs in post-infarcted hearts.

Abbreviations

sema 3A: Semaphorin 3A; VAs: Ventricular arrhythmias; NE: Norepinephrine; MI: Myocardial infarction; NGF: Nerve growth factor; LV: Left ventricle.; GFP: Green fluorescent protein; RNAi: RNA interference; DsRNA: Double-stranded RNA; siRNA: Small interference RNA; oligo: Oligonucleotide; shRNA: Short hairpin RNA; BCA: Bicinchoninic acid; PVDF: Polyvinylidene fluoride; LAD: Left anterior descending; ECG: Electrocardiogram; PES: Programmed electrical stimulation; GAPDH: Glyceraldehyde-3-phosphate dehydrogenase; TH: Tyrosine hydroxylase; MAP: Mean arterial blood pressure; P-V: Pressure-volume; LVESP: LV end-systolic pressure; LVEDP: LV end-diastolic pressure; dP/dtmax: Systolic pressure increment; dP/dtmin: Diastolic pressure decrement; EDV: End-diastolic volume; ESV: End-systolic volume; EF: Ejection fraction; CHAT: Choline acetyltransferase; HPLC: High performance liquid chromatography; Ach: Acetylcholine; Ito: Transient outward current; IK1: Inward rectifier current; HBV: Heart rate variability; BRS: Baroreflex sensitivity; HRR: Heart rate recovery.

Competing interests

The authors and funders declare that they have no competing interests.

Authors' contributions

The contributions of individual authors to this paper were as follows. Conceived and designed the experiments: SY HH. Performed the experiments: HH YX MX WC YW Xinran Li JY YN SY. Analyzed the data: HH YX. Contributed reagents/materials/analysis tools: Xiaolu Li. Wrote the paper: HH. All authors read and approved the final manuscript.

Acknowledgements

The work was supported by the National Natural Science Foundation of China (NSFC, 81070088), Doctoral Fund of Ministry of Education of China (20130131110069),Science and Technology Development Planning of Shandong Province (2013GGB14056, 2015GSF118022) and Independent Innovation foundation for Jinan Science and Technology Development Planning (201311020) and the Shandong Taishan Scholarship (Suhua Yan). The funders had no role in study design, data collection and analysis, decision to publish, or preparation of the manuscript.

References

1. Exner DV. Noninvasive risk stratification after myocardial infarction: rationale, current evidence and the need for definitive trials. Can J Cardiol. 2009;25:21A–7.
2. Kuriachan V, Exner DV. Role of risk stratification after myocardial infarction. Curr Treat Options Cardiovasc Med. 2009;11(1):10–21.
3. Ieda M, Fukuda K. Cardiac innervation and sudden cardiac death. Curr Cardiol Rev. 2009;5(4):289.
4. Yan SH, Hu HS, Wang XL, Xing QC, Wang Q, Shi CW, et al. Effects of prolonged metoprolol treatment on neural remodeling and inducible ventricular arrhythmias after myocardial infarction in rabbits. Int J Cardiol. 2007;117(3):317–22.
5. Wang Y, Liu J, Suo F, Hu HS, Xue M, Cheng WJ, et al. Metoprolol–mediated amelioration of sympathetic nerve sprouting after myocardial infarction. Cardiology. 2013;126(1):50–8.
6. Chen PS, Chen LS, Cao JM, Sharifi B, Karagueuzian HS, Fishbein MC. Sympathetic nerve sprouting, electrical remodeling and the mechanisms of sudden cardiac death. Cardiovasc Res. 2001;50(2):409–16.
7. Liu YB, Wu CC, Lu LS, Su MJ, Lin CW, Lin SF, et al. Sympathetic nerve sprouting, electrical remodeling, and increased vulnerability to ventricular fibrillation in hypercholesterolemic rabbits. Circ Res. 2003;92(10):1145–52.
8. Vaseghi M, Shivkumar K. The role of the autonomic nervous system in sudden cardiac death. Prog Cardiovasc Dis. 2008;50(6):404.
9. Pruvot E, Thonet G, Vesin JM, van Melle G, Seidl K, Schmidinger H, et al. Heart rate dynamics at the onset of ventricular tachyarrhythmias as retrieved from implantable cardioverter–defibrillators in patients with coronary artery disease. Circulation. 2000;101(20):2398–404.
10. Malfatto G, Facchini M, Sala L, Branzi G, Bragato R, Leonetti G. Relationship between baseline sympatho-vagal balance and the autonomic response to cardiac rehabilitation after a first uncomplicated myocardial infarction. Ital Heart J. 2000;1(3):226–32.
11. Nguyen BL, Li H, Fishbein MC, Lin SF, Gaudio C, Chen PS, et al. Acute myocardial infarction induces bilateral stellate ganglia neural remodeling in rabbits. Cardiovasc Pathol. 2012;21(3):143–8.
12. Cao JM, Chen LS, KenKnight BH, Ohara T, Lee MH, Tsai J, et al. Nerve sprouting and sudden cardiac death. Circ Res. 2000;86(7):816–21.
13. Govoni S, Pascale A, Amadio M, Calvillo L, D'Elia E, Cereda C, et al. NGF and heart: Is there a role in heart disease? Pharmacol Res. 2011;63(4):266–77.
14. Hu H, Xuan Y, Wang Y, Xue M, Suo F, Li X, et al. Targeted NGF siRNA delivery attenuates sympathetic nerve sprouting and deteriorates cardiac dysfunction in rats with myocardial infarction. PLoS One. 2014;9(4), e95106.
15. Goshima Y, Sasaki Y, Yamashita N, Nakamura F. Class 3 semaphorins as a therapeutic target. Expert Opin Ther Targets. 2012;16(9):933–44.
16. Ieda M, Kanazawa H, Kimura K, Hattori F, Ieda Y, Taniguchi M, et al. Sema3a maintains normal heart rhythm through sympathetic innervation patterning. Nat Med. 2007;13(5):604–12.
17. Hashimoto H, Ino H, Koda M, Murakami M, Yoshinaga K, Yamazaki M, et al. Regulation of semaphorin 3A expression in neurons of the rat spinal cord and cerebral cortex after transection injury. Acta Neuropathol. 2004;107(3):250–6.
18. Jiang SX, Whitehead S, Aylsworth A, Slinn J, Zurakowski B, Chan K, et al. Neuropilin 1 directly interacts with Fer kinase to mediate semaphorin 3A-induced death of cortical neurons. J Biol Chem. 2010;285(13):9908–18.
19. Chen RH, Li YG, Jiao KL, Zhang PP, Sun Y, Zhang LP, et al. Overexpression of sema3a in myocardial infarction border zone decreases vulnerability of ventricular tachycardia post-myocardial infarction in rats. J Cell Mol Med. 2013;17(5):608–16.
20. Nakano Y, Chayama K, Ochi H, Toshishige M, Hayashida Y, Miki D, et al. A nonsynonymous polymorphism in Semaphorin 3A as a risk factor for human unexplained cardiac arrest with documented ventricular fibrillation. PLoS Genet. 2013;9(4), e1003364.
21. Ichim CV, Wells RA. Generation of high-titer viral preparations by concentration using successive rounds of ultracentrifugation. J Transl Med. 2011;9(1):1–8.
22. Saal KA, Koch JC, Tatenhorst L, Szego EM, Ribas VT, Michel U, et al. AAV. shRNA-mediated downregulation of ROCK2 attenuates degeneration of dopaminergic neurons in toxin-induced models of Parkinson's disease in vitro and in vivo. Neurobiol Dis. 2015;73:150–62.
23. Nguyen T, El Salibi E, Rouleau JL. Postinfarction survival and inducibility of ventricular arrhythmias in the spontaneously hypertensive rat effects of ramipril and hydralazine. Circulation. 1998;98(19):2074–80.
24. Lee TM, Chen CC, Hsu YJ. Differential effects of NADPH oxidase and xanthine oxidase inhibition on sympathetic reinnervation in postinfarct rat hearts. Free Radic Biol Med. 2011;50(11):1461–70.
25. Schmittgen TD, Livak KJ. Analyzing real-time PCR data by the comparative CT method. Nat Protoc. 2008;3(6):1101–8.
26. Kakinuma Y, Akiyama T, Sato T. Cholinoceptive and cholinergic properties of cardiomyocytes involving an amplification mechanism for vagal efferent effects in sparsely innervated ventricular myocardium. FEBS J. 2009;276(18):5111–25.
27. Li W, Knowlton D, Van Winkle DM, Habecker BA. Infarction alters both the distribution and noradrenergic properties of cardiac sympathetic neurons. Am J Physiol Heart Circ Physiol. 2004;286(6):H2229–36.
28. Hayashi M, Nakashima T, Taniguchi M, Kodama T, Kumanogoh A, Takayanagi H. Osteoprotection by semaphorin 3A. Nature. 2012; 485(7396):69–74.
29. Zipes DP, Rubart M. Neural modulation of cardiac arrhythmias and sudden cardiac death. Heart Rhythm. 2006;3(1):108.
30. Chen LS, Zhou S, Fishbein MC, CHEN PS. New perspectives on the role of autonomic nervous system in the genesis of arrhythmias. J Cardiovasc Electrophysiol. 2007;18(1):123–7.
31. Lymperopoulos A. Physiology and pharmacology of the cardiovascular adrenergic system. Front Physiol. 2013;4.
32. Parrish DC, Alston EN, Rohrer H, Hermes SM, Aicher SA, Nkadi P, et al. Absence of gp130 in dopamine β-hydroxylase-expressing neurons leads to autonomic imbalance and increased reperfusion arrhythmias. Am J Physiol Heart Circ Physiol. 2009;297(3):H960–7.
33. Hasan W. Autonomic cardiac innervation: development and adult plasticity. Organogenesis. 2013;9(3):176.
34. Kimura K, Ieda M, Fukuda K. Development, maturation, and transdifferentiation of cardiac sympathetic nerves. Circ Res. 2012;110(2):325–36.
35. Chao MV. Neurotrophins and their receptors: a convergence point for many signalling pathways. Nat Rev Neurosci. 2003;4(4):299–309.
36. Sun SQ, Wang XT, Qu XF, Li Y, Yu Y, Song Y, et al. Increased expression of myocardial semaphorin 3A in isoproterenol-induced heart failure rats. Chinese Med J-Beijing. 2011;124(14):2173.
37. Marks AR, Priori S, Memmi M, Kontula K, Laitinen PJ. Involvement of the cardiac ryanodine receptor/calcium release channel in catecholaminergic polymorphic ventricular tachycardia. J Cell Physiol. 2002;190(1):1–6.
38. Baker KE, Curtis MJ. Left regional cardiac perfusion in vitro with platelet-activating factor, norepinephrine and K+ reveals that ischaemic arrhythmias are caused by independent effects of endogenous 'mediators' facilitated by interactions, and moderated by paradoxical antagonism. Br J Pharmacol. 2004;142(2):352–66.
39. Wen HZ, Jiang H, Li L, Xie P, Li JY, Lu ZB, et al. Semaphorin 3A attenuates electrical remodeling at infarct border zones in rats after myocardial infarction. Tohoku J Exp Med. 2011;225(1):51–7.
40. Naccarella F, Lepera G, Rolli A. Arrhythmic risk stratification of post–myocardial infarction patients. Curr Opin Cardiol. 2000;15(1):1–6.
41. Tang XQ, Tanelian DL, Smith GM. Semaphorin3A inhibits nerve growth factor-induced sprouting of nociceptive afferents in adult rat spinal cord. J Neurosci. 2004;24(4):819–27.
42. Reed M, Robertson C, Addison P. Heart rate variability measurements and the prediction of ventricular arrhythmias. QJM. 2005;98(2):87–95.

4

Thromboembolic events, bleeding, and drug discontinuation in patients with atrial fibrillation on anticoagulation

Oliver Königsbrügge[1]*(iD), Alexander Simon[2], Hans Domanovits[2], Ingrid Pabinger[1] and Cihan Ay[1,3]

Abstract

Background: The clinical practice of stroke prevention in atrial fibrillation (AF) with direct oral anticoagulants (DOACS) differs from anticoagulation in randomized trial patients. We investigated the risk of thromboembolism, bleeding, and drug discontinuation in a hospital-based real-world setting.

Methods: All-comer patients with non-valvular AF were recruited into a registry at an academic tertiary care center. After informed consent, patients underwent a personal structured interview including medical history, past and current anticoagulation, and returned for follow-up after 6–12 months.

Results: The registry comprised 282 patients (42% women, median age 71 years) with a median CHA2DS2-Vasc-Score of 4 (25. to 75. percentile 2.5–5), who were prospectively followed 285 days in median. At inclusion, 118 patients took vitamin-K-antagonists, 33 dabigatran, 87 rivaroxaban, 30 apixaban, 5 low-molecular-weight heparin, and 9 were on no anticoagulant. Occurrence of stroke (rate 2.8/100 patient-years), was associated with prior stroke (hazard ratio [HR] 18.5, 95% confidence interval 2.16–159), increased HbA1c (HR per 1% increase 1.71, 1.20–2.45) and borderline significantly associated with vascular disease (HR 8.33, 0.97–71.3). Further we observed a high rate of major bleeding (2.8/100 patient-years), clinically relevant non-major bleeding (4.1/100 patient-years), and venous thromboembolism (2.8/100 patient-years). Anticoagulation was discontinued by 80 patients (36.9/100 patient-years), and diabetes (HR 2.31, 1.32–4.02), history of bleeding (HR 2.51, 1.44–4.37) and elevated leucocyte count (HR per 1G/l increase 1.02, 1.00–1.05) were associated with increased risk of discontinuation.

Conclusions: In this hospital-based registry, patients with atrial fibrillation had an increased risk of thromboembolic events despite anticoagulation. The low drug persistence may be attributable to distinct comorbid conditions and bleeding complications.

Keywords: Atrial fibrillation, Anticoagulation, Tertiary healthcare, Stroke, Hemorrhage, Medication persistence

Background

The increased risk of stroke and systemic embolism in patients with non-valvular atrial fibrillation (AF) can be attenuated with continuous oral anticoagulation treatment [1]. Direct oral anticoagulants (DOACs), including the direct thrombin inhibitor dabigatran and the direct factor Xa inhibitors rivaroxaban, apixaban, and edoxaban, have shifted the paradigm of anticoagulation treatment from routine drug monitoring and dose adjustment to a one-size-fits-all strategy, and changed clinical practice of oral anticoagulation. Real-world data have confirmed the efficacy and safety of DOACs for stroke prevention [2, 3]. However, in a hospital-based patient population with AF, comorbid conditions, comedications and surgical interventions may complicate treatment with anticoagulant drugs, which has not been specifically addressed in previous real-world investigation.

* Correspondence: oliver.koenigsbruegge@meduniwien.ac.at
[1]Department of Medicine I, Clinical Division of Hematology & Hemostaseology, Medical University of Vienna, Währinger Gürtel 18-20, A-1090 Vienna, Austria
Full list of author information is available at the end of the article

Furthermore, there is still concern that the ease of drug administration and clinical management with DOACs may not guarantee better persistence on treatment in a real-world setting. Drug persistence is defined as the total time a patient stays on a prescribed medication and reduced persistence increases the risk of stroke [4, 5]. In the randomized controlled trials that led to the licensing of DOACs for stroke prevention in AF, 20.7%–34.3% of patients receiving DOACs discontinued drug treatment during the study period and 16.6%–34.4% discontinued the control treatment, warfarin [6–9]. However, drug persistence in clinical trials may be completely different from real-world persistence, because there are different incentives for remaining on treatment in real-world patients.

We aimed to examine the characteristics of non-valvular AF patients in a hospital-based setting and investigate risk factors for occurrence of thromboembolic events, bleeding episodes and drug persistence while on anticoagulant treatment, as well as reasons for drug discontinuation.

Methods

Patients

Patients with non-valvular AF referred to the Clinical Division of Hematology and Hemostaseology were recruited into a hospital-based, prospective registry from July 2013 to May 2016. Inclusion criteria were confirmed diagnosis of AF by a 12-channel, resting electrocardiogram (ECG), willingness to comply with study procedures, and written informed consent. The study has approval of the local ethics committee. There were no exclusion or selection criteria concerning anticoagulation treatment, medical history, risk of stroke, or bleeding. After obtaining informed consent for study participation, a study investigator performed a personal structured interview with each patient, recorded the medical history and a detailed anticoagulation history. Patients returned for voluntary, scheduled follow-up visits 6 and 12 months after recruitment.

Baseline assessment of patient characteristics

All baseline patient data was recorded from personal interviews and verified against medical records. The structured interview included a detailed medical history, especially concerning prior thromboembolic events, and a detailed record of previous periods of anticoagulation treatment and associated complications. During baseline data collection, a history of vascular disease was defined as arterial disease of any degree including coronary heart disease, peripheral artery disease, and carotid artery disease. Cancer was defined as any history of malignancy or active malignancy at study inclusion with the exception of basalioma. Patients were anticoagulation naive at baseline if they had not received continuous anticoagulation treatment previously for longer than 3 months. The baseline kidney function was calculated on the grounds of the estimated glomerular filtration rate (eGFR) and isotope-dilution mass spectrometry (IDMS) traceable serum creatinine levels using the Modification of Diet in Renal Disease (MDRD) equation. The risk of stroke was assessed with the CHA_2DS_2-Vasc score and the risk of bleeding with the HAS-BLED score.

Definition of events during prospective observation

Bleeding outcomes were classified according to the recommendations of the Scientific and Standardization Committee of the International Society of Thrombosis and Hemostasis. Major bleeding was defined as clinically overt bleeding with fatal outcome, involvement of a critical anatomic site, fall in hemoglobin concentration of more than 2 g/dl, transfusion of >2 units of whole blood or packed red blood cells, or leading to permanent disability [10]. Clinically relevant non-major (CRNM) bleeding was defined as overt bleeding not meeting criteria for major bleeding but requiring medical intervention, hospitalization, temporary interruption or delayed dosing of anticoagulation, pain, or impairment of daily activities [11]. Minor bleeding was defined as any other bleeding not meeting the above criteria. Venous thromboembolism (VTE) was defined as objectively confirmed deep vein thrombosis (DVT) or pulmonary embolism (PE). Stroke was defined as the sudden onset of a distinct focal neurologic deficit in a location consistent with the territory of a major cerebral artery and conclusive imaging evidence. In the absence of imaging evidence, but conclusive neurological symptoms confirmed by a specialist in neurology, we recorded a transient ischemic attack (TIA). All events were internally validated according to the criteria listed above.

Definition of anticoagulation persistence

Drug persistence was defined as the time in weeks from the initiation of anticoagulation until discontinuation of treatment [12]. Only patients who initiated anticoagulation at the time of recruitment were included in the persistence analysis. The percentage of patients remaining on the baseline anticoagulant was calculated for 6 and 12 months as well as the annualized discontinuation-rate. The end of anticoagulation persistence was defined as the permanent cessation of anticoagulation treatment or switching from one anticoagulant to a different anticoagulant, but did not include pausing anticoagulation treatment for a limited time of less than 1 month.

Statistical methods

Baseline patient characteristics of the registry cohort were described as absolute and relative frequencies or with median and 25th to 75th percentile, respectively for categorical and continuous data. The baseline group comparisons between DOAC and vitamin-K-antagonist

(VKA) patients were calculated with the Mann–Whitney-U test for categorical parameters or the chi^2 test for continuous variables. An asymptotic two-sided p-value of smaller than 0.05 was considered statistically significant. The risks of stroke, TIA, or systemic embolism, bleeding, and drug discontinuation were calculated with the univariable Cox proportional hazards model. All calculations were performed with SPSS (Windows Version 23.0; IBM Corp., Armonk, NY, http://www.ibm.com). Risk of discontinuation was only calculated with patients who initiated a new anticoagulation therapy at study inclusion.

Results

Baseline registry characteristics

The registry includes 282 patients (118 [42%] women, 164 [58%] men) with ECG-confirmed diagnosis of AF and a median age of 71 years (25th to 75th percentile 65 – 77 years). At baseline, 118 patients (41.8%) were on VKA, 33 patients (11.7%) on dabigatran, 87 (30.9%) on rivaroxaban, 30 (10.6%) on apixaban, 5 patients (1.8%) on long-term low-molecular-weight heparin (LMWH) and 9 patients (3.2%) did not take any anticoagulant drug. The baseline characteristics of the full registry and respective to groups of patients on each anticoagulant are shown in Table 1. DOACs were more frequently prescribed to patients with more recently diagnosed AF and to patients previously naïve to anticoagulation treatment (Table 1). Patients with history of CRNM or major bleeding, with age between 65–75 years were also more frequently on DOAC treatment. Patients older than 75 years were more often on VKA, while patients on DOACs, especially rivaroxaban and apixaban, tended to have lower hemoglobin and hematocrit levels than patients on VKA. Patients with lower eGFR, however, tended to take VKA (Table 1).

Prospective outcomes

Prospective follow-up was available for 269 patients and 13 patients (4.6%) were lost to follow-up. The median observation time was 285 days (227–405 days) (minimum 1 day, maximum 966) for a total of 217 patient-years of observation time. During follow-up, 6 (2.2%) cardioembolic events occurred (4 ischemic strokes, 1 TIA, 1 systemic embolism), corresponding to an event-rate of 2.8 per 100 patient-years. Of these events, 4 occurred while on VKA, 1 while on rivaroxaban, and 1 while on triple therapy with VKA.

In univariable Cox regression, patients with a history of stroke, TIA, or systemic embolism had an 18-fold increased risk of a new stroke, TIA or systemic embolism (hazard ratio [HR] 18.5, 95% confidence interval [CI] 2.16–159, $p = 0.008$), patients with vascular disease had a borderline significant 8.3-fold increased risk of stroke (HR 8.3, 95% CI 0.97–71.3, $p = 0.05$), and for every 1%

increase in HbA1c the risk of stroke increased 1.7-fold (95% CI 1.20–2.45, $p = 0.003$) (Table 2). For every one point added to the CHA2DS2-Vasc score the risk of stroke doubled (HR 2.06, 95% CI 1.27–3.35, $p = 0.004$). One myocardial infarction occurred while on VKA, and 6 VTE events occurred (4 DVT, 2 PE), corresponding to an event-rate of 2.8 per 100 patient-years. One VTE event occurred while on rivaroxaban therapy, 2 during rivaroxaban pause, 1 during VKA treatment, 1 during VKA pause, and 1 after discontinuation of rivaroxaban. Major bleeding events occurred in 6 patients (3 intraocular hemorrhages, 2 intraabdominal bleedings with massive blood loss and/or transfusions, 1 subdural hematoma) and CRNM bleeding events occurred in 9 patients (5 gastrointestinal [GI] bleeds, 4 other bleeds requiring hospitalization). The event rate for major bleeding was 2.8 per 100 patient-years and for CRNM bleeding 4.1 per 100 patient-years. Minor bleeding events occurred in 43 patients and 15 patients died during follow-up of causes unrelated to atrial fibrillation or anticoagulation. The results of our analysis revealed no statistically significant risk factor for bleeding that occurred during follow-up.

Anticoagulation persistence

The median persistence was 32 weeks (25th to 75th percentile: 12 to 46 weeks) and 80 patients (29.7%) discontinued the anticoagulation therapy, which they had received at baseline. This corresponds to a rate of discontinuation of 36.9 per 100 patient-years. After 6 months, the overall drug persistence of the baseline anticoagulant was 76.7% and after 12 months further reduced to 54.7%. There was no difference in the persistence between patients receiving DOACs and VKA (Fig. 1). The most frequent reasons for discontinuing anticoagulation were patient-reported end of AF and permanent return to sinus rhythm (20%), emergence of a new contraindication for current anticoagulation treatment (15%) (e.g. mechanical heart valve), physician's recommendation (12.5%), and occurrence of major or CRNM bleeding events (11.3%) (Table 3). The choice for an alternative anticoagulant after discontinuation of the baseline anticoagulant drug was evenly distributed between VKA, rivaroxaban, apixaban or no anticoagulant at all (Table 3). In regression analysis, patients with diabetes had a 2.3-fold increased risk of discontinuation (95% CI 1.32 to 4.02), patients with history of bleeding had a 2.5-fold increased risk (95% CI 1.44 to 4.37) and per 1 G/l increase in leucocyte count the risk of discontinuation increased by 2% (HR = 1.02, 95% CI 1.00 to 1.05).

Discussion

In this analysis of a real-world, tertiary-care, hospital-based registry of patients with atrial fibrillation, the rate

Table 1 Baseline cohort characteristics

Characteristic	Full cohort (N = 282)	VKA (N = 118)	Dabigatran (N = 33)	p*	Rivaroxaban (N = 87)	p*	Apixaban (N = 30)	p*
Age	71 (65–77)	73 (67–79)	73 (68–77)	0.8	71 (66–75)	0.1	71 (64–75)	**0.04**
Female sex	116 (43.1)	47 (41.6)	11 (34.4)	0.5	30 (37.0)	0.5	22 (75.9)	**0.001**
BMI	27.0 (24.5–30.4)	27.3 (24.9–31.2)	27.3 (25.0–31.0)	0.7	27.0 (24.0–31.1)	0.5	26.9 (22.2–28.3)	0.09
Type of AF								
Recently diagnosed	52 (18.4)	10 (8.5)	8 (24.2)	**0.04**	16 (18.4)	0.2	13 (43.3)	**<0.001**
paroxysmal	131 (46.5)	60 (50.8)	10 (30.3)	**0.05**	42 (49.4)	0.8	12 (40.0)	0.3
persisting	19 (6.7)	9 (7.6)	1 (3.0)	0.4	7 (8.6)	0.7	1 (3.3)	0.5
permanent	80 (28.4)	39 (33.1)	14 (42.4)	0.3	22 (27.2)	0.4	4 (13.3)	**0.04**
Time since AF diagnosis, years	4 (1–8)	4 (2–9)	5 (0.1–9)	0.5	3 (1–10)	0.1	2 (0–6)	**0.01**
History of electrical cardioversion	83 (30.9)	40 (35.4)	10 (31.3)	0.7	21 (25.9)	0.2	9 (31.0)	0.7
History of ablation	35 (13.0)	15 (13.3)	5 (15.6)	0.7	13 (16.0)	0.6	1 (3.4)	0.1
Family history of AF	33 (12.3)	13 (11.5)	3 (9.4)	0.7	10 (12.3)	0.9	7 (24.1)	0.08
Medical history								
Congestive heart failure	81 (30.1)	34 (30.1)	13 (40.6)	0.3	24 (29.6)	0.9	8 (27.6)	0.8
Hypertension	227 (84.4)	99 (87.6)	30 (93.8)	0.3	65 (80.2)	0.2	26 (89.7)	0.8
Age ≥ 75 years	98 (36.4)	53 (46.9)	13 (40.6)	0.5	23 (28.4)	**0.009**	8 (27.6)	0.06
Age 65–74 years	114 (42.4)	41 (36.3)	14 (43.8)	0.4	43 (53.1)	0.02	13 (44.8)	0.4
Diabetes	81 (28.7)	31 (27.4)	10 (31.3)	0.4	22 (27.2)	0.7	8 (27.6)	0.9
Stroke / TIA / systemic embolism	55 (20.4)	22 (19.5)	7 (21.9)	0.8	20 (24.7)	0.4	4 (13.8)	0.5
Vascular disease	96 (35.7)	41 (36.3)	13 (40.6)	0.7	28 (34.6)	0.8	11 (37.6)	0.9
CHA$_2$DS$_2$-VASC Score	4 (2.5–5)	4 (3–5)	4 (3–5)	0.9	3 (2–5)	0.3	4 (3–4.5)	0.4
HAS-BLED Score	2 (1–3)	2 (1–2)	2 (1–3)	0.7	2 (1–3)	0.2	2 (1–3)	0.5
Abnormal liver or kidney function	52 (19.3)	24 (21.2)	5 (15.6)	0.5	18 (22.2)	0.9	5 (17.2)	0.6
CRNM bleeding	13 (4.8)	1 (0.9)	2 (6.3)	0.06	4 (4.9)	0.08	4 (13.8)	**0.001**
Major bleeding	10 (3.7)	1 (0.9)	5 (15.6)	**<0.001**	4 (4.9)	0.08	0	0.6
Venous thromboembolism	22 (8.2)	7 (6.2)	3 (9.4)	0.5	9 (11.1)	0.2	3 (10.3)	0.4
Cancer	58 (21.6)	19 (16.8)	9 (28.1)	0.2	19 (23.5)	0.3	6 (20.7)	0.6
OAC-naïve at baseline	18 (6.7)	4 (3.5)	2 (6.3)	0.5	6 (7.4)	0.2	4 (13.8)	**0.03**
Aspirin comedication	58 (21.6)	23 (20.4)	5 (15.6)	0.6	19 (23.5)	0.6	6 (20.7)	0.9
Clopidogrel comedication	14 (5.2)	9 (8.0)	2 (6.3)	0.7	3 (3.7)	0.2	0	0.1
Baseline laboratory parameters								
Platelet count	214 (176–264)	211 (180–251)	203 (172–239)	0.4	215 (174–286)	0.3	238 (177–275)	0.4
Hemoglobin	13.2 (11.8–14.4)	13.5 (12.5–14.8)	13.2 (11.8–15.2)	0.3	12.7 (11.4–14.1)	**0.002**	12.8 (11.0–14.1)	**0.05**
Hematocrit	39.5 (35.1–42.8)	40.3 (37.4–43.9)	39.5 (34.9–42.6)	0.2	38.5 (33.6–41.0)	**0.001**	38.8 (33.9–41.2)	**0.03**
Leucocyte count	6.8 (5.7–8.5)	6.8 (5.7–7.9)	7.0 (6.0–8.6)	0.3	6.9 (5.7–8.9)	0.3	6.4 (5.2–7.9)	0.3
eGFR (ml/min/1.73 m^2)	65.2 (53.3–79.6)	60.4 (49.5–74.3)	71.2 (58.4–91.8)	**0.03**	66.8 (56.2–82.1)	**0.01**	65.8 (56.6–73.1)	0.2

Footnote: * Mann–Whitney-U test or chi^2 p-value for asymptomatic two-sided difference between respective DOAC group and VKA group, statistically significant p-values in bold print

Abbreviations: AF atrial fibrillation, VKA Vitamin-K-antagonist, BMI body-mass-index, TIA transient ischemic attack, CRNM bleeding clinically relevant non-major bleeding, OAC oral anticoagulation, eGFR estimated glomerular filtration rate

of cardioembolic events (2.8 per 100 patient-years) was higher than in the randomized controlled trials for stroke prevention in AF. In RE-LY, ROCKET-AF, ARIS-TOTLE and ENGAGE-AF-TIMI48, 1.6–2.2% of patients randomized to warfarin and 1.11–2.04% for patients randomized to the study drugs had strokes or systemic embolisms per year [6–9]. The stroke-rate in our study was also higher than in other data sets of real-world AF

Table 2 Univariable Cox regression analysis of risk factors for the outcomes stroke, bleeding, and drug discontinuation

Characteristic	Hazard of stroke, TIA, systemic embolism ($N = 269$)		Hazard of CRNM or major bleed ($N = 269$)		Hazard of anticoagulant discontinuation ($N = 144$)	
	Hazard ratio (95% confidence interval)	p-value	Hazard ratio (95% confidence interval)	p-value	Hazard ratio (95% confidence interval)	p-value
Age[a]	0.98 (0.90–1.06)	0.59	1.03 (0.97–1.09)	0.30	0.99 (0.96–1.02)	0.54
Female sex	6.45 (0.75–55.2)	0.09	0.95 (0.36–2.56)	0.93	1.01 (0.59–1.75)	0.96
BMI[a]	0.96 (0.81–1.13)	0.63	1.00 (0.92–1.10)	0.96	0.99 (0.94–1.04)	0.65
Medical history						
Congestive heart failure	2.00 (0.40–9.94)	0.40	1.15 (0.42–3.18)	0.78	1.28 (0.73–2.23)	0.39
Hypertension	24.2 (0.00–999)	0.60	23.8 (0.01–999)	0.42	0.60 (0.28–1.28)	0.18
Diabetes	2.42 (0.49–12.0)	0.28	1.13 (0.39–3.27)	0.82	2.31 (1.32–4.02)	**0.003**
Stroke/TIA/systemic embolism	18.5 (2.16–159)	**0.008**	0.76 (0.22–2.69)	0.67	0.76 (0.38–1.53)	0.44
Vascular disease	8.33 (0.97–71.3)	0.05	0.62 (0.21–1.82)	0.39	1.16 (0.67–2.00)	0.61
CHA$_2$DS$_2$–VASC Score[a]	2.06 (1.27–3.35)	**0.004**	1.03 (0.77–1.37)	0.85	1.05 (0.90–1.21)	0.57
History of bleeding	0.85 (0.10–7.27)	0.88	1.17 (0.33–4.15)	0.81	2.51 (1.44–4.37)	**0.001**
HAS-BLED Score[a]	1.61 (0.90–2.87)	0.11	1.18 (0.77–1.80)	0.45	1.14 (0.92–1.42)	0.22
Venous thromboembolism	2.26 (0.26–19.4)	0.46	0.87 (0.11–6.64)	0.89	1.29 (0.51–3.26)	0.59
Active cancer/history of cancer	0.04 (0.00–330)	0.48	1.24 (0.35–4.40)	0.74	1.15 (0.62–2.12)	0.66
OAC-naïve at baseline	0.05 (0.00–999)	0.69	0.94 (0.12–7.23)	0.95	0.78 (0.31–1.97)	0.60
Baseline laboratory parameters (hazard ratios per 1 unit increase)						
Platelet count[a]	1.00 (0.99–1.01)	0.71	1.00 (0.99–1.01)	0.60	1.00 (0.99–1.00)	0.34
Hemoglobin[a]	0.80 (0.52–1.22)	0.29	1.05 (0.81–1.37)	0.71	0.89 (0.79–1.02)	0.08
Hematocrit[a]	0.95 (0.81–1.11)	0.51	1.01 (0.91–1.11)	0.86	0.96 (0.92–1.01)	0.11
Leucocyte count[a]	1.02 (0.91–1.13)	0.77	0.82 (0.63–1.06)	0.12	1.02 (1.00–1.05)	**0.041**
eGFR[a]	0.97 (0.93–1.01)	0.17	0.98 (0.96–1.01)	0.21	1.01 (1.00–1.02)	0.27
HbA1c[a]	1.71 (1.20–2.45)	**0.003**	1.13 (0.75–1.72)	0.54	1.31 (0.87–1.98)	0.20

Legend: *BMI* body-mass index, *TIA* transient ischemic attack, *VKA* vitamin-K-antagonist, *OAC* oral anticoagulant, *eGFR* estimated glomerular filtration rate, 999 as the upper bound of the 95% confidence interval signifies an abbreviation of a very wide confidence interval, p-values in bold font represent statistically significant findings, [a] the hazard ratios for continuous variables are given as per 1 unit increase: age in years, BMI in kg/m^2, platelet count in G/l, hemoglobin in g/dl, hematocrit in %, leucocyte count in G/l, eGFR in ml/min/1.73 m^2, HbA1c in rel.%, and D-dimer in μg/ml

patients. Graham et al. reported a stroke rate of 1.1 per 100 patient years for dabigatran and 1.4 for warfarin in a database of US Medicare patients [13]. Korenstra et al. found a rate of stroke of 0.8% per year for VKA and 1.0% per year for dabigatran outpatients [14], and Hecker et al. reported an event rate of 2.0 per 100 patient-years in rivaroxaban patients in daily-care [15]. In a recent report from the GARFIELD-AF registry, the rate of stroke was 1.25 per 100 patient-years [16]. Not surprisingly, these cohorts had lower frequencies of risk factors for strokes, including a prior history of stroke, a history of vascular disease, diabetes and a decreased CHA2DS2-Vasc Score, compared to our cohort. This is confirmation that a stroke risk evaluation is clinically meaningful in a hospital-based setting. We also observed a rate of myocardial infarction of 0.5 per 100 patients-years and a rate of VTE of 2.8 per 100 patient-years. Firstly, it is interesting that a cohort reported by Beyer-Westendorf et al. from a population of primary-care AF patients with similar baseline stroke risk factors and

similar stroke rate had no VTE events at all [2]. Thus, the risk of VTE in AF patients, especially when medically ill or frail, should not be neglected. Secondly, a closer inspection of the circumstances under which VTE events occurred, revealed that the majority occurred during temporary pausing of the anticoagulation therapy. Thus, VTE events may have been avoidable with a proper bridging strategy or minimizing of the anticoagulation pause. We would like to interpret this signal as a call to action on emphasizing educational programs on safe and efficacious anticoagulation management during interventions, operations, and hospitalizations.

Major bleeding events occurred with a rate of 2.8 per 100 patient-years and CRNM bleeding events with a rate of 4.1 per 100 patient-years. The rate of major or CRNM bleeding events was, however, not elevated in our cohort compared to some other real-world registries despite a median age of 71 years and a history of severe bleeding complications in 8.5% of patients. This may be an indication that bleeding risk evaluation in medically ill

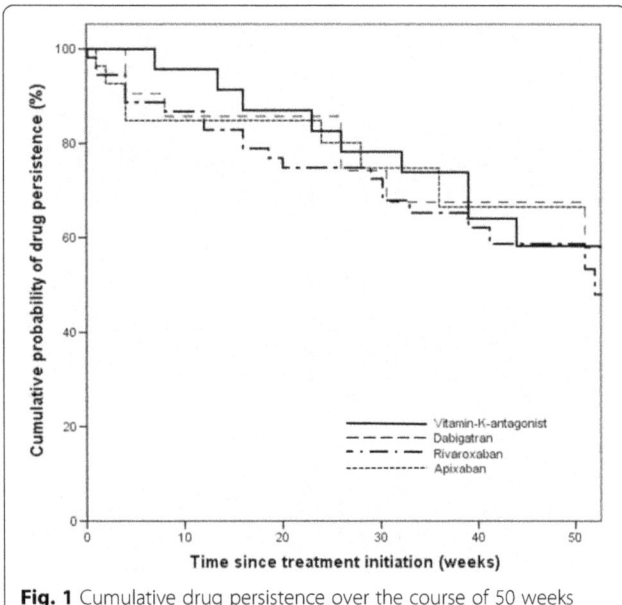

Fig. 1 Cumulative drug persistence over the course of 50 weeks

frequency in this cohort is nonetheless surprising and may warrant more awareness among physician who treat patients with anticoagulation.

We further investigated persistence on anticoagulation treatment in this registry and found that 80 patients (29.7%) discontinued their baseline anticoagulation over the course of the follow-up, which translates to a discontinuation rate of 36.9 per 100 patient-years. The majority, 69 of them, switched to a different anticoagulant agent, but 11 patients discontinued anticoagulation treatment altogether. We found that after 6 months the drug persistence on the baseline anticoagulant agent was 76.7% and after 12 months further reduced to 54.7%. The overall persistence in the registry is lower than in some previous reports. While in the pre-DOAC era, discontinuation frequency had been 26–28% [17, 18], Beyer-Westendorf et al. reported a persistence rate of 81.5% in patients on treatment with rivaroxaban after a median treatment time of 544 days [19]. The most frequent reason for discontinuation of anticoagulation treatment in our registry was permanent return to sinus rhythm. This group of patients is perceived as a low-risk group and especially after successful ablation treatment, anticoagulation treatment is oftentimes discontinued in clinical practice [20]. There is, however, no evidence supporting a discontinuation of anticoagulation in patients reporting a permanent return to sinus rhythm, because AF may be asymptomatic in nature.

patients may be different from the general population and that bleeding assessment tools, such as the HAS-BLED score, should be updated to the DOAC era. Three patients, without diabetes or previous history of intraocular or retinal bleeding, suffered from symptomatic, intraocular hemorrhage during follow-up. Bleeding in this atypical site has previously been reported in trials on anticoagulation in AF patients [7], but the high

Moreover, we identified novel patient characteristics that decrease anticoagulation persistence. A history of bleeding, although not a risk factor for occurrence of major or CRNM bleeding was a strong risk factor for discontinuation and the composite of all bleeding events was the second most frequent reason for anticoagulation discontinuation. Further, patients with diabetes and increased leucocyte count had increased risk of discontinuation. These patients had to discontinue their baseline anticoagulation treatment predominately for emerging chronic medical issues, such as deterioration of kidney function, coronary heart and peripheral artery disease, and for safety considerations because of initiation of antiplatelet medication.

Table 3 Reasons for discontinuation of first choice anticoagulant and frequency of alternative choice anticoagulants (N = 80)

	Frequency (%)
Reason for discontinuation	
Patient-reported permanent return to sinus rhythm	16 (20.0)
Contraindication	12 (15.0)
Physician's recommendation	10 (12.5)
Difficulty reaching INR 2–3 (VKA only)	9 (11.3)
Major or clinically-relevant non-major bleed	9 (11.3)
Thromboembolism	6 (7.5)
Minor bleeding	5 (6.3)
Renal insufficiency	3 (1.1)
Patient's wish	3 (1.1)
other	7 (8.8)
Alternative choice anticoagulant	
Vitamin-K-Antagonist	16 (20.0)
Dabigatran	8 (10.0)
Rivaroxaban	16 (20.0)
Apixaban	18 (22.5)
LMWH (long-term)	5 (6.3)
None	17 (21.3)

Although our registry was not intended for a direct comparison of the persistence between different anticoagulants, our data allow a cautious analysis of drug persistence on VKA and on DOACs. Patients receiving DOACs were younger, had a higher frequency of previous bleeding and had more frequently a recent diagnosis of AF. Nevertheless, patients receiving DOACs did not have inferior drug persistence compared to patients receiving VKA. In studies in German and UK primary care settings, patients on treatment with DOACs even had better drug persistence than patients on VKA [21, 22]. The benefit of DOACs over VKA concerning persistence may have been attenuated in the hospital setting, because treating physicians were more cautious in the use of DOACs when new medical complications emerged.

This present investigation was not without limitations. Patients were not randomized to anticoagulation treatment, which may have led to a selection bias in the distribution of comorbidities between DOAC patients and VKA patients. For example, those patients who remained on VKA treatment during the observation time were likely long-time VKA users with a stable management of the international-normalized ratio (INR) and personal positive experience with VKA use. The study was not suitable for assessing time in therapeutic range because INR values in between follow-up visits were not captured. Analysis of safety or efficacy between drug classes were also not permissible because there was no randomization to anticoagulation treatment. Patients were referred to the outpatient clinic for the purposes of study inclusion and not based on any selection criteria such as high risk of bleeding or stroke. There may however be an inherent selection bias in the small sample size. The low sample size further led to wide confidence interval in the logistic regression analysis. Members of the registry staff did not actively prescribe medications or suggest drug discontinuation, nor did they influence the choice of DOAC. However, in cases of adverse events, patients were encouraged to seek the advice of a physician who is independent from the registry. We were unable to analyze if drug persistence was a risk factor for occurrence of thromboembolic outcomes, because the follow-up was too short to allow statistical inference. Low adherence to anticoagulant prescription is potentially associated with increased risk of thromboembolism, but is notoriously difficult to capture and was not assessed in our investigation. There was no independent adjudication of study outcomes, but we validated outcomes internally according to criteria stated in the methods section. However, the data quality was ensured by performing all patient interviews in person with overall very good patient compliance to study procedures and a low dropout rate (4.8%).

Conclusion

Patients with AF in this hospital setting had increased risk of thromboembolism and bleeding, which was mediated by the presence of comorbid conditions, especially a history of prior cardiovascular or cerebrovascular diseases. Further, anticoagulation treatment was frequently discontinued due to bleeding or thromboembolic complications, but also due to reasons such as permanent return to sinus rhythm, patient opinion or physician's advice. The risk of thromboembolism in the group of hospital-patients should not be underestimated and patients should be encouraged to utilize follow-up visits specifically concerning anticoagulation treatment in the first year after anticoagulation initiation.

Abbreviations
AF: Atrial fibrillation; CI: 95% confidence interval; CRNM bleeding: Clinically-relevant non-major bleeding; DOACs: Direct oral anticoagulants; DVT: Deep vein thrombosis; ECG: Electrocardiogram; eGFR: Estimated glomerular filtration rate; HR: Hazard ratio; IDMS: Isotope-dilution mass spectrometry; INR: International normalized ratio; LMWH: Low-molecular-weight heparin; MDRD: Modification of diet in renal disease equation; PE: Pulmonary embolism; TIA: Transient ischemic attack; VKA: Vitamin-K-antagonist; VTE: Venous thromboembolism

Acknowledgements
We would like to thank all clinical collaborators who contributed patients, especially Johanna Gebhart, Johannes Thaler, Julia Riedl, Giora Meron, Martin Frossard, Florian Thalhammer and Guido Gualdoni.

Funding
The study was supported by unrestricted grants from Bayer Austria and Daiichi Sankyo Austria, who did not play any role in the design of the study, the collection, analysis, or interpretation of data nor in writing the manuscript.

Authors' contributions
OK conceived the study, compiled and analyzed data, and wrote the manuscript; AS interpreted data, revised the manuscript for intellectual content, and approved the manuscript for submission; HD interpreted data, revised the manuscript for intellectual content, and approved the manuscript for submission; IP interpreted data, revised the manuscript for intellectual content, and approved the manuscript for submission; CA conceived the study, analyzed data, and revised the manuscript for intellectual content and approved the manuscript for submission. All authors read and approved the final manuscript.

Competing interests
O. Königsbrügge has received honoraria for lectures from Bayer and Sanofi. A. Simon has no conflicts to disclose. H. Domanovits has given lectures for Bayer, Boehringer-Ingelheim, and Daiichi-Sankyo. I. Pabinger has received honoraria from Bayer, Daiichi-Sankyo and Boehringer-Ingelheim for occasional lectures and advisory board meetings. C. Ay has received honoraria for lectures and advisory board meetings from Bayer, Daiichi-Sankyo, Pfizer, Bristol-Myers Squibb, Boehringer-Ingelheim and Sanofi.

Author details
[1]Department of Medicine I, Clinical Division of Hematology & Hemostaseology, Medical University of Vienna, Währinger Gürtel 18-20, A-1090 Vienna, Austria. [2]Department of Emergency Medicine, Medical University of Vienna, Vienna, Austria. [3]Department of Medicine, Thrombosis and Hemostasis Program, McAllister Heart Institute, University of North Carolina at Chapel Hill, Chapel Hill, NC, USA.

References
1. Hart RG, Palacio S, Pearce LA. Atrial Fibrillation, Stroke, and Acute Antithrombotic Therapy: Analysis of Randomized Clinical Trials. Stroke. 2002;33:2722–7.
2. Beyer-Westendorf J, Ebertz F, Förster K, Gelbricht V, Michalski F, Köhler C, et al. Effectiveness and safety of dabigatran therapy in daily-care patients with atrial fibrillation Results from the Dresden NOAC Registry. Thromb Haemost. 2015;113:1247–57.
3. O'Brien EC, Kim S, Thomas L, Fonarow GC, Kowey PR, Mahaffey KW, et al. Clinical Characteristics, Oral Anticoagulation Patterns, and Outcomes of Medicaid Patients With Atrial Fibrillation: Insights From the Outcomes Registry for Better Informed Treatment of Atrial Fibrillation (ORBIT-AF I) Registry. J Am Heart Assoc. 2016;5:e002721.
4. Yao X, Abraham NS, Alexander GC, Crown W, Montori VM, Sangaralingham LR, et al. Effect of Adherence to Oral Anticoagulants on Risk of Stroke and Major Bleeding Among Patients With Atrial Fibrillation. J Am Heart Assoc. 2016;5:1–12.

5.　Palomäki A, Mustonen P, Hartikainen JEK, Nuotio I, Kiviniemi T, Ylitalo A, et al. Underuse of anticoagulation in stroke patients with atrial fibrillation - the FibStroke Study. Eur J Neurol. 2016;23:133–9.

6.　Connolly SJ, Ezekowitz MD, Yusuf S, Eikelboom J, Oldgren J, Parekh A, et al. Dabigatran versus warfarin in patients with atrial fibrillation. N Engl J Med. 2009;361:1139–51.

7.　Patel M, Mahaffey K, Garg J, Pan G, Singer DE, Hacke W, et al. Rivaroxaban versus warfarin in nonvalvular atrial fibrillation. N Engl J Med. 2011;365:883–91.

8.　Granger CB, Alexander JH, McMurray JJV, Lopes RD, Hylek EM, Hanna M, et al. Apixaban versus warfarin in patients with atrial fibrillation. N Engl J Med. 2011;365:981–92.

9.　Giugliano RP, Ruff CT, Braunwald E, Murphy SA, Wiviott SD, Halperin JL, et al. Edoxaban versus warfarin in patients with atrial fibrillation. N Engl J Med. 2013;369:2093–104.

10.　Schulman S, Kearon C. Definition of major bleeding in clinical investigations of antihemostatic medicinal products in non-surgical patients. J Thromb Haemost. 2005;3:692–4.

11.　Kaatz S, Ahmad D, Spyropoulos AC, Schulman S. Definition of clinically relevant non-major bleeding in studies of anticoagulants in atrial fibrillation and venous thromboembolic disease in non-surgical patients: Communication from the SSC of the ISTH. J Thromb Haemost. 2015;13:2119–26.

12.　Cramer JA, Roy A, Burrell A, Fairchild CJ, Fuldeore MJ, Ollendorf DA, et al. Medication compliance and persistence: Terminology and definitions. Value Heal. 2008;11:44–7.

13.　Graham DJ, Reichman ME, Wernecke M, Zhang R, Southworth MR, Levenson M, et al. Cardiovascular, Bleeding, and Mortality Risks in Elderly Medicare Patients Treated With Dabigatran or Warfarin for Nonvalvular Atrial Fibrillation. Circulation. 2015;131:157–64.

14.　Korenstra J, Wijtvliet EPJ, Veeger NJGM, Geluk CA, Bartels GL, Posma JL, et al. Effectiveness and safety of dabigatran versus acenocoumarol in "real-world" patients with atrial fibrillation. Europace. 2016;18:1319–27.

15.　Hecker J, Marten S, Keller L, Helmert S, Michalski F, Werth S, et al. Coagulation and Fibrinolysis Effectiveness and safety of rivaroxaban therapy in daily-care patients with atrial fibrillation Results from the Dresden NOAC Registry. Thromb Haemost. 2016;1155:1–11.

16.　Bassand J-P, Accetta G, Camm AJ, Cools F, Fitzmaurice DA, Fox KAA, et al. Two-year outcomes of patients with newly diagnosed atrial fibrillation: results from GARFIELD-AF. Eur Heart J. 2016;37:2882–89.

17.　Fang MC, Go AS, Chang Y, Borowsky LH, Pomernacki NK, Udaltsova N, et al. Warfarin discontinuation after starting warfarin for atrial fibrillation. Circ Cardiovasc Qual Outcomes. 2010;3:624–31.

18.　Hylek EM, Evans-Molina C, Shea C, Henault LE, Regan S. Major hemorrhage and tolerability of warfarin in the first year of therapy among elderly patients with atrial fibrillation. Circulation. 2007;115:2689–96.

19.　Beyer-Westendorf J, Förster K, Ebertz F, Gelbricht V, Schreier T, Göbelt M, et al. Drug persistence with rivaroxaban therapy in atrial fibrillation patients - Results from the Dresden non-interventional oral anticoagulation registry. Europace. 2015;17:530–8.

20.　Nührich JM, Kuck KH, Andresen D, Steven D, Spitzer SG, Hoffmann E, et al. Oral anticoagulation is frequently discontinued after ablation of paroxysmal atrial fibrillation despite previous stroke: data from the German Ablation Registry. Clin Res Cardiol. 2015;104:463–70.

21.　Beyer-Westendorf J, Ehlken B, Evers T. Real-world persistence and adherence to oral anticoagulation for stroke risk reduction in patients with atrial fibrillation. Europace. 2016;18:1150–7.

22.　Martinez C, Katholing A, Wallenhorst C, Freedman SB. Therapy persistence in newly diagnosed non-valvular atrial fibrillation treated with warfarin or NOAC: A cohort study. Thromb Haemost. 2016;115:31–9.

5

Global Bi-ventricular endocardial distribution of activation rate during long duration ventricular fibrillation in normal and heart failure canines

Qingzhi Luo[†], Qi Jin[†], Ning Zhang, Yanxin Han, Yilong Wang, Shangwei Huang, Changjian Lin, Tianyou Ling, Kang Chen, Wenqi Pan and Liqun Wu[*]

Abstract

Background: The objective of this study was to detect differences in the distribution of the left and right ventricle (LV & RV) activation rate (AR) during short-duration ventricular fibrillation (SDVF, <1 min) and long-duration ventricular fibrillation VF (LDVF, >1 min) in normal and heart failure (HF) canine hearts.

Methods: Ventricular fibrillation (VF) was electrically induced in six healthy dogs (control group) and six dogs with right ventricular pacing-induced congestive HF (HF group). Two 64-electrode basket catheters deployed in the LV and RV were used for global endocardium electrical mapping. The AR of VF was estimated by fast Fourier transform analysis from each electrode.

Results: In the control group, the LV was activated faster than the RV in the first 20 s, after which there was no detectable difference in the AR between them. When analyzing the distribution of the AR within the bi-ventricles at 3 min of LDVF, the posterior LV was activated fastest, while the anterior was slowest. In the HF group, a detectable AR gradient existed between the two ventricles within 3 min of VF, with the LV activating more quickly than the RV. When analyzing the distribution of the AR within the bi-ventricles at 3 min of LDVF, the septum of the LV was activated fastest, while the anterior was activated slowest.

Conclusions: A global bi-ventricular endocardial AR gradient existed within the first 20 s of VF but disappeared in the LDVF in healthy hearts. However, the AR gradient was always observed in both SDVF and LDVF in HF hearts. The findings of this study suggest that LDVF in HF hearts can be maintained differently from normal hearts, which accordingly should lead to the development of different management strategies for LDVF resuscitation.

Keywords: Ventricular Fibrillation, Activation Rate, Heart Failure

Background

Frequency analysis using the fast Fourier transform (FFT) has been widely used to characterize features of ventricular fibrillation (VF). Electrical and optical mapping experiments in previous animal and human studies have evaluated the spatiotemporal distribution of the activation rate (AR) during VF and have provided

mechanistic insight into the organization of VF, thereby improving our understanding of the initiation and maintenance of this complex arrhythmia [1–7]. The regional frequency characteristics may be related to a fixed anatomic myocardial substrate and dynamic physiological factors such as refractory periods [8]. It has also been postulated that the fastest activating region drives fibrillation throughout the rest of the myocardium by giving rise to activation fronts that propagate into the more slowly activating regions.

The activation of VF changes as it continues, which raises the possibility that the relative importance of

* Correspondence: wuliqun89@aliyun.com
[†]Equal contributors
Department of Cardiology, Shanghai Ruijin Hospital, Shanghai Jiao Tong University School of Medicine, No. 197, Ruijin Er Road, Shanghai 200025, People's Republic of China

different arrhythmogenic mechanisms changes. It has been proposed that defibrillation mechanisms and efficacy may differ in different pathological animal models during different stages of VF [9]. Panfilov et al. reported that the excitation frequency is an important index in VF that can reflect the underlying myocardial pathophysiology; it may also be predictive of the defibrillation threshold [10]. Previous studies have reported that the dynamics of VF in heart failure (HF) hearts differ from those in normal hearts, with a substantial decrease in AR [3, 11]. The aim of this study was to determine the distribution of AR across two fibrillating global ventricular endocardium samples at different stages in normal and HF canine hearts. We hypothesized that as the duration of VF continued, there would be quantifiable regional AR varieties in the inter-ventricles and/(or) intra-ventricles.

Methods

Pacemaker implantation

Twelve beagles (11 ± 1.2 kg) were divided into two groups. Six dogs were selected to create the HF model, and the other six dogs served as the control group. A pacemaker (Kappa 710, Medtronic, Minneapolis, Minnesota, USA) was implanted in a subcutaneous pocket and attached to a pacing lead (5076, Medtronic, Minneapolis, Minnesota, USA) in the RV apex under fluoroscopic visualization via the right external jugular vein. When the surgery was completed, the dogs were given antibiotics, after which they underwent rapid ventricular pacing at 240 beats per minute for three to 4 weeks. Then, echocardiography was performed to confirm that the HF model was successfully established. Rapid pacing was maintained until a day before the electrophysiological mapping study.

Animal preparation

Each animal was injected intramuscularly with ketamine (10 mg/kg) and tropine (0.04 mg/kg) for anesthetic induction. Anesthesia was maintained intravenously with propofol (8–16 mg/kg/h), and the animals were ventilated in a restrained, dorsally recumbent position. To determine the adequacy of the anesthesia, ventilation and oxygenation, the arterial blood pressure, blood gases, cardiac electrical activity, body temperature and serum electrolytes were monitored, and interdigital reflexes were tested throughout the entire study. After the completion of the data collection, the animals were euthanized with an intravenous injection of potassium chloride. The hearts were exposed through a median sternotomy and supported in a pericardial sling. A catheter (model 80,993, IBI, St. Jude Medical, Saint Paul, Minnesota, USA) was inserted for defibrillation with the negative electrode in the RV apex and the positive electrode in the superior vena cava (Fig. 1).

Bi-ventricular endocardial mapping

A multielectrode basket (Constellation Catheter, model US8031U, Boston Scientific, Natick, MA, USA) was introduced through the left carotid artery into the LV. Another basket catheter was inserted through the right jugular vein into the RV. Each catheter contained eight splines each with eight (8 × 8) electrodes approximately 2 mm apart. These two catheters were used to map the ventricular endocardium simultaneously (Fig. 1). A detailed description of this technique was presented in our earlier report [9].

VF induction and AR analysis

VF was induced by a 30 Hz stimulation delivered (MicroPace III, EPS 320 Cardiac stimulator) through one of the basket electrodes. Four VF episodes were induced in each animal. The first three VF episodes were

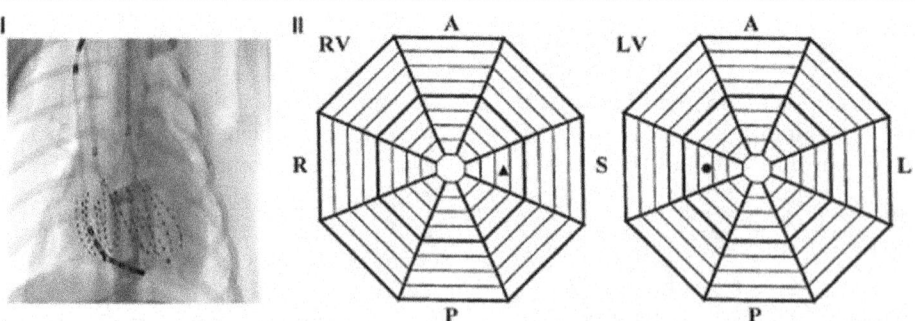

Fig. 1 Global electrical mapping of the RV and LV endocardium. Panel I shows a fluoroscopic image of a posterior–anterior view of two basket catheters in the LV and RV and the RV defibrillation catheter. Panel II shows the basket orientation in the LV and RV. R, right free wall; A, anterior free wall; L, left free wall; P, posterior free wall; and S, septum. Apical electrodes are placed toward the center of the display, and basal electrodes are located near the periphery

recorded for 20 s as a short-duration (SDVF) episode before being halted by a 400–600 V biphasic shock (6/4 ms) delivered from a defibrillator electrode. The last VF episode was allowed to continue for at least 3 min (long-duration VF, LDVF), and the animal was not resuscitated. The first 20 s of VF data during this LDVF episode served as the fourth SDVF episode. There were no significant differences in the VF parameters among multiple short VF episodes. Additionally, the AR distribution did not depend on the basket electrodes used to induce VF. The two 64-electrodes of the basket catheter and the six limb-ECG leads were recorded with a 160-channel cardiac data acquisition system. The AR was estimated through FFT analysis of VF at each electrode of the basket catheter and the six limb leads of the body ECG for a 2 s interval beginning 20 s after VF induction. The frequency with the highest power between 1 and 20 Hz was taken as the AR.

Statistical analysis

To ascertain how the AR in different ventricular regions varied during VF, the endocardium of the two ventricles were divided into 8 zones according the display of the basket electrode (Fig. 1). We defined the lower half of the basket as the apex and the upper half as the base. Data are given as the mean ± SD. Analysis of variance was used to test for significant differences among the mean AR of the zones for the VF episodes, followed by a Fisher's protected least significance difference to determine which zones differed significantly. To determine the difference between the apex and the base of the RV, LV in AR during VF, the data were analyzed for significance using a paired t test. A value of $P<0.05$ was considered significant.

Results

HF model

There was unambiguous evidence (tachypnea, lethargy and ascites) of myocardial systolic dysfunction in the HF group but not in the control animals. The LV ejection fraction for the HF canines was substantially decreased (63 ± 5.3% vs. 29.5 ± 8.2%, $P < 0.0001$), accompanied by significant increases in the LV end-diastolic dimension and LV end-systolic dimension.

Regional distribution of VF AR in the control group

In the control group, the LV activated faster than the RV (12 ± 0.3 vs. 11.6 ± 0.3, $P = 0.04$) in the first 20 s. However, there was no significant difference in the AR between LV and RV after 20 s. There was a dramatic decrease in AR between 20 s and 90 s, after which it declined smoothly. At 3 min, there was no significant difference between the LV and RV (5.23 ± 0.20 vs. 5.27 ± 0.11, $P = 0.27$) (Fig. 2). When analyzing the

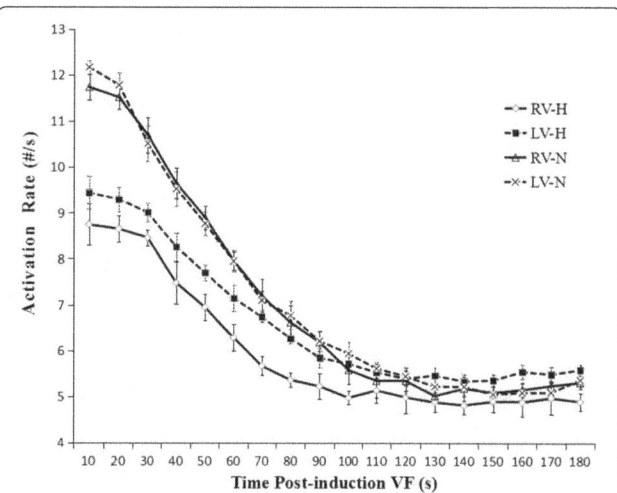

Fig. 2 Evolution of the AR during VF. In the control group, there was only an AR gradient between the ventricles within the first 20 s. In contrast, in the HF group, there was a detectable bi-ventricular AR gradient for the entire VF duration. From 90 s to the end of analysis at 3 min of VF, neither the RV or LV in the HF hearts activated differently than those of the control animals. (LV-N: left ventricle in the normal group; LV-H: left ventricle in the HF group; RV-N: right ventricle in the normal group; RV-H: right ventricle in the HF group.) See the text of the article for additional details

distribution of AR within LV, the posterior wall of the LV activated the fastest (I in Fig. 3a), while the anterior wall was the slowest (II in Fig. 3a), with a 7% difference between the fastest and the slowest activating regions (5.50 ± 0.54 vs. 5.09 ± 0.24, $P = 0.024$). When analyzing the distribution of AR within the RV, the posterior wall activated the fastest (I in Fig. 3b), while the anterior wall was the slowest (I in Fig. 3b), with an 11% difference between the fastest and the slowest activating regions (5.55 ± 0.13 vs. 4.95 ± 0.29, $P<0.001$) (Fig. 4). Additionally, the apical wall activated faster than the basal wall in both ventricles of the normal hearts with LV apex>LV base(5.54 ± 0.20 vs. 4.97 ± 0.12, $P<0.01$); and RV apex>RV base (5.38 ± 0.19 vs. 4.92 ± 0.25, $P<0.01$) (Fig. 5a).

Regional distribution of the VF AR in the HF group

In the HF group, a detectable AR gradient always existed between the two ventricles, with the LV activating more quickly than the RV after VF induction. In the first 20 s interval, the LV activated faster than the RV (9.4 ± 1.15 vs. 8.7 ± 1.1, $P = 0.02$). At 3 min, the LV still activated more quickly than the RV (5.54 ± 0.76 vs. 5.08 ± 0.66, $P = 0.004$) (Fig. 2). When analyzing the distribution of AR within LV, the septum of the LV activated the fastest (I in Fig. 3c), while the anterior wall activated the slowest (II in Fig. 3c), with a 7% difference between the fastest and the slowest activating regions (5.75 ± 0.49 vs. 5.33 ± 0.25, $P = 0.016$). When analyzing the distribution of the AR within the RV, the septum of the RV was

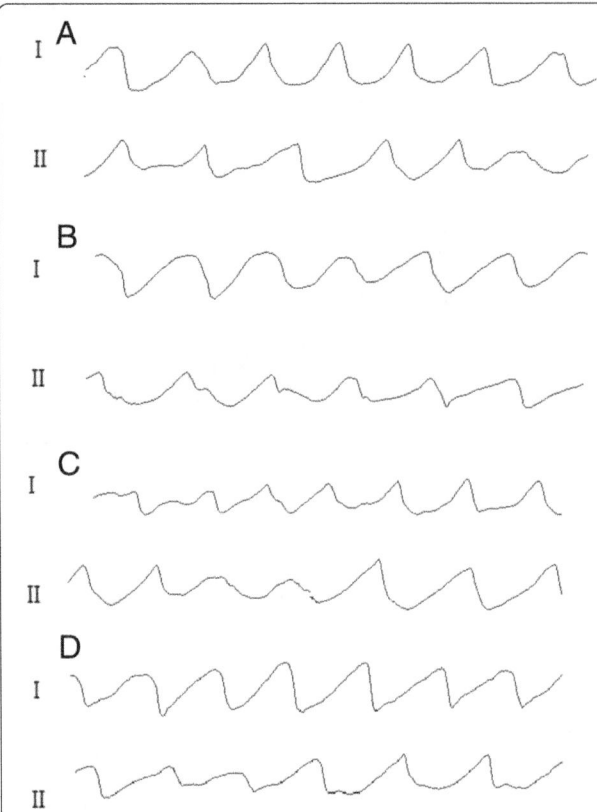

Fig. 3 Snapshots of activation during VF in one normal and one HF-affected dog at the 3 min LDVF. Recordings of VF activation from one control heart are shown in Fig. 3a and b, with Fig. 3a I representing the posterior wall and II representing the anterior wall of the LV. In Fig. 3b, I indicates the posterior wall, and II indicates the anterior wall of RV; as shown, the posterior wall activates faster than the anterior wall. Recordings of VF activation from one HF-affected animal are shown in Fig. 3c and d. Figure 3c I shows the septal wall, and II shows the anterior wall of the LV. Figure 3d I shows the septal wall, and II indicates the anterior wall of the RV; the septal wall activates faster than the anterior wall

HF group relative to the normal canine hearts (0.66 ± 0.18 vs. 0.40 ± 0.22, $P = 0.015$). Additionally, the LV-RV AR gradient was greater at the beginning than at the end of the entire VF episode in the HF group (0.66 ± 0.18 vs. 0.45 ± 0.21, $P = 0.009$) (Fig. 2). Third, the activation of VF differed between the two groups at the 3 min LDVF. In the control group, the posterior of the LV activated fastest, while the anterior wall activated the slowest. In the HF group, the septum of the LV was activated the fastest, while the anterior wall was activated more slowly (Fig. 4).

Discussion

The major findings of this study are as follows. (1) In the control group, the LV activated slightly faster than the RV in the first 20 s, after which there was no difference in the AR between the LV and RV. At 3 min of LDVF, the posterior of the LV activated fastest, while the anterior activated the slowest. The apical part activated faster than the basal part in the bi-ventricles. (2) In the HF group, there was always a noticeable LV-RV AR gradient, with the LV activating more quickly than the RV. At 3 min of LDVF, the septum of the LV activated fastest, while the anterior activated the slowest. Similarly, the apical part activated faster than the basal parts in the bi-ventricles. (3) In both groups, the AR decreased dramatically for the first 90 s, after which it declined more smoothly. (4) The AR of both the RV and LV in the HF group were slower than those in normal hearts for the first 90 s. From 90 s to the end of the analysis at 3 min of VF, neither the RV nor LV in HF hearts was activated differently from the bi-ventricles of the control animals.

Possible mechanism of VF maintenance within 3 min

Data from previous animal studies suggest that one or two primary wavefronts located in the regions with the fastest AR drive the rest of the heart and that these regions, rather than the entire myocardium, are responsible for the maintenance of VF [12].

In the control group of this study, the overall wavefront direction of the bi-ventricles was from the apex to the base and from the posterior to the anterior at 3 min of LDVF. Previous studies have shown that the posterior LV activates faster than the anterior LV during VF in swine and that VF wavefronts tend to move from the posterior to the anterior. These reports are consistent with our findings [6, 13]. Therefore, if such a rotor is present, a possible site for a mother rotor is around the insertion of the posterior papillary muscle, which is located at the intersection of the posterior LV posterior wall and the posterior septum. This scenario may give rise to additional wavefronts that traverse the more slowly activating portion of the LV and the RV. Kim et al. [14] reported that the geometry of the ventricular

found to be activated the fastest (I in Fig. 3d), while the anterior wall was found to be activated more slowly (II in Fig. 3d), with an 11% difference between the fastest and the slowest activating regions (5.50 ± 0.11 vs. 4.88 ± 0.20, $P<0.001$) (Fig. 4). In addition, a significant AR gradient was observed between the apical and basal portions of both ventricles in the HF hearts, with LV apex>LV base (5.77 ± 0.20 vs 5.30 ± 0.10, $P<0.01$); and RV apex>RV base (5.27 ± 0.31 vs 5.04 ± 0.30, $P<0.01$) (Fig. 5b).

Differences in the AR distribution between the normal and failing hearts

There were several differences between the two groups. First, relative to normal hearts, the AR of the HF group was much slower in the first 90 s, and a significant LV-RV AR gradient was always present. Second, at the first 20 s interval, there was a clear LV-RV AR gradient in the

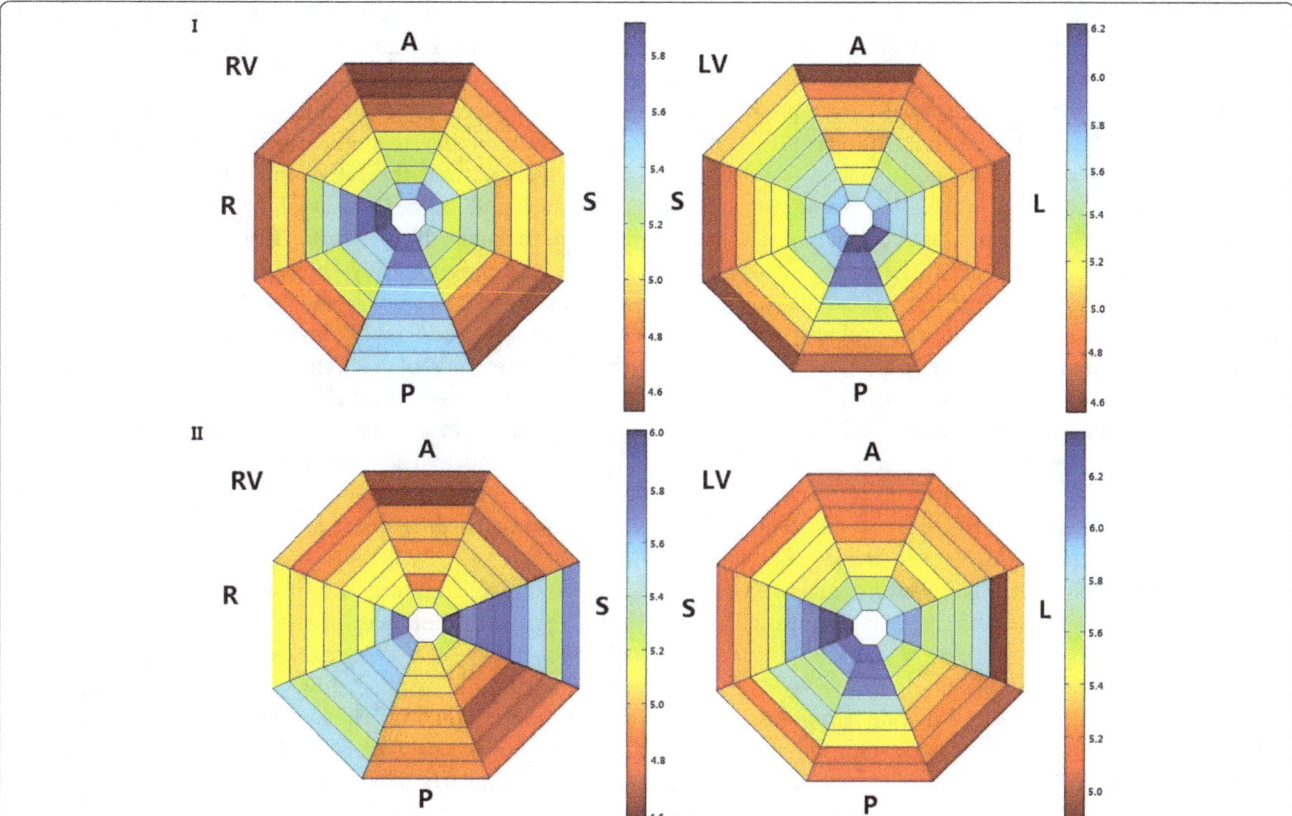

Fig. 4 3 min LDVF regional AR distribution in the RV and LV in one normal and one HF animal. Figure 4 I shows the regional AR distribution of the two ventricles in the control group for the 3 min LDVF. In the LV, the posterior wall activates before the anterior wall. In the RV, the posterior wall also activates before the anterior wall. Figure 4 II represents the regional AR distribution of the RV and LV in the HF group for the 3 min LDVF. In the LV, the septal tissue activates the fastest, while the anterior wall activates the slowest. In the RV, the septal tissue activates the fastest, while the anterior wall activates the slowest. The colors represent the AR of the 64-basket electrodes according to the time scale shown to the right (blue represents the fastest activation and red represents the slowest activation)

wall and the anatomical structures, such as the posterior papillary muscle, influences the wave breaks and the maintenance of VF. Moreover, Pak et al. [15] demonstrated that ablation targeting the posterior papillary muscle reduces the potential for induction of VF,

suggesting that eliminating the anchoring site might prevent sustained reentry and VF. The VF AR differences between the fastest and slowest regions in the present study were not large; Zaitsev et al. [16] and Samie et al. [17] reported larger differences in the AR between the

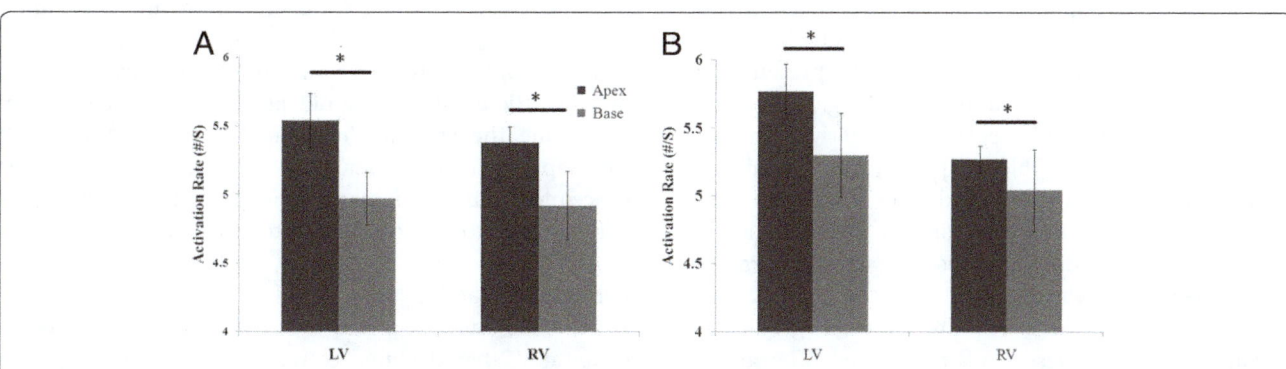

Fig. 5 Three-minute LDVF AR distribution of the apical and basal portions of the bi-ventricles. Figure 5**a** represents the apex-base AR differences in the control group, with the apex activating faster than the base in the LV (*$P<0.01$) and RV (*$P<0.01$). Figure 5**b** shows the apex-base AR differences in the HF group, with the apex activating faster than the base in the LV (*$P<0.01$) and RV (*$P<0.01$)

fastest and slowest regions. Therefore, it is not known if these smaller AR differences are sufficient to support the mother rotor hypothesis. However, in human VF, rotors are not stable temporally and spatially over greater surfaces; these high-frequency regions thus require further study regarding VF maintenance.

In the HF group at the 3 min LDVF, we demonstrated that the AR of RV was much slower than the LV and that the septum of the LV activated more rapidly than any other portion of the LV or the RV, indicating that if there existed a mother rotor, it was probably located in the septum. This hypothesis is supported by the findings of Ikeda et al., who studied endocardial activation patterns during VF, in which the septum was found to have more wavelet numbers and a shorter cycle length than the other portions of the LV and RV [18]. It has been proposed that a smaller critical mass is required to maintain VF in the septum. All these observations suggest the possibility that the septum may serve as a possible source for the dominant region during VF in HF canines.

Inter-ventricular differences in the endocardial AR

Rogers et al. [19] described the activation differences between the RV and LV during VF in normal porcine hearts, suggesting that there is a quantifiable difference between the LV regions, showing more wavefronts and activations than the RV. Umapathy et al. reported that the LV has a larger dominant frequency span than the RV [5]. The presence of spatially distributed gradients in the density of the inward rectifier current (I_{k1}), with the left ventricular myocytes showing significantly weaker inward-directed rectification than the right ventricular myocytes, has been postulated to play crucial roles in the LV-RV gradients of excitation frequency during VF [20, 21]. In our study, we found that the AR of the LV differed from that of the RV for the first 20 s, but it did not show strong differences during the rest of the process. One possible explanation of the different findings is that the mapping methods have varied between different studies. For example, Rogers et al. recorded only parts of the epicardium, while in the present study, recordings were instead acquired via the global endocardial mapping of the two ventricles. Otherwise, since VF activations were not stable temporally and spatially over greater surfaces, these contradictory results might be explained by the spatial averaging of the excitation frequencies, which reduce the discriminatory characteristics between the regions.

In the HF dogs, there was always an AR gradient between the bi-ventricles as VF progressed. The gradient indicated that these regions participated in different ways in different animal models. For previous studies with diseased hearts, Huang et al. [11] demonstrated

that VF in the setting of HF was significantly different from that in control dogs during VF. Their study showed that VF had a lower peak dV/dt, a slower AR, a significantly lower reentry occurrence, and an increased block occurrence relative to the VF in the controls. Moreno et al. [3] showed that the HF group had a lower dominant frequency and higher levels of organization during VF than in normal sheep hearts. Consistent with previous studies, the present study showed a slower AR in the HF animals. Everett et al. [22] showed that different ventricular substrates produced by different animal models altered the characteristics of VF. Thus, different mechanisms of VF might be present in the LV, which could contribute to the differences in the AR gradient distribution during VF between the normal and HF models.

Intra-ventricular differences in the endocardial regional AR

The findings from our study demonstrated that there were regional differences in the different portions of the LV and RV, with some regions activating rapidly and other regions activating slowly. We observed a significant tendency for the VF wavefronts to spread from the apex toward the base of both the LV and RV in the normal and HF hearts. However, Nanthakumar et al. [4] did not find a significant direction from apex to base, suggesting that the epicardial base had the highest peak frequency. Earlier studies have revealed that there was no significant difference in the dominant frequency span between LV free wall and septum. In this study, the posterior wall of the LV activated the fastest in the control group, which seemed to coincide with the posterior papillary muscle. In the HF dogs, the septum of the LV activated the most rapidly, suggesting that the septum might be the source of the wave fronts. The differences in these results can be explained by differences in the species studied, differences in the heart sizes, differences in the animal models, and different effects between the isolated hearts and the intact hearts. From our analysis, the spatial differences in AR cannot be entirely explained by underlying fixed intrinsic anatomical changes or electrophysiological properties of the myocardium. It has been predicted that dynamic physiological factors may determine the regional frequency characteristics [2, 8]. The rapid dynamic increase in the wavefronts and other descriptors during VF may be independent of any underlying change to the intrinsic state of the heart.

Clinical implications

A previous study reported that the incidence of out-of-hospital VF has declined compared with asystole as the initially recorded rhythm [23]. Cardiac pump failure without an arrhythmic event is suspected to be one of the factors. Although the AR of both the RV and the LV in the HF group were slower than those of normal hearts during the first 90 s interval, neither the RV nor the LV in the HF hearts were activated differently from the bi-ventricles in the control animals from 90 s to the end of analysis at 3 min of VF. Additionally, no LDVF episode was terminated within 3 min in HF hearts in the present study. Therefore, further study should be performed to detect whether LDVF in failing hearts is converted to asystole earlier than in normal hearts.

In the clinical setting, patients with preexisting HF are typically assumed to have a lower chance of successful cardiopulmonary resuscitation. The findings of this study indicate that LDVF is maintained differently in HF hearts than it is in normal hearts. Various intra- and inter-ventricular areas were activated differently during LDVF under the condition of HF. Some areas might be triggered by early or delayed after-depolarization with increased AR. Thus, in addition to electrical shock, other treatments, including agents that inhibit triggered activities and pacing, could potentially improve the outcomes of cardiopulmonary resuscitation in such patients.

Study limitations
The limitations of this study are as follows. First, although the global bi-ventricular endocardium was simultaneously mapped, our mapping technology could not detect the micro-reentry at the endocardium. The basket electrodes were widely spaced, such that the fine details of the endocardial activation sequence were not identified. Second, transmural mappings were not performed. Therefore, this study could not detect the presence of a transmural AR gradient between the epicardium and endocardium during VF.

Conclusion
Estimates of the distribution of VF AR are not uniform across the endocardium. A global bi-ventricular endocardial AR gradient was observed in the first 20 s of SDVF but was not observed in LDVF in normal hearts. However, the AR gradient was always present in both SDVF and LDVF in the HF hearts. The findings of this study suggest that the LDVF in the HF hearts is maintained differently from normal hearts, which accordingly leads to different recommended management strategies during LDVF resuscitation.

Abbreviations
AR: Activation rate; FFT: Fast Fourier transform; HF: Heart failure; LDVF: Long-duration ventricular fibrillation; LV: Left ventricle; LV-H: Left ventricle in the HF group; LV-N: Left ventricle in the normal group; RV: Right ventricle; RV-H: Right ventricle in the HF group; RV-N: Right ventricle in the normal group; SDVF: Short-duration ventricular fibrillation; VF: Ventricular fibrillation

Acknowledgments
Not applicable.

Funding
This work was supported in part by the Chinese National Natural Science Foundation (Grants 81,470,450, 81,470,451, and 81,270,260) and the Shanghai Municipal Education Commission-Gaofeng Clinical Medicine Grant 20,161,404.

Authors' contribution
QZL and QJ conducted the electrophysiological mapping studies, performed the statistical analysis and drafted the manuscript. NZ and YXH conducted the mapping study. YLW, SWH and CJL collected the data. TYL and WQP participated in the study design. KC participated in its design and helped revised the language writing. LQW conceived of the study, participated in its design and coordination, and helped to correct the manuscript. All authors reviewed and approved of the final version of the manuscript.

Competing interests
The authors declare that they have no competing interests.

References
1. Choi B-R, Nho W, Liu T, Salama G. Life span of ventricular fibrillation frequencies. Circ Res. 2002;91(4):339–45.
2. Valderrábano M, Yang J, Omichi C, et al. Frequency analysis of ventricular fibrillation in swine ventricles. Circ Res. 2002;90(2):213–22.
3. Moreno J, Zaitsev AV, Warren M, et al. Effect of remodelling, stretch and ischaemia on ventricular fibrillation frequency and dynamics in a heart failure model. Cardiovasc Res. 2005;65(1):158–66.
4. Nanthakumar K, Huang J, Rogers JM, et al. Regional differences in ventricular fibrillation in the open-chest porcine left ventricle. Circ Res. 2002; 91(8):733–40.
5. Umapathy K, Masse S, Sevaptsidis E, et al. Regional frequency variation during human ventricular fibrillation. Med Eng Phys. 2009;31(8):964–70.
6. Newton JC, Johnson PL, JUSTICE R, Smith WM, Ideker RE. Estimated global epicardial distribution of activation rate and conduction block during porcine ventricular fibrillation. J Cardiovasc Electrophysiol. 2002;13(10):1035–41.
7. Clayton RH, Holden AV. Effect of regional differences in cardiac cellular electrophysiology on the stability of ventricular arrhythmias: a computational study. Phys Med Biol. 2003;48(1):95.
8. Choi B-R, Liu T, Salama G. The distribution of refractory periods influences the dynamics of ventricular fibrillation. Circ Res. 2001;88(5):e49–58.
9. Jin Q, Zhou J, Zhang N, et al. Defibrillation threshold varies during different stages of ventricular fibrillation in canine hearts. Heart Lung Circ. Feb 2013; 22(2):133–40.
10. Panfilov I, Lever NA, Smaill BH, Larsen PD. Ventricular fibrillation frequency from implanted cardioverter defibrillator devices. Europace. 2009;11(8):1052–6.
11. Huang J, Rogers JM, Killingsworth CR, et al. Improvement of defibrillation efficacy and quantification of activation patterns during ventricular fibrillation in a canine heart failure model. Circulation. 2001;103(10):1473–8.
12. Tabereaux PB, Dosdall DJ, Ideker RE. Mechanisms of VF maintenance: wandering wavelets, mother rotors, or foci. Heart Rhythm. 2009;6(3):405–15.
13. Huang J, Walcott GP, Killingsworth CR, Melnick SB, Rogers JM, Ideker RE. Quantification of activation patterns during ventricular fibrillation in open-chest porcine left ventricle and septum. Heart Rhythm. 2005;2(7):720–8.
14. Kim Y-H, Garfinkel A, Ikeda T, et al. Spatiotemporal complexity of ventricular fibrillation revealed by tissue mass reduction in isolated swine right ventricle. Further evidence for the quasiperiodic route to chaos hypothesis. J Clin Investig. 1997;100(10):2486.
15. Pak HN, Kim YH, Lim HE, et al. Role of the posterior papillary muscle and purkinje potentials in the mechanism of ventricular fibrillation in open chest dogs and Swine: effects of catheter ablation. J Cardiovasc Electrophysiol. 2006;17(7):777–83.
16. Zaitsev AV, Berenfeld O, Mironov SF, Jalife J, Pertsov AM. Distribution of excitation frequencies on the epicardial and endocardial surfaces of fibrillating ventricular wall of the sheep heart. Circ Res. 2000;86(4):408–17.
17. Samie FH, Jalife J. Mechanisms underlying ventricular tachycardia and its transition to ventricular fibrillation in the structurally normal heart. Cardiovasc Res. 2001;50(2):242–50.
18. Ikeda T, Kawase A, Nakazawa K, et al. Role of structural complexities of septal tissue in maintaining ventricular fibrillation in isolated, perfused canine ventricle. J Cardiovasc Electrophysiol. 2001;12(1):66–75.

19. Rogers JM, Huang J, Pedoto RW, Walker RG, Smith WM, Ideker RE. Fibrillation is more complex in the left ventricle than in the right ventricle. J Cardiovasc Electrophysiol. 2000;11(12):1364–71.

20. Samie FH, Berenfeld O, Anumonwo J, et al. Rectification of the background potassium current a determinant of rotor dynamics in ventricular fibrillation. Circ Res. 2001;89(12):1216–23.

21. Pandit SV, Kaur K, Zlochiver S, et al. Left-to-right ventricular differences in I KATP underlie epicardial repolarization gradient during global ischemia. Heart Rhythm. 2011;8(11):1732–9.

22. Everett TH, Wilson EE, Foreman S, Olgin JE. Mechanisms of ventricular fibrillation in canine models of congestive heart failure and ischemia assessed by in vivo noncontact mapping. Circulation. 2005;112(11):1532–41.

23. Cobb LA, Fahrenbruch CE, Olsufka M, Copass MK. Changing incidence of out-of-hospital ventricular fibrillation, 1980-2000. JAMA. 2002;288(23):3008–13.

6

MicroRNA profiling in the left atrium in patients with non-valvular paroxysmal atrial fibrillation

Jiangang Wang[1*], Shiqiu Song[1], Changqing Xie[2], Jie Han[1], Yan Li[1], Jiahai Shi[3], Meng Xin[1], Jun Wang[1], Tiange Luo[1], Xu Meng[1] and Bo Yang[4]

Abstract

Background: We aimed to identify the miRNA expression profiles in left atrial appendage, with the intention of identifying miRNAs that were significantly associated with non-valvular paroxysmal AF.

Methods: The RNA samples were isolated from healthy controls (n = 5) and patients with atrial fibrillation (n = 8). To confirm the findings obtained by analyzing the miRNA profile, we measured the expression of selected miRNAs in the entire cohort by quantitative PCR.

Results: Ten specific miRNAs were found to be differentially expressed between atrial fibrillation and healthy controls with more than a 2-fold change (P < 0.05). Consistent with the data obtained for the profile, expression levels of miRNA-155, miRNA-146b-5p and miRNA-19b were significantly increased in patients with atrial fibrillation. Interestingly, levels of miRNA-146b-5p and miRNA-155, which are known to be associated with inflammation, were independently and positively associated with left atrium dimension, atrial fibrillation duration and high sensitivity C-reactive protein levels. By using four Databases (TargetScan, miRanda, Starbase Clip-seq and miRDB) to perform target gene prediction, there were four genes were related to the inflammatory response and fibrosis, and three others encoding cardiac ion channel proteins. As a result of TaqMan qPCR and Western analysis, the relative mRNA and protein expression level of three target genes (DIER-1, TIMP-4 and CACNA1C) were significantly lower in the atrial fibrillation group than that in the healthy control group.

Conclusions: Expression of inflammation-associated miRNAs is significantly up-regulated in the left atrial appendage of patients with non-valvular paroxysmal atrial fibrillation, which may play a significant role in electrical and structural remodeling.

Background

MiRNAs are endogenous ~23 nt RNAs that play important gene-regulating roles in animals and plants by pairing to the messenger RNAs (mRNAs) of protein-coding genes to direct their post-transcriptional regulation [1, 2]. Therefore, measuring miRNA expression can be useful for gene regulation studies at systems-level, especially when miRNA measurements are combined with mRNA profiling and other genome-scale data. Also, it is reported that miRNAs are unusually well-preserved in a range of biological specimens. This has led to considerable interest in the development of miRNAs as biomarkers for diverse molecular diagnostic applications, including in the treatment of

* Correspondence: wangjiangang7545@126.com
[1]Department of Cardiac Surgery, Beijing Anzhen Hospital, Capital Medical University, Beijing 100029, P.R. China
Full list of author information is available at the end of the article

cancer, cardiovascular diseases, autoimmune diseases and forensics [3–5]. Accordingly, miRNA profiling has become an area of interest for researchers and investigators working in various areas of biology and medicine [6].

Atrial fibrillation (AF) is the most common sustained cardiac rhythm disorder, and is increasing in prevalence and incidence [7, 8]. With the recent and rapid strides in the field of miRNA research, investigators have begun to appreciate the roles of mRNAs in the cardiovascular system [9]. Several studies have reported the direct involvement of miRNAs in controlling the cardiac excitability and arrhythmogenesis in specific pathophysiological conditions [10–12]. A group of miRNAs (such as miR-1 and miR-328) have been shown to regulate the genes encoding cardiac ion channel proteins and other relevant genes. Some of these miRNAs have been shown to be involved in AF, and some are considered to have the potential to regulate AF based on their target genes [13–15]. However, since most of the specimens have been obtained from patients with valvular AF, from previous studies one cannot distinguish whether the findings reveal inherent characteristics of the atria themselves or are due to underlying valvular heart diseases.

AF is as a complex electrical phenotype involving complex factors beyond electrophysiology. AF may have distinct underlying mechanisms, and different miRNAs might be involved in different types of AF. Currently, there is a growing body of evidence suggesting that a specifically altered pattern of miRNA expression in atrial tissue and plasma is associated with AF [16–20]. However, the miRNA signature in AF, particularly in non-valvular AF, is still unknown. Here we aimed to identify the miRNA expression profiles in left atrial appendage (LAA), with the intention of identifying miRNAs that were significantly associated with non-valvular paroxysmal AF (PAF).

Methods
A detailed description of Methods is available in the Additional file 1.

Results
Study population
A total of 47 subjects were studied. LAAs were obtained from 30 patients with PAF. The mean age was 48.5 ± 7.2 years, and 63 % were males. The time since the first diagnosis of AF was ≈ 2 years. The mean left atrial diameter (LAD) was 53.1 ± 2.2 mm. The HC group consisted of seventeen dumped LAA samples obtained from transplant donors following heart transplantation. The HC group consisted of 13 males and 4 females; their mean age was 33 ± 1.3 years. The clinical characteristics of the 2 study populations are summarized in Additional file 2.

MiRNA profiles in AF patients versus healthy controls
To determine the levels of miRNAs in LAA in patients with non-valvular PAF, we performed miRNA profiling in 8 patients with AF and in 5 HCs (Additional file 3 and Additional file 4). The miRNA expression profiles of AF and HCs were compared. The levels of miRNAs profoundly differed between patients and HCs, as illustrated in the heat map diagram shown in Fig. 1a. Quantification revealed that 10 miRNAs were differentially expressed between the patients and HCs with more than 2-fold change ($P < 0.05$). These miRNAs were miR-155, miR-146b-5p, miR-19b, miR-142-3p, miR-486-5p, miR-223, miR-193b, miR-519b-3p, miR-301b and miR-193a-5p.

The RT-PCR analysis confirmed the significant up-regulation of miR-155, miR-146b-5p, miR-19b, miR-142-3p, miR-486-5p, miR-223, miR-193b, miR-519b-3p and miR-301b, and significant down-regulation of miR-193a-5p (Fig. 1b). In particular, miR-155, miR-146b-5p, and miR-19b demonstrated the most pronounced changes among the 10 differentially expressed miRNAs. These qRT-PCR results confirmed the miRNA microarray results and indicated the potential roles of miRNAs in the progression of AF.

To confirm the findings of the miRNA profile analysis, we measured the expression of selected miRNAs in the entire cohort (n = 47) by using TaqMan quantitative PCR (qPCR). As shown in Fig. 2, the expression of predominantly inflammation-associated miRNAs such as miR-146b-5p, miR-19b, and miR-155 [21–23] were significantly increased in patients with AF.

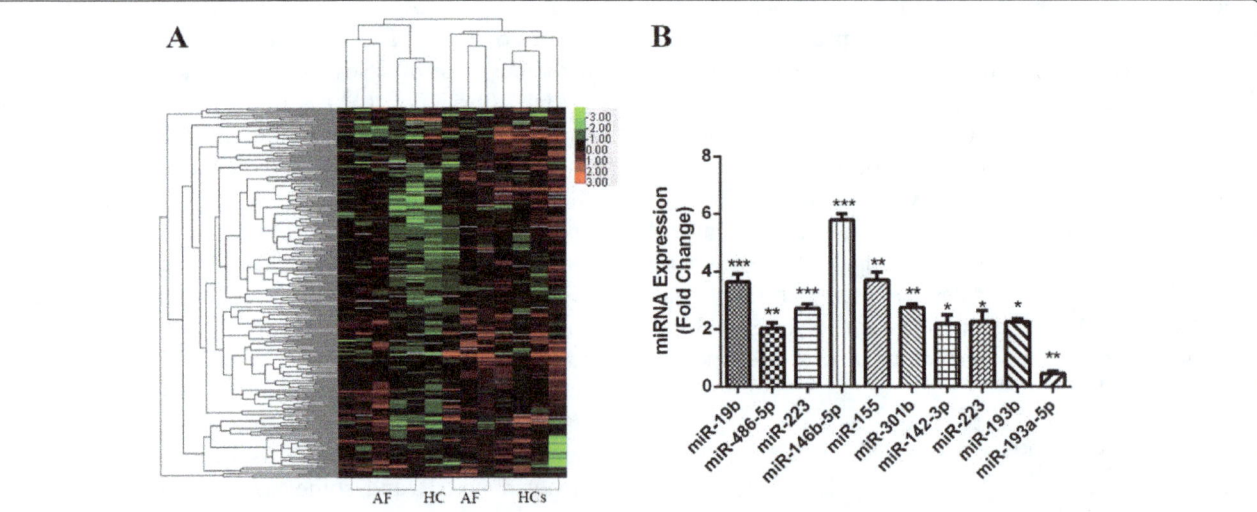

Fig. 1 Profile of miRNAs in patients with atrial fibrillation versus health controls. **a** Heat map diagram t. **b** qRT-PCR verification of the miRNA expression profile in atrial fibrillation. ***$P < 0.001$; **$P < 0.01$; *$P < 0.05$

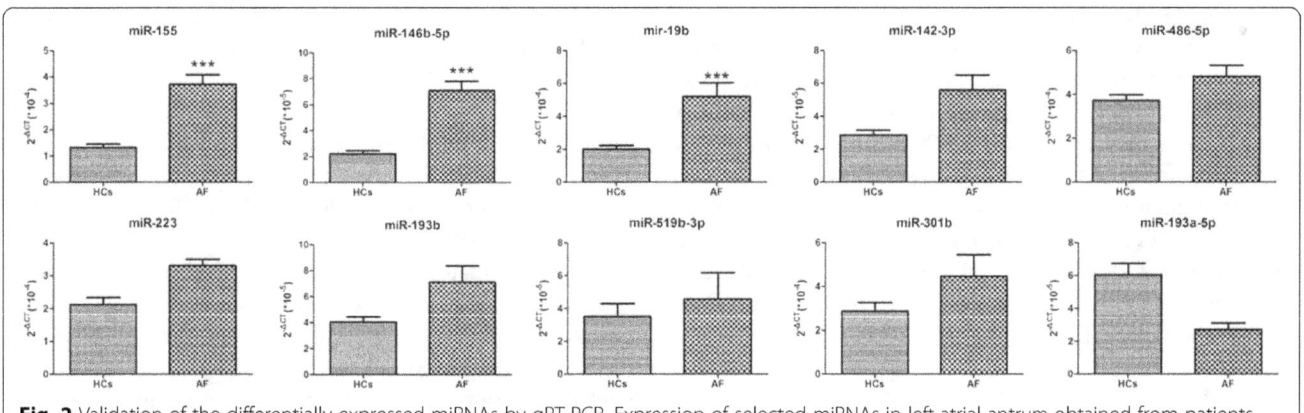

Fig. 2 Validation of the differentially expressed miRNAs by qRT-PCR. Expression of selected miRNAs in left atrial antrum obtained from patients with atrial fibrillation (n = 30) and health controls (n = 17), as determined by TaqMan PCR. *** $P < 0.001$; ** $P < 0.01$; * $P < 0.05$

Correlation between miRNAs expression and AF

To determine the factors that influence the levels of miRNAs, we analyzed the association between miRNAs and the baseline characteristics of the patients. There were significant positive correlations between the expression of miR-146b-5p and miR-155, and AF patients' LAD, plasma levels of high sensitivity C-reactive protein (hsCRP) and AF duration, respectively (Fig. 3). Interestingly, the LAD, AF duration and hsCRP levels are considered to be predictors of increased risk for the AF recurrence [24, 25].

To verify whether the up-regulation of these inflammation-associated miRNAs is the main factor for recurrence of AF, we analyzed the expression of miRNAs in patients with sinus rhythm (SR group) and in patients who had recurrence of AF (AF group) in our original cohort after 2 year follow-up (Additional file 5). As shown in the table, the miRNA-155 and miR-146b expression levels, LAD, hsCRP levels, and AF duration were found to significantly predict recurrence in the univariate regression models. However, in multivariate analysis only miRNA-155 [Hazard Ratio [HR], 1.113; $P = 0.037$) and miR-146b-5p (HR, 1.646; $P = 0.030$) expression levels, LAD (HR, 1.036; $P = 0.039$) and AF duration (HR, 1.216; $P = 0.044$) were found to significantly predict the recurrence of AF.

MiRNAs expression profile is correlated with genes that are involved in AF

Given the fact that miRNA is involved in post-transcriptional regulation, we endeavored to determine whether there is was correlation between the levels of miRNAs expression and their target genes involved in the pathogenesis of AF. We performed target prediction for miRNAs by using 4 Databases (TargetScan, miRanda, Starbase Clip-seq and miRDB) and identified the genes, based on the similar prediction by at least the 3 of the 4 databases. We found that at least 7 genes were related to AF. Among these, 4 genes were related to the inflammatory response and fibrosis, and three others encoding cardiac ion channel proteins (Additional file 6).

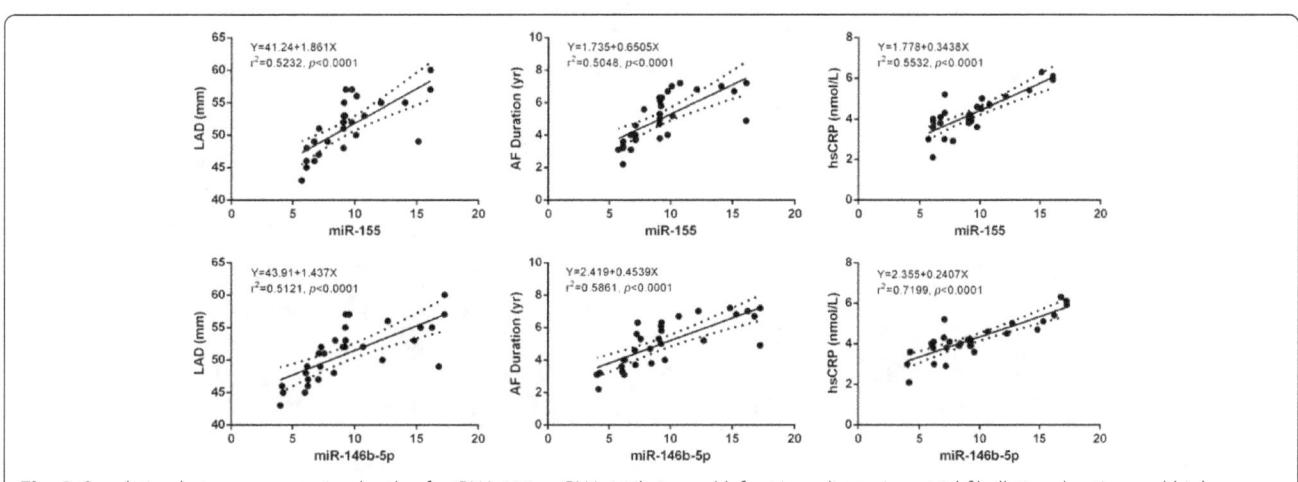

Fig. 3 Correlation between expression levels of miRNA-155, miRNA-146b-5p and left atrium dimension, atrial fibrillation duration and high sensitivity C-reactive protein

MRNA and protein expression of target gene

To determine whether those seven predicted target genes were involved in non-valvular PAF, we measured those expression of mRNA and protein in the entire cohort (n = 47). As a result of TaqMan qPCR, the relative mRNA expression level of the DIER-1, TIMP-4 and CACNA1C were significantly lower in the AF group than that in the HC group (Fig. 4a). As a result of Western blotting analysis, the DIER-1, TIMP-4 and CACNA1C protein expression were also significantly lower in AF group than in HC group (Fig. 4b).

Discussion

The most important results of our study may be summarized as follows: 1. Expression levels of miR-155, miR-146b-5p and miR-19b were significantly increased in patients with non-valvular PAF compared with HCs. 2. Levels of miR-146b-5p and miR-155, which are known to be associated with inflammation, were independently and positively associated with LAD, AF duration and hsCRP levels. 3. On multivariate analysis only miR-155 and miR-146b-5p

expression levels, LAD, and AF duration were found to significantly predict AF recurrence after procedure.

Co-morbidities might affect miRNAs expression

This study provides the first profiling of miRNAs in patients with non-vavular PAF and HCs. We found that in the LAA miR-155, miR-146b-5p and miR-19b are aberrantly up-regulated in patients with AF compared with HCs. A group of miRNAs regulate genes encoding cardiac ion channel proteins and other relevant genes, and several studies have reported the direct involvement of miRNAs in controlling cardiac excitability and arrhythmogenesis in certain pathological conditions [12]. Some such miRNAs have been shown to be directly involved in AF, and some are considered to have the potential to regulate AF based on their target genes. However, to our knowledge, earlier investigations verified the regulation of miRNAs in the atrial tissue from patients with valvular AF and other co-morbidities in non-AF patients (such as coronary heart disease). Therefore, from those studies it would not possible

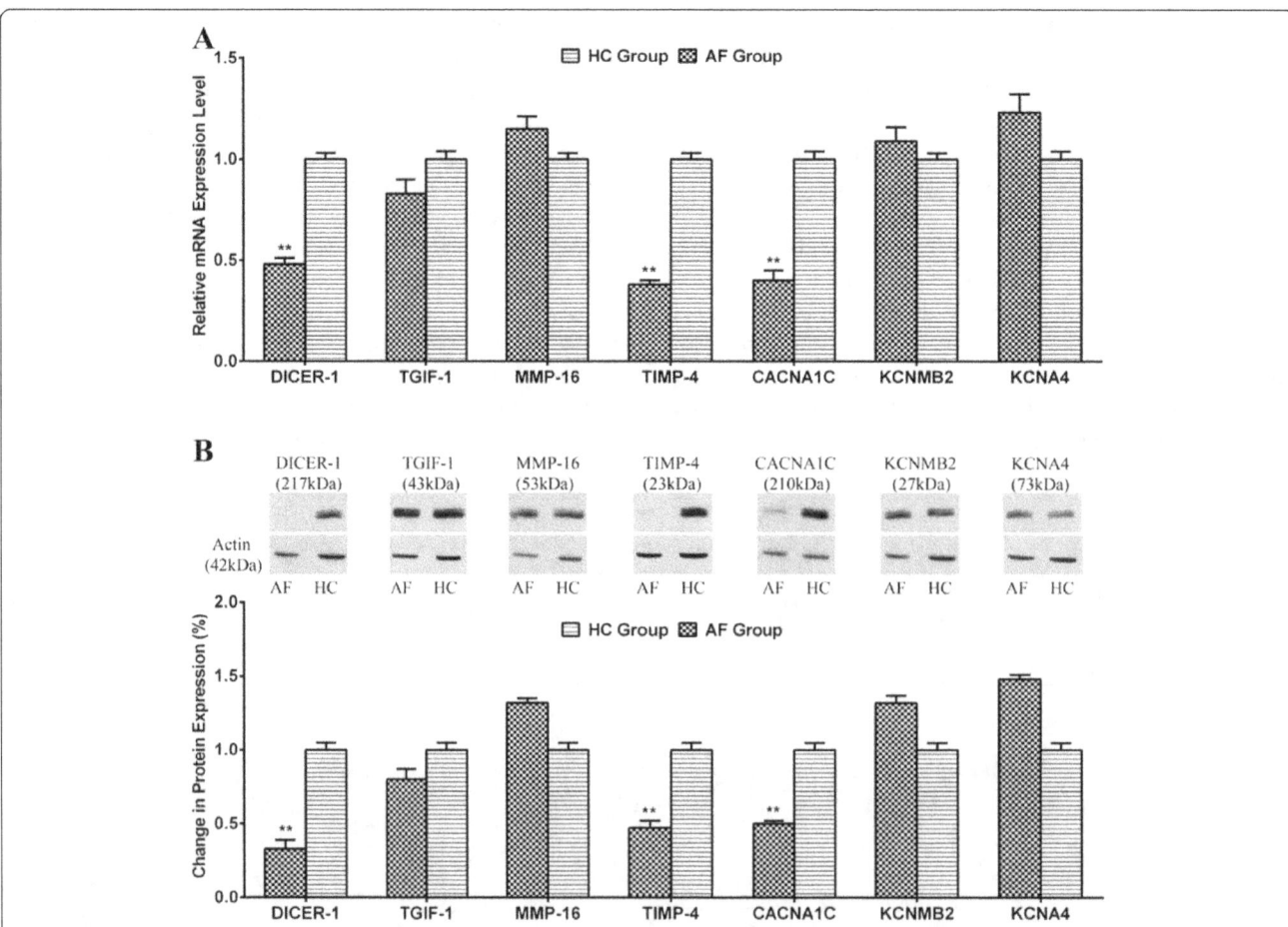

Fig. 4 Expression level of target genes in the atrial fibrillation (AF) group (n = 30) and healthy control (HC) group (n = 17). **a** The relative mRNA expression level of the target genes as determined by TaqMan PCR. **b** Protein expression of the target genes using the Western blot. ***P < 0.001; **P < 0.01; *P < 0.05

to deduce whether pre-existing heart diseases already influenced the expression of miRNAs.

Previous studies have reported that expression of miR-NAs such as miR-1, miR-328 and miR-499 are altered in valvular AF patients, but it did not significantly change in our study [13–15]. This variation in the findings, compared with other studies, may be attributed to the differences in the tissues that were sampled (LAA in the current study versus left atrial tissue in the other previous studies) and the heterogeneity of human myocardial samples. AF is a multifaceted electrical phenotype involving complex factors beyond electrophysiology and can occur in a variety of pathological settings. The different types of AF have distinct underlying mechanisms, and different miRNAs might be involved. The results of Cooley and Xiao et al. showed that the presence of valvular heart disease in AF influenced miRNA expression patterns in both left and right atria [16, 17].

Morphological and electrophysiological differences have been demonstrated between theright atria and left atria, which at least in part, may reflect different mechanisms involved in AF between the right atria and left atria. Thus, it is not surprising that AF-associated miRNAs of the right atria may differ from those of the left atria. A recent study compared the potential differences of AF-associated miRNAs in the RA and LA from rheumatic mitral valve disease patients. They have found the different distributions of AF-associated miRNAs in the right atrial appendage and LAA from rheumatic mitral valve disease patients. This may reflect different miRNA mechanisms in AF between the RA and LA. 26 But for the non-valvular AF, AF substrate in the left atria is related to AF initiation and maintenance, which plays an important role to initiate and perpetuate AF. And the potential difference of AF-associated miRNAs between right atria and left atria are still unknown due to lack of the RA and LA sample availability.

In our study miR-155, miR-146b-5p, and miR-19b were significantly up-regulated in non-valvular PAF patients. Most important, we also found significantly higher levels of expression of miR-155 and miR-146b-5p were independently associated with LAD, AF duration and hsCRP levels. However, only miR-155 and miR-146b expression level, LA dimension and AF duration were found to significantly predict AF recurrence in multivariate analysis.

Role of LAA in maintaining AF

Less invasive AF ablation procedures have been developed due to increasing knowledge about the pathophysiology of AF and due to the development of ablation devices, which replace the original 'cut-and-sew' technique for scarification [26, 27]. Wolf et al. developed an off-pump procedure, in which the pulmonary veins (PVs) are isolated, ganglionic plexus are ablated, and the LAA is amputated through a bilateral thoracotomy [26]. The LAA is derived from the primordial left atrium, which is formed mainly by the adsorption of the primordial PVs and their branches. This similar embryological origin suggests that the LAA may initiate AF like the PVs. This could explain the potential and active role of LAA as an underestimated source of AF. In our study, miRNAs profiling in LAA provided very compelling evidence, which illustrated the potential of miRNAs as a new mechanism for non-valvular PAF.

MiRNAs and cardiac remodeling

Interestingly, miR-155, which is reported to be involved in cardiovascular diseases, showed the largest increases in our AF patients compared with HCs. miR-155 might directly influence arrhythmia outcomes by targeting critical ion channel gene expression, including CACNA1C and KCNA4, which encode the cardiac L-type Ca^{2+} channel (I_{CaL}) α1c and the initial component of the transient outward potassium current (I_{to1}), respectively. And our results showed that the expression of the CACNA1C was significantly lower in the AF group than the HC group, not only for the protein level, but also the mRNA level. Moreover, miR-155 up-regulation may also play a role in inflammation [21]. In fact, emphasis has been given to miR-155 because it represents a typical multifunctional miRNA [28]. Even though the mechanism that regulates miRNA function and expression has not been completely understood, the information presently available (i.e. over expression in AF patients) allows us to recognize miR-155 as a gene of potentially paramount clinical importance in AF diagnosis and treatment. It is reasonable to speculate that evaluation of mRNA-155 in tissues or biological fluids might be utilized as a biochemical parameter for AF detection and prognosis.

MiR-146, is also thought to be a mediator of inflammation along with miR-155 [29]. The expression of miR-146 is up-regulated by inflammatory factors such as interleukin 1 and tumor necrosis factor [22]. miR-146 regulates a number of targets, which are mostly involved in Toll-like receptor pathways that bring about a cytokine response as part of the innate immune system [30]. Recently, miR-146b-5p was reported to be up-regulated in AF patients, which is consistent with our findings [18]. Potential targets of miR-146b-5p include TGIF1, MMP16 and TIMP4 that are reported to be regulated in cardiomyocyte fibrosis, and these might be expected to contribute to AF by promoting fibrosis, an established AF substrate [31]. This possibility remains to be investigated. Our results showed that the expression of the TIMP-4 was significantly lower in the LAA of the AF group than in that of the HC group, not only for the protein level, but also the mRNA level.

MiR-19b also takes part in inflammatory responses enhancing or repressing pro-inflammatory mediators' expression [23]. It positively regulates Toll-like receptor signaling with DICER-1 deletion and miRNA depletion. The miR-19b is an important protagonist in this phenomenon, regulating positively the NF-kB activity [23]. The miRNA depletion inhibits cytokines production by NF-kB. Also, it is directly involved in the modulation of several NF-kB signaling negative regulators expression, indicating the importance of miR-19b on NF-kB signaling. This miRNA has not been extensively studied, but our data suggests a possible role of this miRNA in the pathology of AF, which is yet to be identified.

Study limitations
One of the limitations of the present study is that at this point we are unable to provide molecular insights for the cause of miRNA dysregulation in non-valvular PAF. The levels of miRNAs may be affected by multiple factors such as the change in expression in the tissue, the release of the miRNAs by the cells and the stability of miRNAs. Secondly, the exact targets and pathways by which alterations in miRNAs cause AF remain elusive. Although our analysis has indicated some potential genes and pathways that are involved in AF, it is difficult to estimate the actual false-positive rate of the overall target prediction. A better understanding of the biological significance of these broad, but often subtle, changes in miRNA expression that are found in AF patients could be achieved with the development of novel experimental models, in which the levels of one or more miRNAs could be precisely manipulated.

Conclusions
The present study provides the first insight into the levels of miRNAs in the LAA in patients with non-valvular PAF. While previous studies have demonstrated reliable measurement of miRNAs, our study specifically addressed the levels and regulation of ionic, inflammatory and fibrotic derived miRNAs and shows, specific miRNAs which may be involved in both electrical and structural remodeling of the fibrillating atria. However, these data further need to be confirmed in larger clinical population. Furthermore, the mechanisms underlying the dysregulation, and as well as the putative impact of the changes in miRNAs levels in the physiology or pathophysiology, remains to be elucidated.

Abbreviations
AF: Atrial fibrillation; FDR: False discovery rate; HCs: Healthy controls; HR: Hazard Ratio; LAA: Left atrial appendage; LAD: Left atrial diameter or dimension; mRNAs: Messenger RNAs; PAF: Paroxysmal atrial fibrillation; QPCR: Quantitative PCR; RT-PCR: Real time PCR; SR: Sinus rhythm.

Competing interests
The authors declare that they have no competing interests.

Authors' contributions
JW conceived of the study, and participated in its design and coordination and drafted the manuscript. SS drafted the manuscript. CX participated in its design. JH and YL collected the specimen. JS, MX, JW, and TL carried out the molecular biological studies. BY revised the draft. XM conceived of the study, and participated in its design and coordination. All authors read and approved the final manuscript.

Authors information
The first two authors are co-first authors.

Acknowledgments
We thank Dr. José Jalife, from Center for Arrhythmia Research, University of Michigan, for his constructive comments to this study. This study was supported by the National Natural Science Foundation of China (Grant No. 81370294).

Author details
[1]Department of Cardiac Surgery, Beijing Anzhen Hospital, Capital Medical University, Beijing 100029, P.R. China. [2]Department of Internal Medicine, Vidant Medical Center, Broody School of Medicine, East Carolina University, Greenville, North Carolina 27834, USA. [3]Department of Cardiothoracic Surgery, Affiliated Hospital of Nantong University, Nantong 226001, China. [4]University of Michigan Cardiovascular Center, University of Michigan, Ann Arbor, Michigan 48109, USA.

References
1. Lee RC, Feinbaum RL, Ambros V. The C. elegans heterochronic gene lin-4 encodes small RNAs with antisense complementarity to lin-14. Cell. 1993;75:843–54.
2. Bartel DP. MicroRNAs: genomics, biogenesis, mechanism, and function. Cell. 2004;116:281–97.
3. Slack FJ, Weidhaas JB. MicroRNA in cancer prognosis. N Engl J Med. 2008;359:2720–2.
4. Tili E, Michaille JJ, Costinean S, Croce CM. MicroRNAs, the immune system and rheumatic disease. Nat Clin Pract Rheumatol. 2008;4:534–41.
5. Matkovich SJ, Wang W, Tu Y, Eschenbacher WH, Dorn LE, Condorelli G, et al. MicroRNA-133a protects against myocardial fibrosis and modulates electrical repolarization without affecting hypertrophy in pressure-overloaded adult hearts. Circ Res. 2010;106:166–75.
6. Pritchard CC, Cheng HH, Tewari M. MicroRNA profiling approaches and considerations. Nat Rev Genet. 2012;13:358–69.
7. Fuster V, Ryden LE, Cannom DS, Crijns HJ, Curtis AB, Ellenbogen KA, et al. ACCF/AHA/HRS focused updates incorporated into the ACC/AHA/ESC 2006 guidelines for the management of patients with atrial fibrillation: a report of the American College of Cardiology Foundation/American Heart Association Task Force on practice guidelines. Circulation. 2011;2011(123):e269–367.
8. Lip GY, Tse HF, Lane DA. Atrial fibrillation. Lancet. 2012;379:648–61.
9. Callis TE, Wang DZ. Taking microRNAs to heart. Trends Mol Med. 2008;14:254–60.
10. Yang B, Lin H, Xiao J, Lu Y, Luo X, Li B, et al. The muscle-specific microRNA miR-1 regulates cardiac arrhythmogenic potential by targeting GJA1and KCNJ2. Nat Med. 2007;13:486–91.
11. Zhao Y, Ransom JF, Li A, Vedantham V, Von DM, Muth AN, et al. Dysregulation of cardiogenesis, cardiac conduction, and cell cycle in mice lacking miRNA-1-2. Cell. 2007;129:303–17.
12. Kim GH. MicroRNA regulation of cardiac conduction and arrhythmias. Transl Res. 2012;161:381–92.
13. Girmatsion Z, Biliczki P, Bonauer A, Wimmer-Greinecker G, Scherer M, Moritz A, et al. Changes in microRNA-1 expression and IK1 up-regulation in human atrial fibrillation. Heart Rhythm. 2009;6:1802–9.
14. Lu Y, Zhang Y, Wang N, Pan Z, Gao X, Zhang F, et al. MicroRNA-328 contributes to adverse electrical remodeling in atrial fibrillation. Circulation. 2010;122:2378–87.

15. Ling TY, Wang XL, Chai Q, Lau TW, Koestler CM, Park SJ, et al. Regulation of the SK3 channel by microRNA-499-Potential role in atrial fibrillation. Heart Rhythm. 2013;10:1001–9.

16. Xiao J, Liang D, Zhang Y, Liu Y, Zhang H, Liu Y, et al. MicroRNA expression signature in atrial fibrillation with mitral stenosis. Physiol Genomics. 2011;43:655–64.

17. Cooley N, Cowley MJ, Lin RC, Marasco S, Wong C, Kaye DM, et al. Influence of atrial fibrillation on microRNA expression profiles in left and right atria from patients with valvular heart disease. Physiol Genomics. 2012;44:211–9.

18. Liu Z, Zhou C, Liu Y, Wang S, Ye P, Miao X, et al. The expression levels of plasma micoRNAs in atrial fibrillation patients. PLoS One. 2012;7:e44906.

19. Nishi H, Sakaguchi T, Miyagawa S, Yoshikawa Y, Fukushima S, Saito S, et al. Impact of microRNA expression in human atrial tissue in patients with atrial fibrillation undergoing cardiac surgery. PLoS One. 2013;8:e73397.

20. Yeh YH, Kuo CT, Lee YS, Lin YM, Nattel S, Tsai FC, et al. Region-specific gene expression profiles in the left atria of patients with valvular atrial fibrillation. Heart Rhythm. 2013;10:383–91.

21. O'Connell RM, Taganov KD, Boldin MP, Cheng G, Baltimore D. MicroRNA-155 is induced during the macrophage inflammatory response. Proc Natl Acad Sci U S A. 2007;104:1604–9.

22. Yamasaki K, Nakasa T, Miyaki S, Ishikawa M, Deie M, Adachi N, et al. Expression of MicroRNA-146a in osteoarthritis cartilage. Arthritis Rheum. 2009;60:1035–41.

23. Gantier MP, Stunden HJ, McCoy CE, Behlke MA, Wang D, Kaparakis-Liaskos M, et al. A miR-19 regulon that controls NF-κB signaling. Nucleic Acids Res. 2012;40:8048–58.

24. Marchese P, Bursi F, Delle DG, Malavasi V, Casali E, Barbieri A, et al. Indexed left atrial volume predicts the recurrence of non-valvular atrial fibrillation after successful cardioversion. Eur J Echocardiogr. 2011;12:214–21.

25. Cai L, Yin Y, Ling Z, Su L, Liu Z, Wu J, et al. Predictors of late recurrence of atrial fibrillation after catheter ablation. Int J Cardiol. 2013;164:82–7.

26. Wolf RK, Schneeberger EW, Osterday R, Miller D, Merrill W, Flege Jr JB, et al. Video-assisted bilateral pulmonary vein isolation and left atrial appendage exclusion for atrial fibrillation. J Thorac Cardiovasc Surg. 2005;130:797–802.

27. Robertson JO, Lawrance CP, Maniar HS, Damiano Jr RJ. Surgical techniques used for the treatment of atrial fibrillation. Circ J. 2013;77:1941–51.

28. Faraoni I, Antonetti FR, Cardone J, Bonmassar E. miR-155 gene: a typical multifunctional microRNA. Biochim Biophys Acta. 2009;1792:497–505.

29. Rebane A, Akdis CA. MicroRNAs: Essential players in the regulation of inflammation. J Allergy Clin Immunol. 2013;132:15–26.

30. Sheedy FJ, O'Neill LA. Adding fuel to fire: microRNAs as a new class of mediators of inflammation. Ann Rheum Dis. 2008;67(3):iii50–5.

31. Fan D, Takawale A, Lee J, Kassiri Z. Cardiac fibroblasts, fibrosis and extracellular matrix remodeling in heart disease. Fibrogenesis Tissue Repair. 2012;5:15.

7

Transesophageal vs. intracardiac echocardiographic screening in patients undergoing atrial fibrillation ablation with uninterrupted rivaroxaban

A. Tsyganov[1][*][†] ⓘ, A. Shapieva[1][†], V. Sandrikov[2], S. Fedulova[2], S. Mironovich[1], A. Dzeranova[2] and E. Lyan[3]

Abstract

Background: Patients with atrial fibrillation (AF) routinely undergo different imaging modalities for the evaluation of the left atrial (LA) appendage to rule out thrombus prior to the AF ablation procedure. Recently, uninterrupted novel oral anticoagulants were introduced for patients undergoing atrial fibrillation (AF) ablation to minimize the peri-procedural thromboembolism risk. We performed a retrospective analysis to evaluate the safety of uninterrupted rivaroxaban and whether transesophageal (TEE) or intracardiac echocardiography (ICE) is necessary for patients undergoing AF ablation.

Methods: Data from 332 consecutive patients (42% females, aged 64 ± 11 years) with AF undergoing either TEE (*n* = 115) prior to catheter ablation or ICE (*n* = 217) for the detection of LA thrombus were analyzed. All patients were on uninterrupted rivaroxaban during, and for at least, 4 weeks before the procedure. Heparin bolus was administered in all patients before transseptal puncture to maintain a target activated clotting time of >350 s.

Results: A total of 277 patients (80.4%) had paroxysmal AF. The average CHA2DS2VASc score was 2.11 ± 0.91 in the TEE group and 2.46 ± 0.61 in the ICE group. The CHA2DS2VASc score was ≥2 in 64 (55.7%) and 214 (98.6%) patients in the TEE and ICE groups, respectively. The left atrial appendage was adequately visualized in all cases. None of the patients have an identifiable LA thrombus either in the TEE group or the ICE group. One (0.3%) thromboembolic periprocedural stroke occurred in a patient with long-standing persistent AF in the TEE group.

Conclusions: This study illustrates that performing AF ablation with ICE guidance on uninterrupted rivaroxaban for at least 4 weeks even without TEE is feasible and safe.

Keywords: NOAC, Transesophageal echocardiography, ICE, Atrial fibrillation, Catheter ablation

Background

Radiofrequency catheter isolation of pulmonary veins has evolved into a cornerstone strategy in the treatment of symptomatic atrial fibrillation (AF) [1]. The procedural complexity and its operator dependency expose patients to a significant number of potential complications [2]. Periprocedural cerebrovascular events are a recognized complication [3]. The presence of left atrial (LA) thrombi is considered to be an absolute contraindication for interventions in the LA, because of increased risk of clot dislodgement and subsequent thromboembolic event with catheter manipulation during the ablation procedure. Many strategies have been developed to reduce the incidence of periprocedural stroke in patients undergoing ablation for AF. These include routine periprocedural anticoagulation as well as transesophageal echocardiography (TEE) immediately prior to the procedure to rule out the presence of LA thrombus [4–7].

The main purpose of our study was to evaluate the safety of uninterrupted novel oral anticoagulants (NOAC) in patients presenting for the AF ablation. Secondly, we identified the incidence of LA thrombi in

* Correspondence: tsyganov.alexey@gmail.com
†Equal contributors
[1]Cardiac Electrophysiology Department, Petrovsky National Research Centre of Surgery, Abrikosovsky per. 2, Moscow 119991, Russia
Full list of author information is available at the end of the article

patients with uninterrupted NOAC despite 4 weeks of therapeutic anticoagulation and determined whether pre-procedural TEE should be recommended in all patients.

Methods

Patient selection

We retrospectively analyzed 332 consecutive patients treated with NOAC who were referred to two centers between September 2013 and October 2016. All patients had documented symptomatic AF and underwent radiofrequency catheter ablation for AF with uninterrupted rivaroxaban. Baseline demographic and clinical characteristics, including age, gender, BMI, hypertension, diabetes mellitus, coronary artery disease, and congestive heart failure, were recorded for all patients. Data related to the diagnosis of AF, including AF pattern, oral anticoagulation, and previous interventions, was also recorded. Risk stratification for thromboembolism and bleeding was performed based on the CHA2DS2-VASc and HAS-BLED score, respectively. Creatinine clearance was estimated by Cockcroft-Gault eq. A 2D transthoracic echocardiogram was carried out on all patients to estimate left ventricular ejection fraction and any structural heart diseases.

This study was approved by the Institutional Review Board of Petrovsky National Research Centre of Surgery (IRB No. 130/1).

Transesophageal echocardiography

TEE was performed (iE33, Philips Medical Systems, MA, US) and interpreted by an experienced echocardiographer for the presence or absence of the LA thrombus. A thrombus was considered to be present if a mass detected in the LA appendage or other sites appeared to be distinct from the underlying endocardium in more than one imaging plane and was not caused by pectinate muscles.

Intracardiac echocardiography

ICE was performed by using a 10F AcuNav phased-array probe (Siemens AG, Germany) connected to a Vivid *i* system (General Electric, IL, US), and advanced through the left femoral vein. The catheter was initially positioned in the right atrium and then was rotated to visualize whole left atrium including the appendage. It was then curved and advanced into the right ventricle next to the pulmonic artery for a better visualization of the left atrial appendage. In some cases, the ICE probe was advanced into the coronary sinus, and LA appendage imaging was performed (Fig 1). Moreover, ICE was used during the procedure for the identification of procedure-related complications.

Procedure protocol

All patients received 20 mg of rivaroxaban 4 weeks prior to the procedure without discontinuation in the intraprocedural period. The LAA visualization approach was

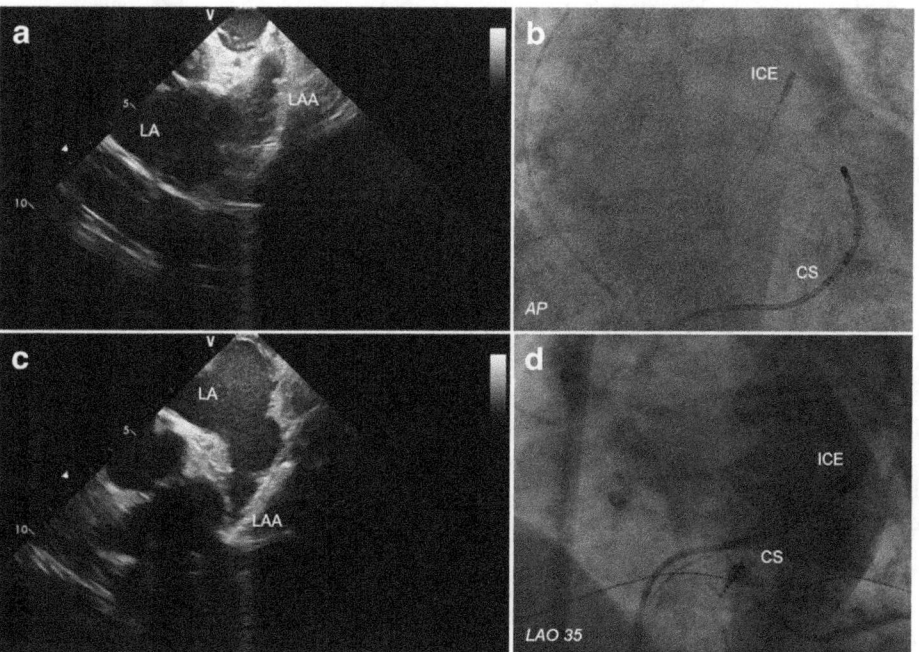

Fig. 1 The upper row is demonstrating an example of the intracardiac echocardiographic image of the left atrial appendage from the pulmonary artery (**a**), and a fluoroscopic view of the intracardiac echocardiography probe in the pulmonary artery (**b**). The lower row is demonstrating an example of the intracardiac echocardiographic image of the left atrial appendage from the coronary sinus (**c**), and a fluoroscopic view of the intracardiac echocardiography probe in the coronary sinus (**d**)

chosen by the operator, thus neither in the TEE nor the ICE group, we did not use both modalities. All ablation procedures were performed under deep sedation. A bolus of heparin (100 IU/L) was administered immediately after vascular access before double transseptal puncture. Anticoagulation therapy was continued throughout the procedure with a targeted activated clotting time (ACT) above 350 s. The ACT was repeated every 20–30 min, and additional bolus was administrated to maintain target ACT. Transseptal sheaths were continuously flushed with heparinized saline (2000 IU/L) 180 ml per hour. A 3D map of the LA geometry was created using the Carto 3 navigation system (Biosense Webster Inc., CA, US). Continuous point-by-point ablation using a 3.5 mm irrigated open-tip catheter (ThermoCool SmartTouch D-F curve, Biosense Webster Inc., CA, US) was used to create a pulmonary vein antrum lesion set in all patients. For patients with long-standing persistent AF were performed additional linear ablation across the LA roof, in the mitral valve isthmus or LA anteroseptal region, and in the cavotricuspid isthmus. The cavotricuspid line was applied in patients with previously reported or observed typical atrial flutter. In the case of spontaneous induction of atypical atrial flutter, an activation map had been constructed, and ablation of the zone of interest was done. A deflectable circular mapping catheter (Lasso 2515, Biosense Webster inc., CA, US) was used for verification of the pulmonary veins isolation and line conduction block. At the end of the procedure, if pulmonary vein isolation (PVI) alone or plus linear did not achieve sinus rhythm, electrical cardioversion was performed.

All complications within the first 48 h after the ablation procedure were included in this study. All patients were recommended to continue rivaroxaban for at least 3 months or long-life after discharge if the CHA2DS2-VASc score was 0 or ≥1, respectively.

Data analysis

Continuous variables were expressed as the mean ± standard deviation. Categorical variables were expressed as absolute numbers and percentages. Differences between means among groups were compared using the Student t test for continuous variables and with the nonparametric χ2 test or Fisher exact test when appropriate for categorical variables. A p value less than 0.05 was considered significant. SPSS software version 20.0 (IBM, NY, US) was used for statistical analysis.

Results

Patient characteristics

A total of 115 patients (37 females, mean age 57.4 ± 11.5 years) underwent TEE prior to catheter ablation, and 217 patients (103 female, mean age 67.6 ± 8.3 years) underwent ICE during the procedure

without prior TEE. Patients in the ICE group tended to be older, having higher BMI and LA size, and more often suffer from hypertension and diabetes mellitus, while the incidence of coronary artery disease was lower. The average CHA2DS2VASc tended to be higher in the ICE group, but HAS-BLED scores were similar in both groups. However, the CHA2DS2VASc score was ≥2 only in 64 (55.7%) patients in the TEE group versus 214 (98.6%) patients in the ICE group. Two hundred and sixty-seven patients (80.4%) had paroxysmal AF, 56 patients (16.9%) had persistent AF, and 9 patients (2.7%) had long-persistent AF. Thirty-eight patients underwent a redo procedure after the previous PVI. Three patients had a concomitant atypical atrial flutter before the procedure. In one patient, atypical atrial flutter was observed during the procedure.

The left atrial appendage was adequately visualized in all cases. None of the patients have an identifiable LA thrombus either in the TEE group or ICE group.

Baseline characteristics of the study population are summarized in Table 1.

Clinical outcomes

PVI was achieved in all patients. In nine patients with long-standing, persistent AF, linear ablation was performed. A total of 37 patients underwent the cavotricuspid isthmus ablation. All patients with atypical atrial

Table 1 Demographic patient data

	TEE group	ICE group	p-value
Paroxysmal	71 (61,7%)	196 (90,3%)	<0.001
Persistent	38 (33%)	18 (8,3%)	<0.001
Long-standing persistent	6 (5,3%)	3 (1,4%)	0.042
Age, years	57.4 ± 11.5	67.6 ± 8.3	<0.001
BMI	28.6 ± 4.5	29.7 ± 4.6	0.044
Coronary artery disease	27 (23.5%)	1 (0.4%)	<0.001
Hypertension	78 (67.8%)	210 (96.8%)	<0.001
Diabetes mellitus	11 (9.6%)	65 (29.9%)	<0.001
Congestive heart failure	16 (13.9%)	22 (10.1%)	0.312
Previous stroke or TIA	1 (0.8%)	0 (0%)	0.951
Left atrial size, mm	41.9 ± 6.2	43.4 ± 3.7	0.006
LV EF, %	58.9 ± 8.3	60.2 ± 7.7	0.194
Creatinine clearance, ml/min	108.81 ± 32.76	112.06 ± 24.05	0.092
CHA2DS2-VASc score	2.09 ± 0.91	2.46 ± 0.61	0.048
0	23 (20%)	1 (0.4%)	<0.001
1	28 (24.3%)	2 (0.9%)	<0.001
≥2	64 (55.7%)	214 (98.6%)	<0.001
HAS-BLED	0.85 ± 0.89	0.96 ± 0.84	0.071

Data are presented as mean ± SD

AF atrial fibrillation, *BMI* body mass index, *TIA* transient ischemic attack, *TEE* transesophageal echocardiogram, *ICE* intracardiac echocardiography, *LV EF* left ventricular ejection fraction

flutter were successfully mapped and ablated; of which, two had peri-mitral, one had peri-venous, and the other one had right atrial upper loop re-entry flutter. The mean procedure time was 101.5 ± 15.1 in the TEE group and 110.8 + 12.4 min in the ICE groups (p = 0.78).

One (0.3%) thromboembolic event occurred in a patient on uninterrupted 20 mg daily rivaroxaban. The patient had the persistent type of atypical atrial flutter after previous PVI and cavotricuspid isthmus ablation. His CHA2DS2-VASc score was equal to 2. He underwent the repeat procedure for PVI and linear ablation for right atrial upper loop re-entry flutter. The sinus rhythm was restored during linear ablation in the right atrium between the superior and inferior vena cava. The day after the procedure, the patient had an acute stroke with right temporal hemianopia. Magnetic resonance imaging revealed an acute infarction in the left parietal lobe.

A total of 6 (1.8%) patients had bleeding complications. Two (0.6%) major bleeding complications were pericardial effusion with cardiac tamponade, managed by percutaneous pericardial drainage with no sequelae. Four patients (1.2%) who had minor bleeding complications suffered a groin hematoma. No patient with groin hematoma required intervention.

Discussion

Periprocedural screening of intracardiac thrombi and optimal anticoagulation strategy plays an important role in the prevention of thromboembolic complications associated with AF ablation. NOAC were developed as an alternative to vitamin K antagonist for prevention of thromboembolism in patients with AF. In the RELY study, the rate of LA thrombus detection among patients undergoing TEE before cardioversion was 1.2% and 1.8% for patients on dabigatran 150 mg and 110 mg, respectively. However, continuous treatment with NOAC for >3 weeks before cardioversion was less than 80%. TEE data were available in 86 patients on apixaban in the ARISTOTLE study, and none of them had LA thrombus. In the ROCKET AF study, no TEE data were collected to assess rates of LA thrombus among patients on rivaroxaban undergoing cardioversions or catheter ablation of AF [8–10]. In recent studies, the use of NOAC has been shown to be safe and effective in preventing bleeding and thromboembolic complications during uninterrupted periprocedural anticoagulation for AF ablation procedure [11–13].

At present TEE is considered the gold standard in detecting LA thrombi, with a high degree of sensitivity and specificity complying 97% and 100%, respectively [14]. Although an invaluable diagnostic tool, TEE is also a relatively invasive procedure with inherent risk. Major TEE-related complication rates range from 0.2% to 0.5%. Mechanical injury to the gastrointestinal tract can lead to life-threatening complications. The risk of significant gastrointestinal bleeding is estimated between 0.02% and 1.0% [15, 16]. Moreover, TEE may be associated with increased rates of false positive results, associated with artifacts, pectinate muscles, or "smoke" in the LA appendage [17]. However, several studies have shown that AF ablation can be performed without TEE screening when patients are anticoagulated with NOAC [12, 18]. In a prospective multicenter trial, Di Biase et al. showed that AF ablation procedure in patients on uninterrupted NOAC is feasible and safe without TEE, including patients with high risk for stroke (the average CHA2DS2-VASc score was 3.0 ± 1.3) [19]. In that study, all patients underwent ablation procedure under ICE guidance. There was no case-detected thrombus in the LA. Our study, in which an uninterrupted strategy with rivaroxaban was also used, showed no thromboembolic complications in the ICE group, thus confirming the conclusion of Di Biase's study. However, in a recent study, Frenkel et al. showed 3.4% of the LA thrombosis in the uninterrupted NOAC (rivaroxaban and apixaban) cohort were screened with TEE [20].

In a Task Force survey, approximately 50% of members performed TEE in all patients undergoing AF ablation, regardless of the stroke risk [21]. In many electrophysiology laboratories, ICE is used to assist in transseptal puncture and catheter navigation. Moreover, it can also be used for LA imaging when TEE is unequivocal or impossible to perform [22]. In the Action-Ice I Study, Baran et al. showed that ICE could be used safely and effectively for the evaluation of the LA appendage in patients undergoing AF ablation [23]. ICE allows proper visualization of the LA appendage in 85% to 88% of all cases. In most cases, the standard right atrial view does not provide adequate, consistent visualization of the LA appendage. The ICE catheter, when placed in locations that are more proximate to the LA appendage, such as the pulmonary artery or the coronary sinus, improves sensitivity and specificity in detecting the LA appendage thrombus [23, 24]. To the best our knowledge, the likelihood of obtaining satisfactory LA appendage visualization in different imaging planes by an experienced electrophysiologist is nearly 100%. In this study, we did not estimate other thrombogenic milieus, such as a spontaneous echo contrast or LA appendage flow velocity, for two reasons. First, it did not influence the decision to perform the ablation procedure, and there is no consensus that any TEE variable other than the LA thrombus is associated with the occurrence of periprocedural thromboembolic events [25].

The risk of the LA thrombi in patients who are fully anticoagulated with NOAC is very low, but it still exists especially in high-risk patients with CHA_2DS_2-VASc score ≥ 2. Furthermore, despite periprocedural anticoagulation and

TEE or ICE, thromboembolic events can happen in AF patients. In our series, only one patient from the TEE group suffered from a periprocedural stroke, and unfortunately, the incidence and clinical predictors of such complication in patients undergoing AF ablation are not fully understood. Finally, our study adds evidence to the periprocedural management field of AF ablation procedure, illustrating the safety of this procedure in high-risk patients who have been on uninterrupted NOAC for at least four weeks. Use of ICE allows dismissing TEE, as well as avoiding a small, but existing risk of thromboembolic complications associated with AF ablation.

Limitations

The major limitation of our study is its retrospective nature. Thus, the approach of LA visualization was neither randomized nor systematic, but instead a reflection of the choices of the operator. Only rivaroxaban was included; therefore, it is difficult to generalize for the entire class of NOAC. The majority of patients in the ICE group had paroxysmal AF, in which the stroke risk is already minimized as compared to the non-paroxysmal population, that reflects the biased allocation of study participants. Also, ablation strategy and experience could influence thromboembolic events during the procedure regardless of TEE or ICE screening. Most importantly, this study was underpowered to provide statistically rigorous results, and was thus, exploratory in nature.

Conclusions

Our study illustrates that ICE may become a useful clinical tool for LA assessment in patients undergoing AF ablation. Moreover, AF ablation with ICE guidance on uninterrupted rivaroxaban for at least 4 weeks without TEE is feasible and safe.

Abbreviations

ACT: Activated clotting time; AF: Atrial fibrillation; ICE: Intracardiac echocardiography; LA: Left atrium; NOAC: Novel oral anticoagulants; PVI: Pulmonary vein isolation; TEE: Transesophageal echocardiography

Acknowledgements

Not applicable.

Funding

Not applicable.

Authors' contributions

AT and AS made substantial contributions to conception and study design, analysis, and interpretation of data and manuscript drafting. SM, SF, and AD performed collection and assembly of data. VS and EL have been involved in drafting the manuscript and revising it critically for important intellectual content. All authors read and approved the final manuscript.

Competing interests

The authors declare that they have no competing interests.

Author details

[1]Cardiac Electrophysiology Department, Petrovsky National Research Centre of Surgery, Abrikosovsky per. 2, Moscow 119991, Russia. [2]Department of Clinical Physiology, Radiology and Diagnostic Imaging, Petrovsky National Research Centre of Surgery, Abrikosovsky per. 2, Moscow, Russia. [3]Cardiac Electrophysiology Department, Mechnikov North-West State Medical University, Kirochnaya ul. 41, Saint Petersburg 191015, Russia.

References

1. Kirchhof P, Benussi S, Kotecha D, Ahlsson A, Atar D, Casadei B, et al. 2016 2016 ESC guidelines for the management of atrial fibrillation developed in collaboration with EACTS. Eur Heart J. 2016;37:2893–962.
2. Deshmukh A, Patel NJ, Pant S, Shah N, Chothani A, Mehta K, et al. In-hospital complications associated with catheter ablation of atrial fibrillation in the United States between 2000 and 2010: analysis of 93 801 procedures. Circulation. 2013;128:2104–12.
3. Scherr D, Sharma K, Dalal D, Spragg D, Chilukuri K, Cheng A, et al. Incidence and predictors of periprocedural cerebrovascular accident in patients undergoing catheter ablation of atrial fibrillation. J Cardiovasc Electrophysiol. 2009;20:1357–63.
4. Kanj MH, Wazni O, Fahmy T, Thal S, Patel D, Elay C, et al. Pulmonary vein antral isolation using an open irrigation ablation catheter for the treatment of atrial fibrillation: a randomized pilot study. J Am Coll Cardiol. 2007;49:1634–41.
5. Ren JF, Marchlinski FE, Callans DJ, Gerstenfeld EP, Dixit S, Lin D, et al. Increased intensity of anticoagulation may reduce risk of thrombus during atrial fibrillation ablation procedures in patients with spontaneous echo contrast. J Cardiovasc Electrophysiol. 2005;16:474–7.
6. Bruce CJ, Friedman PA, Narayan O, Munger TM, Hammill SC, Packer DL, et al. Early heparinization decreases the incidence of left atrial thrombi detected by intracardiac echocardiography during radiofrequency ablation for atrial fibrillation. J Interv Card Electrophysiol. 2008;22:211–9.
7. Di Biase L, Burkhardt J, Santangeli P, Mohanty P, Sanchez J, Horton R, et al. Periprocedural stroke and bleeding complications in patients undergoing catheter ablation of atrial fibrillation with different anticoagulation management: results from the role of Coumadin in preventing Thromboembolism in Atrial fibrillation (AF) patients undergoing catheter ablation (COMPARE) randomized trial. Circulation. 2014;25:2638–44.
8. Nagarakanti R, Ezekowitz MD, Oldgren J, Yang S, Chernick M, Aikens TH, et al. Dabigatran versus warfarin in patients with atrial fibrillation: an analysis of patients undergoing cardioversion. Circulation. 2011;123:131–6.
9. Flaker G, Lopes RD, Al-Khatib SM, Hermosillo AG, Hohnloser SH, Tinga B, et al. Efficacy and safety of apixaban in patients after cardioversion for atrial fibrillation: insights from the ARISTOTLE trial. J Am Coll Cardiol. 2014;63:1082–7.
10. Piccini JP, Stevens SR, Lokhnygina Y, Patel MR, Halperin JL, Singer DE, et al. Outcomes after cardioversion and atrial fibrillation ablation in patients treated with rivaroxaban and warfarin in the ROCKET AF trial. J Am Coll Cardiol. 2013;61:1998–2006.
11. Imamura K, Yoshida A, Takei A, Fukuzawa K, Kiuchi K, Takami K, et al. Dabigatran in the periprocedural period for radiofrequency ablation of atrial fibrillation: efficacy, safety, and impact on duration of hospital stay. J Interv Card Electrophysiol. 2013;37:223–31.
12. Di Biase L, Lakkireddy D, Trivedi C, Deneke T, Martinek M, Mohanty S, et al. Feasibility and safety of uninterrupted periprocedural apixaban administration in patients undergoing radiofrequency catheter ablation for atrial fibrillation: results from a multicenter study. Heart Rhythm. 2015;6:1162–8.
13. Cappato R, Marchlinski FE, Hohnloser SH, Naccarelli GV, Xiang J, Wilber DJ, et al. Uninterrupted rivaroxaban vs. uninterrupted vitamin K antagonists for catheter ablation in non-valvular atrial fibrillation. Eur Heart J. 2015;36:1805–11.
14. Koca V, Bozat T, Akkaya V, Sarikamis C, Turk T, Vural H, et al. Left atrial thrombus detection with multiplane transesophageal echocardiography: an echocardiographic study with surgical verification. J Heart Valve Dis. 1999;8:63–6.
15. Daniel W, Erbel R, Kasper W, Visser C, Engberding R, Sutherland G, et al.

Safety of transesophageal echocardiography: a multicenter survey of 10,419 examinations. Circulation. 1991;83:817–21.

16. Lennon MJ, Gibbs NM, Weightman WM, Leber J, Ee HC, Yusoff IF. Transesophageal echocardiography - related gastrointestinal complications in cardiac surgical patients. J Cardiothorac Vasc Anesth. 2005;19:141–5.

17. Klein A, Murray R, Grimm R. Role of transesophageal echocardiography-guided cardioversion of patients with atrial fibrillation. J Am Coll Cardiol. 2001;37:691–704.

18. Balouch M, Ipek EG, Chrispin J, Bajwa RJ, Zghaib T, Berger RD. Trends in Transesophageal Echocardiography Use, Findings, and Clinical Outcomes in the Era of Minimally Interrupted Anticoagulation for Atrial Fibrillation Ablation. JACC Clin Electrophysiol 2016. doi:10.1016/j.jacep.2016.09.011.

19. Di Biase L, Briceno D, Trivedi C, Mohanty S, Gianni C, Burkhardt J, et al. Is transesophageal echocardiogram mandatory in patients undergoing ablation of atrial fibrillation with uninterrupted novel oral anticoagulants? Results from a prospective multicenter registry. Heart Rhythm. 2016;13:1197–202.

20. Frenkel D, D'Amato SA, Al-Kazaz M, Markowitz SM, Liu SF, Thomas G, et al. Prevalence of left atrial thrombus detection by transesophageal echocardiography: a comparison of continuous non-vitamin K antagonist oral anticoagulant versus warfarin therapy in patients undergoing catheter ablation for atrial fibrillation. JACC: Clin Electrophysiol. 2016;2:295–303.

21. Calkins H, Kuck KH, Cappato R, Brugada J, Camm AJ, Chen SA, et al. 2012 HRS/EHRA/ECAS expert consensus statement on catheter and surgical ablation of atrial fibrillation: recommendations for patient selection, procedural techniques, patient management and follow-up, definitions, endpoints, and research trial design. J Interv Card Electrophysiol. 2012;33:171–257.

22. Tsyganov A, Petru J, Skoda J, Sediva S, Hala P, Weichet J, et al. Anatomical predictors for successful pulmonary vein isolation using balloon-based technologies in atrial fibrillation. J Interv Card Electrophysiol. 2015;44:265–71.

23. Baran J, Stec S, Pilichowska-Paszkiet E, Zaborska B, Sikora-Frac M, Krynski T, et al. Intracardiac echocardiography for detection of thrombus in the left atrial appendage comparison with transesophageal echocardiography in patients undergoing ablation for atrial fibrillation: the action-ice I study. Circ Arrhythm Electrophysiol. 2013;6:1074–81.

24. Saksena S, Sra J, Jordaens L, Kusumoto F, Knight B, Natale A, et al. A prospective comparison of cardiac imaging using intracardiac echocardiography with transesophageal echocardiography in patients with atrial fibrillation: the intracardiac echocardiography-guided cardioversion helps interventional procedures study. Circ Arrhythm Electrophysiol. 2010;3:571–7.

25. Chilukuri K, Mayer S, Scherr D, Dalal D, Abraham T, Henrikson C, et al. Transoesophageal echocardiography predictors of periprocedural cerebrovascular accident in patients undergoing catheter ablation of atrial fibrillation. Europace. 2010;11:1543–9.

8

Findings of transoesophageal echocardiogram in appropriately anticoagulated patients with persistent atrial fibrillation prior to planned cardioversion

Jūratė Barysienė[1,2], Aistė Žebrauskaitė[1,2]* , Dovilė Petrikonytė[1,2], Germanas Marinskis[1,2], Sigita Aidietienė[1,2] and Audrius Aidietis[1,2]

Abstract

Background: To evaluate a diagnostic value of transoesophageal echocardiogram (TEE) in appropriately anticoagulated patients with a non-valvular atrial fibrillation (AF) and to establish possible additional indications for TEE; to evaluate the incidence of left atrial (LA) thrombi in appropriately anticoagulated patients in daily clinical practice.

Methods: This retrospective study analyses data of 432 patients who had been anticoagulated by means of oral anticoagulants (OACs) prior to planned cardioversion during the period from 2012 to 2015. Thromboembolic (TE) and bleeding risks were assessed using CHA2DS2-VASc and HAS-BLED scores. Transthoracic and transoesophageal echocardiograms were evaluated. TE complications during 30 days after discharge were assessed.

Results: 432 patients were selected, aged from 22 to 89 years (mean 65.0 ±11.5), 277 (64.1%) males and 155 (35.9%) females, 306 (70.8%) on warfarin and 126 (29.2%) on non-vitamin K antagonist oral anticoagulants (NOAC). Mean CHA2DS2-VASc score was 3.5 ±1.5. TEE was performed for 120 (27.8%) patients, more frequently for patients on NOACs and for ones with III° LA enlargement.
TEE revealed LA thrombi in seven (5.8%) of the patients. In warfarin and NOACs groups thrombi were revealed in five (7.0%) and two (4.1%) patients, respectively. TEE did not reveal any thrombi in patients with normal left ventricular (LV) function; however, thrombi were found in two (6.1%) patients with slightly decreased LV function, and in five (17.9%) patients with markedly decreased LV function.
In patients with decreased left ventricular ejection fraction (LVEF) thrombi in LA were found more frequently than in patients with normal and slightly decreased LVEF (17.9% vs 2.2%, p=0.008). CHA2DS2-VASc score of all 7 patients was ≥5. None of the patients after cardioversion had TE complications 30 days after discharge.

Conclusions: The risk of LA thrombi in patients prepared for scheduled cardioversion in line with the guidelines is low. Higher risk of thrombi was present in patients with decreased LVEF (≤40%), CHA2DS2-VASc ≥5. In order to assess more accurately indications to perform TEE for appropriately anticoagulated patients prior to scheduled cardioversion a study with larger number of patients is required.

Keywords: Atrial fibrillation, Non-vitamin K antagonist oral anticoagulants, Anticoagulation, Cardioversion, Transoesophageal echocardiogram, Thromboembolism

* Correspondence: zebrauskaite.aiste@gmail.com
[1]Centre of Cardiology and Angiology, Vilnius University Hospital Santariskiu Clinics, 2 Santariškių St., LT -08661 Vilnius, Lithuania
[2]Clinic of Cardiovascular Diseases, Faculty of Medicine, Vilnius University, 21 Čiurlionio St., LT-03101 Vilnius, Lithuania

Background

Atrial fibrillation (AF) is the most common long-lasting supraventricular arrhythmia [1]. In order to improve the condition of patients suffering from symptomatic persistent AF, restoration of sinus rhythm (SR) can be performed.

Ischemic stroke is the most common complication of AF, with the risk remaining high if prophylaxis of thromboembolic (TE) complications is not administered. AF is the cause of every fourth/fifth ischemic stroke and mortality of these strokes is two times higher in comparison with other types of ischemic stroke [1, 2].

Oral anticoagulants (OACs) may reduce the risk of AF related ischemic stroke by 60 – 80%. The risk of TE complications increases during restoration of SR [1]. The incidence of TE events in patients who were not treated with OACs before restoration of SR ranges from 5 to 7% [3], while in patients appropriately prepared for scheduled cardioversion, the incidence of these complications can be decreased to 1.0% [4, 5].

To prevent TE complications before scheduled SR restoration vitamin K antagonists (VKA) [1, 6] or non-vitamin K antagonist oral anticoagulants (NOACs) are administered [1, 6]. Transoesophageal echocardiogram (TEE) for detection of intracardiac thrombi can be performed in order to assess the efficacy of anticoagulation therapy or as an alternative for treatment with OACs [1, 6].

Furthermore, changes of pharmacogenomics of drugs action are more frequent in patients taking VKA. Actually, only two thirds of the patients on warfarin achieve the therapeutic international normalized ratio (INR) interval for > 64% of period required [7].

Therefore, the duration of preparation for scheduled cardioversion lasts from two to three months [8, 9]. The action of NOACs is stable, dosage is simple, preparation for scheduled SR restoration is shorter. On the other hand, some patients do not comply even with this simplified NOAC administering schedule [10]. This is why physicians have doubts concerning the reliability of anticoagulation before scheduled cardioversion and they perform additional TEE.

The aims of this retrospective study are to evaluate the expedience of TEE before cardioversion in patients properly anticoagulated with OACs suffering from persistent non-valvular AF; to assess the incidence of detection of intracardiac thrombi; to evaluate risk factors of thrombi formation, and to establish additional indications for administering TEE before scheduled SR restoration procedure.

What's new?

In patients with atrial fibrillation appropriately prepared with oral anticoagulants for scheduled cardioversion, risk of thromboembolic complications remains below 1.0%, with the incidence of asymptomatic left atrium thrombi up to 7.7% [11, 12]. The aim is to establish clinical criteria of appropriately anticoagulated patients who are at higher risk of thromboembolic complications and for whom transoesophageal echocardiogram would be beneficial before sinus rhythm restoration.

The higher risk of cardiac thrombi is in patients with decreased left ventricular ejection fraction (≤40%), CHA2DS2-VASc ≥ 5.

Methods

This retrospective study was performed at the Centre of Cardiology and Angiology at Vilnius University Hospital Santariskiu Clinics and included patients who were ≥18 years old, suffering from non-valvular AF and who were prepared for scheduled SR restoration using OACs.

During the period from October 2012 to November 2015, 2940 patients underwent scheduled electrical cardioversion. 2987 patients underwent TEE; this number included 567 patients with persistent non-valvular AF who were prepared for direct current cardioversion (DCC) using OACs; 432 patients were properly anticoagulated and included into this study. The data were obtained from Hospital electronic database, out-patient and in-patient case files. The study was approved by local Bioethics committee.

AF without moderate or high degree stenosis of mitral valve or presence of mechanical valve prosthesis was considered to be non-valvular. Prior to scheduled cardioversion, the patients for ≥3 weeks used NOACs (dabigatran, rivaroxaban, apixaban) or warfarin, maintaining documented INR 2.0-3.0, for not less than 3 subsequent weeks. Individual dosing of NOAC drugs was done according to recommendations. Since it is difficult to confirm directly that patients are indeed taking NOACs properly, we considered to have patients' verbal confirmation and signature in hospital file confirming that she/he did not miss the dosage.

The following criteria were evaluated: patient age, sex, body mass index (BMI), concomitant diseases (arterial hypertension (AH), diabetes mellitus (DM), heart failure (HF), former stroke or transient ischemic attack (TIA), coronary artery disease (CAD). The risk of ischemic stroke and systemic embolism was evaluated using CHA2DS2-VASc scale [13], the risk of bleeding was assessed using HAS-BLED scale [14].

Left ventricular hypertrophy (LVH), size of left atrium (LA) and left ventricular ejection fraction (LVEF) were assessed using trans-thoracic echocardiography. LVH was diagnosed if interventricular septum and posterior left ventricle (LV) wall thickness equaled or exceeded 11 mm [15]. The size of LA was assessed according to atrial volume in 4-chamber view: no enlargement 22–58 ml, I° enlargement 59–68 ml, II° enlargement

69–78 ml, III° enlargement ≥79 ml [15]. LV systolic function was evaluated by LVEF: normal ≥50%, slightly decreased 41–49%, decreased ≤40% [16]. TEE was performed in 120 patients. TEE was performed more frequently for patients on NOACs because of insufficient confidence and experience of physicians with these drugs, also because it was not possible to check the effect of the drug. The decision to perform TEE was made on the assumption of the physicians that expected risk of TE complications was higher. HF or III° LA enlargement, especially their combination, were considered as main factors influencing decision to perform TEE. All patients were studied using Philips iE33 ultrasound machine. All TEE images obtained in each patient were recorded as movie images on a digital media for display and evaluation in real time. TEE images of the LA and left atrium appendage (LAA) were evaluated in the horizontal (0°) plane and in the plane at rotation of the imaging sector (0°–180°) during continuous visualization of the LAA. Thrombus was defined as an echo-dense, well-circumscribed, uniformly consistent mass with a texture different from that of the LAA wall. If thrombi were present, DCC was not performed.

All the study patients for whom scheduled DCC was performed were interviewed by phone 30 days after restoration of SR, in order to reveal TE complications.

Statistical analysis. The data were processed using SPSS 20 and Microsoft Excel software, Pearson's chi square tests were applied and standard deviations (SD) were calculated for the mean values.

Results

The total number of the patients with non-valvular AF prepared for scheduled SR restoration using OACs was 567. Appropriate anticoagulation was not achieved in 135 patients and the data of these patients were not included into subsequent analysis. Appropriate anticoagulation for scheduled DCC was achieved in 432 patients and the data of these patients were analyzed. The scheme of patients distribution is shown in Fig. 1.

The age of the patients ranged from 22 to 89 years, mean age was 65.1 ± 11.5 years. There were 277 (64.1%) male and 155 (35.9%) female patients. The mean age of male and female patients was 61.8 ± 11.9 and 70.5 ± 8.1 years, respectively.

The majority of the patients were suffering from AH (92.4%), HF (76.4%) and CAD (50.5%). Decreased LV systolic function was present in 18.3% and LA enlargement was observed in 83.1% of the patients. The distribution of the patients in accordance with demographic data, stroke, TE and bleeding risk, echocardiography findings and concomitant diseases is presented in Table 1.

Warfarin and NOACs were administered for 306 (70.8%) and 126 (29.2%) patients, respectively. In NOACs group 74 (58.7%) patients were on dabigatran, 39 (31.0%) were on rivaroxaban and 13 (10.3) were on apixaban.

Warfarin was administered for the patients in whom the risk of TE complications and bleeding was higher (CHA2DS2-VASc 3.6 (SD ± 1.6) vs 3.4 (SD ± 1.5), $p = 0.058$); HAS-BLED ≥ 3 (5.6% vs 4.8% $p = 0.08$).

For males and elderly (>75 years) patients NOACs were administered more frequently (30.3% vs 27.1%, $p = 0.27$ and 25.4% vs 20.3%, $p = 0.27$, respectively). In patients with good LV systolic function, administration of NOACs was more frequent (61.1% vs 46.4%, $p < 0.001$) and when LV EF was ≤ 40% administration of warfarin was more common (21.2% vs 11.1%, $p < 0.001$). When there was no LA enlargement, NOACs were administered more frequently (25.4% vs 13.4%, $p = 0.008$), but if LA was enlarged treatment by warfarin was usually preferred (74.6% vs 86.6%, $p = 0.008$). Patients with the history of stroke or TIA were prepared for restoration of SR with warfarin more frequently (6.9% vs 1.6%, $p = 0.013$). Almost one-third of the patients properly prepared for SR restoration (n = 120, 27.8%) underwent TEE before the procedure. This investigation was more frequently performed for the patients treated with NOACs (n = 49, 38.9% vs n = 71, 23.2%, $p < 0.001$). Detailed characteristics of the groups of the patients are presented in Table 2.

The total score of CHA2DS2-VASc, HAS-BLED and patient age had no influence on decision to perform TEE (see Table 3). TEE was performed more frequently for patients with enlargement of LA III° (32.5% vs 21.8%, $p = 0.01$) and suffering from HF (81.7 vs 74.4%, $p = 0.068$).

TEE revealed LA thrombi in 7 (5.8%) patients, in 5 males and 2 females (71.4% and 28.6%, respectively). In these patients SR was not restored, treatment with OACs was continued. The patients' age ranged from 44 to 84 years (mean age 64.1 ± 14.9). CHA2DS2-VASc score in these patients ranged from 5 to 7 points. Thrombi were found in 2 (6.1%) of patients with slightly decreased LV function and in 5 (17.9%) of patients with markedly decreased LV function. In patients with decreased LVEF thrombi in LA were found more frequently than in patients with normal and slightly decreased LVEF (17.9 vs 2.2%, $p = 0.008$). Decreased LV systolic function and CHA2DS2-VASc score ≥5 were observed in all male patients. In both female patients LV systolic function was slightly decreased and CHA2DS2-VASc score was 6. Thrombi were detected in 5 (7.0%) patients of warfarin group and in 2 patients (4.1%) of NOACs group. The duration of the preparation period for the scheduled restoration of SR in patients with LA thrombi in warfarin group was longer in comparison

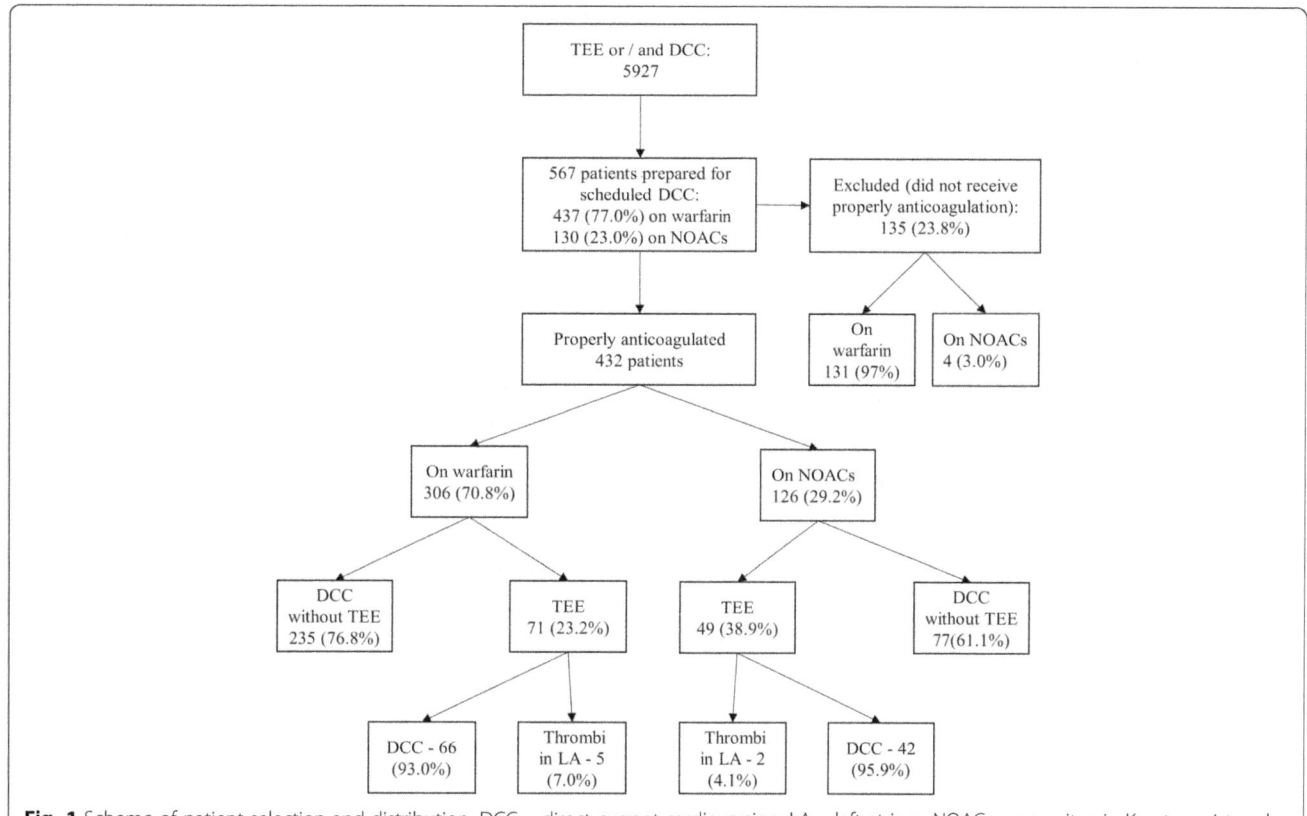

Fig. 1 Scheme of patient selection and distribution. DCC – direct current cardioversion, LA – left atrium, NOACs – non-vitamin K antagonist oral anticoagulants, TEE - transoesophageal echocardiography

with the period in NOACs group (2 – 24 months, mean 11.4 months vs 3 – 8 weeks, mean 6 weeks). A previous history of LA thrombi was found in two male patients, and SR was restored after prolonged anticoagulagion and repeated TEE. After the next AF relapse, TEE revealed LA thrombi again, anticoagulation was prolonged and TEE repeated. One patient did not have LA thrombi, SR was restored and the patient is waiting for LA appendage closure. Another patient still has LA thrombi, and permanent AF was diagnosed. For other 3 patients TEE was repeated after 1 and 3 months, thrombi in LA remained and permanent AF with OAC treatment and rate control was continued. For 2 patients TEE was repeated after 1 month, thrombi in LA resolved and SR was restored, with no TE complications 30 days after cardioversion. In both groups the presence of thrombi did not depend on the grade of LA enlargement.

An interview by phone was performed 30 days after restoration of SR. There were no TE complications in patients four weeks after discharge.

Discussion

The aim of our study was to assess the diagnostic value of TEE in patients with non-valvular AF anticoagulated according to guidelines, and to establish possible additional indications for TEE and to evaluate incidence of

LA thrombi in properly anticoagulated patients in daily clinical practice. In our study this incidence is similar to other studies' data, in which thrombi in LA were found for 3.6–7.7% patients properly anticoagulated with warfarin before scheduled cardioversion [11, 12]. We found LA thrombi in 7.0% patients in warfarin group and 4.1% in NOACs group, we cannot state that risk of thromboembolism is higher in the warfarin group, because the number of these patients is small and because of mentioned selection bias. It should be noted that the number of patients on warfarin was larger and the duration of preparation for scheduled DCC of patients in whom LA thrombi were revealed lasted longer, in comparison with those in NOACs group, with duration ranging from 2 to 24 months (mean 11 months) vs 3-8 weeks (mean 6 weeks), respectively. The prolonged duration of preparation possibly had an influence on thrombi formation as well.

It is not obligatory to perform TEE for patients properly prepared for DCC by OACs [1, 6]. However, if a physician has any concerns regarding compliance to OAC treatment, or for other reasons that may influence the formation of intracardiac thrombi before scheduled DCC, it is reasonable to perform TEE [6, 17]. In RE-LY study the duration of dabigatran administration before scheduled DCC was ≥3 weeks. In the group of patients

Table 1 Distribution of the patients according to demographic data, echocardiography findings, stroke, thromboembolic and bleeding risk stratification, concomitant diseases

	Patients (n, %)	Warfarin group (n, %)	NOACs group (n, %)
Male	277 (64.1%)	193 (63.1%)	84 (66.7%)
Female	155 (35.9%)	113 (36.9%)	42 (33.3%)
Age, years ± SD	65.1 ± 11.5	64.6 ± 11.1	64.9 ± 12.5
CHA$_2$DS$_2$-VASc value ± SD	3.5 ± 1.5	3.6 ± 1.6	3.4 ± 1.5
HAS-BLED value ± SD	0.9 ± 0.9	1.1 ± 0.9	0.9 ± 0.9
HF	330 (76.4%)	238 (77.8%)	92 (73.0%)
AH	399 (92.4%)	280 (91.5%)	119 (94.4%)
CAD	216 (50.0%)	164 (53.6%)	52 (41.3%)
Previous stroke or TIA	23 (5.3%)	21 (6.9%)	2 (1.6%)
DM	54 (12.5%)	41 (13.4%)	13 (10.3%)
BMI 18.5 – 24.9 kg/m^2	59 (14.5%)	39 (13.5%)	20 (16.8%)
BMI 25.0 – 29.9 kg/m^2	138 (33.9%)	95 (33.0%)	43 (36.1%)
BMI ≥30 kg/m^2	209 (51.4%)	153 (53.0%)	56 (47.0%)
LVH	29 (6.7%)	19 (6.2%)	10 (7.9%)
LVEF ≥50%	219 (50.7%)	142 (46.4%)	77 (61.1%)
LVEF 41–49%	134 (31.0%)	99 (32.4%)	35 (27.8%)
LVEF ≤40%	79 (18.3%)	65 (21.2%)	14 (11.1%)
No LA enlargement	73 (16.9%)	41 (13.4%)	32 (25.4%)
I° LA enlargement	126 (29.2%)	91 (29.7%)	35 (27.8%)
II° LA enlargement	126 (29.2%)	94 (30.7%)	32 (25.4%)
III° LA enlargement	107 (24.8%)	80 (26.1%)	27 (21.4%)
Total	432 (100%)	306 (70.8%)	126 (29.2%)

BMI body mass index, *CAD* coronary artery disease, *DM* diabetes mellitus, *HF* heart failure, *LA* left atrial, *LVEF* left ventricular ejection fraction, *LVH* left ventricle hypertrophy, *NOACs* non-vitamin K antagonist oral anticoagulants, *SD* standard deviation, *TIA* transient ischemic attack

Table 2 Distribution of the patients in accordance with decision to perform TEE, with demographic data, thromboembolic and bleeding risk stratification, echocardiography findings and concomitant disease

	TEE performed (n, %)	TEE not performed (n, %)
Male	77 (64.2%)	200 (64.1%)
Female	43 (35.8%)	112 (35.9%)
On warfarin	71 (23.2%)	235 (76.8%)
On NOACs	49 (38.9%)	77 (61.1%)
Mean age, years ± SD	63.5 ± 11.1	65.2 ± 11.6
CHA$_2$DS$_2$-VASc value ± SD	3.5 ± 1.5	3.6 ± 1.6
HAS-BLED value ± SD	1.1 ± 1.0	1.0 ± 0.8
HF	98 (81.7%)	232 (74.4%)
AH	113 (94.2%)	288 (91.7%)
CAD	54 (45.0%)	162 (51.9%)
Previous stroke or TIA	8 (6.7%)	15 (4.8%)
DM	16 (13.3%)	38 (12.2%)
BMI <25 kg/m^2	13 (11.1%)	47 (16.2%)
BMI 25,0 – 29,9 kg/m^2	47 (40.2%)	91 (31.4%)
BMI ≥30 kg/m^2	60 (49.6%)	152 (52.4%)
LVH	7 (5.8%)	22 (7.1%)
LVEF ≥50%	59 (49.2%)	160 (51.3%)
LVEF 41–49%	33 (27.5%)	105 (33.7%)
LVEF ≤40%	28 (23.3%)	47 (15.1%)
No LA enlargement	19 (15.8%)	54 (17.3%)
I° LA enlargement	24 (20.0%)	102 (32.7%)
II° LA enlargement	38 (31.7%)	88 (28.2%)
III° LA enlargement	39 (32.5%)	68 (21.8%)
Total	120 (27.8%)	312 (72.2%)

BMI body mass index, *CAD* coronary artery disease, *DM* diabetes mellitus, *HF* heart failure, *LA* left atrial, *LVEF* left ventricular ejection fraction, *LVH* left ventricle hypertrophy, *NOACs* non-vitamin K antagonist oral anticoagulants, *SD* standard deviation, *TEE* transoesophageal echocardiography, *TIA* transient ischemic attack

who received 110 mg of dabigatran twice daily, TEE was performed for 25.5%. LA thrombi were detected in 1.8% of these patients. In the group of patients who received 150 mg of dabigatran twice daily, TEE was performed in 24.1% of the cases and LA thrombi were detected in 1.2% of the patients [18]. In ARISTOTLE study, for patients prepared for scheduled DCC with apixaban, TEE was performed for 36.6% of the patients and no LA thrombi were found. However, the treatment duration prior to restoration of SR was long (251 ± 248 days) [19]. The question whether the treatment with NOACs lasting from 3 to 4 weeks is sufficient to prepare the patient for scheduled DCC remains an object for discussion. The study of dabigatran demonstrated that preparation for scheduled DCC for 4 weeks is safe [20] but the problem of compliance with the treatment still remains. The half-life of NOACs (about 12 hours) is markedly shorter in comparison with warfarin; therefore, missing of a dose at the appropriate time results in the rapid decrease of

anticoagulation action. The patients comply with the treatment of NOACs better than these on warfarin, but the accuracy of use of preparations is not clear. During a one-year period of observation, 47.5% of the patients receiving NOACs compared to 40.2% of the patients on warfarin, complied with the treatment for 80% of observation period (p < 0.001) [10]. In order to assure appropriate use of the drug, more strict control is required. This is why additional TEE is being performed, even in patients properly prepared with OACs for planned SR restoration [1, 6, 9]. We did not find any relationship between the decision to perform TEE and the estimated CHA2DS2-VASc score. The age of the patient was not considered as a decisive factor to carry out TEE. Approximately half of the patients (49.2%) who underwent TEE were younger than 65 years.

Table 3 Distribution of patients who had and did not have TEE, in accordance with CHA$_2$DS$_2$-VASc and HAS-BLED risk scores

	CHA$_2$DS$_2$-VASc score								
	0	1	2	3	4	5	6	7	8
TEE was performed (n, %)	0 0%	9 7.5%	26 21.7%	23 19.2%	32 26.7%	19 15.8%	8 6.7%	3 2.5%	0 0%
TEE was not performed (n, %)	5 1.6%	21 6.7%	65 20.8%	58 18.6%	74 23.7%	55 17.6%	27 8.7%	6 1.9%	1 0.3%
	HAS-BLED score								
	0	1	2	3	4				
TEE was performed (n, %)	42 35.0%	42 35.0%	26 21.7%	7 5.8%	3 2.5%				
TEE was not performed (n, %)	95 30.4%	140 44.9%	64 20.5%	12 3.8%	1 0.3%				

TEE transoesophageal echocardiography

In our study, more than a half of the patients (55.2%) were obese (BMI ≥30 kg/m^2). Obesity increases the risk of development of a new AF, the incidence of AF relapses and the risk of development of permanent AF. In obese patients with AF, the decrease of the weight reliably decreases the incidence of AF relapses and total duration of the episodes [21]; on the other hand, there are controversial data if obese patients with AF have an increased risk of TE events. According to our data, this factor had no influence on the incidence of AF relapses, the decision to perform TEE, or the detection of heart chamber thrombi.

Male and elderly patients received NOACs more frequently in our study. Warfarin was more frequently administered to the patients with a higher risk of TE complications and history of stroke or TIA. The incidence of NOACs administration was higher for patients with normal systolic LV function, without LA enlargement, while patients with decreased LVEF or LA enlargement received warfarin more frequently.

The majority of patients (73.9%; $p = 0.087$) with a high risk of bleeding (HAS-BLED ≥3) used warfarin. For patients who had a high TE risk (CHA2DS2-VASc ≥6) only warfarin was administered. Warfarin was more frequently administered to the patients suffering from CAD, possibly because of ESC 2015 Guidelines recommending exclusive prescription of warfarin as a part of triple anticoagulation therapy after acute coronary syndromes or scheduled percutaneous transluminal coronary angioplasty. TEE was performed in NOACs group more frequently, in comparison with the warfarin group (38.9 vs 23.2%).

In the study performed by Zylla et al. [17] 643 patients with non-valvular AF and prepared for scheduled DCC by VKA and NOACs were evaluated. TEE was performed for all study subjects. The mean CHA2DS2-VASc score was 4. LA thrombi were detected in 10.6% of the patients and the incidence of thrombi was higher in the warfarin group (17.8 vs 3.9%). In patients for whom TEE revealed thrombi they had a higher CHA2DS2-VASc score (4–5 points in 49%), larger LA or suffered from LV systolic dysfunction. The incidence of thrombi detected was higher in patients treated by VKA with intra-cardiac devices (pacemakers, defibrillators), suffering from CAD. The patients in NOACs group were younger, had a lower CHA2DS2-VASc score, less dilated LA, and better LV systolic function; the incidence of NOACs administration was lower for patients with intra-cardiac devices implanted. The data of our study are quite similar. LA thrombi were revealed in 7 (5.8%) of patients properly prepared using OACs for SR restoration. We found out that the mean CHA2DS2-VASc score was 3.5, but the sample of patients with 4 points was the largest (24.5%). In the case when the CHA2DS2-VASc score was ≥6, only warfarin was administered. The patients on NOACs were younger in our study and they also had less concomitant diseases. However, in patients >75 years old NOACs were administered more frequently, possibly because of difficulties in monitoring INR while administering warfarin, and INR lability.

Similarly, to the data of Zylla et al. [17], in our study the incidence of LA thrombi was higher in warfarin group. Patients in whom intracardiac thrombi were revealed had a higher CHA2DS2-VASc score, and decreased LV systolic function. In two patients who had history of LA thrombi TEE revealed newly formed ones. Both of these patients were on warfarin and their CHA2DS2-VASc score was 6.

The risk of TE complications in the event of markedly decreased LV systolic function (LV EF < 35%) in females is two times higher, in comparison with the risk in males [22]. However, the incidence of thrombi in males, according to our data, is two times higher.

In our study, an interview by phone 30 days after restoration of SR showed no TE complications.

This retrospective study was based on everyday clinical practice and demonstrated that even for patients properly prepared for SR restoration, TEE was performed quite extensively. The risk of thrombi formation, when the patient is prepared by OACs for restoration of SR and adequate anticoagulation is achieved, is low but still remains. Therefore, in all cases the risk for a patient should be evaluated individually.

Limitations

The number of patients in whom LA thrombi have been identified is small (n = 7). It is necessary to perform larger studies of properly anticoagulated patients to make firm conclusions.

Conclusions

The risk of LA thrombi in patients who are prepared for scheduled SR restoration according to guidelines is low. The higher risk of cardiac thrombi was present in patients with decreased LVEF (≤40%), CHA2DS2-VASc ≥5. A larger number of patients is required, in order to assess more precise TEE indications for properly anticoagulated patients prior to scheduled cardioversion.

Abbreviations

AF: Atrial fibrillation; AH: Arterial hypertension; BMI: Body mass index; CAD: Coronary artery disease; DCC: Direct current cardioversion; DM: Diabetes mellitus; HF: Heart failure; INR: International normalized ratio; LA: Left atrium; LAA: Left atrial appendage; LV: Left ventricle; LVEF: Left ventricular ejection fraction; LVH: Left ventricular hypertrophy; NOAC: Non-vitamin K antagonist oral anticoagulants; OACs: Oral anticoagulants; SD: Standard deviation; SR: Sinus rhythm; TE: Thromboembolic; TEE: Transoesophageal echocardiogram; TIA: Transient ischemic attack; VKA: Vitamin K antagonists

Acknowledgements

None.

Funding

No funding was received to carry out this study.

Authors' Contributions

The study conception and design – JB, GM, AA. Acquisition of data – AZ, DP. Analysis and interpretation of data – JB, AZ, AA. Drafting of the manuscript – JB, AZ, AA, GM. Critical revision – GM, AA. All the participants have made themselves familiar with the manuscript and gave their approval of the final draft of the manuscript.

Competing interests

The authors declare they have no competing interests.

References

1. Kirchhof P, Benussi S, Kotecha D, Ahlsson A, Atar D, Casadei B, et al. 2016 ESC Guidelines for the management of atrial fibrillation developed in collaboration with EACTS. Eur Heart J. 2016;37(38):2893–962.
2. Vidaillet H, Granada JF, Chyou PH, Maassen K, Ortiz M, Pulido JN, et al. A population-based study of mortality among patients with atrial fibrillation or flutter. Am J Med. 2002;113(5):365–70.
3. Collins LJ, Silverman DI, Douglas PS, Manning WJ. Cardioversion of Nonrheumatic Atrial Fibrillation. Circulation. 1995;92(2):160–3.
4. Arnold AZ, Mick MJ, Mazurek RP, Loop FD, Trohman RG. Role of prophylactic anticoagulation for direct current cardioversion in patients with atrial fibrillation or atrial flutter. J Am Coll Cardiol. 1992;19(4):851–5.
5. Bjerkelund CJ, Orning OM. The efficacy of anticoagulant therapy in preventing embolism related to D.C. electrical conversion of atrial fibrillation. Am J Cardiol. 1969;23(2):208–16.
6. Heidbuchel H, Verhamme P, Alings M, Antz M, Diener H-C, Hacke W, et al. Updated European Heart Rhythm Association Practical Guide on the use of non-vitamin K antagonist anticoagulants in patients with non-valvular atrial fibrillation. Eur Eur Pacing Arrhythm Card Electrophysiol J Work Groups Card Pacing Arrhythm Card Cell Electrophysiol Eur Soc Cardiol. 2015;17(10):1467–507.
7. Shafeeq H, Tran TH. New Oral Anticoagulants for Atrial Fibrillation. Pharm Ther. 2014;39(1):54–64.
8. Bushoven P, Linzbach S, Vamos M, Hohnloser SH. Optimal Anticoagulation Strategy for Cardioversion in Atrial Fibrillation. Arrhythmia Electrophysiol Rev. 2015;4(1):44–6.
9. Ryman J, Frick M, Frykman V, Rosenqvist M. Duration of warfarin sodium therapy prior to electrical cardioversion of atrial fibrillation. J Intern Med. 2003;253(1):76–80.
10. Yao X, Abraham NS, Alexander GC, Crown W, Montori VM, Sangaralingham LR, et al. Effect of Adherence to Oral Anticoagulants on Risk of Stroke and Major Bleeding Among Patients With Atrial Fibrillation. J Am Heart Assoc. 2016;5(2), e003074.
11. Seidl K, Rameken M, Drögemüller A, Vater M, Brandt A, Schwacke H, et al. Embolic events in patients with atrial fibrillation and effective anticoagulation: value of transesophageal echocardiography to guide direct-current cardioversion. Final results of the Ludwigshafen Observational Cardioversion Study. J Am Coll Cardiol. 2002;39(9):1436–42.
12. Fukuda S, Watanabe H, Shimada K, Aikawa M, Kono Y, Jissho S, et al. Left atrial thrombus and prognosis after anticoagulation therapy in patients with atrial fibrillation. J Cardiol. 2011;58(3):266–77.
13. Lip GYH, Nieuwlaat R, Pisters R, Lane DA, Crijns HJGM. Refining clinical risk stratification for predicting stroke and thromboembolism in atrial fibrillation using a novel risk factor-based approach: the euro heart survey on atrial fibrillation. Chest. 2010;137(2):263–72.
14. Pisters R, Lane DA, Nieuwlaat R, de Vos CB, Crijns HJGM, Lip GYH. A novel user-friendly score (HAS-BLED) to assess 1-year risk of major bleeding in patients with atrial fibrillation: the Euro Heart Survey. Chest. 2010;138(5):1093–100.
15. Recommendations for Cardiac Chamber Quantification by Echocardiography in Adults: An Update from the American Society of Echocardiography and the European Association of, Cardiovascular Imaging. Eur Heart J Cardiovasc Imaging. 2016;17(4):412.
16. Ponikowski P, Voors AA, Anker SD, Bueno H, Cleland JGF, Coats AJS, et al. 2016 ESC Guidelines for the diagnosis and treatment of acute and chronic heart failure. Eur Heart J. 2016;18(8):891–975.
17. Zylla MM, Pohlmeier M, Hess A, Mereles D, Kieser M, Bruckner T, et al. Prevalence of intracardiac thrombi under phenprocoumon, direct oral anticoagulants (dabigatran and rivaroxaban), and bridging therapy in patients with atrial fibrillation and flutter. Am J Cardiol. 2015;115(5):635–40.
18. Nagarakanti R, Ezekowitz MD, Oldgren J, Yang S, Chernick M, Aikens TH, et al. Dabigatran versus warfarin in patients with atrial fibrillation: an analysis of patients undergoing cardioversion. Circulation. 2011;123(2):131–6.
19. Flaker G, Lopes RD, Al-Khatib SM, Hermosillo AG, Hohnloser SH, Tinga B, et al. Efficacy and safety of apixaban in patients after cardioversion for atrial fibrillation: insights from the ARISTOTLE Trial (Apixaban for Reduction in Stroke and Other Thromboembolic Events in Atrial Fibrillation). J Am Coll Cardiol. 2014;63(11):1082–7.
20. Johansson A-K, Juhlin T, Engdahl J, Lind S, Hagwall K, Rorsman C, et al. Is one month treatment with dabigatran before cardioversion of atrial fibrillation sufficient to prevent thromboembolism? Eur Eur Pacing Arrhythm

Card Electrophysiol J Work Groups Card Pacing Arrhythm Card Cell Electrophysiol Eur Soc Cardiol. 2015;17(10):1514–7.

21. Abed HS, Wittert GA, Leong DP, Shirazi MG, Bahrami B, Middeldorp ME, et al. Effect of weight reduction and cardiometabolic risk factor management on symptom burden and severity in patients with atrial fibrillation: a randomized clinical trial. JAMA. 2013;310(19):2050–60.

22. Dries DL, Rosenberg YD, Waclawiw MA, Domanski MJ. Ejection Fraction and Risk of Thromboembolic Events in Patients With Systolic Dysfunction and Sinus Rhythm: Evidence for Gender Differences in the Studies of Left Ventricular Dysfunction Trials. J Am Coll Cardiol. 1997;29(5):1074–80.

9

Atrial time and voltage dispersion are both needed to predict new-onset atrial fibrillation in ischemic stroke patients

Daniel Cortez[1,2*†] , Maria Baturova[1,3,4†], Arne Lindgren[5,6], Jonas Carlson[1], Yuri V. Shubik[4], Bertil Olsson[1] and Pyotr G. Platonov[1,7]

Abstract

Background: Atrial fibrillation (AF) is a known risk factor for ischemic stroke. Electrocardiographic predictors of AF in population studies such as the Framingham Heart Study, as well as in hypertensive patients have demonstrated a predictive value of the P-wave duration for development of AF. QRS vector magnitude has had a predictive value in ventricular arrhythmia development. We aimed to assess the value of the three-dimensional P-wave vector magnitude and its relationship to P-wave duration for prediction of new-onset AF after ischemic stroke.

Methods: First-ever ischemic stroke patients without AF at inclusion in the Lund Stroke Register were included. Measurements of P wave duration (Pd), QRS duration, corrected QT interval, and PQ interval were performed automatically using the University of Glasgow 12-lead ECG analysis algorithm. The P-wave vector magnitude (Pvm) was calculated automatically as the square root of the sum of the squared P-wave magnitudes in leads V6, II and one half of the P-wave amplitude in V2 ($\sqrt{PV6^2 + PII^2 + (0.5*PV2)^2}$), based on the P-wave magnitude (Pvm) as defined by the visually transformed Kors' Quasi-orthogonal method.

Results: The median age was 73 (IQR 63–80) years at stroke onset (135 males, 92 females). Multivariate predictors of new-onset atrial fibrillation included age > 65 years, hypertension, and Pd/Pvm. A cut-off value of 870 ms/mV gave sensitivity, specificity, positive and negative predictive values of 51, 79, 30 and 87%, respectively. The Pd/Pvm was the only ECG predictor of AF with a significant multivariate hazard ratio of 2.02 (95% CI 1.18 to 3.46, $p = 0.010$).

Conclusion: P-wave dispersion as measured by the Pd/Pvm was the only ECG parameter measured which independently predicted subsequent AF identification in a cohort of stroke patients. Further prospective studies in larger cohorts are needed to validate its clinical usefulness.

Keywords: Atrial fibrillation, Ischemic stroke, P-wave vector magnitude, P-wave duration

Background

Atrial fibrillation (AF) is a known risk factor for ischemic stroke [1]. A high prevalence of AF is noted in ischemic stroke patients [1]. The impact of ischemic stroke on the risk of subsequent development of AF is only beginning to become clear [2, 3]. Information on development of new AF in ischemic stroke patients using ECG monitoring has been seldom reported until recently [4–6]. Clinical cardiovascular risk scoring tools such as the $CHADS_2$ and CHA_2DS_2-VASc have demonstrated association with development of first-ever AF during 2-year and 10-year follow-up time frames in recent studies [7–9].

Electrocardiographic predictors of AF in populations such as the Framingham Heart Study, as well as in hypertensive patients have demonstrated a predictive value of the p-wave duration for development of AF [10, 11]. This parameter, however, was not predictive in ischemic stroke patients during a 10-year follow-up [9]. However P-wave axis change has not been assessed nor has P-wave vector

---

* Correspondence: dr.danielcortez@gmail.com
†Equal contributors
[1]Department of Cardiology, Clinical Sciences, Lund University, Lund, Sweden
[2]Electrophysiology Department, Penn State Milton S. Hershey Medical Center, Hershey, USA
Full list of author information is available at the end of the article

magnitude in this population, as the P-wave axis normally corresponds to 60 degrees with similar variability in the frontal plane to the QRS axis with more variability in the transverse and sagittal planes [12]. In regards to voltage assessment, the P-wave terminal force in V_1 of >0.04 mm/s (PTFV1) has also not reliably been predictive of AF in this same population [8]. Recently, another P-wave time measure, the prolongation of the P-wave duration (Pd) >120 ms along with biphasic morphology in the inferior leads or in aVF and III along with notched p-wave in II, known as advanced inter-atrial block, has been shown to have predictive value for development of atrial fibrillation in ischemic stroke patients [13]. In a 10-year follow-up in ischemic stroke patients, the QRS duration (QRSd) has only had very modest results for predicting AF in ischemic stroke patients [8]. Thus, to date only one useful time-dependent independent 12-lead electrocardiographic predictor for AF in ischemic stroke patients has shown its value (advanced inter-atrial block), whereas no voltage-dependent measures have been tested.

Vectorcardiographic (VCG) principles (3-dimensional parameters, derived from a 12-lead electrocardiogram) have provided additional diagnostic [14, 15] and prognostic [16–20] information, building upon the traditional 12-lead ECG. Dispersion of ventricular depolarization, as measured by the QRS vector magnitude has had predictive value in ventricular arrhythmia development pre-operatively and peri-operatively in patients with congenital heart disease, independent of QRSd [21, 22]. Furthermore, a low P-wave amplitude in lead I is associated with displaced conduction and clinical recurrence of paroxysmal AF post-radiofrequency ablation [23]. A low 3-dimensional P-wave vector magnitude (Pvm), however, has not been assessed in any known cohorts based on the 12-lead ECG or otherwise. Also, this potentially useful tool, which gives the magnitude of the p-wave in 3-dimensional space has yet to be employed for the prediction of AF. Given the relationship between P-wave amplitude and ventricular depolarization duration, further assessment into time-duration and amplitude interrelationship is warranted. To date no relationship of atrial voltage to time duration have been assessed for prediction of AF. Furthermore, P-wave time duration per voltage assessment has therefore also not been assessed in predicting AF in ischemic stroke patients or otherwise.

We aimed to assess the value of the three-dimensional P-wave vector magnitude (Pvm) and its relationship to P-wave duration for prediction of new-onset AF after ischemic stroke.

Methods
Study cohort
The original study population originated from the Lund Stroke Register (LSR) and comprised 336 consecutive first-ever ischemic stroke patients included in LSR between March 1, 2001 and February 28, 2002 as it had been described previously [8]. At enrollment in the LSR, 109 ischemic stroke patients had AF detected by ECG screening, medical records review or record linkage with the Swedish National Patient Register as described previously [8] and were excluded from this analysis. All patients enrolled signed written consents. The present study sample therefore comprised of 227 first-ever ischemic stroke patients (median age 73 years at stroke onset (interquartile range 25–75% (IQR 63–80), 92 females) without known AF at inclusion in the LSR. We followed up all study subjects until October 17, 2011, the date when the information from the Swedish National Patient Register was obtained. Informed consent was obtained from all participants included in the LSR. The study was approved by the Lund University Ethics Committee.

Baseline ECG and clinical assessment
Medical records of all study subjects were analyzed for history of cardiac failure, hypertension, diabetes mellitus, transient ischemic attack (TIA) and ischemic heart disease at baseline. Cardiovascular risk profiles measured by $CHADS_2$ and CHA_2DS_2-VASc scales [8] were evaluated for the time of inclusion in the LSR in the acute phase when the index ischemic stroke had just occurred.

Sinus rhythm ECG recordings obtained at stroke admission with median time from stroke event to ECG registration 0 day (IQR 0–2 days) were extracted from the regional electronic database (GE MUSE, GE Healthcare, MegaCare) and processed offline. The measurements of Pd, QRSd, corrected QT interval (QTc), PQ interval were performed automatically using the University of Glasgow 12-lead ECG analysis algorithm [24]. The Pvm was calculated automatically as the square root of the sum of the squared P-wave magnitudes in leads V6, II and one half of the P-wave amplitude in V2 ($\sqrt{PV6^2 + PII^2 + (0.5^*PV2)^2}$), based on the P-wave magnitude as defined by the visually transformed Kors' Quasi-orthogonal method [25, 26]. Please see Figs. 1 and 2. The Pd/Pvm was defined as the Pduration/Pvm and was calculated from the data above automatically utilizing MATLAB R2013b (The MathWorks, Inc., Natick, MA, USA) for Linux.

P wave duration, QRS duration, corrected QT interval and PQ interval were measured in ms. Corrected QT was calculated using Bazett's formula: QTc = QT/√R-R interval. Pvm was calculated in microvolts. Negative P-wave terminal force in lead V_1 was also calculated as described previously [8].

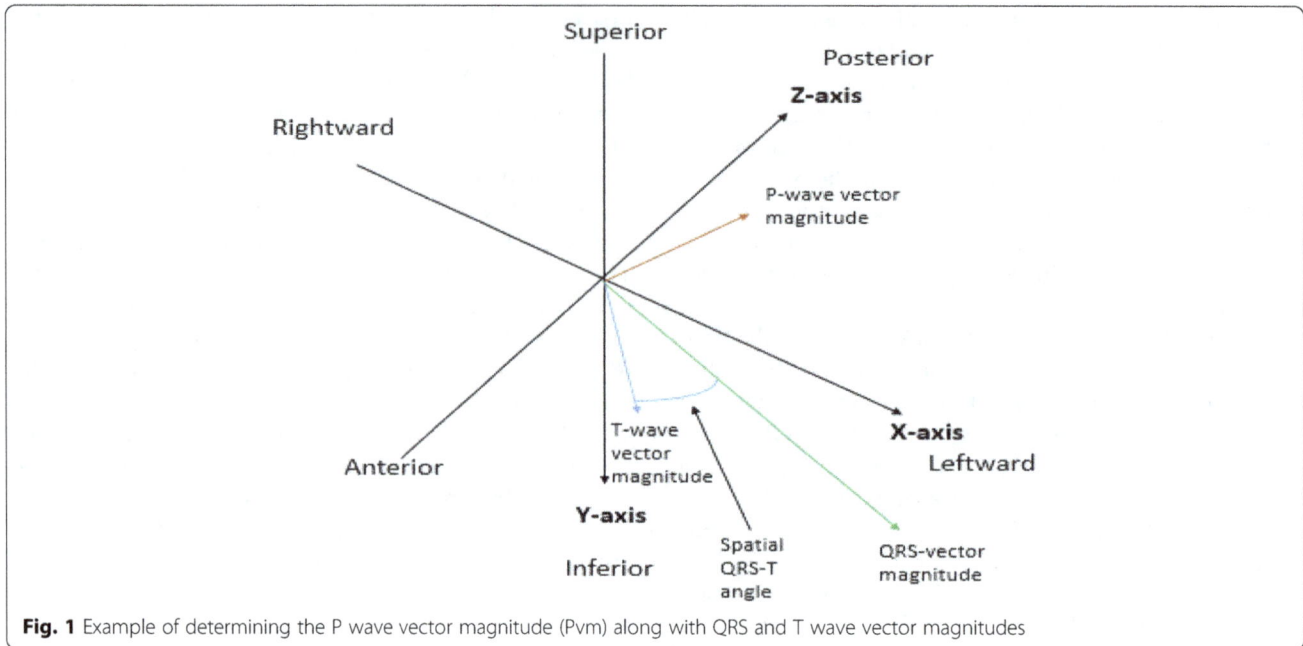

Fig. 1 Example of determining the P wave vector magnitude (Pvm) along with QRS and T wave vector magnitudes

Ascertainment of new-onset AF during follow-up

New onset AF was assessed during the follow-up period starting from the date of enrollment until the end of follow-up or date of death. AF documentation was based on information obtained from the regional electronic ECG archive which contains all ECG recordings taken in the hospital's local catchment area and also by linkage with national registers: the Swedish Patient Register and the Swedish Causes of Death Register. All available ECG recordings for all study subjects from the date of enrollment until the end of follow-up in 2011 were reviewed for the presence of AF by a trained cardiologist (MB). On surface ECG, AF was defined as a rhythm disorder which lasted sufficiently long for a 12-lead ECG to be recorded, with irregular RR intervals, indistinct P waves and atrial cycle length of 200 ms where distinct atrial activity was visible on surface ECG [27].

The Swedish Patient Register is administered by the Swedish National Board of Health and Welfare and includes data on main and secondary diagnoses at

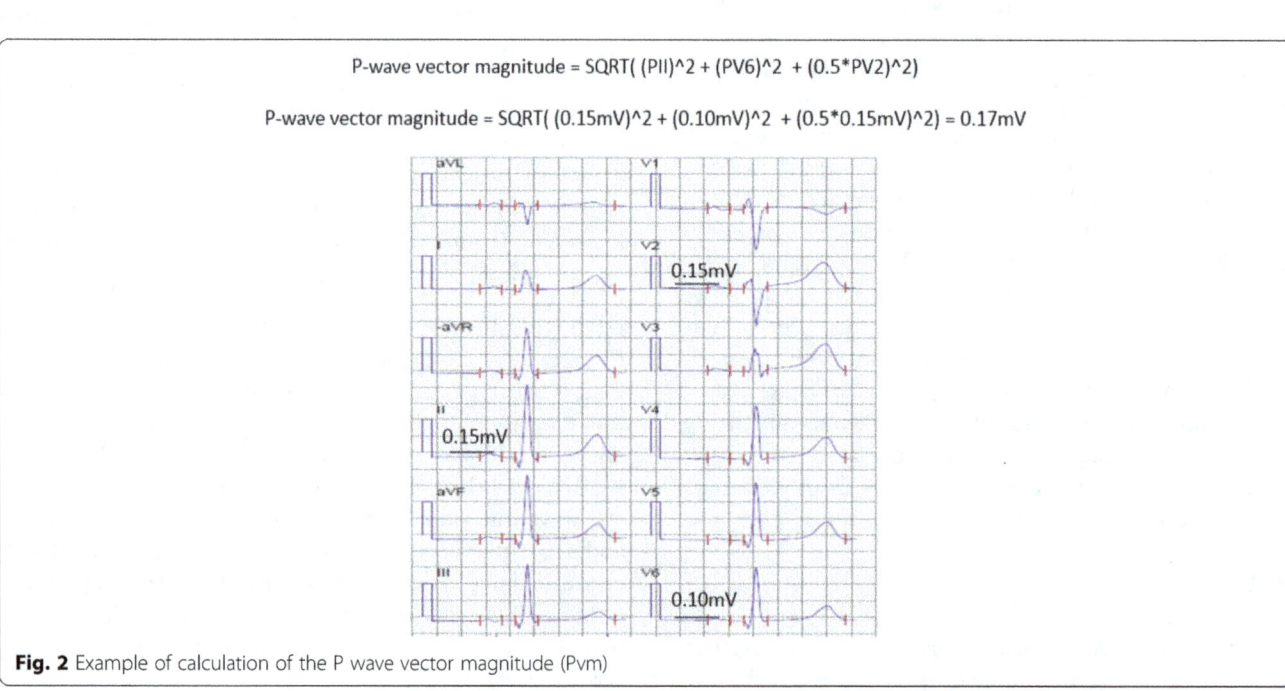

Fig. 2 Example of calculation of the P wave vector magnitude (Pvm)

discharge from all public hospitals in Sweden starting in 1987. The register uses International Classification of Disease (ICD) codes with the 10th edition (ICD-10) used from 1997 and until today. The Cause of Death Register is also provided by the Swedish National Board of Health and Welfare and contains information (since 1961) from death records, including underlying causes of death and up to 20 contributory causes of death coded to the current edition (ICD-10). The presence of the ICD-10 code I48 in the Swedish national registers identified AF diagnosis with high specificity and modest sensitivity as we showed recently in a validation study on patients with ischemic stroke enrolled in the LSR [2].

Statistical methods

Baseline clinical characteristics were compared between stroke patients who developed AF during follow-up and those who remained AF-free using chi-square or Fisher's exact test for categorical variables and Student's t-test versus Mann–Whitney U-testing, as appropriate, for continuous variables with an approximately normal distribution or alternatively non-parametric tests, as appropriate. Parametric data are presented as mean ± standard deviation, whereas non-parametric data are presented as median (interquartile range). For log linearity, each variable was categorized into quartiles where applicable and plotted to assess linearity of the quartiles. The primary outcome in this study was defined as occurrence of AF. Subjects who did not develop AF during the 10-year follow-up were censored at time of death or at end of follow-up.

Cox proportional hazard regression models were used to estimate the adjusted hazard ratios (HR) and their 95% confidence intervals (CI) of new onset AF associated with clinical and ECG covariates. Univariate Cox regression analyses were performed separately for each component of CHA_2DS_2-VASc score and for each ECG parameter. Clinical factors and ECG parameters significantly associated with new onset AF in the univariate analyses were included in a stepwise regression analysis with backward elimination. Our Cox model was adjusted for known significant clinical covariates (known to predispose to AF or known to have a relationship to the Pd/Pvm). The Kaplan-Meier product-limit method was used to generate a survival curve indicating new onset AF during 10-year follow-up after enrollment in LSR. A Kaplan-Meier curve was also used to demonstrate discernible differences at an optimum cut-off for the Pd/Pvm in identifying incidence of new-onset atrial fibrillation. Optimum cut-off was assessed by the receiver operating characteristic (ROC) curve. Cut-off p-values at 0.10 or less were used as entry cut-off values for multivariate analyses. P values of 0.05 were considered significant. All analyses were performed using SPSS Statistics 20 (SPSS Inc., Chicago, Illinois, USA). No reproducibility testing was performed given our fully automatic data processing.

Results

Baseline characteristics of all study subjects at time of enrollment are presented in Table 1. At baseline 227 were fulfilled inclusion criteria and were included in the analysis.

Table 1 Baseline clinical characteristics of stroke patients without or with subsequent development of atrial fibrillation

Parameter	Stroke (N=227)	No AF (n=188)	AF (n=39)	P-value
Age, years	73 [63 to 80]	73 [61 to 80]	73 [69 to 80]	0.072
Male sex (%)	135 (59%)	114 (61%)	21 (54%)	0.693
Heart Failure	7 (3%)	4 (2.1%)	3 (7.7%)	0.218
Hypertension (%)	130 (57%)	101 (53.7%)	29 (74.4%)	0.012
Diabetes (%)	35 (15%)	26 (13.8%)	9 (23.7%)	0.210
Vascular disease (%)	95 (42%)	77 (41.0%)	18 (46.2%)	0.560
TIA (%)	49 (22%)	45 (23.9%)	4 (10.3%)	<0.001
New-onset atrial fibrillation	39 (17%)	0 (0.0%)	39 (100.0%)	<0.001
Median time to AF onset/end follow-up	3.2 [1.3 to 5.9])	9.7 [4.3 to 10.1]	2.9 [1.2 to 6.4]	<0.001
P duration	116 [106 to 126]	116 [106 to 122]	118 [111 to 131]	0.224
QRSd	78 [68 to 90]	86 [78 to 94]	88 [75 to 99]	0.880
Pvm	0.16 [0.13 to 0.20]	0.16 [0.13 to 0.20]	0.13 [0.11 to 0.19]	0.006
P duration/Pvm	711 [560 to 893]	694 [547 to 862]	801 [586 to 1046]	0.009

Data presented as Median [Interquartile range]
All patients had no evidence of AF in the immediate acute phase after stroke onset
AF atrial fibrillation, *TIA* transient ischemic attack, *QRSd* QRS duration, *Pvm* P-wave vector magnitude

Detection of new onset atrial fibrillation (10-year follow-up)
The median time for follow-up was 9.4 years [IQR 6.1–9.9], 115 (51%) stroke patients died. Complete follow-up data were available for 112 (49%) of the stroke patients. In total, 2588 ECG's were reviewed with a median number of ECG recordings per person of four (IQR 1–9) [8]. New onset atrial fibrillation was found in 39 (17%) of the stroke patients (Hazard ratio 1.49, 95% confidence interval 0.09–2.35, p = 0.121) as previously reported [2, 8]. The median time to AF onset was 3.2 (IQR 1.3 to 5.9) years.

ECG and clinical predictors of new onset atrial fibrillation after ischemic stroke
On ECGs obtained in the acute phase after stroke onset, the median QRSd was 96 ms (IQR 88–108), the median duration of the P wave was 116 ms (IQR 106–124), and the median PQ interval was 169 ms (IQR 152–188). The median Pvm was 0.15 mV (IQR 0.13 to 0.20) and the median Pd/Pvm was 737 ms/mV (IQR 581 to 955).

Table 2 depicts univariate and multivariate predictors of new-onset atrial fibrillation in stroke patients. Significant univariate predictors of new-onset atrial fibrillation included age > 65 years, presence of hypertension, heart failure, QRSd, and Pd/Pvm (Table 2). No standard ECG characteristics including P-wave duration, QRS duration or negative P-wave terminal force in lead V1 or QRSd were significantly associated with new-onset AF during follow-up. Independent predictors of new-onset atrial fibrillation were instead Pvm/Pd and those parameters considered a moderator of Pvm/Pd including age > 65 years, hypertension, and heart failure (Table 2) [28]. The C-statistic for the model was 0.71 (95% CI 0.61 to 0.82).

The area under the ROC curve value for the Pd/Pvm was 0.63 (0.55 to 0.71, p = 0.013). At an optimal cut-off value of 870 ms/mV the sensitivity, specificity, positive and negative predictive values were 51, 79, 40 and 89%, respectively (optimized for highest negative predictive value given the ECG the screening value of the ECG). A Kaplan-Meier curve based on this cut-off value (Fig. 3) provided a p-value of <0.001 for differentiation between survival curves for the risk of development AF during 10-year follow-up after first-ever ischemic stroke. Sub-analyses of patients who do not meet any of the independent predictors (ie. without hypertension, who were less than 65 years of age, did not have heart failure and had a Pd/Pvm of less than 870 ms/mV), did had a 93.2% chance of not developing atrial fibrillation. The positive predictive value for development of AF was 27.9% in a patient without hypertension, who were less than 65 years of age and did not have heart failure, but with a Pd/Pvm of less than 870 ms/mV.

Discussion
Our study demonstrates that a measure of P-wave dispersion by duration and voltage assessment from the standard 12-lead ECG, taken during hospital admission for ischemic stroke, in the form of Pd/Pvm can predict new-onset AF during follow-up while neither P-wave duration nor P-wave terminal force in lead V_1 were significantly associated with subsequent AF occurrence. The relation of Pd/Pvm to new-onset AF remained independent after adjustment for other clinical parameters.

Presence of AF
As previously reported, by the end of the 10-year follow-up AF was detected in 15% of our initially AF-free

Table 2 Clinical electrocardiographic predictors of new-onset atrial fibrillation during 10-year follow-up of ischemic stroke patients without known atrial fibrillation at their index stroke

Univariate Cox regression analysis			Multivariate Cox regression analysis	
Parameter	Hazard ratio (95% CI)	P-value	Hazard ratio (95% CI)	P-value
Age > 65 years	2.88 (1.20 to 6.89)	0.018	1.04 (1.02 to 1.07)	0.001
Hypertension	3.45 (1.40 to 3.49)	0.007	3.21 (1.35 to 7.67)	0.008
Heart failure	4.04 (1.24–13.18)	0.020	2.72 (1.08 to 6.83)	0.033
Diabetes	1.83 (0.87 to 3.87)	0.111		
Male gender	1.22 (0.50 to 1.59)	0.459		
Stroke group	1.391 (0.855 to 2.263)	0.184		
P duration	1.02 (0.96 to 1.05)	0.105		
QRS duration	1.02 (1.00 to 1.04)	0.025	1.01 (1.00 to 1.02)	0.354
PQ interval	1.00 (0.99 to 1.01)	0.966		
Pvm	1.001 (0.994 to 1.009)	0.751		
P duration/Pvm	2.320 (1.367 to 3.938)	0.002	2.02 (1.18 to 3.46)	0.010
P terminal force V1	1.00 (95% CI 1.00–1.00)	0.142		

Pvm p-wave vector magnitude, *95% CI* 95% confidence interval

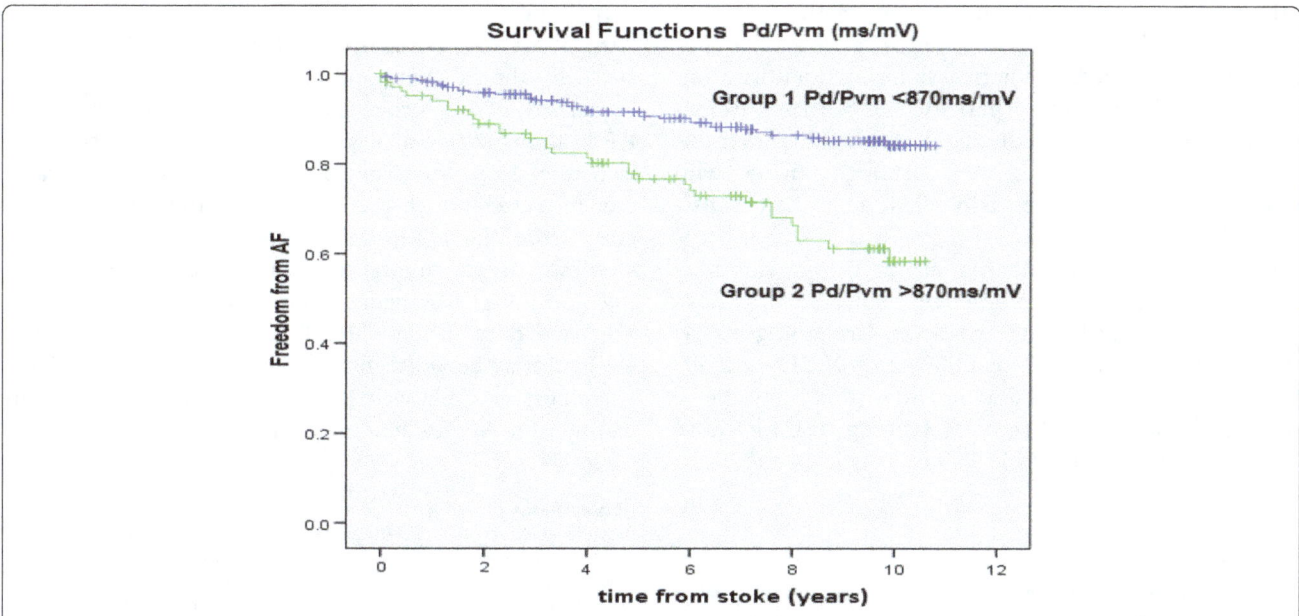

Fig. 3 Kaplan-Meijer survival curve from stroke onset to atrial fibrillation detection for p wave duration/p-wave vector magnitude (Pd/Pvm) at a cut-off of 870 milliseconds/millivolt (ms/mV), log rank p-value <0.001

subjects, which corresponds to the reported AF incidence for an aging population of 18% in those older than 85 years by the end of a 7-year follow-up and 17% of those 65–74 years by the end of a 6-year follow-up [9, 29]. Compared with studies based on only ECG screening, studies that employed implantable devices generally have shown higher AF detection rates - of up to 28–30% in patients with ischemic stroke or TIA, as well as in those with risk factors for ischemic stroke [30–32].

Clinical parameters

We previously reported that in the same cohort age > 65 years, presence of hypertension or heart failure showed a univariate as well as multivariate predictive relation to subsequent AF onset during a 10-year follow-up period [8]. Clinical parameters we found significant in previous analyses were used in the Cox modeling in the current analysis [8, 28].

P-wave duration divided by 3-dimensional p-wave vector magnitude (Pd/Pvm)

Previous literature mostly has focused on P-wave duration as a predictive tool for new-onset atrial fibrillation with some success in non-ischemic stroke populations [10, 11]. Although in the subgroup of those <60 years of age, the overall P-wave duration yielded a non-significant HR (1.15, 95% CI 0.90 to 1.47). It has also been shown that maximum P wave duration at the upper fifth percentile was associated with long-term AF risk in an elderly community-based cohort [11]. In hypertensive patients the P-wave duration independently

predicted the development of new-onset atrial fibrillation [11]. However, in a recent publication of our cohort, no significant predictive value was found for the P-wave duration as a predictor for new-onset AF [8]. In another study, prolonged P-wave duration and advanced interatrial block in particular have shown an association with AF [13]. Furthermore, PTFV1 was not found to be a reproducibly significant predictor of AF [9]. In patients with recurrent atrial fibrillation after catheter ablation, low voltage in lead I (<0.01 mV) was associated with recurrence of AF [21]. Our results demonstrate that atrial voltage dispersion, as measured by Pvm is not in itself alone associated with the development of AF. However, our study is the first to show that atrial time duration versus voltage dispersion (Pd/Pvm) is a potentially clinically useful predictive measure which can be obtained by the ECG alone. Pvm has also shown predictive value for atrial arrhythmias in patients with congenital heart disease, and in particular tetralogy of Fallot patients undergoing pulmonary valve replacements [28]. In this same study Pvm inversely correlated with higher right atrial pressure, left and right ventricular ejection fractions, QRSd, and older age [28]. In the above publication Pvm was predictive of organized right atrial arrhythmias (intra-atrial re-entrant tachycardia and typical flutter), thus in the more disorganized left atrial arrhythmia (AF), it appears time dispersion across the left atrium must also be taken into account. A risk score based on the above parameters might be helpful in ruling out those at risk for atrial fibrillation, and furthermore can be automatically calculated, however further reproducibility with other ECG systems and automated methods would be required. Our study also demonstrated a high specificity and negative predictive value for identification of AF in ischemic stroke patients but with low sensitivity and positive predictive values. This demonstrates that in our cohort although those who develop AF cannot necessarily all be identified (sensitivity 51%) and the value of a Pd/Pvm > 870 ms/mV does not necessarily identify all of those who may develop AF (positive predictive value 30%). Those who do not develop AF, however, are going to be those who have a Pd/Pvm <870 ms/mV. Thus if effectively reproduced independently, this may be a reasonable and cost-effective screening test for those at risk for developing AF.

Limitations

This study was retrospective and did not use a prespecified AF screening protocol, thus the number of ECG's available during follow-up analysis was lower in subjects without detected AF. This may represent an underestimation of AF in patients with asymptomatic AF, given their lack of need to contact health care providers. Also, the ECG search utilized in this study was limited to Southern Sweden's Skania region, thus other ECG's possibly performed outside of the Skania region were unavailable for review. Therefore, if a patient was mobile and sought healthcare elsewhere, these ECG's would not be included. Other prolonged data monitoring such as via implantable devices (e.g. loop recorders) were not available for data analysis. Our data was, however obtained via linkage with the Swedish Patient Register, which for each specific treatment occasion contains up to 20 contributory diagnoses per patient, suggesting that if observed, AF would have been registered in the Patient register. Also, during a 10-year follow-up after stroke a number of confounders such as inability to detect all episodes of AF and lack of reported events such as transient ischemic attacks or other parameters in the CHA_2DS_2-VASc score calculation as well as degree of heart failure, which may not have been taken into account. This is also inherently a limitation of Registry data along with lack of atrial size/volume data, which have been shown to be predictors of atrial fibrillation [32, 33]. Furthermore, the Cox model assumes constant effect over time, which may not be complete accurate for every single parameter. Our results need to be viewed in light of these possible confounders. Also the analysis was a post-hoc analysis performed on a prospectively this prospectively enrolled cohort, thus limitations exist regarding assessment of Pd/Pvm compared to other parameters.

Conclusion

Atrial time dispersion over voltage magnitude, as measured by the Pd/Pvm, appears to have some usefulness in risk stratifying stroke patients for risk of subsequent AF in the post-hoc analysis of an observational study on ischemic stroke survivors. It was the only ECG parameter measured which predicted new-onset AF independently from the clinical covariates. Further prospective studies in larger cohorts, including investigation regarding non-invasive imaging parameter directly compared, are needed to validate its clinical usefulness, however, Pd/Pvm may be worth further investigation for potential usefulness as a relatively simple and easily available clinical tool for AF prediction after ischemic stroke.

Abbreviations

AF: Atrial fibrillation; ECG: Electrocardiogram; ICD: Internal cardiac defibrillator; LSR: Lund Stroke Register; ms: millisecond; mV: millivolt; Pd: P-wave duration (milliseconds); PTFV1: P-wave terminal force in V_1 of >0.04 mm/s; Pvm: P-wave vector magnitude (millivolts); QRSd: QRS duration; ROC: Receiver operating characteristic curve; TIA: Transient ischemic attack

Acknowledgements

Not applicable.

Funding

This work was supported by the Swedish National Health Service, Donation funds at Skåne University Hospital, Lund, Sweden, the Swedish Heart-Lung Foundation (20140734), the Swedish Research Council (K2010-61X-20,378-04-3), Region Skåne, the Freemasons Lodge of Instruction EOS in Lund, King Gustaf V and Queen Victoria's Foundation, Lund University, Sparbanksstiftelsen Färs & Frosta, the Swedish Stroke Association, and the Swedish Institute.

Authors' contributions

DC made substantial contributions to data conception, design, analysis and interpretation; he wrote the manuscript. MB was responsible for the data collection, and was thoroughly involved in drafting the manuscript. JC was responsible for the data, analysis and interpretation; he was involved in drafting the manuscript. AL made substantial contributions to conception, design, analysis and interpretation of data; was responsible for manuscript revision. YS was responsible for manuscript revision. BO made substantial contributions to conception, design, and manuscript revision. PP made substantial contributions to conception, design, data acquisition, analysis and interpretation; he was involved in drafting and revising the manuscript; agreed to be accountable for all aspects of work in ensuring that any questions related to accuracy or integrity are appropriately investigated and resolved. All authors read and approved the final manuscript.

Competing interests

The authors declare that they have no competing interests.

Author details

[1]Department of Cardiology, Clinical Sciences, Lund University, Lund, Sweden. [2]Electrophysiology Department, Penn State Milton S. Hershey Medical Center, Hershey, USA. [3]St. Petersburg University Clinic, St. Petersburg, Russia. [4]Cardiology Research, Clinical and Educational Center, St. Petersburg State University, St. Petersburg, Russia. [5]Department of Neurology and Rehabilitation Medicine, Skane University Hospital, Lund, Sweden. [6]Department of Clinical Sciences Lund, Neurology, Lund University, Lund, Sweden. [7]Arrhythmia Clinic, Skåne University Hospital, Lund, Sweden.

References

1. Friberg L, Hammar N, Pettersson H, Rosenqvist M. Increased mortality in paroxysmal atrial fibrillation: report from the Stockholm cohort-study of atrial fibrillation (SCAF). Eur Heart J. 2007;28:2346–53.

2. Baturova MA, Lindgren A, Shubik YV, Olsson SB, Platonov PG. Atrial fibrillation in patients with ischaemic stroke in the Swedish national patient registers: how much do we miss? Europace. 2014;16:1714–9.

3. Sanna T, Diener HC, Passman RS, Di Lazzaro V, Berstein RA, Morillo CA, et al. Cryptogenic stroke and underlying atrial fibrillation. N Engl J Med. 2014;370: 2478–86.

4. Jabaudon D, Sztajzel J, Sievert K, Landis T, Sztajzel R. Usefulness of ambulatory 7-day ECG monitoring for the detection of atrial fibrillation and flutter after acute stroke and transient ischemic attack. Stroke. 2004;35(7): 1647–51.

5. Stahrenberg R, Weber-Kruger M, Seegers J, Edelmann F, Lahno R, Haase B, et al. Enhanced detection of paroxysmal atrial fibrillation by early and prolonged continuous Holter monitoring in patients with cerebral ischemia presenting in sinus rhythm. Stroke. 2010;41:2884–8.

6. Brachmann J, Morillo CA, Sanna T, Di Lazzaro V, Diener HC, Bernstein RA, et al. Uncovering atrial fibrillation beyond short-term monitoring in cryptogenic stroke patients: three-year results from the cryptogenic stroke and underlying atrial fibrillation trial. Circ Arrhythm Electrophysiol. 2016;9:1.

7. Henriksson KM, Farahmand B, Asberg S, Terent A, Edvardsson N. First-ever atrial fibrillation documented after hemorrhagic or ischemic stroke: the role of the CHADS(2) score at the time of stroke. Clin Cardiol. 2011;34:309–16.

8. Baturova MA, Lindgren A, Calrson J, Shubik YV, Olsson SB, Platonov PG. Predictors of new onset atrial fibrillation during 10-year follow-up after first-ever ischemic stroke. Int J Cardiol. 2015;199:248–52.

9. Zuo ML, Liu S, Chan KH, Lau KK, Chong BH, Lam KF, et al. The CHADS2 and CHA2DS2-VASc scores predict new occurrence of atrial fibrillation and ischemic stroke. J Interv Card Electrophysiol. 2013;37:47–54.

10. Magnani JW, Johnson VM, Sullivan LM, Gorodeski EZ, Schnabel RB, Lubitz SA, et al. Wave duration and risk of longitudinal atrial fibrillation in persons ≥ 60 years old (from the Framingham heart study). Am J Cardiol. 2011;107: 917–21.

11. Ciaroni S, Cuenoud L, Bloch A. Clinical study to investigate the predictive parameters for the onset of atrial fibrillation in patients with essential hypertension. Am Heart J. 2000;139:814–9.

12. Bonow RO, Mann DL, Zipes DP, Libby P. Braunwald's heart disease. A textbook of cardiovascular medicine. 9th ed. New York: W.B. Saunders Company; 2011.

13. Martinez-Selles M, Baranchuk A, Elosua R, Bayes de Luna A, O'Neal WT, Kamel H, et al. Advanced interatrial block and ischemic stroke: the atherosclerosis risk in communities study. Neurology. 2016;87:352–6.

14. Triola B, Olson MB, Reis SE, Rautaharju P, Merz CN, Kelsey SF, et al. Electrocardiographic predictors of cardiovascular outcome in women: the National Heart, Lung, and Blood Institute-sponsored women's ischemia syndrome evaluation (WISE) study. J Am Coll Cardiol. 2005;46:51–6.

15. Voulgari C, Tentolouris N, Moyssakis I, Dilaveris P, Gialafos E, Papadogiannis D, et al. Spatial QRS-T angle: association with diabetes and left ventricular performance. Eur J Clin Investig. 2006;36:608–13.

16. Borleffs CJ, Scherptong RW, Man SC, van Welsenes GH, Bax JJ, van Erven L, et al. Predicting ventricular arrhythmias in patients with ischemic heart disease: clinical application of the ECG-derived QRS-T angle. Circ Arrhythm Electrophysiol. 2009;2:548–54.

17. de Torbal A, Kors JA, van Herpen G, Meij S, Nelwan S, Simoons ML, et al. The electrical T-axis and the spatial QRS-T angle are independent predictors of long-term mortality in patients admitted with acute ischemic chest pain. Cardiology. 2004;101:199–207.

18. Kardys I, Kors JA, van der Meer IM, Hofman A, van der Kuip DA, Witteman JC. Spatial QRS-T angle predicts cardiac death in a general population. Eur Heart J. 2003;24:1357–64.

19. Rautaharju PM, Ge S, Nelson JC, Marino Larsen EK, Psaty BM, Furberg CD, Zhang ZM, et al. Comparison of mortality risk for electrocardiographic abnormalities in men and women with and without coronary heart disease (from the cardiovascular health study). Am J Cardiol. 2006;97:309–15.

20. Yamazaki T, Froelicher VF, Myers J, Chun S, Wang P. Spatial QRS-T angle predicts cardiac death in a clinical population. Heart Rhythm. 2005;2:73–8.

21. Cortez D, Ruckdeschel E, McCanta A, Collins K, Sauer W, Kay J, et al. Vectorcardiographic predictors of ventricular arrhythmia inducibility in patients with tetralogy of Fallot. J Electrocardiol. 2015;48:141–4.

22. Cortez D, Barham W, Ruckdeschel E, Sharma N, McCanta AC, von Alvensleben J, et al. Non-invasive predictors of ventricular arrhythmias in patients with tetralogy of Fallot undergoing pulmonary valve replacement. JACC Electrophys. 2017;3:162–70.

23. Park J-K, Park J, Uhm J-S, Joung B, Lee M-H, Pak H-N. Low P-wave amplitude (<0.1mV) in lead I is associated with displaced inter-atrial conduction and clinical recurrence of paroxysmal atrial fibrillation after radiofrequency catheter ablation. Europace. 2016;18:384–91.

24. Macfarlane PW, Devine B, Clark E. The University of Glasgow (Uni-G) ECG analysis program. Comput Cardiol. 2005;32:451–4.

25. Kors JA, van Herpen G, Sitig AC, van Bemmel JH. Reconstruction of the Frank vectorcardiogram from standard electrocardiographic leads. Eur Heart J. 1990; 11:1083–92.

26. Cortez D, Sharma N, Devers C, Devers E, Schlegel TT. Visual transform applications for estimating the spatial QRS-T angle from the conventional 12-lead ECG: Kors is still most frank. J Electrocardiol. 2014;47:12–9.

27. Camm AJ, Kirchhof P, Lip GY, Schotten U, Savelieva I, Ernst S, et al. Guidelines for the Management of Atrial Fibrillation: the task force for the management of Atrial fibrillation of the European Society of Cardiology (ESC). Eur Heart J. 2010;31:2369–429.

28. Cortez D, Barham W, Ruckdeschel E, Sharma N, McCanta AC, von Alvensleben J, et al. Noninvasive predictors of perioperative atrial arrhythmias in patients with tetralogy of Fallot undergoing pulmonary valve replacement. Clin Cardiol. 2017; [Epub ahead of print]

29. Heeringa J, van der Kuip DA, Hofman A, Kors JA, van Herpen G, Stricker BH, et al. Prevalence, incidence and lifetime risk of atrial fibrillation: the Rotterdam study. Eur Heart J. 2006;27(8):949–53.

30. Ziegler PD, Glotzer TV, Daoud EG, Wyse DG, Singer DE, Ezekowitz MD, et al. Incidence of newly detected atrial arrhythmias via implantable devices in patients with history of thromboembolic events. Stroke. 2010;41:256–60.

31. Ziegler PD, Glotzer TV, Daoud EG, Singer MD, Ezekowitz MD, Hoyt RH, et al. Detection of previously undiagnosed atrial fibrillation in patients with stroke risk factors and usefulness of continuous monitoring in primary stroke prevention. Am J Cardiol. 2012;110:1309–14.

32. Kim D, Shim CY, Cho IJ, Kim YD, Nam HS, Chang HJ, et al. Incremental value of left atrial global longitudinal strain for prediction of post stroke atrial fibrillation in patients with acute ischemic stroke. J Cardiovasc Ultrasound. 2016;24:20–7.

33. Baturova MA, Sheldon SH, Carlson J, Brady PA, Lin G, Rabinstein AA, et al. Electrocardiographic and echocardiographic predictors of paroxysmal atrial fibrillation detected after ischemic stroke. BMC Cardiovasc Disord. 2016;16:209.

10

Incidence and timing of potentially high-risk arrhythmias detected through long term continuous ambulatory electrocardiographic monitoring

Matthew D. Solomon[1,2,5*], Jingrong Yang[1], Sue Hee Sung[1], Martha L. Livingston[3], George Sarlas[3], Judith C. Lenane[3] and Alan S. Go[1,2,4]

Abstract

Background: Ambulatory electrocardiographic (ECG) monitoring is the standard to screen for high-risk arrhythmias. We evaluated the clinical utility of a novel, leadless electrode, single-patient-use ECG monitor that stores up to 14 days of a continuous recording to measure the burden and timing of potentially high-risk arrhythmias.

Methods: We examined data from 122,815 long term continuous ambulatory monitors (iRhythm ZIO® Service, San Francisco) prescribed from 2011 to 2013 and categorized potentially high-risk arrhythmias into two types: (1) ventricular arrhythmias including non-sustained and sustained ventricular tachycardia and (2) bradyarrhythmias including sinus pauses >3 s, atrial fibrillation pauses >5 s, and high-grade heart block (Mobitz Type II or third-degree heart block).

Results: Of 122,815 ZIO® recordings, median wear time was 9.9 (IQR 6.8–13.8) days and median analyzable time was 9.1 (IQR 6.4–13.1) days. There were 22,443 (18.3 %) with at least one episode of non-sustained ventricular tachycardia (NSVT), 238 (0.2 %) with sustained VT, 1766 (1.4 %) with a sinus pause >3 s (SP), 520 (0.4 %) with a pause during atrial fibrillation >5 s (AFP), and 1486 (1.2 %) with high-grade heart block (HGHB). Median time to first arrhythmia was 74 h (IQR 26–149 h) for NSVT, 22 h (IQR 5–73 h) for sustained VT, 22 h (IQR 7–64 h) for SP, 31 h (IQR 11–82 h) for AFP, and 40 h (SD 10–118 h) for HGHB.

Conclusions: A significant percentage of potentially high-risk arrhythmias are not identified within 48-h of ambulatory ECG monitoring. Longer-term continuous ambulatory ECG monitoring provides incremental detection of these potentially clinically relevant arrhythmic events.

Keywords: Arrhythmia, Ambulatory monitoring, Diagnostic testing, Electrocardiography

Background

Ambulatory electrocardiographic (ECG) monitoring is the standard of care to screen symptomatic outpatient adults for high-risk ventricular and atrial arrhythmias [1–3]. However, there is marked variation in the technological features and patient compliance among different ECG monitoring systems [4, 5]. Traditional 24-h monitoring devices (i.e., Holter monitors) often do not detect symptomatic or clinically meaningful arrhythmias [6, 7].

Recent technological advances have allowed for higher fidelity recording and larger storage capacities that are able to capture full disclosure ECG recordings beyond the traditional 24- or 48-h monitoring periods. Furthermore, innovative device designs aim to increase patient convenience and patient compliance. Emerging evidence suggests that longer wear times yield greater arrhythmia detection in selected at-risk patients that could impact clinical decision-making and outcomes [8]. Although there has been very limited evaluation of this approach outside of detecting the presence of atrial fibrillation, longer monitoring periods are emerging as a new standard of care for selected patients.

* Correspondence: matthew.d.solomon@kp.org
[1]Division of Research, Kaiser Permanente Northern California, Oakland, CA, USA
[2]Stanford University School of Medicine, Stanford, CA, USA
Full list of author information is available at the end of the article

To understand the applicability in day-to-day clinical practice, we evaluated contemporary results from a novel, long-term ambulatory ECG monitoring system to measure the burden and timing of potentially high-risk arrhythmias, including ventricular tachycardia, high-grade heart block and clinically significant pauses in atrioventricular conduction.

Methods

Data and study population

We analyzed data for all the ZIO® Service long-term continuous ambulatory ECG monitors (ZIO® Service, iRhythm Technologies, Inc., San Francisco, California) that were prescribed from November 2011 to December 2013 (N = 128,401). The ZIO® Patch is a lightweight, lead-wire free, single-patient-use ECG monitor that adheres to the left upper chest and records and stores up to 14 days of continuous, beat-to-beat ECG. Patients have the option of pressing a trigger button on the device and filling out a log to document symptomatic events during their wear duration, which allows for symptom-rhythm correlation in the ECG report. After a patient completes their 14-day recording, the ZIO® Patch is removed from the chest and mailed to iRhythm Technologies, Inc., where the up to 14-day single-channel recording is analyzed using a combination of proprietary algorithms and review by Certified Cardiac Technicians (CCT). The findings are then reported to the ordering physician in a report that includes information on several standard arrhythmias, including atrial fibrillation and flutter, ventricular tachycardia, supraventricular tachycardia, atrioventricular pauses, heart block, atrial and ventricular ectopic beats, and other identified arrhythmias. All components of the device are recycled after data downloading. Further details on the ZIO® Service and its analytic algorithms have been described previously [5, 9].

We applied standard quality control techniques to assemble a cleaned, analytic dataset of basic patient information and detailed information on detected arrhythmias. This included removing outliers that contained likely erroneous data, including records with heart rates >300 beats or <20 per minute, along with excluding patients <18 years old, records with start times outside our study dates, and records with wear-time or analyzable-time of less than 24 h. Analyzable time was calculated as the amount of time that the ECG patch was recording (enrollment period) minus the amount of time of unanalyzable ECG signal due to artifact.

Outcomes

We categorized potentially high-risk arrhythmias into two types: (1) ventricular arrhythmias, including nonsustained and sustained ventricular tachycardia; and (2) bradyarrhythmias including sinus pauses >3 s, atrial fibrillation pauses >5 s, and high grade heart block including Mobitz Type II or third-degree heart block. Sustained ventricular tachycardia (VT) included VT that lasted greater than 30 s. Mobitz II heart block and third degree heart block were identified by the manufacturer according to their FDA-cleared algorithms and 100 % data curation and quality review by CCT's trained in advanced arrhythmia detection. Symptomatic pauses were defined as a pause (greater than 3 s for sinus rhythm and greater than 5 s for those in atrial fibrillation) that occurred within 45 s of a patient trigger.

Statistical analysis

All analyses were performed at the Kaiser Permanente Northern California Division of Research using SAS statistical software, version 9.3 (Cary, N.C.). Continuous variables were reported as means with standard deviations and categorical variables as frequencies and proportions. We calculated the proportion and associated 95 % confidence interval of patients with each arrhythmia overall and the cumulative yield per additional day of monitoring. We used chi-squared tests to compare the proportion of high-risk arrhythmias detected at 1-, 2-, and 7-days versus 14-days.

A research exemption was obtained from the institutional review board of the Kaiser Foundation Research Institute given that the analyses were completed on a fully de-identified dataset provided by iRhythm Technologies, Inc, and therefore no formal ethics approval was required for this study.

Results

Study sample and distribution of wear and analyzable time

During the study period, we identified 122,815 eligible ZIO® Patch records contributed by 122,454 unique patients (Fig. 1). The overall mean wear time was 9.6 ± 4.0 days, and more than 25 % of the recorders were worn for at least 13.8 days. Analyzable time was similar, with 25 % of recorders containing greater than 13 days of analyzable time.

Cumulative detection of potentially high-risk arrhythmias

Of the 122,815 eligible records, there were 22,443 (18 %) with nonsustained VT, 238 (0.2 %) with sustained VT, 1766 (1.4 %) with sinus pauses >3 s, 521 (0.4 %) with AF pauses >5 s, 249 (0.2 %) with symptomatic pauses and 1468 (0.4 %) with high-grade heart block (Table 1). Overall, ventricular arrhythmias were more prevalent than bradyarrhythmias, although this was driven by the large burden of episodes of nonsustained VT.

More than half (53 %) of the recorders were worn by women; but for nearly all arrhythmias except symptomatic pauses, there were more detected arrhythmias

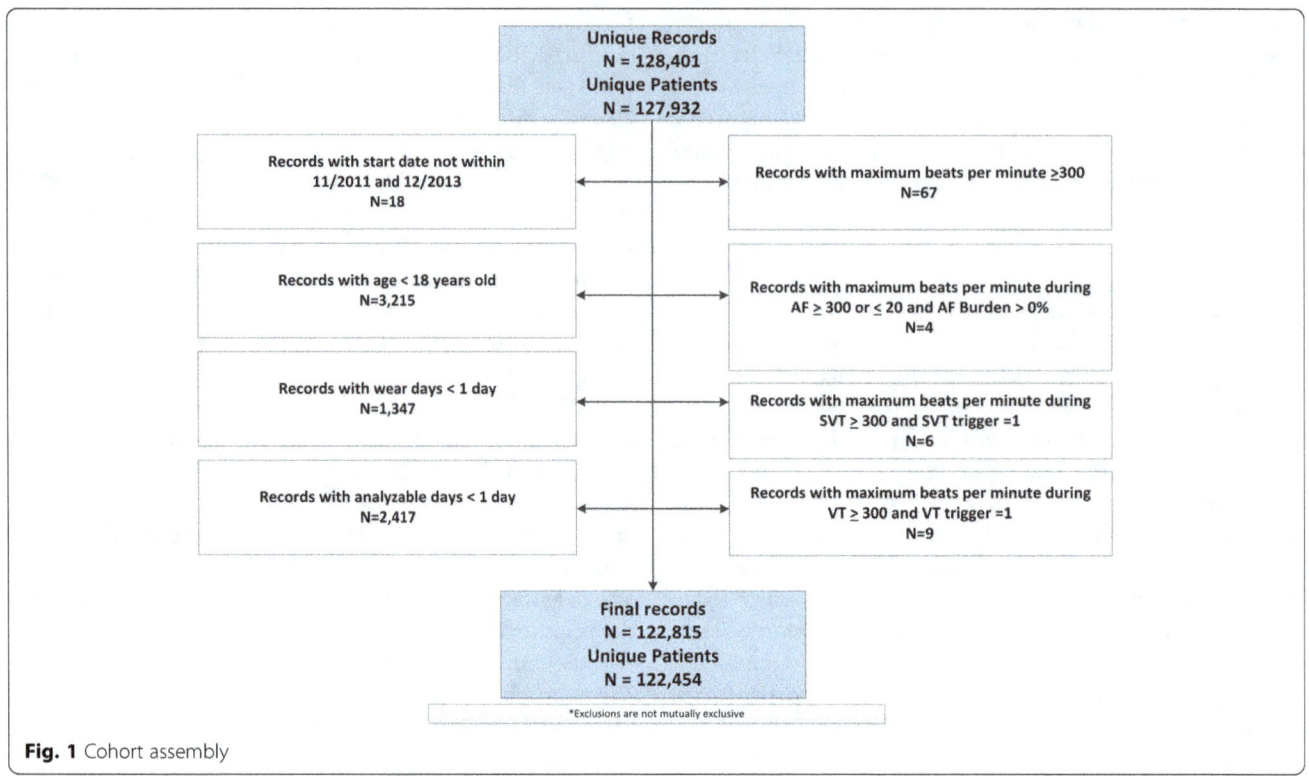

Fig. 1 Cohort assembly

among men than women. Although nearly half (49.8 %) of the analyzed patients were for patients aged less than 65 years old, the majority of all detected arrhythmias were among patients aged 65 years or older.

Timing of detection of potentially high-risk arrhythmias
For the detection of ventricular arrhythmias, there was a marked increase in arrhythmia detection over the course of the 14-day monitors (Fig. 2). For sustained VT, only

52.5 % of the total identified arrhythmias were identified at 24 h, and approximately two-thirds (65.5 %) were identified by 48 h. Most arrhythmias were identified by 7 days (92.9 %), but the additional 7 days of monitoring between 7 and 14 days yielded an additional 7.1 % of these potentially lethal arrhythmias. A similar trend was seen for the more common non-sustained VT, with 23.4, 38.0, and 79.4 % of all non-sustained VT being identified by 1, 2, and 7 days respectively. These trends were

Table 1 Characteristics of 122,815 eligible continuous ambulatory ECG monitoring records between November 2011 and December 2013

Characteristics	Overall	Non-sustained ventricular tachycardia	Sustained ventricular tachycardia	Sinus pause	Atrial fibrillation pause	Symptomatic pause	High-grade heart block[a]
	$N = 122,815$	$N = 22,443$	$N = 238$	$N = 1,766$	$N = 521$	$N = 249$	$N = 1,468$
Age, years, N (%)							
< 65	61,170 (49.8)	7,787 (34.7)	102 (42.9)	497 (28.1)	88 (16.9)	60 (24.1)	481 (32.8)
65–79	42,469 (34.6)	9,596 (42.8)	102 (42.9)	735 (41.6)	272 (52.2)	133 (53.4)	582 (39.7)
≥ 80	19,176 (15.6)	5,060 (22.6)	34 (14.3)	534 (30.2)	161 (30.9)	56 (22.5)	405 (27.6)
Women, N (%)	65,081 (53.0)	8,316 (37.1)	59 (24.8)	698 (39.5)	238 (45.7)	131 (52.6)	571 (38.9)
Wear Days							
Mean (Standard Deviation)	9.6 (4.0)	10.8 (3.5)	10.7 (3.4)	10.7 (3.7)	11.1 (3.4)	10.9 (3.5)	10.4 (3.7)
Median (IQR)	9.9 (6.8–13.8)	12.9 (7.1–13.9)	12.1 (7.1–13.9)	12.9 (7.0–14.0)	13.0 (7.3–14.0)	12.9 (7.1–14.0)	12.1 (7.0–13.9)
Analyzable Days							
Mean (Standard Deviation)	9.2 (3.9)	10.4 (3.5)	10.1 (3.4)	10.2 (3.7)	10.5 (3.3)	10.3 (3.4)	9.9 (3.7)
Median (IQR)	9.1 (6.4–13.1)	11.8 (7.0–13.6)	11.3 (6.9–13.4)	11.8 (6.9–13.6)	12.1 (7.1–13.6)	11.7 (7.0–13.5)	10.9 (6.8–13.5)

[a]Included Mobitz II heart block and third-degree heart block

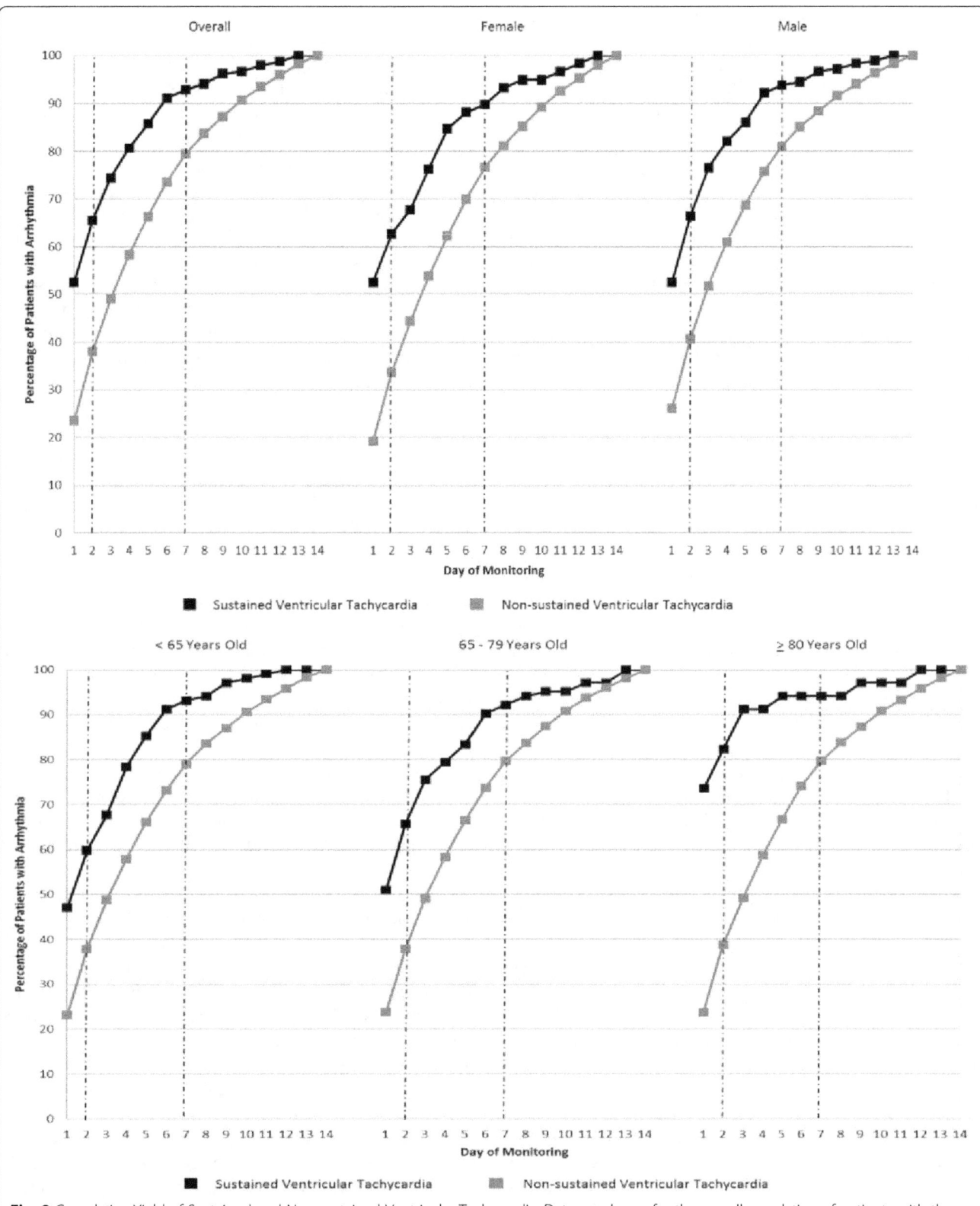

Fig. 2 Cumulative Yield of Sustained and Non-sustained Ventricular Tachycardia. Data are shown for the overall population of patients with the arrhythmia and stratified by age and gender

similar for both men and women and across all age ranges, although sustained VT was detected earlier among very elderly patients (aged 80 years and older).

The detection of potentially high risk bradyarrhythmias was similarly enhanced with longer monitoring periods (Fig. 3). The difference in bradyarrhythmia yield between 1-, 2- and 7-days was substantial. For the most common bradyarrhythmia, sinus pauses >3 s ($N = 1766$), 31.7 % of the total detected arrhythmias were found within 1 day, 46.6 % within 2 days, and 83.1 % within 3 days of monitoring. Similar trends were observed for the other bradyarrhythmias, and these trends were consistent for both genders and across age categories. The diagnostic yields at 2 days versus 7 days for ventricular arrhythmias and bradyarrhythmias were significantly different from each other in the overall populations ($P < 0.01$).

Discussion

Within a very large, contemporary study analyzing nearly 123,000 long-term continuous ambulatory cardiac monitors that were prescribed between 2011 and 2013, we found a moderate burden of potentially high-risk arrhythmias, including both ventricular arrhythmias and bradyarrhythmias. Patient compliance with extended monitoring was high, with at least 25 % of patients achieving greater than 13 days of continuous monitoring. For all arrhythmias examined, longer monitoring times significantly increased the yield of detected arrhythmias. While the gains in arrhythmia yield were particularly marked in the first 7 days of monitoring, it is notable that the gains continued to increase from days 7 to 14. The relatively high wear and analyzable time for the longer term continuous monitors suggests that outpatient ECG monitoring using this approach is feasible and can have significant yield of clinically important arrhythmias beyond atrial fibrillation. Our study examined a more recent time period than prior investigations of long-term continuous monitors [5, 9] and suggests that changes in the device technology and accumulated operator experience may have resulted in improved patient compliance.

Prior research suggests that traditional 24-h Holter monitoring is not sufficiently long enough to detect many types of arrhythmias [10–13], and recent evidence has demonstrated that longer monitoring may be useful to detect arrhythmias in high-risk patient populations, such as those with a recent history of cryptogenic ischemic stroke [8, 14], although the majority of these studies have focused primarily on finding atrial fibrillation. For example, in a registry of 239 patients who wore 30-day loop recorders after discharge for cryptogenic ischemic stroke, researchers found that 24 % of all detected cases of occult atrial fibrillation were found in the final 10 days of 30-day monitoring (i.e., between days 20 and 30) [14].

Similarly, in a larger controlled trial of a similar patient population where 24-h Holter monitoring was compared to 30-day monitoring, 17 % of all cases of atrial fibrillation were detected in the final week of monitoring [8]. Although conventional wisdom suggests that longer monitoring may be useful for detecting rarer, potentially high-risk arrhythmias, such as ventricular arrhythmias and bradyarrhythmias, there is little empirical evidence on the impact and diagnostic yield of longer continuous monitoring for other clinically meaningful arrhythmias outside of atrial fibrillation. One advantage to the studied technology compared to typical 24- or 48-h Holter monitor systems is its longer continuous wear time up to 14 days, as well as its application without any long wires attached to distant electrodes. For longer monitoring periods, loop or event recorders have typically been the preferred technology, with the main disadvantage being that recordings are only stored if they meet predefined algorithms or for symptomatic triggers. A post-hoc investigation of the patient's rhythm pre-or post-event cannot be done. Implantable loop recorders are occasionally used for very rare arrhythmia events, but these have the same limitations as loop and event monitors and also require a small surgical procedure to implant the device with its attendant risks.

For ventricular arrhythmias, we found that although the majority of arrhythmias are identified in the first 7 days, a significant proportion of arrhythmias were still detected in the 7 to 14-day monitoring window. This was more pronounced for non-sustained VT than sustained VT, with more than 20 % of non-sustained VT being identified in the 7–14 day window. Although we did not have detailed clinical characteristics for our patient population, in high-risk patients, such as those with cardiomyopathy, non-sustained VT can be a high risk marker that may warrant a change in treatment such as the consideration of an implantable cardioverter-defibrillator in certain patient populations (i.e., hypertrophic cardiomyopathy). Depending upon the clinical circumstances, both nonsustained and sustained VT often support the need for further diagnostic testing, such as the evaluation for structural heart disease or for cardiac ischemia. Similarly, although potentially high-risk bradyarrhythmias were less common, if they are not appropriately identified and treated, patients may suffer significant morbidity and excess mortality. The consideration of therapeutic interventions such as permanent pacemaker implantation is recommended by the joint American College of Cardiology, American Heart Association, and Heart Rhythm Society guidelines for the high-risk bradyarrhythmias evaluated in our study [15].

Our study had certain limitations. We did not have data on any changes in clinical management or patient outcomes following monitoring, so we were unable to

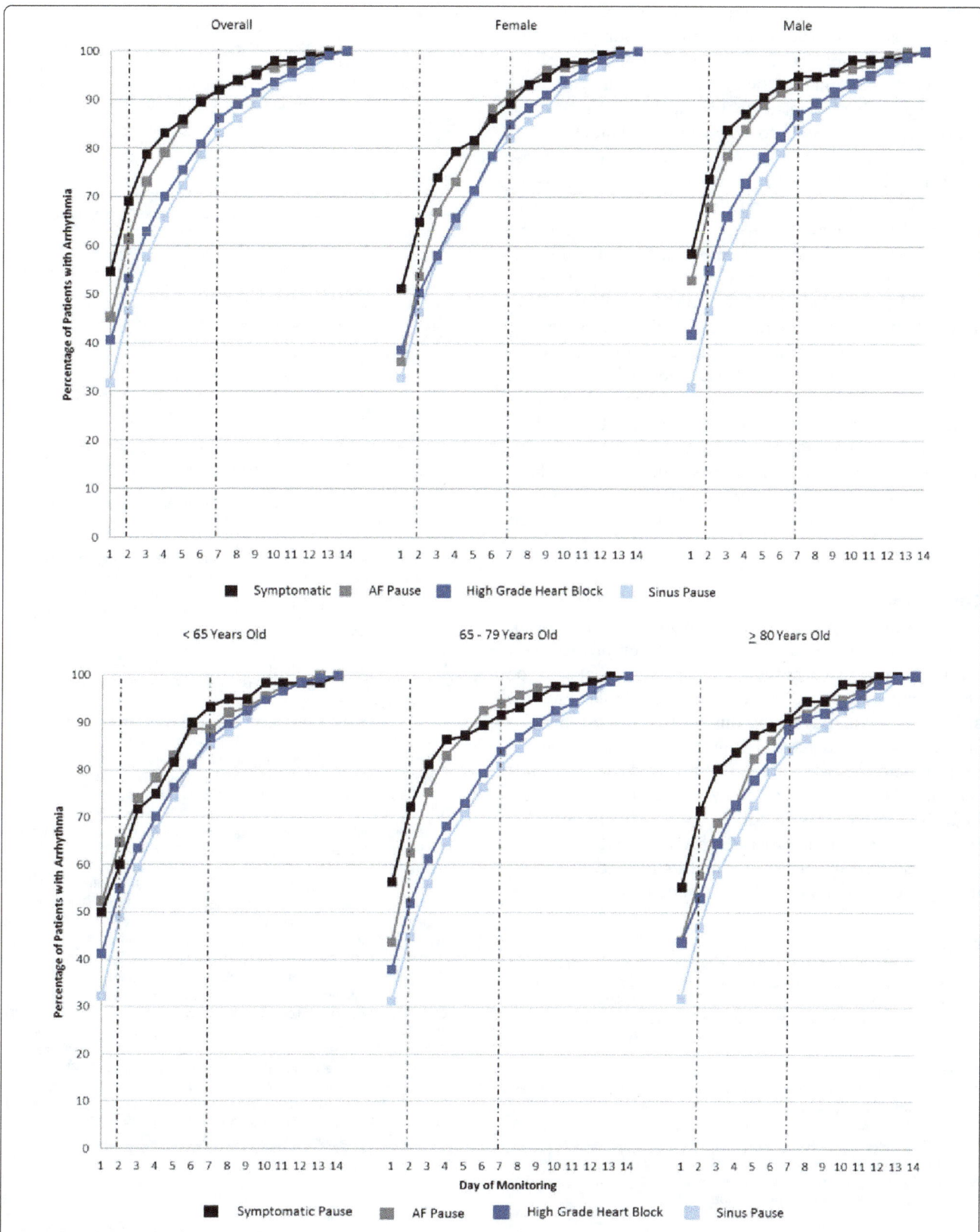

Fig. 3 Cumulative yield of pauses and high grade heart block. Data are shown for the overall population of patients with the arrhythmia and stratified by age and gender. AF = atrial fibrillation

delineate the direct clinical impact from the detection of arrhythmias found from the monitors in our study. We did not have information on all symptomatic triggers, and thus did not analyze the proportion of all symptomatic triggers that correlate to true arrhythmias. Patient information was limited to demographic characteristics, and data were unavailable on patients' comorbidities, which could potentially help further risk stratify patients and allow for predictive modeling to help identify those most at-risk for high-risk arrhythmias. In addition, some bradyarrhythmias, such as asymptomatic sinus and AF pauses, may occur nocturnally in normal subjects. Further, we did not validate the data on the clinical indication for the ordered monitors, and differences among providers' thresholds for ordering the monitors could have an impact on patient selection and arrhythmia yield. Finally, while average wear time was high, at least a quarter of patients wore the device for less than 7 days (25th percentile of 6.8 days), thus artificially reducing the yield of detected arrhythmias from 7 to 14 days. Thus, the actual yield of detected arrhythmias from days 7 to 14 or monitoring may be even higher than we observed.

Conclusion

In sum, our study suggests that longer term monitoring up to 14 days resulted in high patient compliance, and greater detection of high-risk arrhythmias than 24- or 48-h monitoring strategies. We observed similar findings across gender and age subgroups. Although the bulk of arrhythmias were detected within the first 7 days, longer-term monitoring between 7 and 14 days yielded a significant number of likely clinically meaningful, potentially high-risk arrhythmias. Future research should examine the clinical utility of improved high-risk arrhythmia detection in targeted patient groups and its impact on patient management and associated clinical outcomes.

Competing interests

This project was sponsored by a research grant from iRhythm Technologies, Inc., San Francisco, California. Ms Lenane, Ms Livingston, and Mr Sarlas are employees of iRhythm Technologies, Inc., San Francisco, California. The other authors declare that they have no competing interests.

Authors' contributions

All persons who made substantial contributions to the manuscript are listed as authors. MS, AG were responsible for study conception and design. MS, JY, SS, ML, GS, JL, AG were responsible for acquisition of data. MS, AG, SS, ML, GS, JL, were responsible for analysis and interpretation of data. MS drafted the manuscript, and MS, JY, SS, NL, GS, JL, AG were responsible for revising it for important intellectual content. All authors have read and approve the final version of the manuscript.

Funding

This project was sponsored by a research grant from iRhythm Technologies, Inc., San Francisco, California.

Author details

[1]Division of Research, Kaiser Permanente Northern California, Oakland, CA, USA. [2]Stanford University School of Medicine, Stanford, CA, USA. [3]iRhythm Technologies, Inc, San Francisco, CA, USA. [4]Departments of Epidemiology, Biostatistics and Medicine, University of California, San Francisco, CA, USA. [5]Department of Cardiology, Kaiser Permanente Oakland Medical Center, 3600 Broadway, Oakland, CA 94611, USA.

References

1. Crawford MH, Bernstein SJ, Deedwania PC, DiMarco JP, Ferrick KJ, Garson Jr A, et al. ACC/AHA guidelines for ambulatory electrocardiography: executive summary and recommendations. A report of the American College of Cardiology/American Heart Association task force on practice guidelines (committee to revise the guidelines for ambulatory electrocardiography). Circulation. 1999;100(8):886–93.
2. Katritsis DG, Siontis GC, Camm AJ. Prognostic significance of ambulatory ECG monitoring for ventricular arrhythmias. Prog Cardiovasc Dis. 2013;56(2):133–42.
3. Liao J, Khalid Z, Scallan C, Morillo C, O'Donnell M. Noninvasive cardiac monitoring for detecting paroxysmal atrial fibrillation or flutter after acute ischemic stroke: a systematic review. Stroke. 2007;38(11):2935–40.
4. Enseleit F, Duru F. Long-term continuous external electrocardiographic recording: a review. Europace. 2006;8(4):255–66.
5. Barrett PM, Komatireddy R, Haaser S, Topol S, Sheard J, Encinas J, et al. Comparison of 24-hour Holter monitoring with 14-day novel adhesive patch electrocardiographic monitoring. Am J Med. 2014;127(1):95. e11-97.
6. Healey JS, Connolly SJ, Gold MR, Israel CW, Van Gelder IC, Capucci A, et al. Subclinical atrial fibrillation and the risk of stroke. N Engl J Med. 2012;366(2):120–9.
7. Reiffel JA, Schwarzberg R, Murry M. Comparison of autotriggered memory loop recorders versus standard loop recorders versus 24-hour Holter monitors for arrhythmia detection. Am J Cardiol. 2005;95(9):1055–9.
8. Gladstone DJ, Spring M, Dorian P, Panzov V, Thorpe KE, Hall J, et al. Atrial fibrillation in patients with cryptogenic stroke. N Engl J Med. 2014;370(26):2467–77.
9. Turakhia MP, Hoang DD, Zimetbaum P, Miller JD, Froelicher VF, Kumar UN, et al. Diagnostic utility of a novel leadless arrhythmia monitoring device. Am J Cardiol. 2013;112(4):520–4.
10. Seet RC, Friedman PA, Rabinstein AA. Prolonged rhythm monitoring for the detection of occult paroxysmal atrial fibrillation in ischemic stroke of unknown cause. Circulation. 2011;124(4):477–86.
11. Higgins P, MacFarlane PW, Dawson J, McInnes GT, Langhorne P, Lees KR. Noninvasive cardiac event monitoring to detect atrial fibrillation after ischemic stroke: a randomized, controlled trial. Stroke. 2013;44(9):2525–31.
12. Schreiber D, Sattar A, Drigalla D, Higgins S. Ambulatory cardiac monitoring for discharged emergency department patients with possible cardiac arrhythmias. West J Emerg Med. 2014;15(2):194–8.
13. Rothman SA, Laughlin JC, Seltzer J, Walia JS, Baman RI, Siouffi SY, et al. The diagnosis of cardiac arrhythmias: a prospective multi-center randomized study comparing mobile cardiac outpatient telemetry versus standard loop event monitoring. J Cardiovasc Electrophysiol. 2007;18(3):241–7.
14. Flint AC, Banki NM, Ren X, Rao VA, Go AS. Detection of Paroxysmal Atrial Fibrillation by 30-Day Event Monitoring in Cryptogenic Ischemic Stroke: The Stroke and Monitoring for PAF in Real Time (SMART) Registry. Stroke. 2012.
15. Epstein AE, DiMarco JP, Ellenbogen KA, Estes III NA, Freedman RA, Gettes LS, et al. ACC/AHA/HRS 2008 Guidelines for device-based therapy of cardiac rhythm abnormalities: a report of the American College of Cardiology/American Heart Association Task Force on Practice Guidelines (Writing Committee to Revise the ACC/AHA/NASPE 2002 guideline update for implantation of cardiac pacemakers and antiarrhythmia devices): developed in collaboration with the American Association for Thoracic Surgery and Society of Thoracic Surgeons. Circulation. 2008;117(21):e350–408.

11

Rs7193343 polymorphism in zinc finger homeobox 3 (ZFHX3) gene and atrial fibrillation

ChuanNan Zhai[1,2,3], HongLiang Cong[1*], YuJie Liu[1], Ying Zhang[1], XianFeng Liu[1,2], Hao Zhang[1,2] and ZhiJing Ren[1,2]

Abstract

Background: The previous genome-wide studies have shown that rs7193343 single-nucleotide polymorphism (SNP) in zinc finger homeobox 3 (ZFHX3) gene correlate with risk of atrial fibrillation (AF). However, the distribution of this SNP differs significantly among various populations. The present study was to investigate whether combined evidence shows the association between ZFHX3 rs7193343 SNP and the risk of AF in various populations.

Methods: A systematic search of all studies published through Dec 2014 was conducted using the Medline, Embase, WanFang, ScienceDirect, CNKI, and OVID databases. The case-control studies that evaluated an association between rs7193343 SNP and risk of AF were identified. The association between the ZFHX3 rs7193343 SNP and AF susceptibility was assessed using genetic models.

Results: We collected 10 comparisons from six studies for rs7193343 SNP, including 1037 cases and 4310 controls in Asian, 5583 cases and 38215 controls in Caucasian, and then performed an updated meta-analysis and subgroup analysis based on ethnicity. In overall population, the occurrence of AF was found to be associated with T-allelic of rs7193343 SNP in ZFHX3 (OR =1.17, 95% CI 1.10-1.26). In subgroup analysis, we observed there was significant association between T-allele of rs7193343 and risk of AF in Caucasian subgroups (OR =1.20, 95% CI 1.12-1.30), but no statistically significance (OR = 1.07, 95% CI 0.92-1.24) in Asian population.

Conclusion: In Caucasian population, genetic variant rs7193343 SNP is associated with risk of AF in Caucasian population. However, no association is found in Asian population based on the current evidence. Further studies with larger sample size involving case-control populations with multiple ethnics are still required in the future.

Keywords: Atrial fibrillation, Meta-analysis, Zinc finger homeobox 3 gene, Polymorphism, Rs7193343

Background

Atrial fibrillation (AF) is the most common sustained cardiac arrhythmia in clinical practice, and affect individuals suffer from increased rates of stroke, and lead to higher risk of incidence and mortality of cardiovascular disease [1]. The incidence of AF has estimated rate of 0.4–1.0 % which increases with age, in the general population [2, 3]. In 80 people over the age, its prevalence is high at 7.5 % [4, 5]. The factors that increase the risk of developing AF include age, hypertension, heart failure, structural heart diseases, valvular heart disease and a variety of other factors [3, 6]. However, contemporary clinical treatment strategies have only confined curative effects that likely stem from our limited understanding of its potential pathophysiology. Therefore, most medical experts tried to find the significant elements with risk of AF.

Recently, studies have provided unequivocal evidence that AF has the important relevance of genetic factors [7]. AF has been found to occur in large families (monogenic AF) and can be inherited in either an autosomal dominant model or an autosomal recessive [8]. Several

---

* Correspondence: hl_cong@126.com
[1]Department of Cardiology, Tianjin Chest Hospital, Taierzhuang South Road No. 291, Jinnan District, Tianjin, 300350, China
Full list of author information is available at the end of the article

genetic loci, such as loci on chromosome 1q21, 3q21, 5p13, 11p15.5, 12p13, 21q22 and 17q23–q24, have been identified for monogenetic AF [9]. Previous studies shown that the 3 loci most strongly associated with AF occur on chromosomes 4q25 (near PITX2) [10], 16q22 (in ZFHX3) [11], and 1q21 (in KCNN3) [12]. A recent genome-wide association study (GWAS) has also identified variants on chromosome 16q22. The proximate study investigated the role of genetic variants of ZFHX3 (zinc finger homeobox 3) in AF, single-nucleotide polymorphism (SNPs) rs2106261 and rs6499600 showed significant associations, and rs16971436 conferred a borderline significant association with risk of AF in Chinese Han populations [13]. SNP rs7193343 in ZFHX3 gene has been pointed out as marker strongly associated with AF in several different populations [14–16], while other studies assessed the association of rs7193343 with susceptibility of AF, which shown that the association was not statistically significant [14, 16]. Therefore, the results are still in controversy.

Therefore, the aim of the present meta-analysis was to investigate whether combined evidence shows the association between ZFHX3 rs7193343 polymorphism and the risk of AF in various populations, determining whether there was heterogeneity among the studies.

Methods

Search strategy

We performed a systematic search of Medline, Embase, WanFang, ScienceDirect, CNKI, and OVID to identify published epidemiological studies through Dec 2014 that were related to the rs7193343 ZFHX3 polymorphism and AF. The medical subject headings (MeSH; National Library of Medicine, Bethesda, Maryland) "zinc finger homeobox 3", "genetic polymorphism", "atrial fibrillation", and the free-text words "ZFHX3" or "rs7193343" were combined. Only studies published in English or in Chinese were included in the present study. Furthermore, the reference lists of all of the full text papers were examined to identify any initially omitted studies. Secondary searches of the grey literature were not performed.

Inclusion and exclusion criteria

Articles from peer-reviewed medical journals were included if they reported on studies using case-control, nested case-control, cross-sectional design, or cohort and provided sufficient data to calculate an odds ratio (OR) and corresponding 95 % confidence interval (CI). After that, comparisons of laboratory methods and overlapping study data were excluded. Using Hardy-Weinberg equilibrium (HWE), we excluded those studies that contain genotype frequencies that weren't meet criteria in the control groups.

Study selection

Two reviewers independently screened the titles and abstracts for the eligibility criteria. Subsequently, reviewers read the full text of the studies that potentially met the inclusion criteria, and the literature was reviewed to determine final inclusive data. If inclusions have disagreements, we reached a consensus through discussion.

Date extraction

With a standard data extraction form used, two of the authors independently extracted the following data from each full-text report. The data extracted from the candidate studies included the title, authors, published year, number of cases or controls, ethnicity, age, gender, study design, genotyping method, genotype distribution, and frequency of T-allele of the rs7193343 polymorphism in cases or controls. We also examined whether the genotype distributions of the control groups followed HWE [17].

Statistical analysis

Data analysis was conducted using STATA 12.0 (Statacorp, college station, Tex). The association between the ZFHX3 rs7193343 polymorphism and AF susceptibility was assessed under the following genetic models, which were treated as a dichotomous variable, T-allele versus C-allele for allele level comparison.

Between-study heterogeneity was tested using Q statistics, and $P < 0.1$ was considered statistically significant. The Mantel-Haenszel method for fixed effects and the Der-Simonian and Laird method for random effects were used to estimate pooled effects [18]. We used fixed-effects methods if the result of the Q test was not significant. Otherwise, we calculated the pooled ORs and 95% CIs assuming a random-effects model. Fixed effects assume that genetic factors have similar effects on autoimmune disease susceptibility across all studies and that the observed variations between studies are caused by chance alone [19]. The random effects model assumes that different studies may have substantial diversity and assesses both within- and between-study variation [20]. A recently developed measure, I^2, was used to quantify the inconsistency among the studies' results with values of 50 % or higher and the large heterogeneity for values of 75 % or higher [21]. The data are shown as the ORs with 95 %CIs, with two-tailed P-values; statistical significance was set at $P < 0.05$ (two-tailed).

Publication bias was conducted both visually by using a funnel plot and statistically via Begg funnel plots and Egger's bias test, which measures the degree of funnel plot asymmetry [22, 23]. The Begg adjusted rank correlation test was used to assess the correlation between test accuracy estimates and their variances. The deviation of Spearman's rho values from zero provides an estimate of funnel plot asymmetry. Positive values indicate a trend toward higher levels of test accuracy in studies with smaller sample sizes. The Egger's bias test detects funnel plot asymmetry by determining whether the intercept deviates significantly from zero in a regression of the standardized effect estimates against their precision.

Results

Search results

We initially obtained 311 potential articles, and after screened abstract, among which most were excluded for no relevance to our analysis. Eleven articles then were removed because small number cases and unusable data. Finally, five studies [14–16, 24, 25] and a Chinese study [26] including 10 comparisons for rs7193343 that all

adopted observational study design eventually satisfied the eligibility criteria (Fig. 1).

Characteristics of included studies

A total of 10 comparisons from six studies for rs7193343 polymorphism were involved in presence updated meta-analysis containing 6620 cases and 42525 controls (including 1037 cases and 4310 controls in Asian, 5583 cases and 38215 controls in Caucasian) (Table 1). One articles as a brief communication was a multi-centers case-control study including 4 comparisons [14]. However we could not obtain genotype information from the above study. The china study [16] also did not provide genotype data. Although we tried to contract authors of the original

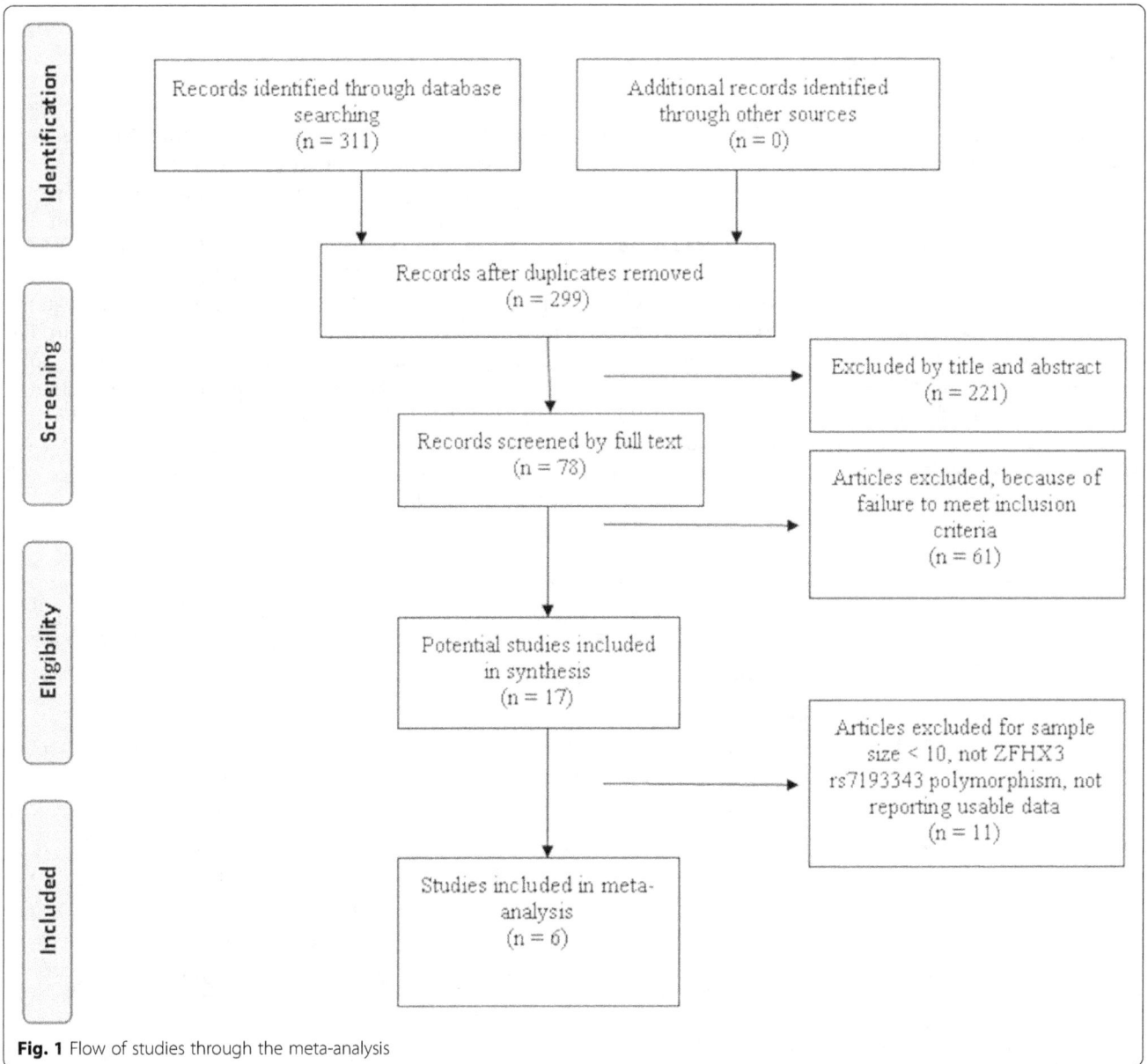

Fig. 1 Flow of studies through the meta-analysis

Table 1 Allele counts for the rs7193343 polymorphism in the included studies

Study	country	Case					Control				
		Genotype [a]			Allele [b] (%)		Genotype [a]			Allele [b] (%)	
		TT	TC	CC	T	C	TT	TC	CC	T	C
DanielF,2009	Iceland	NA	NA	NA	0.229	0.771	NA	NA	NA	0.199	0.801
DanielF,2009	Iceland	NA	NA	NA	0.238	0.762	NA	NA	NA	0.205	0.795
DanielF,2009	Norway	NA	NA	NA	0.177	0.823	NA	NA	NA	0.166	0.834
DanielF,2009	USA	NA	NA	NA	0.183	0.817	NA	NA	NA	0.139	0.861
DanielF,2009	HongKong	NA	NA	NA	0.686	0.314	NA	NA	NA	0.676	0.324
CongL,2011	China	NA	NA	NA	0.320	0.680	NA	NA	NA	0.320	0.680
Marek,2011	Poland	27	128	230	0.222	0.778	28	148	344	0.185	0.815
Wang,2012	China	22	68	12	0.549	0.451	10	66	24	0.430	0.570
Parvez,2013	USA	5	40	57	0.231	0.769	9	62	97	0.217	0.783
Albert,2014	Spanish	10	88	159	0.210	0.790	10	106	263	0.166	0.834

NA not available
[a] Number of [homozygotes of risk allele, TT]/[heterozygotes, TC]/[homozygotes of the other allele, CC]
[b] Risk allele (T-allele or C- allele) frequency

studies, no response got. The characteristics of included studies were shown in Table 2.

Association of rs7193343 polymorphism of ZFHX3 gene with the risk of AF in overall population

As shown in Fig. 2, we used a fixed-effects model to analysis overall studies data of 10 case-control comparisons, performed for meta-analysis and generated a combined allelic OR 1.17 of for risk allele (95 % CI 1.10-1.26), identified no statistics heterogeneity (Q = 7.22, $I^2 = 0.0$ %). These results indicated that there was statistically significant in the association between rs7193343 and AF.

Association of rs7193343 polymorphism of ZFHX3 gene with the risk of AF in subgroups analysis

As shown in Fig. 3, when we restricted to ethnicity subgroup analysis, there was significant association between rs7193343 and the risk of AF in Caucasian subgroups (OR =1.20, 95 %CI 1.12-1.30) in the fixed-effects model, and the result shown no obvious statistics heterogeneity (Q = 2.09, $I^2 = 0.0$ %). Three studies reported the association between rs7193343 polymorphism and AF in Asian population, we used a fixed-effects model analysis because there was no heterogeneity among three studies (Q = 3.18, $I^2 = 37.0$ %), shown no statistically significance (OR = 1.07, 95 %CI 0.92-1.24) (Table 3).

Table 2 Characteristics of included studies

Study,year	ethnicity	Characteristics of controls	Genotyp-ing methods	No.case of total AF	No.case of lone AF	No. of control	age		Gender(M/F)		H W E
							Case	Control	Case	Control	
DanielF,2009	Iceland	Health	HumanHap	2381	NA	33723	NA		NA		Y
DanielF,2009	Iceland	Health	HumanHap	970	NA	1939	NA		NA		Y
DanielF,2009	Norway	Health	HumanHap	722	NA	711	NA		NA		Y
DanielF,2009	USA	Health	HumanHap	735	NA	729	NA		NA		Y
DanielF,2009	HongKong	Health	HumanHap	285	NA	2763	NA		NA		Y
CongL,2011	China	Health	PCR	650	180	1447	58.4(15.9)	59.7(12.2)	398/252	902/545	Y
Marek,2011	Poland	AF[a]	Taqman	410[b]	NA	550[b]	53.3(11.3)	53.1(10.4)	272/128	331/169	Y
Wang,2012	China	Health	PCR	102	NA	100	61.5(12.5)	60.4(9.9)	56/46	52/48	Y
Parvez,2013	USA	AF[a]	PCR	108[b]	NA	184[b]	67(59-72)	66(58-72)	82/26	142/42	Y
Albert,2014	Spanish	Health	Taqman	257	123	379	60.6(11.5)	42.6(15.2)	148/109	193/186	Y

NA not available
AF[a] mean AF recurrence after ablation
[b]mean about the numbers of AF recurrence after ablation

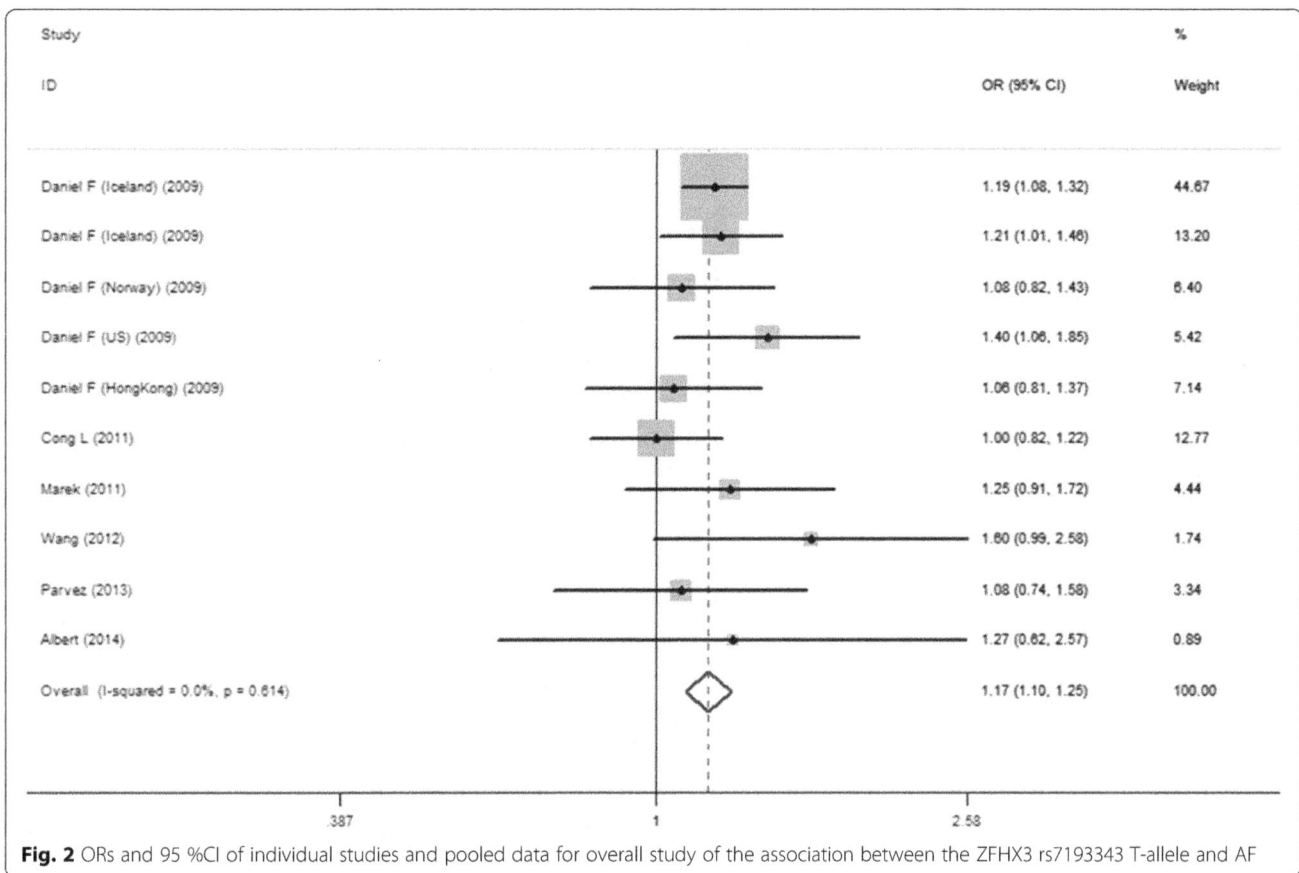

Fig. 2 ORs and 95 %CI of individual studies and pooled data for overall study of the association between the ZFHX3 rs7193343 T-allele and AF

Publication bias

The publication bias test was performed for overall populations. Significant publication bias was shown for overall populations by the Begg rank correlation method (P = 0.47) (Fig. 4) and the Egger weighted regression method (P = 0.76) (Fig. 5).

Discussion

Atrial fibrillation (AF) represents the most serious sustained arrhythmia in the process of clinical diagnosis and treatments. It is the feature of uncoordinated atrial activation. Some studies shown that AF was a important factor with a lifetime risk of one in four for men and women 40 years of age and older [27]. Currently, a number of studies showed that AF was in the relationship of SNPs in genes [13, 28, 29]. A SNP, rs7193343, had been investigated widely. Although several studies demonstrated that rs7193343 polymorphism was associated with occurrence of AF, the results were still in controversy. We, therefore, conducted the present meta-analysis to evaluate the relationship of rs7193343 polymorphism and susceptibility of AF. Thus, we aim to provide objective evidence in the investigation of rs7193343 polymorphism in patients with AF, based on the current published studies.

Recently, a growing body of researches provided the relationship of a variant in the ZFHX3 gene on chromosome 16q22, rs7193343-T and AF in multiple population of different ancestry. However, their conclusions were not consistent. The distribution of genotype of rs7193343 polymorphism in ZFHX3 gene differed significantly among populations. Gudbjartsson et al. [14] expanded a genome-wide association study (GWAS) on atrial fibrillation, they previously identified risk variant on 16q22 rs7193343 associated significantly with AF in samples from Iceland, Norway and US, they also illustrated that the association of SNPs rs7193343-T with AF in Chinese population from Hong Kong, but the result was not significant in this cohort. Furthermore, they found that the T allele of rs7193343 is obviously much more frequent in Chinese descent than the samples of European population. Soon afterwards, the study of Cong L et. al [16] provided the first evidence of a cross-race susceptibility of the 16q22 AF locus in a Chinese Han population, and expanded the association between ZFHX3 and AF to a non-European ancestry population. They carried out a large-scale case-control association study, and identified that ZFHX3 SNP rs7193343 was not associated with AF in the Chinese Han population. Kiliszek et al. [15] identified SNP rs7193343 polymorphism correlated significantly

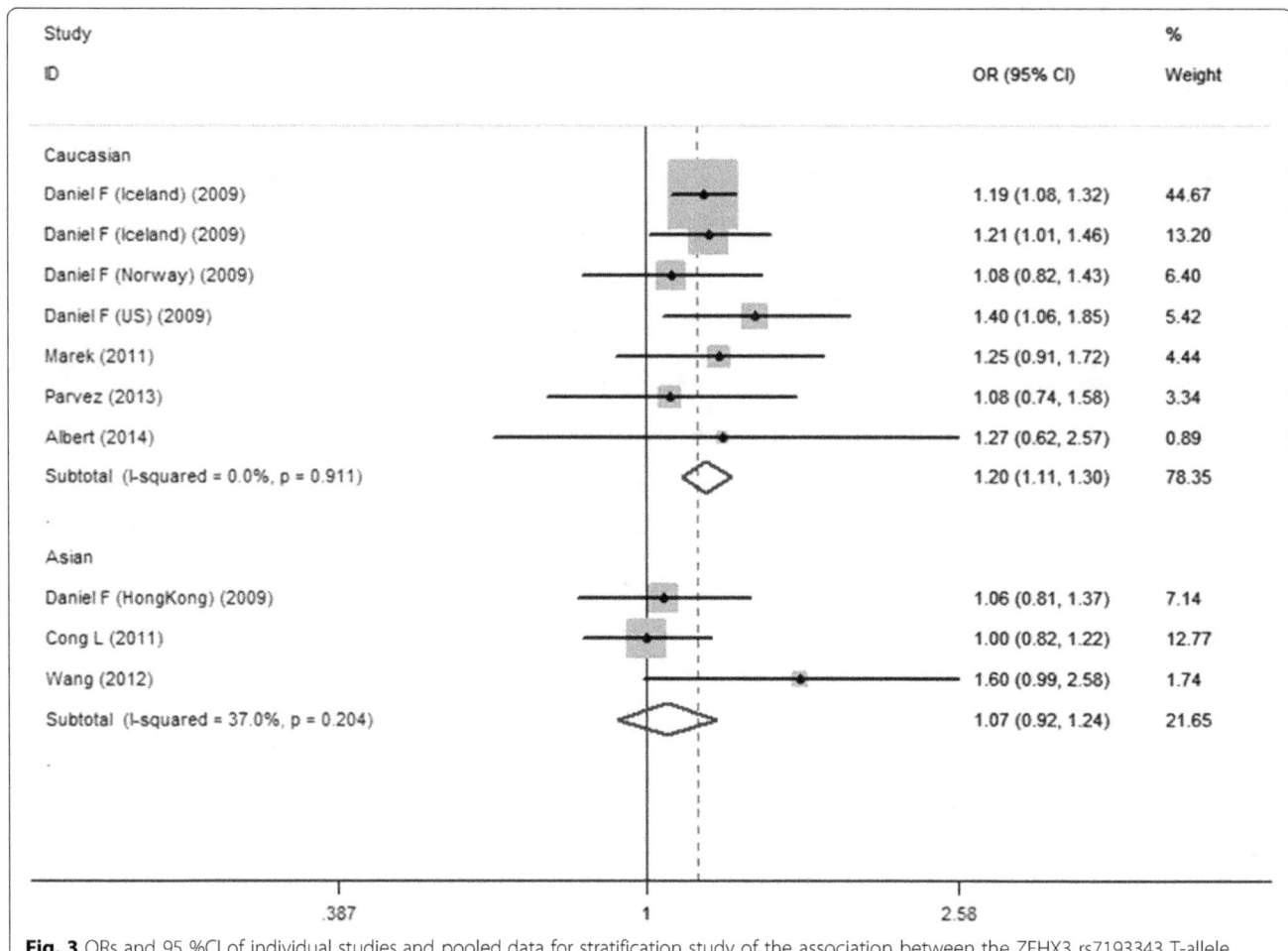

Fig. 3 ORs and 95 %CI of individual studies and pooled data for stratification study of the association between the ZFHX3 rs7193343 T-allele and AF

with AF in Polish patients, and confirmed rs7193343 on chromosome 16q22 that it was an independent marker of AF. Although another study evaluated genomic markers which can predict timing of AF recurrence in patients undergoing elective direct current cardioversion, it did not confirm that rs7193343 has association with early AF recurrence [24].

The present study demonstrated that there was statistically significant in the association between T-allele frequency of rs7193343 and AF in overall population. Interestingly, subgroup analysis was performed according

to the ethnicity, showing significant association between T-allele frequency of rs7193343 and AF in Caucasian population but not in Asian population. Although a previous meta-analysis was conducted recently with positive results [25], no subgroup analysis was performed based on the ethnicity. The heterogeneity originated from ethnicity was of great importance in the pooled results. Thus, it was imperative to update the previous meta-analysis in accordance with ethnicity of individual study. The pooled result based on one kind of ethnicity may be more stable. Although the pooled results in overall

Table 3 Summary ORs and 95% CIs of the rs7193343 polymorphism in ZFHX3 and AF susceptibility

Comparison	Population	Sample size		No. of studies	Type of model	Test of association			Test of heterogeneity		
		Case	Control			OR	95% CI	P value	Q test	P value	I²
T allele versus C allele	Overall	6620	42525	10	Fixed	1.17	1.10-1.26	<0.01	7.22	0.61	0.0 %
	Asian	1037	4310	3	Fixed	1.07	0.92-1.24	0.40	3.18	0.20	37.0 %
	Caucasian	5583	38215	7	Fixed	1.20	1.12-1.30	<0.01	2.09	0.91	0.0 %

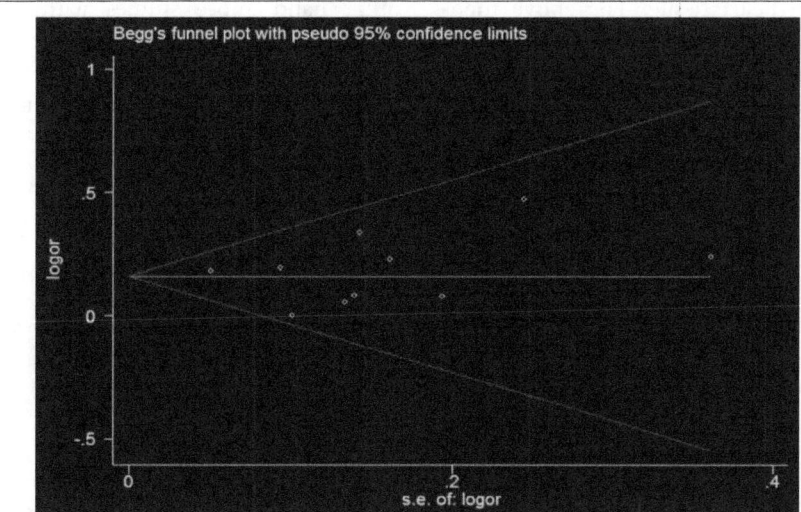

Fig. 4 Funnel plot of studies for the association between the ZFHX3 rs7193343 T-allele and AF in all subjects (Begg rank correlation test, P = 0.47)

population of the present study was consistent with the previous one, there was no statistically significant difference in Asian population. The subgroup analysis is the strengthen of the present meta-analysis.

Rs7193343 is an intronic SNP located in the zinc finger homeobox 3 (ZFHX3) gene (chromosome 16q22) [14]. The variant is also called AT motif-binding factor 1 (ATBF1). The same variant was associated with Kawasaki disease, an inflammatory vasculitis predominantly seen in young children. The gene encodes a transcription factor named Atbf1 that was first described as an enhancer of human a-fetoprotein (AFP) gene expression in the liver [30]. This gene regulates neuronal and muscle differentiation and is a tumor suppressor gene in

several types of cancer [31]. ZFHX3 is expressed in various tissues, including heart, liver, lung, kidney, pituitary gland and brain. Although it is expressed in mouse heart [32], its function in heart tissue is unknown. Atbf1 is required for early transcriptional activation of the gene POU class 1 homeobox 1 (POU1F1) that regulates pituitary cell differentiation and hormone expression in mammals [33]. POU1F1 interacts with the paired-like homeodomain transcription factor 2 (PITX2) to facilitate DNA binding and transcriptional activity, which is of interest because the previously identified AF variants on chromosome 4q25 are located close to PITX2, a gene critical for heart development [34]. Therefore, we speculate there is an association between rs7193343 and

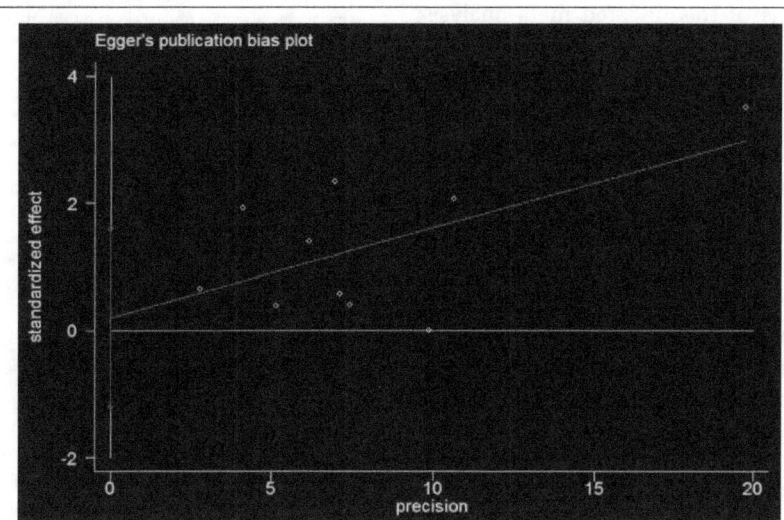

Fig. 5 Funnel plot of studies for the association between the ZFHX3 rs7193343 T-allele and AF in all subjects (Egger weighted regression test, P = 0.76)

expression of ZFHX3 in heart tissue. The above mentioned may be the mechanism of the association between ZFHX3 rs7193343 polymorphism and the risk of AF.

The following potential factors may be account for the different pooled results between the above two ethnical group: (1) inconsistence in genetic background [35], (2) different habits in individual ethnicity [36], (3) environmental factors leading to different susceptibility of AF [37]. Furthermore, we also speculate that the reason why the statistical difference was not significant in Asian population after subgroup analysis may be the limited sample size in this population. Therefore, more studies with large sample size are required to conduct further analysis, especially in Asian population.

Although the results of test for heterogeneity were not significant for subgroup population, heterogeneity cannot be completely resolved. The heterogeneity of included studies includes the following: quality of included studies, gender proportion, age, classification of AF, different genetic background, environmental factors, sampling criteria and cultural difference. The heterogeneity of genetic effects between individual studies may also be caused by the existence of gene-environmental or genetic interaction. In spite of only ten comparisons included, the pooled results may have clinical significance according to the current evidence. Although no publication bias was found in the present study, it is also important to bear in mind that publication bias may exist, since the negative results are less likely to be published. Accordingly, while the results of this meta-analysis should be considered appropriate, the above methodological defects should be considered when interpreting the findings. The present study could provide objective evidence by using genetic meta-analysis approach.

The primary limitations of this updated meta-analysis include the following: (1) the statistical efficacy could be improved by including more studies; (2) Some non-English publications not being included in this study may have caused important studies to be overlooked and publication bias from significant conclusions being more easily published; (3) The genotyping data of SNPs rs7193343 were insufficient, so we were unable to conduct meta-analysis based on the limited studies data; (4) the combined analysis of the results may be affected by the impact of clinical heterogeneity, including the general condition of the cases, habits, medical history, medication compliance and other factors.

Conclusion

Genetic variant rs7193343 is associated with a crucial risk of AF in Caucasian population, whereas SNP rs7193343 is not association with AF in Asian population. This variant could have a clinical utility in estimating AF risk. On the other hand, more studies with great sample size and multiple ethnics are required to determine the significance of rs7193343 SNP between them and to define the effect of the size of T-allele on susceptibility to AF.

Competing interests
The authors declare that they have no conflict of interests.

Authors' contributions
The design of the study was done by HLC. CNZ, YZ and YJL prepare the manuscript and assisted in the study processes. XFL, HZ and ZJR assisted in the data collections. All authors read and approved the final manuscript.

Acknowledgement
The authors thank Professor XM Li and H Zhang for their great advices on researches of the unpublished literature.

Author details
[1]Department of Cardiology, Tianjin Chest Hospital, Taierzhuang South Road No. 291, Jinnan District, Tianjin, 300350, China. [2]Graduate School, Tianjin Medical University, Tianjin 300051, China. [3]Department of Cardiology, Tianjin Gongan Hospital, Xinhua Road No. 162, Heping District, Tianjin, 300042, China.

References
1. Wolf PA, Abbott RD, Kannel WB. Atrial fibrillation as an independent risk factor for stroke: the Framingham Study. Stroke. 1991;22(8):983–8.
2. Feinberg WM, Blackshear JL, Laupacis A, Kronmal R, Hart RG. Prevalence, age distribution, and gender of patients with atrial fibrillation. Analysis and implications Arch Intern Med. 1995;155(5):469–73.
3. Fuster V, Ryden LE, Cannom DS, Crijns HJ, Curtis AB, Ellenbogen KA, et al. ACC/AHA/ESC 2006 guidelines for the management of patients with atrial fibrillation: full text: a report of the American College of Cardiology/American Heart Association Task Force on practice guidelines and the European Society of Cardiology Committee for Practice Guidelines (Writing Committee to Revise the 2001 guidelines for the management of patients with atrial fibrillation) developed in collaboration with the European Heart Rhythm Association and the Heart Rhythm Society. Europace. 2006;8(9):651–745.
4. Stewart S, Hart CL, Hole DJ, McMurray JJ. Population prevalence, incidence, and predictors of atrial fibrillation in the Renfrew/Paisley study. Heart. 2001;86(5):516–21.
5. Go AS, Hylek EM, Phillips KA, Chang Y, Henault LE, Selby JV, et al. Prevalence of diagnosed atrial fibrillation in adults: national implications for rhythm management and stroke prevention: the AnTicoagulation and Risk Factors in Atrial Fibrillation (ATRIA) Study. JAMA. 2001;285(18):2370–5.
6. Perticone F, Sciacqua A, Perticone M, Tassone EJ, Sesti G, Violi F, et al. Clinical risk factors and subclinical target organ damage as predictors of new-onset of atrial fibrillation: The Catanzaro atrial fibrillation project. Int J Cardiol. 2014;177(2):666–8.
7. Andalib A, Brugada R, Nattel S. Atrial fibrillation: evidence for genetically determined disease. Curr Opin Cardiol. 2008;23(3):176–83.
8. Oberti C, Wang L, Li L, Dong J, Rao S, Du W, et al. Genome-wide linkage scan identifies a novel genetic locus on chromosome 5p13 for neonatal atrial fibrillation associated with sudden death and variable cardiomyopathy. Circulation. 2004;110(25):3753–9.
9. Tsai CT, Lai LP, Hwang JJ, Lin JL, Chiang FT. Molecular genetics of atrial fibrillation. J Am Coll Cardiol. 2008;52(4):241–50.
10. Gudbjartsson DF, Arnar DO, Helgadottir A, Gretarsdottir S, Holm H, Sigurdsson A, et al. Variants conferring risk of atrial fibrillation on chromosome 4q25. Nature. 2007;448(7151):353–7.
11. Benjamin EJ, Rice KM, Arking DE, Pfeufer A, van Noord C, Smith AV, et al. Variants in ZFHX3 are associated with atrial fibrillation in individuals of European ancestry. Nat Genet. 2009;41(8):879–81.
12. Ellinor PT, Lunetta KL, Glazer NL, Pfeufer A, Alonso A, Chung MK, et al. Common variants in KCNN3 are associated with lone atrial fibrillation. Nat Genet. 2010;42(3):240–4.

13. Liu Y, Ni B, Lin Y, Chen XG, Fang Z, Zhao L, et al. Genetic polymorphisms in ZFHX3 are associated with atrial fibrillation in a Chinese Han population. PLoS One. 2014;9(7), e101318.

14. Gudbjartsson DF, Holm H, Gretarsdottir S, Thorleifsson G, Walters GB, Thorgeirsson G, et al. A sequence variant in ZFHX3 on 16q22 associates with atrial fibrillation and ischemic stroke. Nat Genet. 2009;41(8):876–8.

15. Kiliszek M, Franaszczyk M, Kozluk E, Lodzinski P, Piatkowska A, Broda G, et al. Association between variants on chromosome 4q25, 16q22 and 1q21 and atrial fibrillation in the Polish population. PLoS One. 2011;6(7), e21790.

16. Li C, Wang F, Yang Y, Fu F, Xu C, Shi L, et al. Significant association of SNP rs2106261 in the ZFHX3 gene with atrial fibrillation in a Chinese Han GeneID population. Hum Genet. 2011;129(3):239–46.

17. Hernandez JL, Weir BS. A disequilibrium coefficient approach to Hardy-Weinberg testing. Biometrics. 1989;45(1):53–70.

18. Robins J, Greenland S, Breslow NE. A general estimator for the variance of the Mantel-Haenszel odds ratio. Am J Epidemiol. 1986;124(5):719–23.

19. Egger M, Smith GD, Phillips AN. Meta-analysis: principles and procedures. BMJ. 1997;315(7121):1533–7.

20. DerSimonian R, Laird N. Meta-analysis in clinical trials. Control Clin Trials. 1986;7(3):177–88.

21. Higgins JP, Thompson SG. Quantifying heterogeneity in a meta-analysis. Stat Med. 2002;21(11):1539–58.

22. Egger M, Davey SG, Schneider M, Minder C. Bias in meta-analysis detected by a simple, graphical test. BMJ. 1997;315(7109):629–34.

23. Begg CB, Mazumdar M. Operating characteristics of a rank correlation test for publication bias. Biometrics. 1994;50(4):1088–101.

24. Parvez B, Shoemaker MB, Muhammad R, Richardson R, Jiang L, Blair MA, et al. Common genetic polymorphism at 4q25 locus predicts atrial fibrillation recurrence after successful cardioversion. Heart Rhythm. 2013;10(6):849–55.

25. Ferran A, Alegret JM, Subirana I, Aragones G, Lluis-Ganella C, Romero-Menor C, et al. Association between rs2200733 and rs7193343 genetic variants and atrial fibrillation in a Spanish population, and meta-analysis of previous studies. Rev Esp Cardiol (Engl Ed). 2014;67(10):822–9.

26. Wang Y, Li Y, Fan J, Xu Y, Chen W, Xiao P, et al. Relationship between rs7193343 polymorphism in the zinc finger homeobox 3 gene and atrial fibrillation. Journal of Clinical Cardiology (China). 2012;28(8):613–7.

27. Lloyd-Jones DM, Wang TJ, Leip EP, Larson MG, Levy D, Vasan RS, et al. Lifetime risk for development of atrial fibrillation: the Framingham Heart Study. Circulation. 2004;110(9):1042–6.

28. Roldan V, Arroyo AB, Salloum-Asfar S, Manzano-Fernandez S, Garcia-Barbera N, Marin F, et al. Prognostic role of MIR146A polymorphisms for cardiovascular events in atrial fibrillation. Thromb Haemost. 2014;112(4):781–8.

29. Orenes-Pinero E, Hernandez-Romero D, Romero-Aniorte AI, Martinez M, Garcia-Honrubia A, Caballero L, et al. Prognostic value of two polymorphisms in non-sarcomeric genes for the development of atrial fibrillation in patients with hypertrophic cardiomyopathy. QJM. 2014;107(8):613–21.

30. Morinaga T, Yasuda H, Hashimoto T, Higashio K, Tamaoki T. A human alpha-fetoprotein enhancer-binding protein, ATBF1, contains four homeodomains and seventeen zinc fingers. Mol Cell Biol. 1991;11(12):6041–9.

31. Berry FB, Miura Y, Mihara K, Kaspar P, Sakata N, Hashimoto-Tamaoki T, et al. Positive and negative regulation of myogenic differentiation of C2C12 cells by isoforms of the multiple homeodomain zinc finger transcription factor ATBF1. J Biol Chem. 2001;276(27):25057–65.

32. Ido A, Miura Y, Watanabe M, Sakai M, Inoue Y, Miki T, et al. Cloning of the cDNA encoding the mouse ATBF1 transcription factor. Gene. 1996;168(2):227–31.

33. Qi Y, Ranish JA, Zhu X, Krones A, Zhang J, Aebersold R, et al. Atbf1 is required for the Pit1 gene early activation. Proc Natl Acad Sci U S A. 2008;105(7):2481–6.

34. Amendt BA, Sutherland LB, Semina EV, Russo AF. The molecular basis of Rieger syndrome. Analysis of Pitx2 homeodomain protein activities. J Biol Chem. 1998;273(32):20066–72.

35. Andreasen L, Nielsen JB, Olesen MS: Genetic Aspects of Lone Atrial Fibrillation: What Do We Know? Curr Pharm Des. 2015;21(5):667–78

36. Suzuki S, Sagara K, Otsuka T, Kano H, Matsuno S, Takai H, et al. Effects of smoking habit on the prevalence of atrial fibrillation in Japanese patients with special reference to sex differences. Circ J. 2013;77(12):2948–53.

37. Etzion Y. A stimulating environment for the atrial kick: spinal cord stimulation can inhibit atrial fibrillation. Heart Rhythm. 2012;9(9):1434–5.

12

Adherence and outcomes to direct oral anticoagulants among patients with atrial fibrillation: findings from the veterans health administration

Ryan T. Borne[1*] (iD), Colin O'Donnell[2], Mintu P. Turakhia[3,4], Paul D. Varosy[1,2], Cynthia A. Jackevicius[5], Lucas N. Marzec[1], Frederick A. Masoudi[1], Paul L. Hess[1,2], Thomas M. Maddox[6] and P. Michael Ho[1,2]

Abstract

Background: The direct oral anticoagulants (DOACs) reduce the risk of stroke in moderate to high-risk patients with non-valvular atrial fibrillation (AF). Yet, concerns remain regarding its routine use in real world practice. We sought to describe adherence patterns and the association between adherence and outcomes to the DOACs among outpatients with AF.

Methods: We performed a retrospective cohort study of patients in the VA Healthcare System who initiated pharmacotherapy with dabigatran, rivaroxaban, or apixaban between November 2010 and January 2015 for non-valvular AF with CHA_2DS_2-VASc score $\geq$ 2. Adherence was determined using pharmacy refill data and estimated by the proportion of days covered (PDC) over the first year of therapy. Clinical outcomes, including all-cause mortality and stroke, were measured at 6 months and used to assess measures of adherence for each DOAC.

Results: A total of 2882 patients were included. Most were prescribed dabigatran (72.7%), compared with rivaroxaban (19.8%) or apixaban (7.5%). The mean PDC was 0.84 ± 0.20 for dabigatran, 0.86 ± 0.18 for rivaroxaban, and 0.89 ± 0.14 for apixaban ($p < 0.01$). The proportion of non-adherent patients, PDC <0.80, was 27.6% for all and varied according DOAC. Lower adherence to dabigatran was associated with higher risk of mortality and stroke (HR 1.07; 1.03–1.12 per 0. 10 decline in PDC).

Conclusions: In a real-world VA population being prescribed anticoagulation for AF, more than one quarter had sub-optimal adherence. Lower adherence was associated with a higher risk of mortality and stroke. Efforts identifying non-adherent patients, and targeted adherence interventions are needed to improve outcomes.

Keywords: Medication adherence, Atrial fibrillation, Direct oral anticoagulants

Background

Atrial fibrillation (AF) is the most common cardiac arrhythmia, with around 5 million new cases each year [1]. Anticoagulation significantly reduces the incidence of clinical stroke and mortality among patients with AF at moderate to high risk of thromboembolic events (CHA_2DS_2-VASc $\geq$2) [2]. Based on the results of multiple randomized controlled trials (RCTs), the direct oral anticoagulants (DOACs) are now frequently used to reduce this risk [3–5]. Additionally, they have demonstrated favorable risk-benefit profiles compared to warfarin with significant reductions in stroke, intracranial hemorrhage, and mortality [6].

While decades of knowledge have demonstrated the safety and efficacy of warfarin, less is known about how the DOACs have been adopted into routine clinical care. Furthermore, concerns remain about DOACs because of their shorter half-lives and the potential for reductions in effectiveness with poor adherence. Because of the lack of laboratory monitoring to assess therapeutic levels, it

* Correspondence: ryan.borne@ucdenver.edu
[1]Division of Cardiology – Campus Box B130, University of Colorado Anschutz Medical Campus, 12631 E. 17th Avenue, Aurora, CO 80045, USA
Full list of author information is available at the end of the article

is important to assess adherence to DOACs and the extent to which it varies by patient characteristics and different DOACs currently available. The VA health care system, being the largest integrated healthcare system with an anticoagulation infrastructure and standard copayments, offers a unique opportunity to examine real-world adherence under ideal conditions.

Accordingly, we evaluated adherence patterns to the three approved DOACs (as of January 2015) and the association between adherence with outcomes among patients with AF and prescribed DOACs in the VA Healthcare System. Specifically, we sought to characterize adherence using portion of days covered (PDC) to dabigatran, rivoraxaban, and apixaban separately. Second, we assessed the patient level factors associated with nonadherence. Finally, we assessed the association between lower adherence and outcomes of stroke and mortality for each of the DOACs.

Methods

Study design

We performed a retrospective cohort study of patients in the VA Healthcare System who initiated pharmacotherapy with dabigatran, rivaroxaban, or apixaban between November 2010 and January 2015 for non-valvular AF with CHA_2DS_2-VASc score ≥ 2. Given its recent approval, edoxaban was not included in this study due to the time during which this analysis was performed. Patients were included who had the earliest DOAC prescription in November 2010 and those who were on warfarin from June, 2006. Patients with AF or atrial flutter were identified from the VA Corporate Data Warehouse medical files through a principal or secondary diagnosis of AF (ICD-9 code 427.3, 427.31, 427.32). Patients could have been taking warfarin previously and switched to a DOAC, or started on a DOAC de novo. Because we were interested in assessing adherence behavior to DOACs, we excluded patients with less than 1 year follow-up after starting a DOAC, patients who initiated a DOAC and then crossed over to warfarin, and patients who were started on 2 or more different DOACs during follow-up.

Medication adherence

Adherence to each DOAC was calculated in the first year of therapy. Adherence was measured using the proportion of days covered (PDC), which is a validated measure previously correlated with DOAC outcomes [3, 4]. The PDC was defined as the number of doses dispensed in relation to the dispensing period. [5, 6] The numerator was based on the prescription fill dates and number of pills dispensed to determine the number of outpatient days for which each DOAC was supplied. Patients were considered

adherent if they achieved a PDC > 80%, a commonly used standard [7]. As a sensitivity analysis, differences in DOAC adherence stratified by prior warfarin use was also evaluated.

Mortality and stroke

We assessed a composite of all-cause mortality and stroke as the primary outcome of interest. Mortality was obtained through the VA Vital Status File, which compiles data from the *Beneficiary Identification Records Locator Subsystem* Death File, VA Medicare Vital Status File, and the Social Security Administration Death Master File. Stroke (ischemic and hemorrhagic) was obtained using previously validated primary or secondary *International Classification of Diseases, 9th Revision, Clinical Modification (ICD-9-CM)* diagnostic codes (346.60, 346.61, 346.62, 346.63, 431, 433.01, 433.11, 433.21, 433.31, 433.81, 433.91, 434.01, 434.11, 434.91, 997.02) [8].

Statistical analysis

Testing for differences in the proportions of dichotomous covariates across the 3 DOAC drugs were calculated with the network algorithm of Mehta and Patel, rather than the less efficient Freeman-Halton extension to 2 × 3 tables of the Fisher exact test. The one-way analysis of variance Savage score was used to test for differences in location for the continuous covariates. A Generalized Estimating Equation (GEE) logistic regression with adjustment for risk factors and a term to adjust for patients clustered within hospitals was used to evaluate the interaction of prior warfarin use vs. de novo treatment with DOAC type and to determine significant risk factors for the outcome of nonadherence. Similarly, a GEE linear model was used to determine the interaction effect of prior warfarin use on PDC at one year.

Cox proportional hazards models adjusted for patient risk factors (heart failure, age, diabetes, stroke/transient ischemic attack, vascular disease, sex, coronary artery disease), and a term for patients within hospital (frailty, a standard statistical term in time to event analyses indicating adjustment for correlated random effects), were used to assess measures of PDC at 6 months and nonadherence at 6 months on the combined endpoint of mortality and/or stroke for each DOAC. The results for mortality and stroke for apixaban were not included due to the low event rate.

All analyses were performed using SAS9.4 TS Level 1 M3 software, © 2002–2012 by SAS Institute Inc., Cary, NC, USA. The Colorado Multiple Institutional Review board approved this study and waiver of informed consent was granted. The authors are solely responsible for the design and conduct, drafting, and editing of this manuscript and its contents.

Results

Over the study period, a total of 10,279 patients were started on DOACs. After excluding patients with less than 1-year follow-up period (n = 3111), those who were prescribed more than 1 DOAC during the study period (n = 872), those who were prescribed warfarin after DOAC initiation (n = 1446) and those with CHA_2DS_2-VASc score < 2 (n = 1968), a total of 2882 patients were included in the analysis (Fig. 1).

Baseline patient characteristics are described in Table 1. The mean age of the cohort was 67.4 ± 9.5, most whom were white (82.7%) and male (96.9%). Co-morbidities included hypertension (88.7%), diabetes mellitus (48.5%), congestive heart failure (29.6%), cerebrovascular disease (11.1%), and prior myocardial infarction (13.6%). The mean and median CHA_2DS_2-VASc score were 2.9 ± 1.1 and 3 (IQR 2–3), respectively. Most patients in the cohort were prescribed dabigatran (72.7%), compared with rivaroxaban (19.8%) or apixaban (7.5%). Differences in patient level characteristics between DOACs were largely similar with significant differences seen in age (mean age among patients prescribed dabigatran 66.9 vs. 73.1 for apixaban), rate of hypertension (89.4% for dabigatran vs. 83.3% for apixaban), and CHA_2DS_2-VASc score (2.89 for dabigatran vs. 3.2 for apixaban).

The mean PDC was 0.84 ± 0.20 for dabigatran, 0.86 ± 0.18 for rivaroxaban, and 0.89 ± 0.14 for apixaban (p < 0.01) (Table 1). The proportion of non-adherent patients, defined as PDC <0.80, was 28.8%, 25.0%, 22.8% respectively (p = 0.05). Adherence using PDC stratified by patients who had previously been on warfarin and those who were started de novo are described in Table 2. There was a statistically significant small difference in PDC between drug types and history of prior warfarin use (P < 0.01). Based on PDC <80% for nonadherence, there was no statistically significant difference between drug types and history of prior warfarin use (P = 0.44).

Table 3 describe factors associated with nonadherence, where an odds ratio of >1 is associated with greater nonadherence and an odds ratio < 1 is associated with greater adherence. Age in years (OR, 0.98; 95% CI, 0.96–0.99; p < 0.01), hypertension (OR, 0.69; 95% CI, 0.49–0.99; p = 0.04), diabetes (OR, 0.57; 95% CI, 0.41–0.79; p < 0.01), and stroke (OR, 0.36; 95% CI, 0.2–0.68; p < 0.01) were associated with greater adherence.

The combined end-point of mortality and/or stroke based on adherence patterns are described in Table 4. The total number of follow-up days was 1,922,857, with mean (SD) and median (IQR) of 667.2 (432.2) and 582 (388, 933), respectively. The overall rate of death and stroke were 17.4% (502) and 1.7% (49), respectively.

Among patients on dabigatran, there was a significant association between lower adherence (per 0.1 decline in PDC measured over the initial 6 months after initiation of therapy) and higher risk of death or stroke; (HR, 1.07; 95% CI, 1.03–1.12; per 0.1 drop in the PDC; p < 0.01; n = 277 total events; death = 253, stroke = 24). Among patients on rivaroxaban, there was a trend for an association between lower adherence at 6 months (per 0.1 decline in PDC) and higher risk of mortality and stroke (HR, 1.07; 95% CI, 0.89–1.28; p = 0.46; n = 25 total events; death = 24, stroke = 1]. In secondary analysis, nonadherence (PDC <80%) at 6 months to dabigatran was associated with increased risk of death or stroke (HR, 1.54; 95% CI, 1.20–1.97; p < 0.01). There was a similar trend for rivaroxaban but it was not statistically significant (HR, 1.74; 95% CI, 0.77–3.94; p = 0.18). Outcomes analyses were not conducted for apixaban due to the small number of events (n = 5).

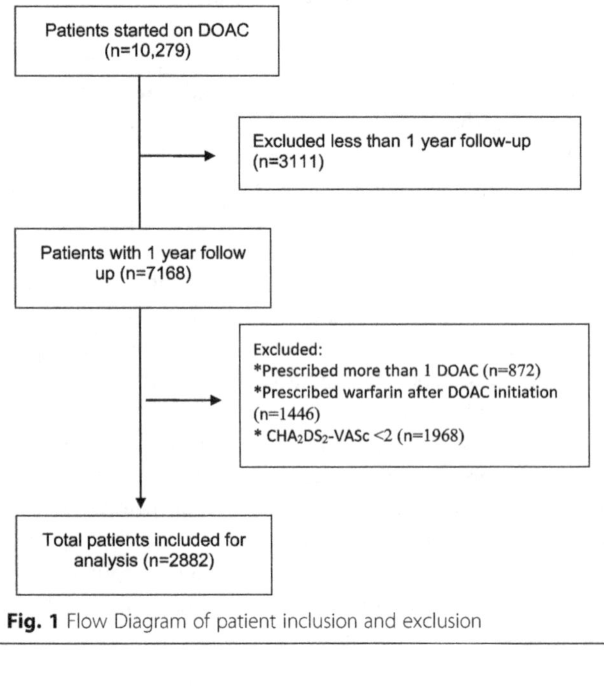

Discussion

Using VHA data from June 2006 to January 2015, we characterized adherence to DOACs and assessed the association between nonadherence and outcomes among patients in the VA Healthcare System. There were three main findings. First, 1 in 4 patients had sub-optimal adherence, which varied slightly based on the DOAC. Second, several patient factors were associated with greater medication adherence, including older age, diabetes, and stroke. Third, nonadherence was associated with adverse outcomes including mortality and stroke for dabigatran, with a similar trend for rivoraxaban.

Fig. 1 Flow Diagram of patient inclusion and exclusion

Table 1 Baseline characteristics among patients being prescribed DOACs

Patient Characteristics	All n = 2882	Dabigatran n = 2096 (72.7%)	Rivaroxaban n = 571 (19.8%)	Apixaban n = 215 (7.5%)	p
Age (mean + SD)	67.4 (9.5)	66.9 (9.3)	67.3 (9.7)	73.1 (8.8)	<0.01
Male (%)	2792 (96.9)	2035 (97.1)	552 (96.7)	205 (95.4)	0.32
White Race (%)	2383 (82.7)	1735 (82.8)	467 (81.8)	181 (84.2)	0.72
Hypertension (%)	2556 (88.7)	1874 (89.4)	503 (88.1)	179 (83.3)	0.03
Congestive Heart Failure (%)	852 (29.6)	624 (29.8)	173 (30.3)	55 (25.6)	0.41
Diabetes Mellitus (%)	1398 (48.5)	1036 (49.4)	270 (47.3)	92 (42.8)	0.15
Cerebrovascular Accident (%)	321 (11.1)	240 (11.5)	63 (11.0)	18 (8.4)	0.41
Prior Myocardial Infarction (%)	391 (13.6)	269 (12.8)	89 (15.6)	33 (15.4)	0.16
Peripheral Arterial Disease (%)	280 (9.7)	201 (9.6)	53 (9.3)	26 (12.1)	0.45
Peripheral Arterial Disease (%)	2.9 (1.1)	2.9 (1.0)	3.0 (1.1)	3.2 (1.2)	<0.01
CHA_2DS_2-VASc (mean + SD)	2.9 (1.1)	2.9 (1.0)	3.0 (1.1)	3.2 (1.2)	<0.01
Adherence					
Mean (SD) pill count per dispensed supply	38.1 (20.9)	38.2 (20.8)	38.2 (22.0)	36.4 (18.7)	<0.01
Proportion of Days Covered (mean + SD)	0.85 (0.19)	0.84 (0.20)	0.86 (0.18)	0.89 (0.14)	<0.01
PDC < 80% n (%)	796 (27.6%)	604 (28.8%)	143 (25.0%)	49 (22.8%)	0.05

Medication nonadherence is a prevalent and growing concern among healthcare providers. Previous investigations have described adherence patterns to dabigatran. Using the Danish National Prescription Registry, Gorst-Rasmussen evaluated 2960 patients started on dabigatran for AF [9]. The mean one-year PDC was 0.84 and about one-quarter of patients were nonadherent (PDC <80%). Among 17,000 patients on dabigatran, PDC among de novo starters were 0.67 and 0.71 for those previously on warfarin [10]. Schulmann interviewed a small cohort of patients (103) and found that 88% of patients were adherent (PDC >80%) to dabigatran [11]. The VA Healthcare System offers a unique opportunity to examine real-world adherence under ideal conditions. It is the largest integrated healthcare system and has specific processes of care by which anticoagulation is safely administered (including anticoagulation clinics and a clinical pharmacist infrastructure). Additionally, copayments are standard across oral anticoagulation agents which does not lead to a differential copayment burden. A previous investigation in the VA population demonstrated that 27.8% of patients on dabigatran for AF were nonadherent, which was also associated with an increased risk for all-cause mortality and stroke [8]. Our findings further this knowledge by demonstrating that nonadherence is common, even among the newer DOACs. Furthermore, these findings are in direct discordance with adherence patterns seen in randomized controlled trials which are generally higher. Differences in adherence patterns between clinical trials and routine clinical practice are multifactorial and include a potential Hawthorne effect for those enrolled in clinical trials and lack of close follow up, high incidence of comorbidities and polypharmacy, and/or financial constraints for those in routine clinical care. Additional research is needed to determine which factors can be targeted to maximize patient outcomes.

Predictors of greater adherence included older age and a history of hypertension, diabetes, and stroke. Factors previously known to be associated with nonadherence include male gender, homelessness, and psychiatric disorders, particularly depression while those associated with greater adherence include high level of education, stability of family background, and affordability to therapy [12–15]. Additionally, treatment of asymptomatic disease is associated with poor adherence [15]. Importantly, cardiovascular disease, such as in some cases of atrial fibrillation, are generally asymptomatic chronic diseases where the perceived benefits of daily medical therapy may not be apparent to patients. Among these patients, physicians should have a heightened awareness of the possibility of poor adherence and consider directly asking patients about their adherence.

Table 2 Adherence patterns among patients previously on warfarin and those started de novo

	Dabigatran	Rivaroxaban	Apixaban	p
De novo (Mean, SD)	0.84 (0.20)	0.87 (0.19)	0.87 (0.15)	<0.01
Prior warfarin use (Mean, SD)	0.84 (0.19)	0.86 (0.18)	0.89 (0.14)	<0.01

Table 3 Predictors of medication nonadherence

Parameter	All Drugs (Dabigatran reference drug) Odds Ratio (95% CI)	Dabigatran Odds Ratio (95% CI)	Rivaroxaban Odds Ratio (95% CI)	Apixaban Odds Ratio (95% CI)
Age	0.98 (0.96, 0.99)	0.99 (0.97, 1.00)	0.96 (0.93, 0.99)	0.97 (0.90, 1.04)
Male	0.85 (0.54, 1.34)	0.85 (0.47, 1.53)	1.58 (0.54, 4.61)	0.26 (0.06, 1.13)
White Race	0.73 (0.59, 0.92)	0.69 (0.53, 0.90)	0.81 (0.48, 1.37)	0.61 (0.23, 1.65)
Hypertension	0.69 (0.49, 0.99)	0.74 (0.47, 1.16)	0.64 (0.27, 1.50)	0.66 (0.17, 2.61)
Congestive Heart Failure	0.74 (0.53, 1.03)	0.91 (0.61, 1.36)	0.52 (0.24, 1.13)	0.28 (0.07, 1.10)
Diabetes Mellitus	0.57 (0.41, 0.79)	0.68 (0.47, 0.97)	0.56 (0.27, 1.14)	0.15 (0.03, 0.67)
CVA	0.36 (0.20, 0.68)	0.47 (0.23, 0.94)	0.29 (0.06, 1.40)	0.11 (0.01, 1.43)
Prior Myocardial Infarction	1.20 (0.96, 1.50)	1.40 (1.07, 1.82)	0.88 (0.55, 1.39)	0.53 (0.18, 1.53)
Peripheral Arterial Disease	0.99 (0.72, 1.36)	0.96 (0.68, 1.34)	1.14 (0.60, 2.17)	1.32 (0.49, 3.54)
CHA_2DS_2-VASc Score	0.88 (0.76, 1.01)	0.81 (0.68, 0.97)	1.09 (0.85, 1.41)	0.81 (0.40, 1.64)

Adherence to DOACs was a significant predictor of outcomes including all-cause mortality and stroke. A similar association of risk of death or stroke was seen among the 27.8% of non-adherent patients on dabigatran, with a hazard ratio of 1.13 (95% CI 1.07–1.19) [8]. Furthermore, prior studies have shown similar associations of risk and nonadherence among patients with coronary artery disease, heart failure, hypertension, and hyperlipidemia [16–19]. For example, among 10,000 patients with diabetes, 21% were non-adherent which was associated with an increased risk for all-cause hospitalization and mortality [16]. These findings suggest that medication nonadherence is common among many chronic illnesses and highly impacts outcomes.

There are a few implications of these findings. First, while adherence was significantly different stratified by DOAC, the absolute difference was very small. Similarly, differences in demographic and co-morbidities associated with nonadherence were small and determining nonadherence to DOACs based on these clinical characteristics may be difficult. This suggests that other mechanisms to detect patients at risk for nonadherence need to be identified, including directly asking patients about adherence or utilizing data systems in which prescription refills, or lack thereof, are recorded and provided in real-time. Further evaluation of such data systems should be

developed to determine if they can successfully be implemented and improve patient adherence. Additionally, it is often thought that adherence to medical therapy improves with simplification; however, we found that adherence to the once daily rivaroxaban did not have better adherence rate. Further studies are needed to evaluate this perception.

Certain factors should be considered in the interpretation of this study. First, our analysis was confined to patients in the VA Healthcare System with the clear majority of patients being white males. Thus, our results may not apply to the broader population of patients being prescribed DOACs. However, the VA provides an opportunity to examine adherence in a closed pharmacy system with highly reliable data sources because refill data for these medications are well captured given the smaller copay in the VA. Second, while we utilized pharmacy databases to capture medication dispensing, there is a lack of distinction between dispensing and consumption, making this type of analysis less reliable at the individual level. However, refill adherence has previously been shown to be an accurate marker of patients' adherence in the VA system [20]. Additionally, direct methods of assessing adherence (i.e. directly observed therapy) have limitations and are not practical for routine clinical use. Third, there were relatively fewer patients on rivaroxaban and apixaban as these are newer to the VA system and their use is dependent on contraindications or previous intolerance to dabigatran. Therefore, broader examination of outcomes is limited due to lack of power given the relatively smaller sample size. Furthermore, longer term outcomes are limited given the exclusion of a large majority of patients who had less than one year follow up. Additionally, the impact of longer duration of follow up on adherence or outcomes was not addressed but should be explored in future analysis. Fourth, direct comparisons between classes of DOACs were not

Table 4 Time fixed analysis for mortality and stroke based on adherence

	Dabigatran HR (95% CI)	p	Rivaroxaban HR (95% CI)	p
PDC 6 month (per 0.1 decline)	1.07 (1.03–1.12)	<0.01	1.07 (0.89–1.28)	0.46
Nonadherence 6 month	1.54 (1.20–1.97)	<0.01	1.74 (0.77–3.94)	0.18

Models were adjusted for demographics and comorbidities (heart failure, age, diabetes, stroke/transient ischemic attack, vascular disease, sex, coronary artery disease)

performed as we are unable to account for unmeasured confounders and selection bias for the determination of which DOAC was selected. Fifth, we did not evaluate the association between adherence and bleeding given the low rate of bleeding events. Sixth, a large portion of patients (1446) were excluded after having been prescribed warfarin after DOAC initiation. The reasons for such were unclear from this study and further evaluation is needed to address reasons for a change in anticoagulation strategies. Finally, our results are likely an overestimation of adherence based on the exclusions. For example, by excluding patients who stopped or did not tolerate a DOAC, we selected a group of patients more likely to adhere to medical therapy and thus increasing the adherence rate beyond what is seen in practice.

Conclusions

This study characterizes adherence patterns and outcomes among patients in the VA Healthcare System using DOACs for AF. First, more than one quarter of patients had sub-optimal adherence with DOACs. While there were differences in adherence between DOAC and patient characteristics, these were not clinically significant. Second, outcomes including all-cause mortality and stroke were associated with medication adherence. Efforts towards identifying non-adherent patients and targeting adherence interventions are needed.

Abbreviations
AF: Atrial fibrillation; DOAC: Direct oral anticoagulant; GEE: Generalized estimating equation; HR: Hazard ratio; IQR: Interquartile range; PDC: Proportion of days covered; RCT: Randomized controlled trial; SD: Standard deviation

Acknowledgements
Not applicable.

Funding
There was no funding for this manuscript.

Authors' contributions
RTB, COD, PMH contributed manuscript writing. RTB, COD, MPT, PDV, CAJ, LNM, FAM, PLH, TMM, and PMH contributed to analysis and interpretation of data and were involved in revising the manuscript critically for important intellectual content and gave final approval of the published version.

Competing interests
PMH is the deputy editor of Circulation: Cardiovascular Quality and Outcomes journal and serves in the steering committee for Janssen, Inc. trial t60 improve adherence to DOACs. There are otherwise no conflicts for all other others pertaining to the work.

Author details
¹Division of Cardiology – Campus Box B130, University of Colorado Anschutz Medical Campus, 12631 E. 17th Avenue, Aurora, CO 80045, USA. ²VA Eastern Colorado Health Care System, Denver, CO, USA. ³Veterans Affairs Palo Alto Health Care System, Palo Alto, CA, USA. ⁴Stanford University School of Medicine, Stanford, CA, USA. ⁵VA Greater Los Angeles Healthcare System, Institute for Clinical Evaluative Sciences, Western University of Health Sciences, Los Angeles, CA, USA. ⁶Washington University School of Medicine, St. Louis, MO, USA.

References
1. Chugh SS, Havmoeller R, Narayanan K, et al. Worldwide epidemiology of atrial fibrillation: a global burden of disease 2010 study. Circulation. 2014; 129(8):837–47.
2. Hart RG, Pearce LA, Aguilar MI. Meta-analysis: antithrombotic therapy to prevent stroke in patients who have nonvalvular atrial fibrillation. Ann Intern Med. 2007;146(12):857.
3. Connolly SJ, Ezekowitz MD, Yusuf S, Eikelboom J, Oldgren J, Parekh A, Pogue J, TE RPAV, Wang S, Alings M, Xavier D, Zhu J, Diaz R, Lewis BS, Darius H, Diener HC, Joyner CD, Wallentin L, RE-LY Steering Committee and Investigators. Dabigatran versus warfarin in patients with atrial fibrillation. N Engl J Med. 2009;361(12):1139.
4. Granger CB, Alexander JH, McMurray JJ, Lopes RD, Hylek EM, Hanna M, Al-Khalidi HR, Ansell J, Atar D, Avezum A, Bahit MC, Diaz R, Easton JD, Ezekowitz JA, Flaker G, Garcia D, Geraldes M, Gersh BJ, Golitsyn S, Goto S, Hermosillo AG, Hohnloser SH, Horowitz J, Mohan P, Jansky P, Lewis BS, Lopez-Sendon JL, Pais P, Parkhomenko A, Verheugt FW, Zhu J, Wallentin L, ARISTOTLE Committees and Investigators. Apixaban versus Warfarin in patients with Atrial fibrillation. N Engl J Med. 2011;365(11):981.
5. Patel MR, Mahaffrey KW, Garg J, Pan G, Singer DE, Hacke W, Breithardt G, Halperin JL, Hankey GJ, Piccini JP, Becker RC, Nessel CC, Paolini JF, Berkowitz SD, Fox KA, Califf RM, ROCKET AF Investigators. Rivaroxaban versus Warfarin in Nonvalvular Atrial fibrillation. N Engl J Med. 2011;365(10):883.
6. Ruff CT, Giugliano RP, Braunwald E, et al. Comparison of the efficacy and safety of new oral anticoagulants with warfarin in patients with atrial fibrillation: a meta-analysis of randomized trials. Lancet. 2014;383(9921):955.
7. Ho PM, Bryson CL, Rumsfeld JS. Medication adherence: its importance in cardiovascular outcomes. Circulation. 2009;119:3028–35.
8. Shore S, Carey EP, Turkhia MP, Jackevicius CA, Cunningham F, Pilote L, Bradley SM, Maddox TM, Grunwald GK, Baron AE, Rumsfeld JS, Varosy PD, Schneider PM, Marzec LN, Ho PM. Adherence to dabigatran therapy and longitudinal patient outcomes: insights from the veterans health administration. Am Heart J. 2014;167:810–7.
9. Gorst-Rasmussen A, Skjoth F, Larsen TB, Rasmussen LH, Lip GYH, Lane DA. Dabigatran adherence in atrial fibrillation patients during the first year after diagnosis: a nation wide cohort study. J Thromb Haemost. 2015;13(4):495–504.
10. Tsai K, Erickson SC, Yang J, Harada AS, Solow BK, Lew HC. Adherence, persistence, and switching patterns of dabigatran etexilate. Am J Manag Care. 2013;19(9):e325–32.
11. Schulman S, Shortt B, Robinson M, Eikelboom JW. Adherence to anticoagulant treatment with dabigatran in a real-world setting. J Thromb Haemost. 2013;11:1295–9.
12. Ho PM, Magid DJ, Shetterly SM, Olson KL, Maddox TM, Peterson PN, Masoudi FA, Rumsfeld JS. Medication nonadherence is associated with a broad range of adverse outcomes in patients with coronary artery disease. Am Heart J. 2008;155(4):772–229.
13. Mochari H, Ferris A, Adigopula S, Henry G, Mosca L. Cardiovascular disease knowledge, medication adherence, and barriers to preventative action in a minority population. Prev Cardiol. 2007;10(4):190–5.
14. Song X, Sander SD, Varker H, Amin A. Patterns and predictors of use of warfarin and other common long-term medications in patients with atrial fibrillation. Am J Cardiovasc Drugs. 2012;12(4):245–53.
15. Osterberg L, Blaschke T. Adherence to medication. N Engl J Med. 2005; 353(5):487–97.
16. Ho PM, Rumsfeld JS, Masoudi FA, McClure DL, Plomondon ME, Steiner JF, Magid DJ. Effect of medication nonadherence on hospitalization and mortality among patients with diabetes mellitus. Arch Intern Med. 2006;166:1863–41.
17. Rasmussen JN, Chong A, Alter DA. Relationship between adherence to evidence-based pharmacotherapy and long-term mortality after acute

myocardial infarction. JAMA. 2007;297:177–86.

18. Spertus JA, Kettelkamp P, Vance C, Decker C, Jones PG, Rumsfeld JS, Messenger JC, Khanal S, Peterson ED, Bach RG, Krumholz HM, Cohen DJ. Prevalence, predictors, and outcomes of premature discontinuation of thienopyridine therapy after drug-eluting stent placement: results from the PREMIER registry. Circulation. 2006;113:2803–9.

19. Hope CJ, Wu J, Tu W, Young J, Murray MD. Association of medication adherence, knowledge, and skills with emergency department visits by adults 50 years or older with congestive heart failure. Am J Health Syst Pharm. 2004;61:2043–9.

20. Hess LM, Raebel MA, Conner DA, et al. Measurement of adherence in pharmacy administrative databases: a proposal for standard definitions and preferred measures. Ann Pharmachother. 2006;40:1280–8.

13

Cost-effectiveness analysis of left atrial appendage occlusion compared with pharmacological strategies for stroke prevention in atrial fibrillation

Vivian Wing-Yan Lee[1*], Ronald Bing-Ching Tsai[1], Ines Hang-Iao Chow[1], Bryan Ping-Yen Yan[2], Mehmet Gungor Kaya[3], Jai-Wun Park[4] and Yat-Yin Lam[2]

Abstract

Background: Transcatheter left atrial appendage occlusion (LAAO) is a promising therapy for stroke prophylaxis in non-valvular atrial fibrillation (NVAF) but its cost-effectiveness remains understudied. This study evaluated the cost-effectiveness of LAAO for stroke prophylaxis in NVAF.

Methods: A Markov decision analytic model was used to compare the cost-effectiveness of LAAO with 7 pharmacological strategies: aspirin alone, clopidogrel plus aspirin, warfarin, dabigatran 110 mg, dabigatran 150 mg, apixaban, and rivaroxaban. Outcome measures included quality-adjusted life years (QALYs), lifetime costs and incremental cost-effectiveness ratios (ICERs). Base-case data were derived from ACTIVE, RE-LY, ARISTOTLE, ROCKET-AF, PROTECT-AF and PREVAIL trials. One-way sensitivity analysis varied by $CHADS_2$ score, HAS-BLED score, time horizons, and LAAO costs; and probabilistic sensitivity analysis using 10,000 Monte Carlo simulations was conducted to assess parameter uncertainty.

Results: LAAO was considered cost-effective compared with aspirin, clopidogrel plus aspirin, and warfarin, with ICER of US$5,115, $2,447, and $6,298 per QALY gained, respectively. LAAO was dominant (i.e. less costly but more effective) compared to other strategies. Sensitivity analysis demonstrated favorable ICERs of LAAO against other strategies in varied $CHADS_2$ score, HAS-BLED score, time horizons (5 to 15 years) and LAAO costs. LAAO was cost-effective in 86.24 % of 10,000 simulations using a threshold of US$50,000/QALY.

Conclusions: Transcatheter LAAO is cost-effective for prevention of stroke in NVAF compared with 7 pharmacological strategies.

Condensed abstract: The transcatheter left atrial appendage occlusion (LAAO) is considered cost-effective against the standard 7 oral pharmacological strategies including acetylsalicylic acid (ASA) alone, clopidogrel plus ASA, warfarin, dabigatran 110 mg, dabigatran 150 mg, apixaban, and rivaroxaban for stroke prophylaxis in non-valvular atrial fibrillation management.

Keywords: Atrial fibrillation, Cost-effectiveness, Left atrial appendage occlusion, Stroke prevention

Abbreviations: AF, Atrial fibrillation; ASA, Acetylsalicylic acid; ICERs, Incremental cost-effectiveness ratios; ICH, Intracranial hemorrhage; LAA, Left atrial appendage; LAAO, Left atrial appendage occlusion; NOACs, Novel oral anticoagulants; NVAF, Non-valvular atrial fibrillation; QALYs, Quality-adjusted life years; TEE, Transesophageal echocardiography; TIA, Transient ischemic attack

* Correspondence: vivianlee@cuhk.edu.hk
[1]School of Pharmacy, Faculty of Medicine, The Chinese University of Hong Kong, 8th Floor, Lo Kwee-Seong Integrated Biomedical Sciences Building, Area 39, Shatin, Hong Kong
Full list of author information is available at the end of the article

Background

Atrial fibrillation (AF) is associated with 4–5 fold increase risk for thromboembolic stroke [1]. Oral anticoagulation therapy with warfarin is the standard therapy for stroke prevention, but is difficult to maintain within the narrow therapeutic range and is under-prescribed in clinical practice. Potential alternatives to warfarin include anti-platelet therapy [2], novel oral anticoagulants (NOACs) such as direct thrombin or factor Xa inhibitors [3, 4] and exclusion of the left atrial appendage (LAA) as a major embolic source [5, 6]. The randomized-controlled WATCHMAN Left Atrial Appendage System for Embolic Protection in Patients with Atrial Fibrillation (PROTECT-AF) trial [5] demonstrated that device occlusion of the LAA orifice by the WATCHMAN device (Boston Scientific, Natick, MA, USA) was non-inferior to warfarin for the prevention of thromboembolic events in NVAF patients. The cost of this device ranges from US$5,770 to US$10,000 depending on the country.

According to recent published economic evaluation studies of LAA compared with warfarin or NOACs, the results indicated that LAA was a cost-effective alternative for stroke prevention in AF patients [7, 8]. However, comprehensive comparison with LAA and each oral anticoagulant should be evaluated to demonstrate significant outcomes. This study estimated the lifetime cost-effectiveness of transcatheter left atrial appendage occlusion (LAAO) for stroke prophylaxis in a hypothetical cohort of 65-year-old patients with non-valvular AF as compared to other pharmacological strategies.

Methods

Decision analytical model

A Markov decision analytic model was used to perform a cost-effectiveness analysis from a US healthcare provider perspective expressed in US dollars. The model was developed using TreeAge Pro Suite 2014 software (TreeAge Software, Inc., Williamstown, MA) for evaluating the long-term costs and effectiveness of treatment strategies for stroke prevention. Outcome measures included quality-adjusted life years (QALYs), lifetime costs and incremental cost-effectiveness ratios (ICERs). All costs and QALYs were discounted at an annual rate of 3 %. The ICERs of < US$50,000 per QALY was considered cost-effective [9].

Model

The model of patients wth AF for stroke prevention was adapted from literature and cardiology consultation [8, 10]. A cohort of 65-year-old patients with non-valvular AF without contraindication to anti-thrombotic therapies was simulated moving between different health states in each Markov cycle of 1 year. The time horizon was lifetime (85 years old). Health states in the model included patient in AF without event, with event before, ischemic stroke (no residual, mild moderate to severe, fatal), transient ischemic attack (TIA), hemorrhage [minor, major, intracranial hemorrhage (ICH), fatal], myocardial infarction (MI), death from vascular cause, and death from all causes. Seven different pharmacological strategies for stroke prevention including acetylsalicyclic acid (ASA) alone (75 to 100 mg), clopidogrel (75 mg) plus ASA, warfarin, dabigatran 110 mg, dabigatran 150 mg, apixaban (5 mg) and rivaroxaban (20 mg) were compared with LAAO. After LAAO, we assumed patients were treated with warfarin for 45 days followed by clopidogrel plus ASA for 180 days, and then lifelong ASA in our study model as in the WATCHMAN trial. There are studies such as the ASA Plavix Feasibility Study with Watchman Left Atrial Appendage Closure Technology (ASAP) study, which used antiplatelet therapy alone after LAAO [5, 11, 12].

Model parameters

Base-case values for analytic model were derived from published randomized studies including Atrial Fibrillation Clopidogrel Trial with Irbesartan for Prevention of Vascular Events (ACTIVE), Randomized Evaluation of Long-Term Anticoagulation Therapy (RE-LY), Apixaban for Reduction in Stroke and Other Throm-boembolic Events in Atrial Fibrillation (ARISTOTLE), Rivaroxaban Once Daily Oral Direct Factor Xa Inhibition Compared with Vitamin K Antagonism for Prevention of Stroke and Embolism Trial in Atrial Fibrillation (ROCKET-AF), Watchman Left Atrial Appendage System for Embolic Protection in Patients With Atrial Fibrillation (PROTECT-AF), and Prospective Randomized Evaluation of the WATCH-MAN LAA Closure Device In Patients with Atrial Fibrillation Versus Long Term Warfarin Therapy (PREVAIL) trials [2–5, 13, 14]. Table 1 summarized the clinical inputs and data sources used in the base-case analysis. Warfarin event rates were pooled warfarin events from RE-LY, ROCKET-AF, and ARISTOTLE trails [3, 4, 13].

Ischemic stroke

The annual ischemic stroke rates were $2 \cdot 8$ %, $1 \cdot 9$ %, $1 \cdot 21$ %, $1 \cdot 34$ %, $0 \cdot 92$ %, $0 \cdot 97$ %, $1 \cdot 34$ % and $0 \cdot 84$ % for ASA alone, clopidogrel plus ASA, warfarin, dabigatran 110 mg, dabigatran 150 mg, apixaban, rivaroxaban, and LAA occlusion, respectively [2–4, 13, 15–18]. Additionally, TIA accounted for 28 % [15, 17] of all neurological ischemic events in this model. The annual ischemic stroke rate of LAA occlusion was pooled by PROTECT-AF and PREVAIL trails [5, 14]. Proportion of 4 sub-classifications of ischemic stroke (no residual, mild, moderate to severe, fatal) varied according to therapy [15, 17].

Table 1 Clinical inputs for base-case value and ranges in decision analytic model

Variable	Base-Case	Range		References
Stroke				
Annual rate of ischemic stroke, %				
Aspirin alone	2·80	2·80	4·50	[2, 18]
Clopidogrel plus aspirin	1·90	1·69	2·11	[2]
Warfarin	1·21	1·05	1·42	[3, 4, 13]
Dabigatran, 110 mg	1·34	1·31	1·55	[3, 15]
Dabigatran, 150 mg	0·92	0·75	1·09	[3, 15]
Apixaban	0·97	0·78	1·19	[13, 16]
Rivaroxaban	1·34	1·07	1·66	[4, 16]
LAA	0·84	0·40	1·10	[5, 14]
Ischemic stroke with clopidogrel plus aspirin or aspirin alone, %				
Fatal (within 30 days)	17·90	10·10	17·90	[17]
Moderate to severe neurologic sequelae	30·00	30·00	41·70	[17]
Mild neurologic sequelae	41·00	34·80	41·00	[17]
No residual neurologic sequelae	11·00	11·00	13·30	[17]
Ischemic stroke with warfarin, dabigatran, apixaban, rivaroxaban or LAA, %				
Fatal (within 30 days)	8·20	5·50	10·90	[15, 17]
Moderate to severe neurologic sequelae	40·20	35·30	45·10	[15, 17]
Mild neurologic sequelae	42·50	37·60	47·40	[15, 17]
No residual neurologic sequelae	9·10	6·20	12·00	[15, 17]
Annual rate of TIA, %	28·00	25·00	33·00	[15, 17]
Hemorrhage				
Annual rate of minor hemorrhage, %				
Aspirin alone	1·40	1·27	1·53	[2]
Clopidogrel plus aspirin	3·50	2·58	4·42	[2]
Warfarin	18·63	11·40	25·80	[3, 4, 13]
Dabigatran, 110 mg	13·20	12·60	13·80	[3, 19]
Dabigatran, 150 mg	14·80	14·20	15·50	[3, 19]
Apixaban	18·10	17·54	19·35	[13]
Rivaroxaban	11·80	10·94	12·88	[4]
LAA (45 days warfarin followed by 180 days clopidogrel and aspirin then lifetime aspirin after LAA)	4·28	3·70	4·86	Assumption
LAA (lifetime aspirin after LAA)	1·40	1·27	1·53	Assumption
Annual rate of major hemorrhage, %				
Aspirin alone	1·00	0·68	1·32	[2]
Clopidogrel plus aspirin	1·50	1·35	1·65	[2]
Warfarin	3·32	3·09	3·57	[3, 4, 13]
Dabigatran, 110 mg	2·87	2·50	3·32	[3, 19]
Dabigatran, 150 mg	3·32	2·89	3·82	[3, 19]
Apixaban	2·13	1·85	2·47	[13]
Rivaroxaban	3·60	3·06	4·08	[4]
LAA (45 days warfarin followed by 180 days clopidogrel and aspirin then lifetime aspirin after LAA)	1·54	1·30	1·77	Assumption
LAA (lifetime aspirin after LAA)	1·00	0·68	1·32	Assumption

Table 1 Clinical inputs for base-case value and ranges in decision analytic model *(Continued)*

Annual rate of ICH, %				
Aspirin alone	0·20	0·19	0·21	[2]
Clopidogrel plus aspirin	0·40	0·24	0·59	[2]
Warfarin	0·75	0·70	0·80	[3, 4, 13]
Dabigatran, 110 mg	0·23	0·14	0·32	[3, 15]
Dabigatran, 150 mg	0·30	0·20	0·40	[3, 15]
Apixaban	0·33	0·24	0·46	[13]
Rivaroxaban	0·50	0·33	0·65	[4]
LAA (45 days warfarin followed by 180 days clopidogrel and aspirin then lifetime aspirin after LAA)	0·37	0·27	0·47	Assumption
LAA (lifetime aspirin after LAA)	0·20	0·19	0·21	Assumption
Annual rate of major hemorrhage as fatal, %				
Aspirin alone	0·20	0·14	0·26	[2]
Clopidogrel plus aspirin	0·30	0·19	0·51	[2]
Warfarin	0·90	0·50	1·80	[3, 4, 13]
Dabigatran, 110 mg	1·22	1·08	1·36	[3]
Dabigatran, 150 mg	1·45	1·33	1·56	[3]
Apixaban	0·37	0·30	0·42	[13]
Rivaroxaban	0·20	0·16	0·40	[4]
LAA (45 days warfarin followed by 180 days clopidogrel and aspirin then lifetime aspirin after LAA)	0·45	0·38	0·51	Assumption
LAA (lifetime aspirin after LAA)	0·20	0·14	0·26	Assumption
Myocardial infarction				
Annual rate of MI, %				
Aspirin alone	0·90	0·77	1·03	[2]
Clopidogrel plus aspirin	0·70	0·53	0·93	[2]
Warfarin	0·78	0·61	1·12	[3, 4, 13]
Dabigatran, 110 mg	0·82	0·61	1·12	[3, 19]
Dabigatran, 150 mg	0·81	0·60	1·09	[3, 19]
Apixaban	0·53	0·40	0·71	[13]
Rivaroxaban	0·91	0·71	1·19	[4]
LAA (45 days warfarin followed by 180 days clopidogrel and aspirin then lifetime aspirin after LAA)	0·76	0·57	1·00	Assumption
LAA (lifetime aspirin after LAA)	0·90	0·77	1·03	Assumption
Pericardial Effusions, %				
Rate of Pericardial effusions				
LAA (within 7 days)	2·07	1·50	2·40	[5, 14]
Success implantation, %				
Rate of LAA device implanted after discontinuing warfarin	0.868	0.8342	0.9018	[18]
Hospitalization				
Annual rate of Hospitalization, %				
Warfarin	20·80	15·5	26·10	[3]
Dabigatran, 110 mg	19·40	13·49	25·32	[3]
Dabigatran, 150 mg	20·20	19·94	20·46	[3]
Apixaban	20·80	15·50	26·10	Assumed equal to Wafarin
Rivaroxaban	20·80	15·50	26·10	Assumed equal to Wafarin

Table 1 Clinical inputs for base-case value and ranges in decision analytic model *(Continued)*

LAA	1·08	0·00	5·00	[5]
Relative Risk of Hospitalization, %				
Warfarin vs. aspirin	1·22	0·64	2·36	[20]
Warfarin vs. clopidogrel plus aspirin	1·22	0·64	2·36	Assumed equal to Aspirin
Death				
Death from vascular cause, %				
Aspirin alone	4·70	4·48	4·92	[2]
Clopidogrel plus aspirin	4·70	4·18	5·26	[2]
Warfarin	2·10	1·71	2·69	[3, 4, 13]
Dabigatran, 110 mg	2·43	2·23	2·63	[3]
Dabigatran, 150 mg	2·28	2·03	2·53	[3]
Apixaban	1·80	1·54	2·10	[13]
All-cause mortality, %				
Aspirin alone	6·60	5·53	7·67	[2]
Clopidogrel plus aspirin	6·40	5·87	7·13	[2]
Warfarin	2·89	0·50	4·13	[3]
Dabigatran, 110 mg	3·75	3·51	3·99	[3]
Dabigatran, 150 mg	3·64	3·28	4·00	[3]
Apixaban	3·52	3·15	3·90	[13]
Rivaroxaban	4.50	4.01	4.99	[4]
LAA	3.20	1.56	4.84	[21]

Hemorrhage

Hemorrhages were classified into 4 categories: minor, major, ICH and fatal (Table 1). The annual rates of ICH were 0·2 %, 0·4 %, 0·75 %, 0·23 %, 0·3 %, 0·33 %, and 0·5 % for ASA alone, clopidogrel plus ASA, warfarin, dabigatran 110 mg, dabigatran 150 mg, apixaban, and rivaroxaban, respectively [2–4, 13, 15]. The rate of ICH after LAAO was 0·37 % for the first year and 0·2 % for the second year onwards. A pro-rata method was used to estimate the event rates for LAAO based on patients' duration of taking ASA, clopidogrel plus ASA, or warfarin therapy (Table 1). We assumed the bleeding rate in the first year after LAAO was lower than warfarin or clopidogrel plus ASA since patients were treated with warfarin for only 45 days followed by clopidogrel plus ASA for 180 days. Bleeding rate from the second year onwards was assumed to be the same as ASA alone [5, 12].

Myocardial infarction

The annual rates of MI was 0·9 % for ASA, 0·7 % for clopidogrel plus ASA, 0·78 % for warfarin, 0·82 % for dabigatran 110 mg, 0·81 % for dabigatran 150 mg, 0·53 % for apixaban, and 0·91 % for rivaroxaban [2–4, 13, 19]. We assumed the rate of MI in the first year after LAAO was lower than warfarin or clopidogrel plus ASA since patients were treated with warfarin for only 45 days followed by clopidogrel plus ASA for 180 days. The rate of MI from the second year onwards was assumed to be the same as ASA alone [5, 12].

Pericardial effusions

The rate of serious pericardial effusions was 2·07 % for patients who received LAAO within 7 days based on the PROTECT-AF and PREVAIL studies [5, 14].

Success rate of LAA occlusion

LAAO success was defined when anticoagulation could be discontinued after implantation of LAAO device. According to published data, the success rate of LAAO was 86.8 % and others were under warfarin therapy in the LAAO strategy [18].

Hospitalization

The rates of hospitalization may be occurred after patients with moderate to severe stroke or pericardial effusions which were obtained from the RE-LY [3], PRO-TECT-AF [5], and the Birmingham Atrial Fibrillation Treatment of the Aged (BAFTA) trial [20]. The hospitalization rates for warfarin, dabigatran 110 mg, dabigatran 150 mg, and LAAO device were 20·8 %, 20·2 %, 19·4 %, and 1·08 %, respectively. The rates of apixaban and rivaroxaban were assumed to be the same as warfarin (Table 1).

Table 2 Health utilities and costs for base-case value and ranges in decision analytic model

Variable	Base-Case	Range		References
Quality of life				
Mean utility score				
Aspirin alone	0·998	0·994	1·0	[10]
Clopidogrel plus aspirin	0·998	0·994	1·0	Assumed equal to Aspirin
Warfarin	0·987	0·953	1·0	[10]
Dabigatran	0·994	0·975	1·0	[17, 19]
Apixaban	0·994	0·975	1·0	Assumed equal to Dabigatran
Rivaroxaban	0·994	0·975	1·0	Assumed equal to Dabigatran
LAA	0·998	0·994	1·0	Assumed equal to Aspirin
Stroke				
Mild neurologic sequelae	0·75	0·75	1·0	[10]
Moderate to severe neurologic				
sequelae	0·39	0·39	1·0	[10]
Myocardial infarction	0·84	0·84	1·0	[23]
Hemorrhage				
Minor hemorrhage	0·8	0·5	0·99	[15–17, 24]
Major hemorrhage	0·8	0·5	0·99	[15–17, 24]
Cost, US$				
Annual cost of medication or device				
Aspirin alone	10·0	5·0	15·0	[10]
Clopidogrel plus aspirin	1,857·0	365·0	2,785.5	[10]
Warfarin	180·0	60·0	270·0	[10]
Dabigatran	3,240·0	2,500·0	4,860	[10]
Apixaban	3,920·1	1960·1	5,880·2	[25]
Rivaroxaban	2,660·9	1,330·4	3,991·3	[25]
LAA	22,500	20,384	24,614	[26], Assumption
Cost of INR + minimal established patient visit	26·0	10·0	39.0	[10]
Short term cost of neurological event				
Moderate to severe ischemic neurological event	14,680·0	6,000·0	25,000·0	[10]
Minor ischemic neurological event	9,200·0	3,500·0	15,000·0	[10]
TIA	7,500·0	3,000·0	12,000·0	[10]
ICH	38,500·0	15,000·0	60,000·0	[10]
Long term cost of neurological event				
Moderate to severe ischemic neurological event	5,400·0	2,000·0	8,000·0	[10]
Minor ischemic neurological event	2,470·0	1,000·0	4,000v0	[10]
TIA	5,700·0	2,000·0	9,000·0	[10]
ICH	7,200·0	3,000·0	12,000·0	[10]
Other costs, US$				[10]
Transesophageal echocardiogram	334.0	167.0	501.0	[27]
Major bleeding without residua	4,400·0	1,500·0	6,000·0	[10]
Minor bleeding	69·0	34·5	200·0	[10]

Table 2 Health utilities and costs for base-case value and ranges in decision analytic model *(Continued)*

Cost of non-stroke, non-hemorrhage death	10,000·0	5,000·0	20,000·0	[10]
MI	17,000·0	5,000·0	50,000·0	[10]
Hospitalization for stroke	80,964·0	40,482·0	121,446·0	Assumption
Hospitalization for pericardial effusions	73,770·0	36,885·0	110,655·0	Assumption

Death

The rates of cardiovascular and all-cause mortality for ASA alone, clopidogrel plus ASA, warfarin, dabigatran 110 mg, dabigatran 150 mg and apixaban were 4·7 % and 6·6 %, 4·7 % and 6·4 %, 2·1 % and 2·89 %, 2·43 % and 3·75 %, 2·28 % and 3·64 %, 1·8 % and 3·52 %, respectively [2–4, 13]. The all-cause mortality rates of rivaroxaban and LAAO were 4.5 % and 3.2 % input the model [4, 21].

Quality of life

Health utilities were obtained from published data (Table 2). The mean utility score was 0·998 for ASA, 0·987 for warfarin [10]. The utility score for dabigatran of 0·994 was based on estimation of previous studies for another direct thrombin inhibitor, ximelagatran [15, 17, 22]. The utility score for dual anti-platelet therapy with clopidogrel plus ASA, and LAAO were assumed to be the same as ASA; otherwise, the utility score for apixaban and rivaroxaban were assumed to be the same as dabigatran in this study.

The mean utility score was 0·75 for mild stroke, 0·39 for moderate to severe stroke [10]. The utility score of MI (0·84) was derived from a nationally representative EQ-5D index scores for a study of chronic conditions in the US [23]. The utility score for minor or major hemorrhage was 0.8 [15–17, 24].

Cost measurement

Direct inpatient and outpatient medical costs were estimated from a healthcare provider perspective (Table 2). The cost data for the base-case and their ranges were based on a two cost-effectiveness studies of stroke prevention in AF patients [10, 25]. These costs included the costs of anti-thrombotic therapy, hemorrhage, neurological ischemia, dyspepsia, or MI. The estimated cost for LAAO procedure was based on the mean charge of US$14,614 for LAA implantation procedure [26] plus the cost of the LAA occluding device of US$7,885 (US$5,770-US$10,000) that led to the total cost in our analysis as US$22,500. Transesophageal echocardiography (TEE) was performed at the time of LAA device implantation and at 45 days, thus the cost of TEE was US$334 [27].

Sensitivity analysis

One-way sensitivity analysis was performed by varying CHADS$_2$ score, HAS-BLED score, time horizons, and different costs of LAA occlusion for all treatment strategies in this study. The stroke rate for patients with AF was increased by CHADS$_2$ score (0–6), which were assumed to be 0·8 %, 2·2 %, 4·5 %, 8·6 %, 10·9 %, 12.3 % and 13.7 %, respectively [18]. The hemorrhage rates were increased by HAS-BLED score (0–5 score), which were assumed to be 1·13 %, 1·02 %, 1·88 %, 3·74 %, 8·7 %, and 12·5 %, respectively [8]. Time horizon was varied from 20 to 5, 10, and 15 years to assess shorter-term cost-effectiveness from a start-age of 65 years. Sensitivity analysis was also performed with lower and higher costs of LAAO. One-way sensitivity analysis illustrated with tornado diagram was used to assess parameter uncertainty and estimate which parameters had the greatest impact in the model. The parameter was identified as sensitive when either the range was the widest or the ICER value was greater than a threshold of US$50,000. The parameters in warfarin and LAAO strategies were pooled from two or more trials (Tables 1 and 2).

Probabilistic sensitivity analysis (PSA) using 10,000 Monte Carlo simulations was conducted to assess parameter uncertainty. The ranges of all parameters were obtained from published studies and calculating formula of 95 % confidence interval (Tables 1 and 2). A beta distribution was used for those parameters between 0 and 1. Cost data were non-negative quantitative data thus applying a gamma distribution.

Results

Base-case analysis

Under base-case conditions, LAAO was considered cost-effective compared with the 7 alternative pharmacological stroke prevention strategies for a hypothetical cohort of 65-year-old patient with non-valvular AF (Table 3 and Fig. 1). In descending sequence, the total costs of all strategies were apixaban ($53,315), rivaroxaban ($51,064), dabigatran 150 mg ($43,946), dabigatran 110 mg ($42,712), LAAO ($37,789), warfarin ($28,090), clopidogrel plus ASA ($26,287) and ASA alone ($12,877), respectively. LAAO was associated with the greatest QALYs (10.99 QALYs), followed by rivaroxaban (9.86 QALYs), warfarin (9.45 QALYs), apixaban (9·40 QALYs), dabigatran 150 mg (9·0 QALYs), dabigatran 110 mg (8.76 QALYs), clopidogrel plus ASA (6·29 QALYs) and ASA alone (6·12 QALYs).

The ICER per QALY gained for LAA occlusion compared with ASA alone, clopidogrel plus ASA and warfarin were $5,115, $2,447 and $6,298, respectively.

Table 3 Lifetime results of total Costs, total QALYs and ICERs for each stroke prevention strategy (start age at 65-year-old patients)

Therapy	Total Discounted Costs, USD	Total Discounted QALYs, Year	Cost per QALY	ICER, vs. Aspirin	ICER, vs. Clopidogrel plus Aspirin	ICER, vs. Warfarin	ICER, vs. LAA Occlusion	ICER, vs. Dabigatran 110 mg	ICER, vs. Dabigatran 150 mg	ICER, vs. Rivaroxaban	ICER, vs. Apixaban	ICER, vs. Next-best strategy
Aspirin	$12,877	6·12	$2,104	—	Dominated[a]	Dominated[a]	Dominated[a]	Dominated[a]	Dominated[a]	Dominated[a]	Dominated[a]	—
Clopidogrel plus aspirin	$26,287	6·29	$4,179	$78,882	—	Dominated[a]	Dominated[a]	Dominated[a]	Dominated[a]	Dominated[a]	Dominated[a]	Extended dominance
Warfarin	$28,090	9·45	$2,972	$4,568	$571	—	Dominated[a]	Dominated[b]	Dominated[b]	Dominated[a]	Dominated[b]	$571
LAA Occlusion	$37,789	10.99	$3,438	$5,115	$2,447	$6,298	—	Dominated[b]	Dominated[b]	Dominated[b]	Dominated[b]	$6,298
Dabigatran 110 mg	$42,712	8.76	$4,876	$11,301	$6,650	Dominated[c]	Dominated[c]	—	Dominated[a]	Dominated[a]	Dominated[a]	Dominated[a]
Dabigatran 150 mg	$43,946	9.00	$4,883	$10,788	$6,516	Dominated[c]	Dominated[c]	$5,142	—	Dominated[a]	Dominated[a]	Dominated[a]
Rivaroxaban	$51,064	9.86	$5,179	$10,210	$6,940	$56,034	Dominated[c]	$7,593	$8,277	—	Dominated[a]	Dominated[a]
Apixaban	$53,315	9.40	$5,672	$12,329	$8,691	Dominated[c]	Dominated[c]	$16,567	$23,423	Dominated[c]	—	Dominated[a]

Abbreviations: LAA left atrial appendage, *ICER* incremental cost-effectiveness ratio, *QALY* quality-adjusted life year, *Extended dominance* the alternative has a higher ICER than a more effective comparator

[a] Less costly and less effective strategy

[b] Less costly but more effective strategy

[c] More costly but less effective strategy

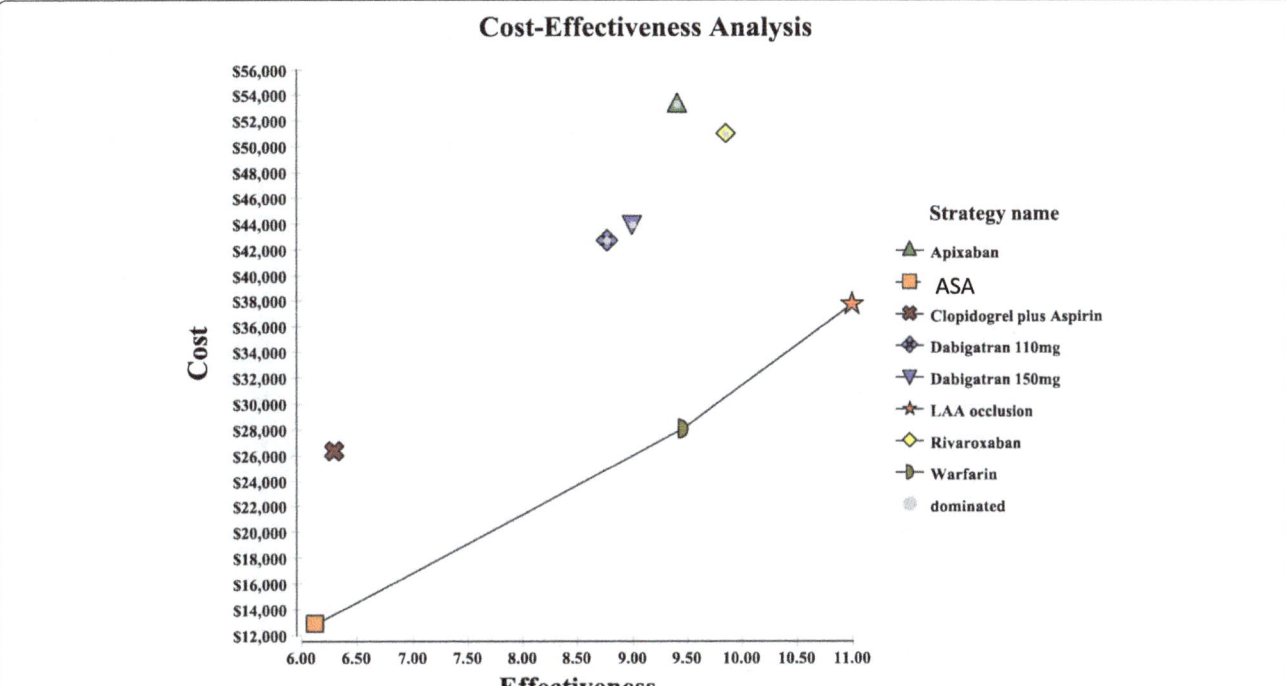

Fig. 1 Shows the result of ICER values in comparison of the next-best strategy, and the black line connected from acetylsalicylic acid (ASA) to LAA occlusion as the cost-effectiveness frontier. The effectiveness is defined as the change of quality adjusted life year (QALY) gained. The cost-effectiveness frontier ran from ASA to warfarin to LAA occlusion and its slope increased when moving from the least costly/least effective alternative (ASA) towards the most costly/most effective alternative (LAA occlusion). Clopidogrel plus ASA was an extended dominance* strategy. LAA occlusion is the next more-effective strategy comparing to warfarin, ICER per QALY gained was US$6,298. Dabigatran 110 mg, dabigatran 150 mg, rivaroxaban, and apixaban were dominated by LAA occlusion because those four alternatives were less effective but more costly than LAA occlusion. *Extended dominance: This refers to the observation when the ICER value for a given strategy is higher than that of the next, more effective, alternative. Clopidogrel plus ASA had a higher ICER value than a more effective alternative (warfarin)

LAAO was dominant (i.e. less costly but more effective) compared to dabigatran 110 mg, dabigatran 150 mg, apixaban, and rivaroxaban.

Sensitivity analysis
Sensitivity analysis demonstrated that LAAO remained cost-effective compared with other strategies when stroke risk was varied from $CHADS_2$ score 0 to 6 (Table 4). In particular, dabigatran 110 mg, dabigatran 150 mg, apixaban and rivaroxaban were dominated by LAAO. When hemorrhage rate was varied by HAS-BLED score from 0 to 5 for anticoagulant drugs in the simulation model, LAAO remained cost-effective compared with each strategy. Varying the time horizon from 20 to 15, 10 and 5 years did not affect the cost-effectiveness of LAAO against all other treatment strategies except for warfarin (ICER: US$74,422) with a short 5 years time horizon. In tornado diagram, the results demonstrated the parameters with greatest impact were all-cause mortality of warfarin (−$32,048–$12,994) and all-cause mortality of LAAO ($3,631–$24,716), respectively (Fig. 2). PSA results demonstrated that the probability of LAAO strategy was the most cost-effective compared with other 7 strategies in

86.24 % of 10,000 Monte Carlo simulations at the threshold of US$50,000/QALY (Fig. 3).

Discussion
Previous study has demonstrated the cost-effectiveness of LAAO, dabigatran and warfarin in the management of NVAF [28]. This was the first comprehensive analysis to compare the cost-effectiveness between seven pharmacological strategies including newer oral anticoagulants and transcatheter LAA occlusion for stroke prevention in NVAF patients. We demonstrated that LAAO was associated with the highest QALYs gained and the lowest ICER per QALY gained compared to 7 other pharmacological regimens in the prevention of AF-related stroke. Sensitivity analysis also demonstrated that LAAO remained cost-effective compared with all 7 alternative strategies across the spectrum of stroke risks, bleeding risk and time horizon.

Atrial fibrillation is a growing problem in an aging society. It causes >50 000 strokes and $12 billion in medical expenditure each year in United States. Warfarin used to be the standard of care in preventing stroke but it is difficult to be used conveniently and safely [29].

Table 4 Sensitivity analysis of total Costs, total QALYs, and ICERs of LAA occlusion compared with each strategy by varying CHADS2 score, HAS-BLED score, time horizons, and LAA occlusion costs

CHADS₂ Score	Aspirin Cost	QALY	Clopidogrel + Aspirin Cost	QALY	Warfarin Cost	QALY	Dabigatran 110 mg Cost	QALY	Dabigatran 150 mg Cost	QALY	Apixaban Cost	QALY	Rivaroxaban Cost	QALY	LAAO Cost	QALY
0 (0·8 %)	$10,117	6·36	$24,998	6·42	$27,027	9·54	$41,569	8·87	$43,685	9·02	$52,949	9·44	$50,966	9·98	$37,567	11.01
1 (2·2 %)	$12,073	6·19	$26,627	6·25	$30,565	9·25	$44,469	8·60	$46,627	8·75	$55,868	9·15	$54,107	9·67	$40,971	10.65
2 (4·5 %)	$15,048	5.93	$29,098	5·99	$35,853	8·81	$48,807	8·20	$51,021	8·34	$60,207	8·71	$58,766	9·19	$46,033	10.11
3 (8·6 %)	$19,710	5·52	$32,949	5·57	$43,894	8·11	$55,412	7·57	$57,698	7·69	$66,749	8·01	$65,765	8·44	$53,661	9.25
4 (10·9 %)	$22,017	5·31	$34,846	5·36	$47,753	7·76	$58,587	7·25	$60,899	7·37	$69,859	7·67	$69,080	8·07	$57,288	8.83
5 (12.3 %)	$23,327	5.19	$35,919	5.24	$49,905	7.57	$60,359	7.07	$62,684	7.18	$71,586	7.47	$70,915	7.86	$59,299	8.59
6 (13.7 %)	$24,571	5.08	$36,937	5.13	$51,922	7.38	$62,021	6.90	$64,357	7.01	$73,198	7.28	$72,626	7.66	$61,177	8.36

ICER, US$ LAAO vs. each strategy

	Aspirin	Clopidogrel + Aspirin	Warfarin	Dabigatran 110 mg	Dabigatran 150 mg	Apixaban	Rivaroxaban	LAAO
Score 0	$5,903	$2,738	$7,170	Dominated	Dominated	Dominated	Dominated	—
Score 1	$6,479	$3,260	$7,433					
Score 2	$7,413	$4,110	$7,831					
Score 3	$9,102	$5,628	$8,568					
Score 4	$10,020	$6,467	$8,911					
Score 5	$10,580	$6,979	$9,210					
Score 6	$11,160	$7,505	$9,444					

HAS-BLED Score	Aspirin Cost	QALY	Clopidogrel + Aspirin Cost	QALY	Warfarin Cost	QALY	Dabigatran 110 mg Cost	QALY	Dabigatran 150 mg Cost	QALY	Apixaban Cost	QALY	Rivaroxaban Cost	QALY	LAAO Cost	QALY
0 (1.13 %)	$12,877	6·12	$26,287	6·29	$36,827	9·40	$62,062	8·64	$61,719	8·88	$72,551	9·30	$69,642	9·78	$38,858	10.98
1 (1.08 %)	$12,877	6·12	$26,287	6·29	$34,333	9·42	$59,791	8·66	$59,450	8·89	$69,999	9·31	$66,679	9·79	$38,552	10.99
2 (1.88 %)	$12,877	6·12	$26,287	6·29	$53,095	9·31	$76,902	8·55	$76,534	8·77	$89,207	9·21	$88,969	9·69	$40,851	10.97
3 (3.74 %)	$12,877	6·12	$26,287	6·29	$88,462	9·09	$109,305	8·35	$108,814	8·55	$125,481	9·02	$130,998	9·50	$45,208	10.95
4 (8.7 %)	$12,877	6·12	$26,287	6.29	$156,713	8·67	$172,530	7·94	$171,469	8·09	$195,786	8·65	$212,146	9·13	$53,713	10.89
5 (12.5 %)	$12,877	6·12	$26,287	6.29	$191,794	8·45	$205,517	7·73	$203,929	7·85	$232,133	8·45	$253,872	8·94	$58,139	10.87

ICER, US$ LAAO vs. each strategy

	Aspirin	Clopidogrel + Aspirin	Warfarin	Dabigatran 110 mg	Dabigatran 150 mg	Apixaban	Rivaroxaban	LAAO
Score 0	$5,346	$2,680	$1,285	Dominated	Dominated	Dominated	Dominated	—
Score 1	$5,272	$2,610	$2,687					
Score 2	$5,768	$3,112	Dominated					
Score 3	$6,694	$4,060	Dominated					
Score 4	$8,561	$5,962	Dominated					
Score 5	$9,529	$6,955	Dominated					

Time horizon	Aspirin Cost	QALY	Clopidogrel + Aspirin Cost	QALY	Warfarin Cost	QALY	Dabigatran 110 mg Cost	QALY	Dabigatran 150 mg Cost	QALY	Apixaban Cost	QALY	Rivaroxaban Cost	QALY	LAAO Cost	QALY
5 years	$6,100	3·47	$12,529	3·50	$6,898	4·02	$17,516	3·94	$17,374	3·97	$20,356	4·03	$17,040	4.08	$24,015	4.25
10 years	$9,788	5·06	$19,929	5·15	$14,876	6·63	$29,508	6·36	$29,707	6·46	$35,233	6·63	$31,205	6.81	$29,026	7.28

Table 4 Sensitivity analysis of total Costs, total QALYs, and ICERs of LAA occlusion compared with each strategy by varying CHADS2 score, HAS-BLED score, time horizons, and LAA occlusion costs (Continued)

15 years	$11,801	5·78	$24,048	5·92	$22,111	8·34	$37,471	7·85	$38,190	8·02	$45,834	8·31	$42,397	8.63	$33,699	9.44
ICER, US$ LAAO vs. each strategy	0 5 years: $22,968		0 5 years: $15,315		5 years: $74,422		5 years: $20,965		05 years: $23,718		5 years: $16,632		5 years: $41,029		—	
	10 years: $8,666		10 years: $4,217		10 years: $21,769		10 years: Dominated		10 years: Dominated		10 years: Dominated		10 years: Dominated			
	15 years: $5,983		15 years: $2,742		15 years: $10,535		15 years: Dominated		15 years: Dominated		15 years: Dominated		15 years: Dominated			
LAAO costs	Cost	QALY	Cost	QALY	Cost	QALY	Cost	QALY	Cost	QALY	Cost	QALY	Cost	QALY	Cost	QALY
Low cost ($20,384)	$12,877	6.12	$26,287	6.29	$28,090	8.76	$42,712	8.76	$43,946	9.00	$53,315	9.40	$51,064	9.86	$36,731	10.99
Base-case ($22,500)	$12,877	6.12	$26,287	6.29	$28,090	8.76	$42,712	8.76	$43,946	9.00	$53,315	9.40	$51,064	9.86	$37,789	10.99
High cost ($24,614)	$12,877	6.12	$26,287	6.29	$28,090	8.76	$42,712	8.76	$43,946	9.00	$53,315	9.40	$51,064	9.86	$38,846	10.99
ICER, US$ LAAO vs. each strategy	Low cost: $4,898		Low cost: $2,222		Low cost: $5,611		Dominated		Dominated		Dominated		Dominated		—	
	Base-case: $5,115		Base-case: $2,447		Base-case: $6,298		Dominated		Dominated		Dominated		Dominated			
	High cost: $5,332		High cost: $2,672		High cost: $6,984		Dominated		Dominated		Dominated		Dominated			

Abbreviations: LAAO left atrial appendage occlusion, *ICER* incremental cost-effectiveness ratio, *QALY* quality-adjusted life year, *CHADS$_2$* congestive heart failure, hypertension, age > 75, diabetes mellitus, and previous stroke/transient ischemic attack, *HAS-BLED* hypertension, abnormal renal/liver function, stroke, bleeding history or predisposition, Labile international normalized ratio, Elderly (>65 years), drugs/alcohol concomitantly, *ICER* calculated as the difference in cost divided by the difference in QALYs for each therapy compared with LAAO strategy, *Dominated* LAAO is less costly but more effective strategy compare with each strategy

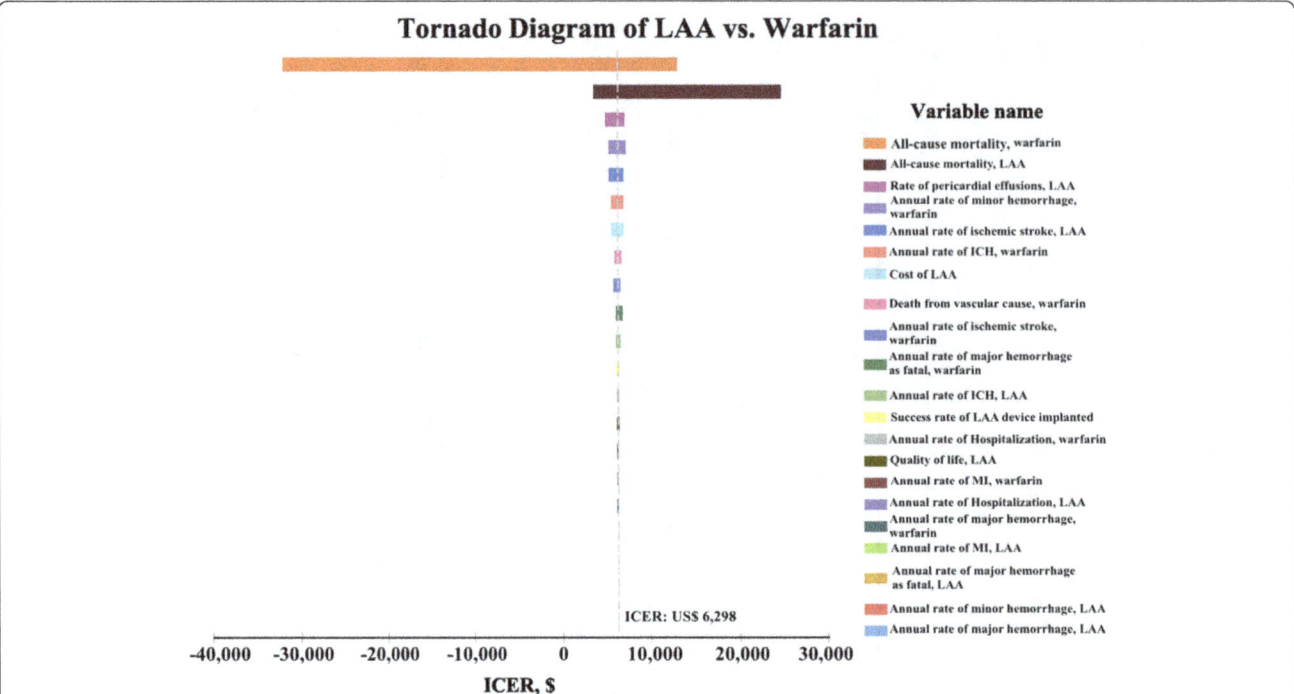

Fig. 2 Shows the Tornado diagram with parameters having the greatest impact on the top. The gray dotted line was the ICER value (US$6,298) of LAA occlusion compared to warfarin with base-case result. The all-cause mortalities of warfarin (variable range: 0.5 to 4.13 %) and LAA occlusion (variable range: 1.8 to 2.7 %) had the greatest impact in the model. Even though the range of ICER values of the two parameters were not greater than the threshold of US$50,000, both parameters could still affect the results in the model. The other parameters assessed were not sensitive to the model's outcomes

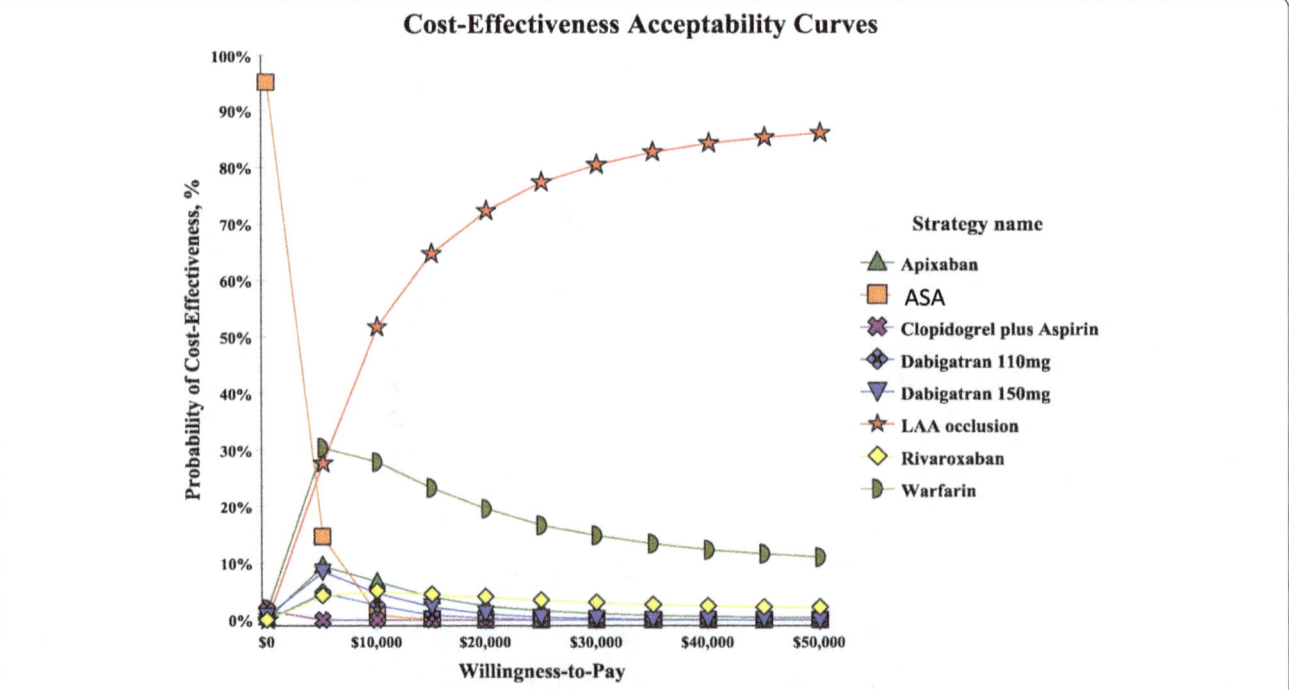

Fig. 3 Shows Cost-effectiveness Acceptability Curves (CEACs) for the probability that LAA occlusion strategy was the most cost-effective compared with other 7 strategies for a range of willingness to pay threshold. Given a maximum acceptable ceiling ratio of US$50,000 per QALY gained, the probability of cost-effectiveness for LAA occlusion strategy was 86.24 %

NOACs may be comparable to warfarin in terms of clinical efficacy but the benefit does not come without risk of bleeding. Transcatheter LAAO potentially reduces both risks of stroke and bleeding associated with long-term anticoagulation and the 2012 European Society of Cardiology Guidelines recommended such intervention can be considered in patients with high stroke risk and contraindications for oral anticoagulants [30]. A few studies attempted to evaluate the cost-effectiveness of these newer stroke preventive strategies. One key analysis based on the RE-LY study [3] showed the ICERs of dabigatran 110 mg and 150 mg compared with warfarin were US$16,147–115,129 and US$39,680–263,543, respectively, which were much higher compared to the ICER for LAAO in our current study. SM Singh, A Micieli and HC Wijeysundera [8] demonstrated LAAO was cost-effective as compared to dabigatran and warfarin but they did not address the impact of other commonly used NOACs and the treatment duration on the cost-effective performance of the device therapy [28]. In current analysis, we demonstrated the superior cost-effectiveness of the device compared to other NOACs, which is independent of stroke risk (CHADS$_2$ score), bleeding risk (HAS-BLED score) and treatment duration (i.e. device strategy was cost-effective even at 5 year follow-up). In particular, LAAO was considered cost-effective comparing to all alternative strategies when HAS-BLED score and CHADS$_2$ score were varied. Considering most adverse events occur during and shortly after device implantation [5, 20], while events with oral anticoagulants develop continuously over time, our findings may provide additional insights in selecting specific therapy for individual patient groups.

Three endovascular LAA occluding devices have been widely used in humans and many other new devices are under pre-clinical evaluation [31]. The PLAATO device was the oldest with reported favorable clinical results up to 5 years but the device has been withdrawn from the market because of financial considerations [32]. PROTECT-AF trial [5] showed the WATCHMAN device was non-inferior to warfarin in reducing ischemic stroke in AF patients with CHADS$_2$ score of ≥1 and the device arm was associated with less hemorrhagic stroke. Early registry results with Amplatzer Cardiac Plug (St Jude Medical Inc, US), consistently reported a high implantation success rate >95 %, implying its wide applicability to AF patients [6, 33]. The longest follow-up data were also shown to demonstrate the promising results with Amplatzer device in AF patients for stroke prevention [33]. While the device therapy addresses both the concerns of inconvenience (no issue with drug interaction, blood monitoring and compliance) and safety (bleeding) associated with long term oral anticoagulant usage, it also has shortcomings in particular procedural-related complications [5, 6, 12, 14] and the risks of having incomplete LAAO and thrombus formation on the device during long-term follow up. The costs of managing these events needed to be studied especially when the device strategy has been widely adopted in in-experienced centers.

Limitations
There are a number of limitations of the current study. Firstly, there was no directly comparative trial between LAAO and oral anticoagulation. Secondly, the base-case values of the current model simulation were derived from individual clinical trials from different countries and healthcare systems with variable costs of management. Thirdly, a number of base-case assumptions were necessary when trial data were lacking. Fourthly, data from randomized clinical trials could not be generalizable to "real world" clinical practice. It should also be noted that only direct medical cost was considered in the analysis. Fifthly, we assumed that warfarin was discontinued after 45 days post LAAO although some patients may require warfarin beyond 45 days when TEE confirmed clots or device leak. Furthermore, the long-term follow-up data for the newer LAAO devices were obtained from a single study with 10-year follow up of Amplatzer left atrial appendage occlusion [33], it may add to model uncertainties and parameter uncertainties in the results, however, sensitivity analyses demonstrated the robustness of study results.

Conclusions
In conclusion, our Markov analytic model demonstrated that transcatheter LAAO was cost-effective compared to ASA alone, clopidogrel plus ASA, warfarin, dabigatran 110 mg, dabigatran 150 mg, rivaroxaban and apixaban for stroke prevention in patients with NVAF.

Acknowledgements
We would like to acknowledge Markus Siebert and Maria Koullick (St. Jude Medical, USA) who gave us invaluable advice regarding healthcare costs for LAA occlusion in the United States.

Authors' contributions
IC and RT analyzed data and prepared report for this project. VL was responsible for study design, interpretation of data and logistics of this project. BY and YYL were responsible for study design and interpretation of data. MGK and JWP provided consultation on study design and interpretation of data. All authors read and approved the final manuscript.

Competing interests
Dr Yat-Yin Lam is the consultant and clinical proctor for St Jude Medical and Boston Scientific LAA occluders. Dr Jai-Wun Park is also the clinical proctor for St Jude Medical LAA occluder. Prof Vivian Lee has received sponsorship from Boehringer Ingelheim (HK) Ltd previously. The remaining authors have no conflicts of interest to declare.

Author details

[1]School of Pharmacy, Faculty of Medicine, The Chinese University of Hong Kong, 8th Floor, Lo Kwee-Seong Integrated Biomedical Sciences Building, Area 39, Shatin, Hong Kong. [2]Department of Medicine and Therapeutics, Faculty of Medicine, The Chinese University of Hong Kong, Prince of Wales Hospital, Shatin, Hong Kong. [3]Department of Cardiology, Erciyes University School of Medicine, Kayseri, Turkey. [4]Charité University Medicine Berlin, Klinikum Coburg, Coburg, Germany.

References

1. Wolf PA, Abbott RD, Kannel WB. Atrial fibrillation as an independent risk factor for stroke: the Framingham Study. Stroke. 1991;22(8):983-8.

2. Active Investigators, Connolly SJ, Pogue J, Hart RG, Hohnloser SH, Pfeffer M, Chrolavicius S, Yusuf S. Effect of clopidogrel added to aspirin in patients with atrial fibrillation. N Engl J Med. 2009;360(20):2066-78.

3. Connolly SJ, Ezekowitz MD, Yusuf S, Eikelboom J, Oldgren J, Parekh A, Pogue J, Reilly PA, Themeles E, Varrone J, et al. Dabigatran versus Warfarin in patients with atrial fibrillation. N Engl J Med. 2009;361:1139-51.

4. Patel MR, Mahaffey KW, Garg J, Pan G, Singer DE, Hacke W, Breithardt G, Halperin JL, Hankey GJ, Piccini JP, et al. Rivaroxaban versus warfarin in nonvalvular atrial fibrillation. N Engl J Med. 2011;365(10):883-91.

5. Holmes DR, Reddy VY, Turi ZG, Doshi SK, Sievert H, Buchbinder M, Mullin CM, Sick P, PA Investigators. Percutaneous closure of the left atrial appendage versus warfarin therapy for prevention of stroke in patients with atrial fibrillation: a randomised non-inferiority trial. Lancet. 2009;374(9689):534-42.

6. Park JW, Bethencourt A, Sievert H, Santoro G, Meier B, Walsh K, Lopez-Minquez JR, Meerkin D, Valdes M, Ormerod O, et al. Left atrial appendage closure with Amplatzer cardiac plug in atrial fibrillation: initial European experience. Catheter Cardiovasc Interv. 2011;77(5):700-6.

7. Reddy VY, Akehurst RL, Armstrong SO, Amorosi SL, Beard SM, Holmes Jr DR. Time to cost-effectiveness following stroke reduction strategies in AF: warfarin versus NOACs versus LAA closure. J Am Coll Cardiol. 2015;66(24):2728-39.

8. Singh SM, Micieli A, Wijeysundera HC. Economic evaluation of percutaneous left atrial appendage occlusion, dabigatran, and warfarin for stroke prevention in patients with nonvalvular atrial fibrillation. Circulation. 2013;127(24):2414-23.

9. Gold MR, Siegel JE, Russell LB, Weinstein MC. Cost-effectiveness in health and medicine. New York: Oxford University Press; 1996.

10. Shah SV, Gage BF. Cost-effectiveness of dabigatran for stroke prophylaxis in atrial fibrillation. Circulation. 2011;123(22):2562-70.

11. Reddy VY, Mobius-Winkler S, Miller MA, Neuzil P, Schuler G, Wiebe J, Sick P, Sievert H. Left atrial appendage closure with the Watchman device in patients with a contraindication for oral anticoagulation: the ASAP study (ASA Plavix Feasibility Study With Watchman Left Atrial Appendage Closure Technology). J Am Coll Cardiol. 2013;61(25):2551-6.

12. Reddy VYMD, Holmes DMD, Doshi SKMD, Neuzil PMDP, Kar SMD. Safety of percutaneous left atrial appendage closure: results from the watchman left atrial appendage system for embolic protection in patients with AF (PROTECT AF) clinical trial and the continued access registry. Circulation. 2011;123(4):417-24.

13. Granger CB, Alexander JH, McMurray JJ, Lopes RD, Hylek EM, Hanna M, Al-Khalidi HR, Ansell J, Atar D, Avezum A, et al. Apixaban versus warfarin in patients with atrial fibrillation. N Engl J Med. 2011;365(11):981-92.

14. Holmes Jr DR, Kar S, Price MJ, Whisenant B, Sievert H, Doshi SK, Huber K, Reddy VY. Prospective randomized evaluation of the watchman left atrial appendage closure device in patients with atrial fibrillation versus long-term warfarin therapy: the PREVAIL trial. J Am Coll Cardiol. 2014;64(1):1-12.

15. Freeman JV, Zhu RP, Owens DK, Garber AM, Hutton DW, Go AS, Wang PJ, Turakhia MP. Cost-effectiveness of dabigatran compared with warfarin for stroke prevention in atrial fibrillation. Ann Intern Med. 2011;154(1):1-11.

16. Harrington AR, Armstrong EP, Nolan Jr PE, Malone DC. Cost-effectiveness of apixaban, dabigatran, rivaroxaban, and warfarin for stroke prevention in atrial fibrillation. Stroke. 2013;44(6):1676-81.

17. O'Brien CL, Gage BF. Costs and effectiveness of ximelagatran for stroke prophylaxis in chronic atrial fibrillation. JAMA. 2005;293(6):699-706.

18. Reddy VY, Doshi SK, Sievert H, Buchbinder M, Neuzil P, Huber K, Halperin JL, Holmes D. Percutaneous left atrial appendage closure for stroke prophylaxis in patients with atrial fibrillation: 2.3-Year Follow-up of the PROTECT AF (Watchman Left Atrial Appendage System for Embolic Protection in Patients with Atrial Fibrillation) Trial. Circulation. 2013;127(6):720-9.

19. Bayard YL, Omran H, Neuzil P, Thuesen L, Pichler M, Rowland E, Ramondo A, Ruzyllo W, Budts W, Montalescot G, et al. PLAATO (Percutaneous Left Atrial Appendage Transcatheter Occlusion) for prevention of cardioembolic stroke in non-anticoagulation eligible atrial fibrillation patients: results from the European PLAATO study. EuroIntervention. 2010;6(2):220-6.

20. Reddy VY, Doshi SK, Sievert H, Buchbinder M, Neuzil P, Huber K, Kar S, Halperin JL, Whisenant B, Swarup V et al.: Long-term PROTECT-AF analysis: Watchman attains efficacy superiority over warfarin in AF. In: Heart Rhythm Society (HRS) 34th Annual Scientific Sessions. Denver, Colorado; May 2013.

21. Gage BF, Cardinalli AB, Owens DK. The effect of stroke and stroke prophylaxis with aspirin or warfarin on quality of life. Arch Intern Med. 1996;156(16):1829-36.

22. Sullivan PW, Ghushchyan V. Preference-Based EQ-5D index scores for chronic conditions in the United States. Med Decis Making. 2006;26(4):410-20.

23. Fryback DG, Dasbach EJ, Klein R, Klein BE, Dorn N, Peterson K, Martin PA. The Beaver Dam Health Outcomes Study: initial catalog of health-state quality factors. Med Decis Making. 1993;13(2):89-102.

24. Thomson R, Parkin D, Eccles M, Sudlow M, Robinson A. Decision analysis and guidelines for anticoagulant therapy to prevent stroke in patients with atrial fibrillation. Lancet. 2000;355(9208):956-62.

25. Centers for Medicare and Medicaid Services (CMS): Hospital Inpatient Prospective Payment Systems for Acute Care Hospitals and the Long Term Care Hospital Prospective Payment System and Proposed Fiscal Year 2015 Rates. In. US: Department of Health and Human services (HHS) 2014: https://www.gpo.gov/fdsys/pkg/FR-2014-05-15/pdf/2014-10067.pdf. Accessed 29 Aug 2016.

26. American Society of Echocardiography. Coding and Reimbursement Newsletter. In.: American Medical Association: 2014. http://asecho.org/wordpress/wp-content/uploads/2014/2006/2014-reimbursement-newsletter-.pdf. Accessed 1 July 2014.

27. Pisters R, Lane DA, Nieuwlaat R, de Vos CB, Crijns HJ, Lip GY. A novel user-friendly score (HAS-BLED) to assess 1-year risk of major bleeding in patients with atrial fibrillation: the Euro Heart Survey. Chest. 2010;138(5):1093-100.

28. Lam YY, Ma TKW, Yan BP. Alternatives to chronic warfarin therapy for the prevention of stroke in patients with atrial fibrillation. Int J Cardiol. 2011;150(1):4-11.

29. Camm AJ, Lip GY, De Caterina R, Savelieva I, Atar D, Hohnloser SH, Hindricks G, Kirchhof P. 2012 focused update of the ESC Guidelines for the management of atrial fibrillation: an update of the 2010 ESC Guidelines for the management of atrial fibrillation. Developed with the special contribution of the European Heart Rhythm Association. Eur Heart J. 2012;33(21):2719-47.

30. Cruz-Gonzalez I, Yan BP, Lam YY. Left atrial appendage exclusion: state-of-the-art. Catheter Cardiovasc Interv. 2010;75(5):806-13.

31. Lam YY, Yip GW, Yu CM, Chan WW, Cheng BC, Yan BP, Clugston R, Yong G, Gattorna T, Paul V. Left atrial appendage closure with AMPLATZER cardiac plug for stroke prevention in atrial fibrillation: initial Asia-Pacific experience. Catheter Cardiovasc Interv. 2012;79(5):794-800.

32. Gage BF, van Walraven C, Pearce L, Hart RG, Koudstaal PJ, Boode BS, Petersen P. Selecting patients with atrial fibrillation for anticoagulation: stroke risk stratification in patients taking aspirin. Circulation. 2004;110(16):2287-92.

33. Nietlispach F, Gloekler S, Krause R, Shakir S, Schmid M, Khattab AA, Wenaweser P, Windecker S, Meier B. Amplatzer left atrial appendage occlusion: single center 10-year experience. Catheter Cardiovasc Interv. 2013;82(2):283-9.

14

Association between hyperuricemia and atrial fibrillation in rural China

Guo-Zhe Sun[1], Liang Guo[1], Jun Wang[1], Ning Ye[1], Xun-Zhang Wang[2] and Ying-Xian Sun[1*]

Abstract

Background: To explore the association between atrial fibrillation (AF) and serum uric acid (SUA) in a general population in rural China.

Methods: From January 2013 to August 2013, we performed a cross-sectional study involving 11,956 permanent residents ≥ 35 years old in the rural Liaoning province of China. All participants completed a questionnaire, had a physical examination, and underwent an electrocardiogram (ECG) and echocardiogram. AF was diagnosed from ECG findings and/or a history of physician-confirmed AF. Blood samples were drawn for laboratory analyses and hyperuricemia was defined as an SUA level > 7.0 mg/dL in men and > 5.7 mg/dL in women, based on the NHANES-III laboratory definition. Logistic regression analyses were performed to estimate the crude and independent associations between hyperuricemia and the prevalence of AF.

Results: A total of 139 participants were diagnosed with AF, of which, 72 were self-reported, 45 were ECG-diagnosed, and 22 were both. There was a higher prevalence of AF in participants with hyperuricemia than those with normal SUA levels (2.4 vs. 1.0 %; $P < 0.001$). The odds ratios (OR) and 95 % confidence intervals (CI) were 2.37 (1.61–3.49) when compared to participants with normal SUA. After adjustment for other cardiovascular and AF risk factors, the independent association remained (OR = 1.94, 95 % CI: 1.26–3.00). Similar associations were observed between SUA as a continuous variable and AF prevalence (adjusted OR = 1.20, 95 % CI: 1.06–1.36). The independent associations were significant in men ($Ps < 0.05$) but not in women ($Ps > 0.05$), although the interaction logistic regression analyses presented these differences as not being statistically significant ($Ps > 0.05$).

Conclusions: SUA is positively associated with the prevalence of AF in rural China.

Background

Atrial fibrillation (AF) is one of the most common cardiac arrhythmias and is associated with overall mortality and mortality from cardiovascular disease [1, 2]. Advancing age, male gender, hypertension, diabetes mellitus, obesity, heart failure, myocardial infarction (MI), and alcohol consumption are the major risk factors for the development of AF [3–6]. The prevalence of AF is expected to increase dramatically over the next few decades as the general population ages and improved cardiovascular therapies keep people with cardiovascular disease alive longer [7]. Identifying all the risk factors for AF will help to create population-based strategies to deal with this serious health problem.

Serum uric acid (SUA) is a risk factor for cerebrovascular and coronary artery disease, as well as for hypertension, metabolic syndrome, and kidney disease [8], though only a few cross-sectional studies in Japan [9], Turkey [10], and China [11–13] have reported a positive association between hyperuricemia and the prevalence of AF. Also, population-based prospective cohorts showed that hyperuricemia was associated with a high risk of AF [14, 15]. However, all of these cross-sectional studies enrolled hospital patients only rather than individuals from the general population. Furthermore, only the study in Japan analyzed the effect of gender on the association between hyperuricemia and AF, reporting that the independent association was observed in women only. Therefore, the current study was designed to explore the association between SUA and AF in a general population from rural China. The study also analyzed the effect of gender on the independent association.

* Correspondence: cmu1h_syx@126.com
[1]Department of Cardiovascular Medicine, The First Hospital of China Medical University, 155 Nanjing Street, Heping, Shenyang, Liaoning 110001, China
Full list of author information is available at the end of the article

Methods

Study population

A representative sample of men and women ≥ 35 years of age from rural areas of Liaoning Province were recruited between January 2013 and August 2013 using a multistage, randomly stratified, cluster-sampling scheme. In particular, three counties (Dawa, Zhangwu, and Liaoyang) were randomly selected from Liaoning Province. One township near a city in each county was randomly selected giving a total of three townships. Six to eight villages from each township were randomly selected to give a total of 26 rural villages. All of the eligible permanent residents aged ≥ 35 years from each village (n = 14,016) were invited to participate in the study, and 11,956 (85.3 %) agreed to do so; women who were pregnant, or people who had cancer or any mental disorders were excluded from the study.

The study was carried out with pre-approval granted by the Ethics Committee of China Medical University (Shenyang, China). Written consent was obtained from all participants after they had been informed of the study's objectives, benefits, medical procedures, and confidentiality safeguards for personal information. In the case of an illiterate participant, written informed consent was obtained from the appropriate legal proxy.

Data collection and measurement

Data were collected during a single clinic visit by cardiologists and trained nurses using a standard questionnaire in a face-to-face interview. All potential investigators had received training on the objectives of the study, how to administer the questionnaire, the standard methods of measurement, the importance of standardization, and study procedures. Only those who earned a perfect score on a post-training test were allowed to participate as study investigators. During data collection, the inspectors received further instructions and support.

Data on demographic characteristics and medical history of AF, MI, hypertension, diabetes mellitus, lifestyle risk factors, and family history of AF were obtained, as described above, by interview with the standardized questionnaire. There was a central steering committee with a subcommittee for quality control that made sure all data were collected according to well-known standards.

According to the American Heart Association, blood pressure (BP) was measured three times at two-minute intervals after at least five minutes of rest using a standardized automatic electronic sphygmomanometer (HEM-907; Omron, Kyoto, Japan). Two doctors checked the calibration of the Omron device every month using a standard mercury sphygmomanometer according to the British Hypertension Society protocol [16]. The participants were advised to avoid caffeinated beverages and to exercise for ≥ 30 min before the measurement. During the measurement, the participants were seated with their arms supported at the level of their hearts. The mean of three BP measurements was calculated and used in all analyses.

Weight and height were measured to the nearest 0.1 kg and 0.1 cm, respectively, with the participants in lightweight clothing without shoes. The body mass index (BMI) was calculated as weight in kilograms divided by the square of the height in meters. Waist circumference (WC) was measured at the umbilicus to the nearest 0.1 cm while the participants were standing following a normal expiration.

Fasting blood samples were collected in the morning after ≥ 8 h of fasting for all participants. Blood samples were obtained from an antecubital vein using BD Vacutainer tubes containing EDTA (Becton, Dickinson and Co., Franklin Lakes, NJ, USA). Serum was subsequently isolated from whole blood, and all serum samples were frozen at –20 °C for testing at a central, certified laboratory. Fasting blood glucose (FBG), total cholesterol (TC), triglycerides (TG), SUA, and other routine blood biochemical indices were analyzed enzymatically on an auto-Analyzer (Olympus AU640; Olympus, Kobe, Japan, or Bayer RA-XT; Bayer Diagnostics, Tarrytown, NY, USA) using kits (Bayer Diagnostics). The laboratory measurements were calibrated and verified following analysis of biochemical indices and the results met the national standards of measurement (CNAS certificate of accreditation No.L0467, quality index U = 0.006 (k = 2)).

Twelve-lead resting, ten-second electrocardiograms (ECGs) were performed on all participants by well-trained cardiologists using an electrocardiography machine (MAC 5500; GE Healthcare, Little Chalfont, Buckinghamshire, UK). The results were analyzed automatically by the MUSE Cardiology Information System (version 7.0.0; GE Healthcare). ECG-based diagnoses of AF were confirmed by at least two independent cardiologists.

Echocardiograms were obtained using a commercially available Doppler echocardiograph (Vivid; GE Healthcare) with a 3.0-MHz transducer. The transthoracic echocardiogram included M-mode, two-dimensional, spectral and color Doppler with subjects in the supine position. Echocardiogram analyses and readings were performed by three doctors specialized in echocardiography, and two other specialists were called in if questions or uncertainty arose. Measurements were performed according to the recommendations of the American Society of Echocardiography. M-mode images were used to measure and calculate the left ventricular ejection fraction (LVEF) [17].

Definitions

AF was diagnosed based on a previous history of AF (previously diagnosed by a physician) and/or evidence of AF on the ECG (absence of consistent P waves, presence of rapid irregular f waves with a frequency of 350–600 beats per minute, and an irregular ventricular response).

Left ventricular hypertrophy diagnosed by ECG (ECG-LVH) was identified using the Cornell Criteria expressed as voltage and QRS duration product: (RaVL + SV3) × QRS duration > 2,440 mm*ms in men and (RaVL + SV3 + 8 mm) × QRS duration > 2,440 mm*ms in women [18]. Left ventricular systolic dysfunction was defined as an LVEF < 0.5 based on M-mode echocardiography. Hyperuricemia was defined as an SUA level > 7.0 mg/dL in men and > 5.7 mg/dL in women, based on the NHANES-III laboratory definitions [19].

Statistical analysis

All statistical analyses were performed using SPSS 17.0 software (SPSS Inc., Chicago, IL, USA). Differences between groups were compared using a two-tailed Student's t-test for continuous variables and a χ^2 test for categorical variables. The age- and gender-specific prevalences of AF among participants with both normal SUA levels and hyperuricemia were calculated, and univariate and multivariate logistic regression analyses were performed to estimate the crude and independent association between SUA and the presence of AF. Interaction regression models were used to test the difference in the association of SUA with AF prevalence between men and women. Data are expressed as odds ratio (OR) and 95 % confidence interval (CI), mean ± standard deviation, or frequency and percentage; a $P < 0.05$ was considered as statistically significant.

Results

Characteristics of the study population

Of the original 11,956 participants, 618 had incomplete data and were excluded from the analysis, leaving a total of 11,338 participants (5,170 men and 6,168 women) with a mean age of 53.8 years. The subjects with hyperuricemia were older than those with normal SUA levels ($P < 0.001$), and there was a higher percentage of men than women in this group ($P < 0.001$) (Table 1). Participants with hyperuricemia had significantly higher WCs, BMIs, systolic and diastolic BPs, FBG, TC, and TG levels (all Ps < 0.001). The hyperuricemia group also had a higher percentage of alcohol drinkers and had a higher prevalence of MI, and ECG-LVH than the normal SUA level group (all Ps < 0.001). The prevalence of AF was significantly higher in participants with hyperuricemia than those with normal SUA ($P < 0.001$).

Prevalence of AF by SUA level

There were 139 participants with AF, and the age-specific prevalence of AF by SUA level is summarized in Fig. 1. Among these AF cases, 72 were self-reported, 45 were ECG-diagnosed, and 22 were both. The prevalence of AF rose steeply with advancing age and was higher in the group with hyperuricemia than in the group with

Table 1 Characteristics of the study population

Variable	Normal SUA level (n = 9,909)	Hyperuricemia (n = 1,429)	P
Age, y	53.7 ± 10.5	54.9 ± 10.9	<0.001
Sex, male	4396 (44.4)	774 (54.2)	<0.001
BMI, kg/m²	24.6 ± 3.6	26.4 ± 3.9	<0.001
WC, cm	81.6 ± 9.6	87.9 ± 9.9	<0.001
SBP, mmHg	141.2 ± 23.4	145.9 ± 23.8	<0.001
DBP, mmHg	81.5 ± 11.5	85.7 ± 12.7	<0.001
FBG, mmol/L	5.88 ± 1.65	6.05 ± 1.47	<0.001
TC, mmol/L	5.18 ± 1.06	5.58 ± 1.23	<0.001
TG, mmol/L	1.53 ± 1.30	2.41 ± 2.34	<0.001
Current smoker	3478 (35.1)	502 (35.1)	0.982
Current drinker	2107 (21.3)	418 (29.3)	<0.001
History of MI	101 (1.0)	30 (2.1)	<0.001
LVEF < 0.5	1126 (11.8)	144 (10.4)	0.131
ECG-LVH	799 (8.1)	215 (15.0)	<0.001
AF	104 (1.0)	35 (2.4)	<0.001
Family history of AF	306 (3.1)	38 (2.7)	0.377

Note: data are expressed as mean ± standard deviation or n (%)
AF atrial fibrillation, BMI body mass index, DBP diastolic blood pressure, ECG-LVH left ventricular hypertrophy detected by electrocardiography, FBG fasting blood glucose, LVEF left ventricular ejection fraction, MI myocardial infarction, SBP systolic blood pressure, SUA serum uric acid, TC total cholesterol, TG triglycerides, WC waist circumference

normal SUA levels at every age. The trends in AF prevalence with age were similar between men and women.

Association between SUA and AF

The association between hyperuricemia and AF was examined by logistic regression analysis (Table 2). Both men and women with hyperuricemia had a higher prevalence of AF than those with normal SUA levels ($P < 0.001$ for men, $P = 0.010$ for women and $P < 0.001$ for total). After adjusting for other cardiovascular and AF risk factors, including age, gender, WC, BMI, systolic and diastolic BP, FBG, TC, TG, smoking, drinking, history of MI, low LVEF, ECG-LVH and familial history of AF, the independent association was significant in men ($P = 0.003$) and in men and women together ($P = 0.003$), but not in women alone ($P = 0.235$). However, $P > 0.05$ was observed for the association of AF with hyperuricemia between men and women. Similar associations were found between SUA as a continuous variable and AF prevalence (Table 3).

Discussion

The results of this study demonstrate that men and women with hyperuricemia in a rural Chinese population have a significantly higher prevalence of AF than those with normal SUA levels. The AF prevalence increases with advancing age in both men and women,

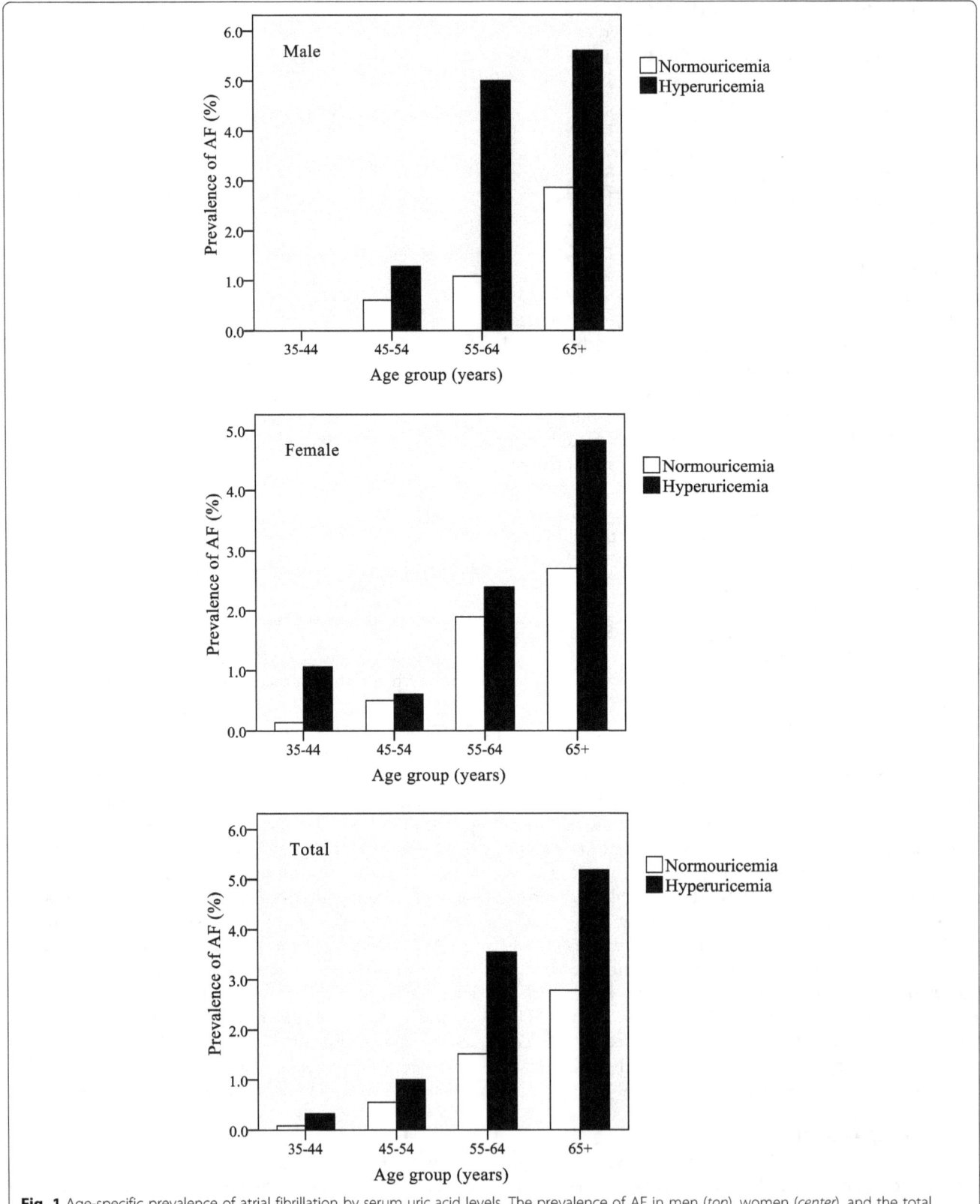

Fig. 1 Age-specific prevalence of atrial fibrillation by serum uric acid levels. The prevalence of AF in men (*top*), women (*center*), and the total population (*bottom*)

Table 2 Hyperuricemia and the prevalence of atrial fibrillation

Group	Total (n)	AF n (%)	Unadjusted model OR (95 % CI)	P	Adjusted model[a] OR (95 % CI)	P
Men						
Normal SUA levels	4,396	44 (1.0)	1	<0.001	1	0.003
Hyperuricemia	774	20 (2.6)	2.62 (1.54–4.48)		2.55 (1.38–4.71)	
Women						
Normal SUA levels	5,513	60 (1.1)	1	0.010	1	0.235*
Hyperuricemia	655	15 (2.3)	2.13 (1.20–3.77)		1.46 (0.78–2.72)	
Total						
Normal SUA levels	9,909	104 (1.0)	1	<0.001	1	0.003
Hyperuricemia	1,429	35 (2.4)	2.37 (1.61–3.49)		1.94 (1.26–3.00)	

AF atrial fibrillation, CI confidence interval, OR odds ratio, SUA serum uric acid

*P = 0.200 for gender difference

[a]Adjusted for age, gender, body mass index, waist circumference, systolic and diastolic blood pressure, fasting blood glucose, total cholesterol and triglyceride levels, smoking, drinking, myocardial infarction, low left ventricular ejection fraction, left ventricular hypertrophy detected by electrocardiography, and family history of AF

but the independent association with SUA is only observed in the total population and in men after adjusting for other cardiovascular risk factors. Our finding that hyperuricemia was positively associated with the AF prevalence in the general population was consistent with previous studies [9–13]. However, in our current study, the independent association was only observed in men but not in women, which was inconsistent with previous findings in Japan [9]. A recent meta-analysis that included both cross-sectional and cohort studies, also reported a positive relationship between SUA and the prevalence of AF [20]. Population-based prospective cohort studies showed that baseline SUA was associated with an increased risk of AF in both genders [14, 15]. It is possible that race and lifestyle influenced the results

Table 3 Serum uric acid levels and the prevalence of atrial fibrillation

Group	Unadjusted model OR (95 % CI)	P	Adjusted model[a] OR (95 % CI)	P
Men				
SUA, per mg/dl	1.30 (1.13–1.50)	<0.001	1.26 (1.08–1.47)	0.004
Women				
SUA, per mg/dl	1.31 (1.11–1.55)	0.002	1.11 (0.92–1.33)	0.291*
Total				
SUA, per mg/dl	1.25 (1.13–1.38)	<0.001	1.20 (1.06–1.36)	0.003

AF atrial fibrillation, CI confidence interval, OR odds ratio, SUA serum uric acid

*P = 0.302 for gender difference

[a]Adjusted for age, gender, body mass index, waist circumference, systolic and diastolic blood pressure, fasting blood glucose, total cholesterol and triglyceride levels, smoking, drinking, myocardial infarction, low left ventricular ejection fraction, left ventricular hypertrophy detected by electrocardiography, and family history of AF

of our study, as Asians and African-Americans have a lower prevalence of AF than other races [21], and our study population consisted of people living exclusively in rural areas, most of whom routinely performed heavy physical labor.

We also tested the difference in the association of SUA with AF between men and women by interaction regression models. However, the effect of gender on the association was not statistically significant with Ps > 0.05. This inconsistency may be due to low AF prevalence and the small sample size. Indeed, the positive association between SUA and AF might also exist in women (even though this might not be statistically significant).

In our current study, AF was diagnosed based on a previous history of physician-diagnosed AF and/or evidence of AF using the ECG. This diagnostic approach has been utilized in previous studies [9, 22]. Self-reported AF history was previously used as a method for the diagnosis of AF. However, it is likely that this approach gave rise to an unintentional bias.

The major clinical risk factors for AF are advancing age, male gender, hypertension, diabetes, obesity, heart failure, valve disease, MI, smoking, and alcohol consumption, but biomarkers such as B-type natriuretic peptide [23, 24] and C-reactive protein [25, 26] also correlate with AF. Systemic inflammation indicated by an elevated level of C-reactive protein is associated with the incidence and persistence of AF [26, 27]. SUA regulates some critical proinflammatory pathways [28] and correlates with several inflammatory markers [29]. Inflammation could cause oxidative damage to the atrium that might contribute to electrical remodeling and increase the incidence of AF [30]. SUA may therefore be another useful biomarker for the condition, though the mechanisms by which SUA influences AF risk are unclear.

A limitation of this study is the cross-sectional design and it is not clear whether lowering SUA levels would also decrease the incidence and prevalence of AF. In addition, the number of people who had hyperuricemia in our study was small, and the prevalence of AF in some subgroups was zero or too small to measure for statistical significance. The association between SUA and AF in our study may also have been affected by confounding risk factors for AF (i.e., hypertension, diabetes, and dislipidemia), which also occur with hyperuricemia. However, results from the univariate and multivariate logistic regression analyses indicate that SUA is an independent risk factor for AF. But, further cohort studies need to be conducted to determine whether reducing SUA levels reduce AF incidence and prevalence.

Conclusions

Men and women in rural China ≥ 35 years of age with hyperuricemia have a significantly higher prevalence of AF than those with normal SUA levels. Hyperuricemia is independently associated with the prevalence of AF after adjusting for various cardiovascular risk factors.

Competing interests
The authors declare that they have no competing interests.

Authors' contributions
GZS collected the data, analyzed and prepared the first draft of the manuscript. LG supervised the data collection and reviewed the manuscript. JW collected the data. NY coordinated the data collection. XZW reviewed the analysis and the manuscript. YXS conceived the study design, reviewed the manuscript and serves as guarantor for the contents of this paper. All authors approved the final version.

Acknowledgments
This study was founded by the National Science and Technology Support Program of China (No. 2012BAJ18B08-7).

Author details
[1]Department of Cardiovascular Medicine, The First Hospital of China Medical University, 155 Nanjing Street, Heping, Shenyang, Liaoning 110001, China. [2]Heart Institute, Cedars Sinai Medical Center, Los Angeles 90048, CA, USA.

References
1. Kannel WB, Abbott RD, Savage DD, McNamara PM. Epidemiologic features of chronic atrial fibrillation: the Framingham study. N Engl J Med. 1982;306:1018–22.
2. Stewart S, Hart CL, Hole DJ, McMurray JJ. A population-based study of the long-term risks associated with atrial fibrillation: 20-year follow-up of the Renfrew/Paisley study. Am J Med. 2002;113:359–64.
3. Benjamin EJ, Levy D, Vaziri SM, D'Agostino RB, Belanger AJ, Wolf PA. Independent risk factors for atrial fibrillation in a population-based cohort. The Framingham Heart Study. JAMA. 1994;271:840–4.
4. Korantzopoulos P, Kolettis TM. Obesity and the risk of new-onset atrial fibrillation. JAMA. 2005;293:1974–5.
5. Schnabel RB, Sullivan LM, Levy D, Pencina MJ, Massaro JM, D'Agostino Sr RB, et al. Development of a risk score for atrial fibrillation (Framingham Heart Study): a community-based cohort study. Lancet. 2009;373:739–45.
6. Djoussé L, Levy D, Benjamin EJ, Blease SJ, Russ A, Larson MG, et al. Long-term alcohol consumption and the risk of atrial fibrillation in the Framingham Study. Am J Cardiol. 2004;93:710–3.
7. Miyasaka Y, Barnes ME, Gersh BJ, Cha SS, Bailey KR, Abhayaratna WP, et al. Secular trends in incidence of atrial fibrillation in Olmsted County, Minnesota, 1980 to 2000, and implications on the projections for future prevalence. Circulation. 2006;114:119–25.
8. Feig DI, Kang DH, Johnson RJ. Uric acid and cardiovascular risk. N Engl J Med. 2008;359:1811–21.
9. Suzuki S, Sagara K, Otsuka T, Matsuno S, Funada R, Uejima T, et al. Gender-specific relationship between serum uric acid level and atrial fibrillation prevalence. Circ J. 2012;76:607–11.
10. Tekin G, Tekin YK, Erbay AR, Turhan H, Yetkin E. Serum uric acid levels are associated with atrial fibrillation in patients with ischemic heart failure. Angiology. 2013;64:300–3.
11. Liu Y, Liu H, Dong L, Chen J, Guo J. Prevalence of atrial fibrillation in hospitalized patients over 40 years old: ten-year data from the People's Hospital of Peking University. Acta Cardiol. 2010;65:221–4.
12. Zhao QY, Yu SB, Huang H, Cui HY, Qin M, Huang T, et al. Serum uric acid levels correlate with atrial fibrillation in patients with chronic systolic heart failure. Chin Med J (Engl). 2012;125:1708–12.
13. Liu T, Zhang X, Korantzopoulos P, Wang S, Li G. Uric acid levels and atrial fibrillation in hypertensive patients. Intern Med. 2011;50:799–803.
14. Nyrnes A, Toft I, Njølstad I, Mathiesen EB, Wilsgaard T, Hansen JB, et al. Uric acid is associated with future atrial fibrillation: an 11-year follow-up of 6308 men and women—the Tromso Study. Europace. 2014;16:320–6.
15. Tamariz L, Agarwal S, Soliman EZ, Chamberlain AM, Prineas R, Folsom AR, et al. Association of serum uric acid with incident atrial fibrillation (from the Atherosclerosis Risk in Communities [ARIC] study). Am J Cardiol. 2011;108:1272–6.
16. O'Brien E, Petrie J, Littler W, de Swiet M, Padfield PL, O'Malley K, et al. The British Hypertension Society protocol for the evaluation of automated and semi-automated blood pressure measuring devices with special reference to ambulatory systems. J Hypertens. 1990;8:607–19.
17. Sahn DJ, DeMaria A, Kisslo J, Weyman A. Recommendations regarding quantitation in M-mode echocardiography: results of a survey of echocardiographic measurements. Circulation. 1978;58:1072–83.
18. Dahlöf B, Devereux RB, Julius S, Kjeldsen SE, Beevers G, de Faire U, et al. Characteristics of 9194 patients with left ventricular hypertrophy: the LIFE study. Losartan Intervention For Endpoint Reduction in Hypertension. Hypertension. 1998;32:989–97.
19. Zhu Y, Pandya BJ, Choi HK. Prevalence of gout and hyperuricemia in the US general population: the National Health and Nutrition Examination Survey 2007–2008. Arthritis Rheum. 2011;63:3136–41.
20. Tamariz L, Hernandez F, Bush A, Palacio A, Hare JM. Association between serum uric acid and atrial fibrillation: a systematic review and meta-analysis. Heart Rhythm. 2014;11:1102–8.
21. Marcus GM, Olgin JE, Whooley M, Vittinghoff E, Stone KL, Mehra R, et al. Racial differences in atrial fibrillation prevalence and left atrial size. Am J Med. 2010;123:375.e1-7.
22. Schnabel RB, Wilde S, Wild PS, Munzel T, Blankenberg S. Atrial fibrillation: its prevalence and risk factor profile in the German general population. Dtsch Arztebl Int. 2012;109:293–9.
23. Patton KK, Ellinor PT, Heckbert SR, Christenson RH, DeFilippi C, Gottdiener JS, et al. N-terminal pro-B-type natriuretic peptide is a major predictor of the development of atrial fibrillation: the Cardiovascular Health Study. Circulation. 2009;120:1768–74.
24. Wang TJ, Larson MG, Levy D, Benjamin EJ, Leip EP, Omland T, et al. Plasma natriuretic peptide levels and the risk of cardiovascular events and death. N Engl J Med. 2004;350:655–63.
25. Cao JJ, Thach C, Manolio TA, Psaty BM, Kuller LH, Chaves PH, et al. C-reactive protein, carotid intima-media thickness, and incidence of ischemic stroke in the elderly: the Cardiovascular Health Study. Circulation. 2003;108:166–70.
26. Aviles RJ, Martin DO, Apperson-Hansen C, Houghtaling PL, Rautaharju P, Kronmal RA, et al. Inflammation as a risk factor for atrial fibrillation. Circulation. 2003;108:3006–10.

27. Issac TT, Dokainish H, Lakkis NM. Role of inflammation in initiation and perpetuation of atrial fibrillation: a systematic review of the published data. J Am Coll Cardiol. 2007;50:2021–8.

28. Kanellis J, Watanabe S, Li JH, Kang DH, Li P, Nakagawa T, et al. Uric acid stimulates monocyte chemoattractant protein-1 production in vascular smooth muscle cells via mitogen-activated protein kinase and cyclooxygenase-2. Hypertension. 2003;41:1287–93.

29. Ruggiero C, Cherubini A, Ble A, Bos AJ, Maggio M, Dixit VD, et al. Uric acid and inflammatory markers. Eur Heart J. 2006;27:1174–81.

30. Carnes CA, Chung MK, Nakayama T, Nakayama H, Baliga RS, Piao S, et al. Ascorbate attenuates atrial pacing-induced peroxynitrite formation and electrical remodeling and decreases the incidence of postoperative atrial fibrillation. Circ Res. 2001;89:E32–8.

15

Thiazolidinedione use and atrial fibrillation in diabetic patients

Zhiwei Zhang[1†], Xiaowei Zhang[1†], Panagiotis Korantzopoulos[2], Konstantinos P. Letsas[3], Gary Tse[4,5], Mengqi Gong[1], Lei Meng[1], Guangping Li[1] and Tong Liu[1*]

Abstract

Background: Accumulating evidence suggests that thiazolidinediones (TZDs) may exert protective effects in atrial fibrillation (AF). The present meta-analysis investigated the association between TZD use and the incidence of AF in diabetic patients.

Methods: Electronic databases were searched until December 2016. Of the 346 initially identified records, 3 randomized clinical trials (RCTs) and 4 observational studies with 130,854 diabetic patients were included in the final analysis.

Results: Pooled analysis of the included studies demonstrated that patients treated with TZDs had approximately 30% lower risk of developing AF compared to controls [odds ratio (OR): 0.73, 95% confidence interval (CI): 0.62 to 0.87, $p = 0.0003$]. This association was consistently observed for both new onset AF (OR =0.77, $p = 0.002$) and recurrent AF (OR =0.41, $p = 0.002$), pioglitazone use (OR =0.56, $p = 0.04$) but not rosiglitazone use (OR =0.78, $p = 0.12$). The association between TZD use and AF incidence was not significant in the pooled analysis of three RCTs (OR =0.77, 95% CI = 0.53–1.12, $p = 0.17$), but was significantly in the pooled analysis of the four observational studies (OR =0.71, $p = 0.0003$).

Conclusions: This meta-analysis suggests that TZDs may confer protection against AF in the setting of diabetes mellitus (DM). This class of drugs can be used as upstream therapy for DM patients to prevent the development of AF. Further large-scale RCTs are needed to determine whether TZDs use could prevent AF in the setting of DM.

Keywords: Atrial fibrillation, Diabetes mellitus, Thiazolidinediones, Pioglitazone, Rosiglitazone, Meta-analysis

Background

Atrial fibrillation (AF) is the most prevalent arrhythmia observed in clinical practice, and is associated with significant morbidity and mortality in the popuation. The burden of AF increases over time mainly due to an aging population and to the increasing prevalence of cardiovascular comorbidities. However, strategies to predict and prevent AF are not fully effective [1]. Diabetes mellitus (DM) is one of the strongest independent risk factors for AF incidence, conferring an approximate 40% higher risk of subsequent AF development [2, 3]. It also predicts the recurrence of AF following a successful direct current cardioversion [4]. Moreover, DM increases the risk of developing stroke, heart failure, and cardiovascular death in patients with AF [5]. Although the exact pathophysiological mechanisms linking DM and AF remain incompletely elucidated, an increasing body of evidence suggests that inflammation and oxidative stress may play an important role [6–8].

Thiazolidinediones (TZDs), a class of peroxisome proliferator-activated receptor-γ (PPAR-γ) agonists, are among the most potent insulin-sensitizing drugs [9]. Apart from their anti-diabetic activity, TZDs display several pleiotropic effects including anti-inflammatory and antioxidant actions that may have potential benefits for AF prevention [10, 11]. However, inconsistent results have been reported regarding TZDs use and AF incidence [12–18]. In light of such conflicting data, we performed a

* Correspondence: liutongdoc@126.com

†Equal contributors

[1]Tianjin Key Laboratory of Ionic-Molecular Function of Cardiovascular Disease, Department of Cardiology, Tianjin Institute of Cardiology, Second Hospital of Tianjin Medical University, No. 23 Pingjiang Road, Hexi District, Tianjin 300211, People's Republic of China

Full list of author information is available at the end of the article

comprehensive meta-analysis to evaluate the present evidence and investigate whether the use of TZDs confers benefits in preventing AF.

Methods

This systematic review was conducted according to the Quality of Reports of Meta-Analyses of Randomized Controlled Trials (QUOROM) recommendations [19] and the guidelines of the Meta-analysis of Observational Studies in Epidemiology Group (MOOSE) [20].

Inclusion criteria

The studies considered for this meta-analysis were either randomized clinical trials (RCTs) or observational studies that investigated the potential effects of TZDs on AF. The inclusion criteria were as follows: *RCTs*: 1) randomized controlled human trials with a parallel design; 2) comparison of TZDs with control; 3) collecting data on new or recurrent AF during follow-up. *Observational Studies*: 1) comparison of TZDs with control; 2) evaluating new or recurrent AF as an outcome. In the studies of interventions with TZDs no limit in the length of follow-up period was set due to the paucity of relevant studies.

Search strategies

A systematic literature search was performed by two investigators (Z. Z. and X. Z.) using the online databases of PubMed and Embase to identify relevant studies published before December 2016. The following key terms were used: "thiazolidinediones", "pioglitazone", "rosiglitazone", "troglitazone", and "atrial fibrillation". Both investigators independently evaluated the search results and

identified potential studies for further assessment. Disagreements were resolved by a third reviewer (T. L.).

Quality assessment and data extraction

As quality scoring in meta-analyses of RCTs and observational studies is controversial, several key points of study quality were assessed according to a critical review checklist of Wynn et al. [21]. The key points of this checklist and quality assessments of included studies are listed in Table 1.

Two investigators (Z. Z. and X. Z.) independently extracted the relevant data using a pre-defined spreadsheets. The extracted data elements of the meta-analysis included information on the inclusion criteria, publication details, study design, follow-up duration, daily dosage of TZDs, definition of AF, methods of AF detection, baseline patient characteristics, the variables of multivariate model used in observational studies and results. Disagreements were resolved through discussion or consensus with a third reviewer (T. L.).

Statistical analysis

Results of the AF outcome are expressed as odds ratio (OR) with 95% confidence interval (CI) for each study using generic inverse-variance method. The hazard ratio value using multivariate Cox proportional hazards model in the primary study was directly considered as OR [22]. Raw event numbers were extracted from the RCTs and adjusted effect estimates from the observational studies to calculate the overall effects. Statistical heterogeneity was assessed by the χ^2 test and quantified by using the I^2 statistic. An $I^2 > 50\%$ is indicative of at least moderate heterogeneity [23]. A random-effects model was used. Subgroup analyses regarding AF subtypes (new onset AF

Table 1 Quality assessments of included studies

Study, year	Study type	Randomisation Method	Blinding	Eligibility criteria reported	Study Population representative of normal practice	Method of follow-up properly defined	Equal follow-up between groups	Was loss to follow-up reported or explained	Prospective recruitment	Consecutive recruitment
PROactive, 2005 [12]	RCT	Randomised permuted blocks	Double	Yes	Yes	Yes	Yes	Yes	Yes	Yes
Anglade, 2007 [13]	Case control	NA	NA	Yes	Yes	Yes	Yes	No loss to follow-up	No	Yes
RECORD, 2009 [14]	RCT	Randompermuted blocks	None	Yes	Yes	Yes	Yes	Yes	Yes	Yes
Gu, 2011 [15]	Cohort	NA	NA	Yes	Yes	Yes	Yes	No loss to follow-up	Yes	Yes
Chao, 2012 [16]	Case control	NA	NA	Yes	Yes	Yes	Yes	No loss to follow-up	No	Yes
Liu, 2014 [17]	RCT	Computer	Double	Yes	Yes	Yes	Yes	No loss to follow-up	Yes	Yes
Pallisgaard, 2016 [18]	Cohort	NA	NA	Yes	Yes	Yes	Yes	No loss to follow-up	Yes	Yes

Abbreviations: *RCT* randomized controlled trial, *NA* not applicable

or recurrent AF), different TZDs (solely pioglitazone or solely rosiglitazone), study designs (RCTs or observational studies), and different follow-up duration (>5 years or ≤5 years) were additionally performed. Sensitivity analysis was done by removing one study at a time and checking the consequent effects on the effect estimate. Publication bias was evaluated using a funnel plot. Two-tailed p values of <0.05 were considered statistically significant. The statistical analysis was performed using the Review Manager (RevMan, version 5.3, Copenhagen: The Nordic Cochrane Centre, The Cochrane Collaboration, 2014).

Results

A total of 346 records were identified initially through our literature search strategy. After careful assessment, seven studies (three RCTs [12, 14, 17] and four observational studies [13, 15, 16, 18]) comprising 130,854 diabetic patients (11,781 in the treatment and 119,073 in the control group) were included in the final meta-analysis (Fig. 1).

Three studies [12, 15, 17] examined the relationship between pioglitazone use and AF, while two other [14, 16] studied rosiglitazone use. The remaining two studies [13, 18] reported data regarding the use of pioglitazone, rosiglitazone and troglitazone. The characteristics of each study are listed in Table 2, and the patients' characteristics in each study are shown in Table 3.

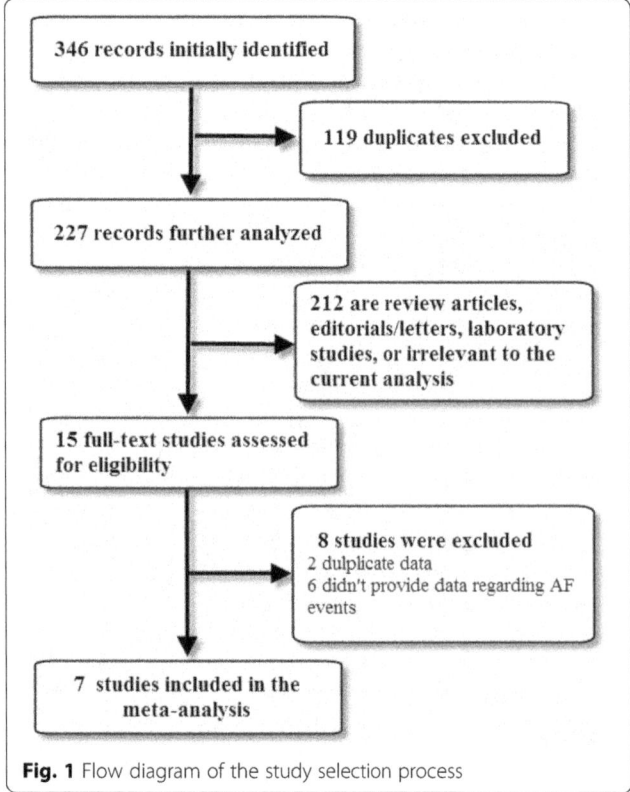

Fig. 1 Flow diagram of the study selection process

Of the seven studies, four [15–18] studies showed that TZDs use attenuated either the risk of new-onset or recurrent AF, whereas the other three [12–14] studies did not indicate a statistically significant difference. Overall, the pooled analysis of the seven included studies suggested that patients treated with TZDs have nearly 30% lower risk of AF compared with controls (OR =0.73, 95% CI = 0.62–0.87, p = 0.0003; Fig. 2). No significant heterogeneity between the individual studies was observed (P = 0.36, I^2 = 9%).

Subgroup analyses according to AF types, different TZDs, follow-up duration, and study designs were subsequently performed (Fig. 2, Table 4). TZDs use was associated with a decrease in the risk of both new-onset [12, 14, 16, 18] (OR =0.77, 95% CI = 0.65–0.91, p = 0.002) and recurrent AF [13, 15, 17] (OR =0.41, 95% CI = 0.24–0.72, 0.002) without any heterogeneity across the studies. Regarding different TZDs, pioglitazone use [12, 15, 17] (OR =0.56, 95% CI = 0.32–0.98, p = 0.04; I^2 = 54%) was associated with a lower risk of AF incidence, whereas rosiglitazone use [14, 16] was not significantly associated with a decreasing AF incidence (OR =0.78, 95% CI = 0.57–1.07, p = 0.12; I^2 = 34%). Regarding the subgroup analysis on different follow-up duration, there was no significant difference between the 3 studies [14, 16, 18] with a follow-up duration >5 years (OR =0.76, 95% CI = 0.63–0.91, p = 0.002; I^2 = 0%) and the 4 studies [12, 13, 15, 17] with a follow-up duration ≤5 years (OR =0.62, 95% CI = 0.41–0.94, p = 0.02; I^2 = 34%). Finally, the pooled analysis of the 4 [13, 15, 16, 18] observational studies showed a strong association between TZDs use and risk reduction of AF (OR =0.71, 95% CI = 0.59–0.85, p = 0.0003; I^2 = 0%), whereas the pooled analysis of the three RCTs showed a non-statistically significant 23% reduction in the odds of developing AF (OR =0.77, 95% CI = 0.53–1.12, p = 0.10; I^2 = 40%).

Besides, due to different pathophysiologic mechanisms of AF, a sensitivity analysis was performed by removing the studies evaluated post-operation AF [13] and post-AF [15] ablation recurrences, no significant differences were found in the heterogeneity (P = 0.44; I^2 = 0%) among the remaining five studies [12, 14, 16–18], and the overall outcome remained the same (OR =0.75, 95% CI = 0.64–0.88, p = 0.0003).

Discussion

The main findings of this comprehensive meta-analysis on 130,854 diabetic patients are the following: i. TZDs may confer protection against AF incidence; ii. the beneficial effects of TZDs were consistently observed in both new onset and recurrent AF; iii. Pioglitazone use was associated with a statistically reduced risk of incident AF, whereas rosiglitazone use showed no statistically significant difference; and iv. the protective effects of TZDs

Table 2 The characteristics of 7 included studies

Study, year	Study population	Patients (n)	Comparators	Daily dosage of TZDs	Follow-up	Definition of AF	Methods of AF detection	The variables of multivariate model
PROactive, 2005 [12]	Patients with type 2 diabetes who had evidence of macrovascular disease	5238	Pioglitazone (n = 2605) vs. placebo (n = 2633)	Titrated from 15 to 45 mg	34.5 months	New-onset AF	NA	NA
Anglade, 2007 [13]	Diabetic patients who underwent CABG and/or valvular surgery	184	Pioglitazone (n = 14), rosiglitazone (n = 24) and troglitazone (n = 2) vs. No TZD (n = 140)	Pioglitazone: average 30 mg Rosiglitazone: average 6 mg, Troglitazone: average 525 mg	30 days	Postoperative AF	NA	NA
RECORD, 2009 [14]	Patients with type 2 diabetes	4447	Rosiglitazone + metformin or sulfonylurea (n = 2220) vs. metformin and sulfonylurea (n = 2227)	Titrated from 4 to 8 mg	5.5 years	New-onset AF	NA	NA
Gu, 2011	Type 2 diabetic patients with paroxysmal AF undergoing catheter ablation	161	Pioglitazone (n = 51) vs. No pioglitazone (n = 99)	30 mg	22.9 ± 5.1 months	Recurrent ATa (AF, AT, AFL)	ECG and Holter recording	Duration of PAF, LAD, treatment with ACEI/ARB
Chao, 2012 [16]	Patients with non-insulin dependent diabetes.	12,065	Rosiglitazone (n = 4137) vs. No rosiglitazone (n = 7928)	NA	63 ± 25 months	New-onset AF	NA	Age, HTN, CAD, chronic renal disease and use of statins or alpha-glucosidase inhibitors
Liu, 2014 [17]	Diabetic patients with the first presence of persistent AF	146	Pioglitazone (n = 70) vs. placebo (n = 76)	30 mg	20.1 months	Recurrent AF	ECG, history of arrhythmia-related symptoms, and Holter monitoring	NA
Pallisgaard, 2016 [18]	Diabetic patients of Danish nationwide registries	108,624	TZD (n = 2658) vs. other second-line antidiabetic drugs (n = 105,966)	NA	12 years	New-onset AF	NA	Age, sex, stroke, HF, all cancer, hyperthyroidism, IHD, COPD, CKD, liver disease, vascular disease, HTN, statin use, prior CABG, and prior PCI

Abbreviations: *AF* atrial fibrillation, *PAF* paroxysmal atrial fibrillation, *ATa* atrial tachyarrhythmias, *AT* atrial tachycardia, *AFL* atrial flutter, *ECG* electrocardiograph, *CABG* coronary artery bypass graft, *TZDs* thiazolidinediones, *LAD* left atrial diameter, *ACEI* angiotensin converting enzyme inhibitor, *ARB* angiotensin receptor blocker, *HTN* hypertension, *CAD* coronary arterial disease, *IHD* ischaemic heart disease, *COPD* chronic obstructive pulmonary disease, *CKD* chronic kidney disease, *PCI* percutaneous coronary intervention, *NA* not applicable

were only observed in the pooled analysis of the observational studies rather than the RCTs.

The PROactive [12] and RECORD [14] RCTs showed that pioglitazone or rosiglitazone use does not provide any benefit in preventing AF incidence among high-risk patients with type 2 DM. However, in these two RCTs, AF was reported as an adverse event rather than a predefined endpoint. Furthermore, these trials displayed a very low AF incidence in both intervention and control groups (1.5–2%), and thus AF detection may be underpowered.

Table 3 Patients characteristics of 7 included studies

Study, year	Design	Age (years) T/C	Male T/C	HF T/C	HTN T/C	CAD T/C	HbA1c (%) T/C	β-blocker T/C	CCB T/C	ACEI/ARB T/C	Statin T/C	Insulin T/C
PROactive, 2005 [12]	RCT	61.9/61.6	67%/66%	NA	75%/76%	48%/48%	7.8/7.9	55%/54%	34%/37%	70%/70%	43%/43%	33.2%/34%
Anglade, 2007 [13]	Nested case control study of patients from the AFIST I, II and III trials	65.8/67.2	72.5%/71.5%	15.0%/18.8%	90.0%/75.7%	NA	NA	75.0%/75.0%	12.5%/21.5%	75.0%/56.9%	77.5%/61.8%	NA
RECORD, 2009 [14]	RCT	58.4/58.5	51.4%/51.7%	0.5%/0.4%	NA	NA	7.9/7.9	22.6%/20.9%	19.1%/21.6%	43.1%/42.1%	18%/19.2%	NA
Gu, 2011	Prospective cohort study	59.6/58.7	52.9%/45.5%	0/0	62.7%/72.7%	5.9%/5.1%	6.2/6.4	35.3%/37.4%	35.3%/28.3%	56.9%/45.5%	13.7%/12.1%	3.9%/2.0%
Chao, 2012 [16]	Nested case control study of patients from NHIRD	53.7/54.1	52.9%/53.6%	4.1%/4.7%	38.1%/44.5%	16.9%/18.4%	NA	45.5%/46.4%	NA	68.6%/68.3%	59%/57.4%	0/0
Liu, 2014 [17]	RCT	60.70/62.25	74.3%/65.8%	0/0	28.6%/30.3%	28.6%/30.3%	6.41/6.19	41.4%/38.2%	20%/17.1%	NA	31.4%/34.2%	NA
Pallisgaard, 2016 [18]	Prospective cohort study	59.59/62.40	56.7%/58.1%	2.3%/4.9%	50.2%/48.4%	NA	NA	31.5%/31.5%	NA	58.8%/55.9%	58.0%/53.0%	NA

Abbreviations: RCT randomized controlled trial, *HF* heart failure, *HTN* hypertension, *CAD* Coronary arterial disease, *HbA1c* haemoglobin A1c, *CCB* calcium channel blocker, *ACEI* angiotensin converting enzyme inhibitor, *ARB* angiotensin receptor blocker, *T/C* thiazolidinediones group/control group, *NA* not applicable

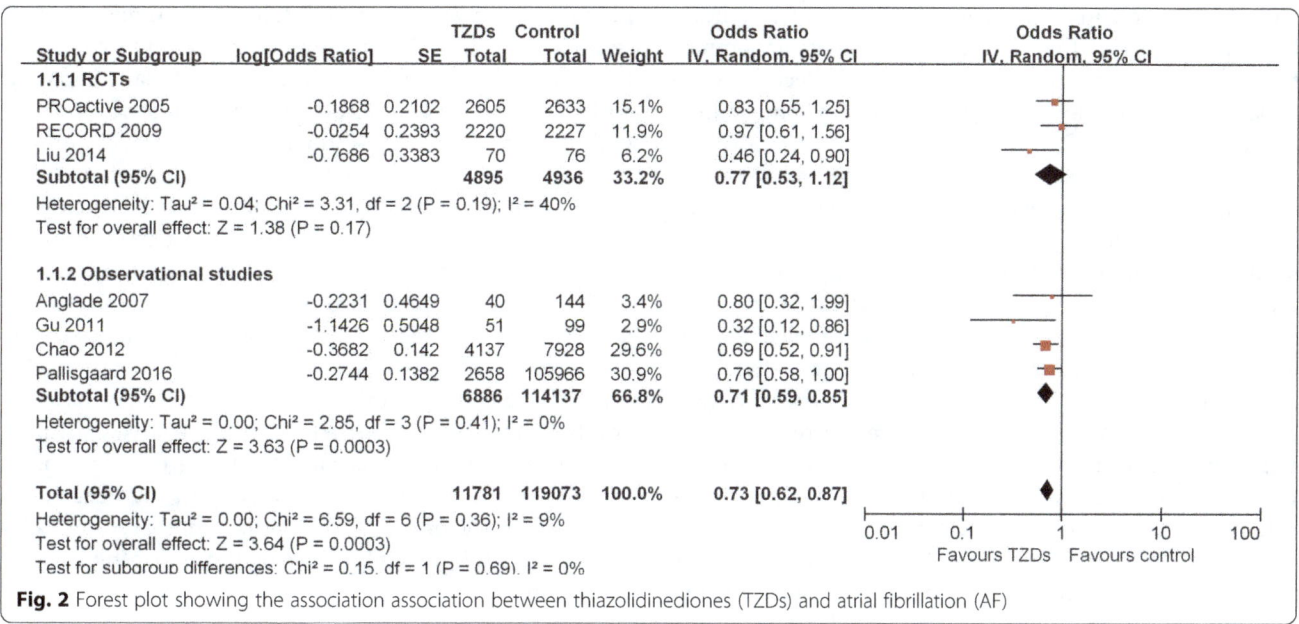

Fig. 2 Forest plot showing the association association between thiazolidinediones (TZDs) and atrial fibrillation (AF)

Moreover, in the present meta-analysis, we observed that pioglitazone use was associated with beneficial effects on AF prevention compared with rosiglitazone use. Similarly, previous study suggested that pioglitazone has a beneficial effect on cardiovascular disease, whereas rosiglitazone seemed to increase cardiovascular risk [24]. By assembling a diabetic cohort of older than 65 years, Winkelmayer et al. [25] demonstrated greater risk of mortality and congestive heart failure among patients who initiated therapy with rosiglitazone compared with pioglitazone, however, there were no differences in their incidences of myocardial infarction or stroke. Previous data [26] also showed similar effects on glycemic control between pioglitazone and rosiglitazone, as well as on other parameters such as C-reactive protein (CRP), plasminogen activator inhibitor-1 and indices of insulin secretion and sensitivity. However, pioglitazone treatment was associated with greater beneficial changes on plasma lipids than rosiglitazone treatment [26], which may partly explain the advantage of pioglitazone in reducing AF incidence.

Recently, the IRIS trial [27] demonstrated that pioglitazone can prevent fatal or nonfatal stroke or myocardial infarction among patients who have insulin resistance along with cerebrovascular disease. However, the underlying mechanism for these beneficial effects of pioglitazone remains incompletely elucidated. AF is a known risk factor of morbidity and mortality by predisposing to strokes and acute coronary syndrome [28]. Thus, it is possible to postulate that pioglitazone reduces the stroke or MI events partly through the reduction of AF burden.

Accumulating evidence supports the role of inflammation and immune response activation in the genesis and perpetuation of AF in different clinical settings, including cardiac surgery, electrical cardioversion and catheter ablation [29]. Oxidative stress has been suggested to play

Table 4 Subgroup analyses of the association between TZDs and AF

Subgroup	Study	Number of studies	Heterogeneity		Meta-analysis		
			I²	P-Value	OR	95% CI	p-Value
AF types	New-onset AF	4	0%	0.64	0.77	0.65–0.91	0.002
	Recurrent AF	2	0%	0.54	0.41	0.24–0.72	0.002
TZDs	Solely pioglitazone	3	54%	0.11	0.56	0.32–0.98	0.04
	Solely rosiglitazone	2	34%	0.22	0.78	0.57–1.07	0.12
Follow-up duration	≤ 5 years	4	34%	0.21	0.62	0.41–0.94	0.02
	> 5 years	3	0	0.47	0.76	0.63–0.91	0.002
Study design	RCTs	3	40%	0.10	0.77	0.53–1.12	0.17
	Observational studies	4	0%	0.41	0.71	0.59–0.85	0.0003

Abbreviations: TZDs thiazolidinediones, AF atrial fibrillation, RCTs randomized controlled trials, OR odds ratio, CI confidence interval

an important role in AF incidence [30]. Numerous studies have demonstrated that TZDs may attenuate inflammation and oxidative stress as well as atrial electrophysiological and structural remodeling in different animal models.

In a ventricular tachypacing-induced CHF rabbit model, Shimano et al. [31] showed that pioglitazone prevents atrial structural remodeling and inhibits AF promotion. Also, similarly to candesartan, pioglitazone suppresses transforming growth factor-β1 (TGF-β1) and tumor necrosis factor-α (TNF-α) expression in atrial tissue, molecules that are inflammatory mediators related to fibrosis-mediated AF incidence [29]. More recently, Kume et al. [32] suggested that pioglitazone effectively attenuates inflammatory profibrotic signals and vulnerability to AF in a pressure overload AF rat model, possibly via its suppression in monocyte chemoattractant protein (MCP-1) expression. PPAR-γ agonists have been shown to attenuate Angiotensin II (Ang II) -induced atrial electrical and structural remodeling in cellular models [33]. These effects are mediated by prevention of ICa-L remodeling by inhibiting CAMP responsive element binding protein (CREB) phosphorylation, as well as by suppression of connective tissue growth factor (CTGF) expression and cell proliferation via inhibiting TGF-β1/Smad2/3 and TGF-β1/tumor necrosis factor receptor associated factor 6 (TRAF6)/TGF-β-associated kinase 1 (TAK1) signaling pathways. In addition, Pioglitazone exhibits beneficial effects on Ang II-induced potassium channel remodeling [34]. More recently, Chen et al. [35] further indicated that pioglitazone inhibits Ang II-induced atrial fibroblasts proliferation through nuclear factor-κB (NF-κB)/TGF-β1/Toll/IL-1 receptor domain-containing adaptor inducing IFN-β (TRIF)/TRAF6 signaling pathway. Additionally, Xu et al. [36] suggested that

pioglitazone prevents age-related arrhythmogenic atrial remodeling and AF incidence by improving heat shock protein (HSP) 70 expression and antioxidant capacity, and by inhibiting the mitochondrial apoptotic signaling pathway. In an alloxan-induced diabetic rabbit model, we have shown that rosiglitazone attenuates arrhythmogenic atrial structural remodeling and AF incidence via anti-inflammatory and antioxidant effects [37]. In keeping with these findings, the IRIS trial found lower CRP levels in the pioglitazone group than in the placebo group. Indeed, increased CRP levels have been associated with greater risk of AF [38].

Finally, the treatment of hyperglycemia may have favorable effects on AF burden. In other words, treatment of DM may ameliorate atrial remodeling [7]. Haemoglobin A1c levels have been associated with the occurrence and recurrence of AF [7, 39, 40], and therefore TZDs may exert their favorable effects through HbA1c level reduction.

Study limitations

The present meta-analysis has potential limitations. Firstly, due to the small number of included studies we analyzed observational studies and RCTs together while 2 included RCTs reported AF as an adverse event rather than a predefined endpoint, and the favorable effects of TZDs use on preventing AF incidence were predominately driven by observational studies, whereas data from the 2 RCTs were unable to draw unanimous conclusion. Secondly, information regarding methods of AF detection, cardiac substrate, ejection fraction and atrial volume were not fully presented in our analysis due to the lack of relative data. Thirdly, the heterogeneous types of patient populations (ranging from uncomplicated type 2

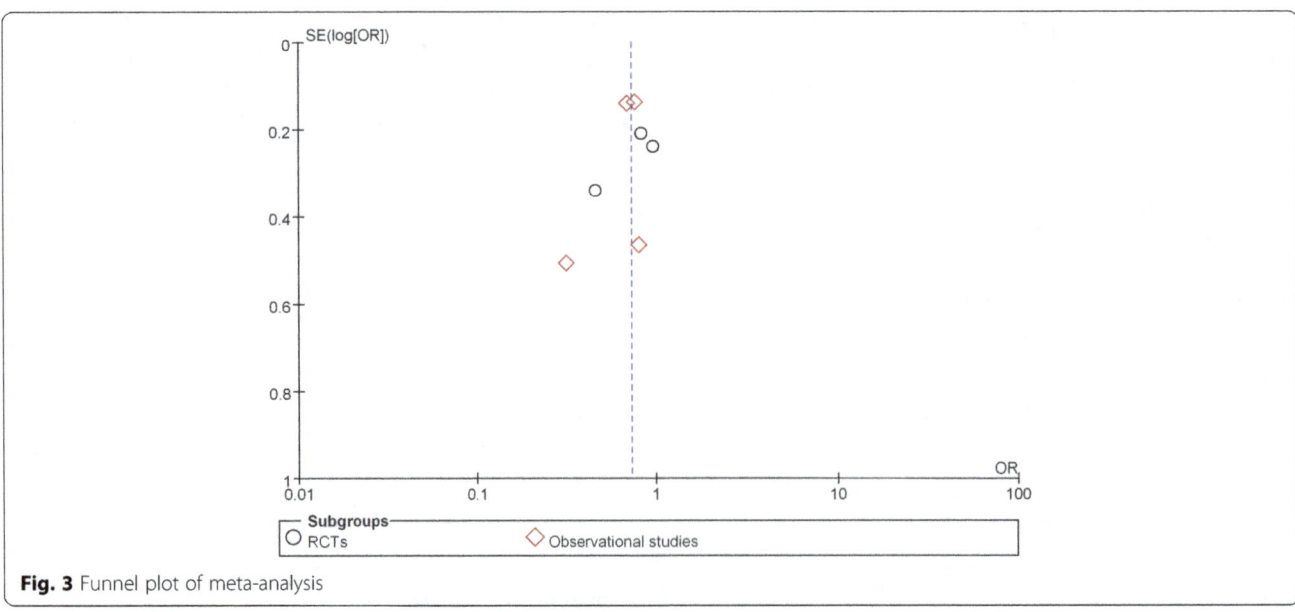

Fig. 3 Funnel plot of meta-analysis

diabetics to post-CABG or post-AF ablation patients) may indicate latent bias in this meta-analysis. Fourthly, "gray" literature (primarily conference abstracts/presentations, ongoing studies, communication with investigators) was not searched. Finally, the results of the funnel plot suggested that publication bias may be present, although the small number of studies made this somewhat difficult to interpret (Fig. 3).

Conclusions

In summary, this meta-analysis suggests that TZDs may be effective in AF prevention in the setting of DM. Therefore, TZDs may be considered as the treatment of choice in diabetic patient with high risk features for AF incidence. Since the overall conclusion was mainly drawn from the observational studies, further large-scale prospective RCTs that assessed AF as a predefined outcome are needed to determine whether TZDs use could prevent AF in the setting of DM.

Abbreviations

AF: Atrial fibrillation; CHF: Congestive heart failure; CI: Confidence interval; CRP: C-reactive protein; DM: Diabetes mellitus; OR: Odds ratio; PPAR-γ: Peroxisome proliferator-activated receptor-γ; RCTs: Randomized clinical trials; TZDs: Thiazolidinediones

Acknowledgments

Not applicable.

Funding

This work was supported by grants (81,570,298, 30,900,618, 81,270,245 to T.L.) from the National Natural Science Foundation of China, Tianjin Natural Science Foundation (16JCZDJC34900 to T.L.).

Authors' contributions

ZZ and ZX participated in study design, searched databases, extracted and assessed data, carried out the statistical analysis and drafted the manuscript. LM and MG performed statistical analyses. TL and GL conceived the design of the study, selected the included studies and drafted the review. KP, KPL and GT revised the manuscript. All authors read and approved the final manuscript.

Competing interests

The authors declare that they have no competing interests.

Author details

[1]Tianjin Key Laboratory of Ionic-Molecular Function of Cardiovascular Disease, Department of Cardiology, Tianjin Institute of Cardiology, Second Hospital of Tianjin Medical University, No. 23 Pingjiang Road, Hexi District, Tianjin 300211, People's Republic of China. [2]First Department of Cardiology, University of Ioannina Medical School, Ioannina, Greece. [3]Second Department of Cardiology, Laboratory of Cardiac Electrophysiology, "Evangelismos" General Hospital of Athens, Athens, Greece. [4]Department of Medicine and Therapeutics, Faculty of Medicine, Chinese University of Hong Kong, Hong Kong, SAR, People's Republic of China. [5]Li KaShing Institute of Health Sciences, Faculty of Medicine, Chinese University of Hong Kong, Hong Kong, SAR, People's Republic of China.

References

1. Chugh SS, Havmoeller R, Narayanan K, Singh D, Rienstra M, Benjamin EJ, et al. Worldwide epidemiology of atrial fibrillation: a global burden of disease 2010 study. Circulation. 2014;129(8):837–47.
2. Huxley RR, Filion KB, Konety S, Alonso A. Meta-analysis of cohort and case-control studies of type 2 diabetes mellitus and risk of atrial fibrillation. Am J Cardiol. 2011;108(1):56–62.
3. Tse G, Lai ET, Tse V, Yeo JM. Molecular and electrophysiological mechanisms underlying cardiac arrhythmogenesis in diabetes mellitus. J Diabetes Res. 2016;
4. Soran H, Younis N, Currie P, Silas J, Jones IR, Gill G. Influence of diabetes on the maintenance of sinus rhythm after a successful direct current cardioversion in patients with atrial fibrillation. QJM. 2008;101(3):181–7.
5. Du X, Ninomiya T, de Galan B, Abadir E, Chalmers J, Pillai A, et al. Risks of cardiovascular events and effects of routine blood pressure lowering among patients with type 2 diabetes and atrial fibrillation: results of the ADVANCE study. Eur Heart J. 2009;30(9):1128–35.
6. Zhang Q, Liu T, Ng CY, Li G. Diabetes mellitus and atrial remodeling: mechanisms and potential upstream therapies. Cardiovasc Ther. 2014;32(5): 233–41.
7. Goudis CA, Korantzopoulos P, Ntalas IV, Kallergis EM, Liu T, Ketikoglou DG. Diabetes mellitus and atrial fibrillation: Pathophysiological mechanisms and potential upstream therapies. Int J Cardiol. 2015;184:617–22.
8. Tse G, Yan BP, Chan YW, Tian XY, Huang Y. Reactive oxygen species, endoplasmic reticulum stress and mitochondrial dysfunction: the link with cardiac arrhythmogenesis. Front Physiol. 2016;7:313.
9. Inzucchi SE, Maggs DG, Spollett GR, Page SL, Rife FS, Walton V, et al. Efficacy and metabolic effects of metformin and troglitazone in type II diabetes mellitus. N Engl J Med. 1998;338(13):867–72.
10. Liu T, Li G. Thiazolidinediones as novel upstream therapy for atrial fibrillation in diabetic patients: a review of current evidence. Int J Cardiol. 2012;156(2):215–6.
11. Liu C, Liu T, Li G. Pioglitazone may offer therapeutic advantages in diabetes-related atrial fibrillation. Int J Cardiol. 2013;168(2):1603–5.
12. Dormandy JA, Charbonnel B, Eckland DJ, Erdmann E, Massi-Benedetti M, Moules IK, et al. Secondary prevention of macrovascular events in patients with type 2 diabetes in the PROactive study (PROspective pioglitAzone clinical trial in macroVascular events): a randomised controlled trial. Lancet. 2005;366(9493):1279–89.
13. Anglade MW, Kluger J, White CM, Aberle J, Coleman CI. Thiazolidinedione use and post-operative atrial fibrillation: a US nested case-control study. Curr Med Res Opin. 2007;23(11):2849–55.
14. Home PD, Pocock SJ, Beck-Nielsen H, Curtis PS, Gomis R, Hanefeld M, et al. Rosiglitazone evaluated for cardiovascular outcomes in oral agent combination therapy for type 2 diabetes (RECORD): a multicentre, randomised, open-label trial. Lancet. 2009;373(9681):2125–35.
15. Gu J, Liu X, Wang X, Shi H, Tan H, Zhou L, et al. Beneficial effect of pioglitazone on the outcome of catheter ablation in patients with paroxysmal atrial fibrillation and type 2 diabetes mellitus. Europace. 2011; 13(9):1256–61.
16. Chao TF, Leu HB, Huang CC, Chen JW, Chan WL, Lin SJ, et al. Thiazolidinediones can prevent new onset atrial fibrillation in patients with non-insulin dependent diabetes. Int J Cardiol. 2012;156(2):199–202.
17. Liu B, Wang J, Wang G. Beneficial effects of pioglitazone on retardation of persistent atrial fibrillation progression in diabetes mellitus patients. Int Heart J. 2014;55(6):499–505.
18. Pallisgaard JL, Lindhardt TB, Staerk L, Olesen JB, Torp-Pedersen C, Hansen ML, et al. Thiazolidinediones are associated with a decreased risk of atrial fibrillation compared with other antidiabetic treatment: a nationwide cohort study. Eur Heart J Cardiovasc Pharmacother; 2016. https://doi.org/10.1093/ ehjcvp/pvw036. [Epub ahead of print].
19. Moher D, Cook DJ, Eastwood S, Olkin I, Rennie D, Stroup DF. Improving the quality of reports of meta-analyses of randomised controlled trials: the QUOROM statement. Quality of reporting of meta-analyses. Lancet. 1999; 354(9193):1896–900.
20. Stroup DF, Berlin JA, Morton SC, Olkin I, Williamson GD, Rennie D, et al. Meta-analysis of observational studies in epidemiology: a proposal for reporting. Meta-analysis of observational studies in epidemiology (MOOSE) group. JAMA. 2000;283(15):2008–12.

21. Wynn GJ, Das M, Bonnett LJ, Panikker S, Wong T, Gupta D. Efficacy of catheter ablation for persistent atrial fibrillation: a systematic review and meta-analysis of evidence from randomized and nonrandomized controlled trials. Circ Arrhythm Electrophysiol. 2014;7(5):841–52.

22. Greenland S. Quantitative methods in the review of epidemiologic literature. Epidemiol Rev. 1987;9:1–30.

23. Higgins JP, Thompson SG, Deeks JJ, Altman DG. Measuring inconsistency in meta-analyses. BMJ. 2003;327(7414):557–60.

24. Simo R, Rodriguez A, Caveda E. Different effects of thiazolidinediones on cardiovascular risk in patients with type 2 diabetes mellitus: pioglitazone versus rosiglitazone. Curr Drug Saf. 2010;5(3):234–44.

25. Winkelmayer WC, Setoguchi S, Levin R, Solomon DH. Comparison of cardiovascular outcomes in elderly patients with diabetes who initiated rosiglitazone vs pioglitazone therapy. Arch Intern Med. 2008;168(21):2368–75.

26. Goldberg RB, Kendall DM, Deeg MA, Buse JB, Zagar AJ, Pinaire JA, et al. A comparison of lipid and glycemic effects of pioglitazone and rosiglitazone in patients with type 2 diabetes and dyslipidemia. Diabetes Care. 2005;28(7): 1547–54.

27. Kernan WN, Viscoli CM, Furie KL, Young LH, Inzucchi SE, Gorman M, et al. Pioglitazone after ischemic stroke or transient ischemic attack. N Engl J Med. 2016;374(14):1321–31.

28. Stewart S, Hart CL, Hole DJ, McMurray JJ. A population-based study of the long-term risks associated with atrial fibrillation: 20-year follow-up of the Renfrew/paisley study. Am J Med. 2002;113(5):359–64.

29. Hu YF, Chen YJ, Lin YJ, Chen SA. Inflammation and the pathogenesis of atrial fibrillation. Nat Rev Cardiol. 2015;12(4):230–43.

30. Korantzopoulos P, Kolettis TM, Galaris D, Goudevenos JA. The role of oxidative stress in the pathogenesis and perpetuation of atrial fibrillation. Int J Cardiol. 2007;115(2):135–43.

31. Shimano M, Tsuji Y, Inden Y, Kitamura K, Uchikawa T, Harata S, et al. Pioglitazone, a peroxisome proliferator-activated receptor-gamma activator, attenuates atrial fibrosis and atrial fibrillation promotion in rabbits with congestive heart failure. Heart Rhythm. 2008;5(3):451–9.

32. Kume O, Takahashi N, Wakisaka O, Nagano-Torigoe Y, Teshima Y, Nakagawa M, et al. Pioglitazone attenuates inflammatory atrial fibrosis and vulnerability to atrial fibrillation induced by pressure overload in rats. Heart Rhythm. 2011;8(2):278–85.

33. Gu J, Liu X, Wang QX, Guo M, Liu F, Song ZP, et al. Beneficial effects of pioglitazone on atrial structural and electrical remodeling in vitro cellular models. J Mol Cell Cardiol. 2013;65:1–8.

34. Gu J, Hu W, Liu X. Pioglitazone improves potassium channel remodeling induced by angiotensin II in atrial myocytes. Med Sci Monit Basic Res. 2014; 20:153–60.

35. Chen XQ, Liu X, Wang QX, Zhang MJ, Guo M, Liu F, et al. Pioglitazone inhibits angiotensin II-induced atrial fibroblasts proliferation via NF-kappaB/ TGF-beta1/TRIF/TRAF6 pathway. Exp Cell Res. 2015;330(1):43–55.

36. Xu D, Murakoshi N, Igarashi M, Hirayama A, Ito Y, Seo Y, et al. PPAR-gamma activator pioglitazone prevents age-related atrial fibrillation susceptibility by improving antioxidant capacity and reducing apoptosis in a rat model. J Cardiovasc Electrophysiol. 2012;23(2):209–17.

37. Liu T, Zhao H, Li J, Korantzopoulos P, Li G. Rosiglitazone attenuates atrial structural remodeling and atrial fibrillation promotion in alloxan-induced diabetic rabbits. Cardiovasc Ther. 2014;32(4):178–83.

38. Liu T, Li G, Li L, Korantzopoulos P. Association between C-reactive protein and recurrence of atrial fibrillation after successful electrical cardioversion: a meta-analysis. J Am Coll Cardiol. 2007;49(15):1642–8.

39. Huxley RR, Alonso A, Lopez FL, Filion KB, Agarwal SK, Loehr LR, et al. Type 2 diabetes, glucose homeostasis and incident atrial fibrillation: the atherosclerosis risk in communities study. Heart. 2012;98(2):133–8.

40. Anselmino M, Matta M, D'Ascenzo F, Pappone C, Santinelli V, Bunch TJ, et al. Catheter ablation of atrial fibrillation in patients with diabetes mellitus: a systematic review and meta-analysis. Europace. 2015;17(10):1518–25.

16

Comparison between CHA$_2$DS$_2$-VASc and the new R$_2$CHADS$_2$ and ATRIA scores at predicting thromboembolic event in non-anticoagulated and anticoagulated patients with non-valvular atrial fibrillation

Rami Riziq-Yousef Abumuaileq[*], Emad Abu-Assi, Andrea López-López, Sergio Raposeiras-Roubin, Moisés Rodríguez-Mañero, Luis Martínez-Sande, Javier García-Seara, Xesús Alberte Fernandez-López, Carlos Peña-Gil and Jose Ramón González-Juanatey

Abstract

Background: Accurate risk stratification is considered the first and most important step in the management of patients with non-valvular atrial fibrillation (NVAF). We compared the performance of the widely used CHA$_2$DS$_2$-VASc and the recently developed R$_2$CHADS$_2$ and ATRIA scores, for predicting thromboembolic (TE) event in either non-anticoagulated or anticoagulated patients with NVAF.

Methods: The non-anticoagulated cohort was comprised of 154 patients, whereas 911 patients formed the cohort of patients on vitamin-K-antagonist. The scores were computed using the criteria mentioned in their developmental cohorts. Measures of performance for the risk scores were evaluated at predicting TE event.

Results: In the non-anticoagulated cohort, 9 TE events occurred during 11 ± 2.7 months. CHA$_2$DS$_2$-VASc showed significant association with TE occurrence: hazard ratio (HR) = 1.58 (95 % confidence interval [95 % IC] 1.01–2.46), but R$_2$CHADS$_2$ and ATRIA did not (HR = 1.23 (95 % CI 0.86–1.77) and 1.20 (95 % CI 0.93–1.56), respectively.

In the anticoagulated cohort, after 10 ± 3 months of follow up, 18 TE events were developed. In that cohort, the three scores showed similar association with TE risk: HR = 1.49 (95 % CI 1.13–1.97), 1.41 (95 % CI 1.13–1.77) and 1.37 (95 % CI 1.12–1.66) for CHA$_2$DS$_2$-VASc, R$_2$CHADS$_2$ and ATRIA, respectively.

In both cohorts, no TE event occurred in patients classified in the low risk category according to CHA$_2$DS$_2$-VASc or R$_2$CHADS$_2$.

Conclusions: In this study of NVAF patients, CHA$_2$DS$_2$-VASc has better association with TE events than the new R$_2$CHADS$_2$ and ATRIA risk scores in the non-anticoagulated cohort. CHA$_2$DS$_2$-VASc and R$_2$CHADS$_2$ can identify patients at truly low risk regardless of the anticoagulation status.

Keywords: Atrial fibrillation, Anticoagulant, Thromboembolism

* Correspondence: drrami2012@hotmail.com
Cardiology Department, University Clinical Hospital, A choupana s/n, 15706, Santiago de Compostela, Spain

Background

Atrial fibrillation (AF) increases the risk of embolic stroke by 5-fold [1]. Effective prevention of thromboembolic events (TE) with oral anticoagulants is the cornerstone of AF management and appropriate TE risk stratification is a critical step in the decision making process regarding this vital issue [2].

The current clinical practice guidelines [3–5] recommend the use of $CHADS_2$ [6] and CHA_2DS_2-VASc [7] risk scores in the effective TE prevention strategy. $CHADS_2$ [6] score was validated and conceived in the year of 2001 with the aim of identifying patients at high risk of TE events. However, patients at low risk according to $CHADS_2$ score continued to have significant annual stroke rate [8, 9], this enhanced the motivation to investigate the significance of other risk factors not included in the $CHADS_2$ score and, in turn, has led to a clinical shift in the paradigm with a new aim to identify "truly low risk" patients using CHA_2DS_2-VASc score [7]. Anyhow, in several studies, $CHADS_2$ and CHA_2DS_2-VASc showed just a moderate discrimination ability to predict TE complications [10, 11], and at least one recently published large cohort study demonstrated an annual ischemic stroke rate of 1.06 % in the group of patients classified in "the true low risk category" according to CHA_2DS_2-VASc [12]. All this could lead to a number of questions and potential avenues for further research.

Recently, and with the aim to improve the ability to predict TE event, two new TE risk scores (i.e. R_2CHADS_2 [13] and ATRIA [14]) have been shown, in their own derivation cohorts, better performance than $CHADS_2$ and CHA_2DS_2-VASc. Really, the two recently proposed risk scores contain new risk factors in their schemes which were not included in the most recommended CHA_2DS_2-VASc score. This fact could qualify them to strongly capture the risk of suffering a future TE event, but little information is available in this regard in independent dataset of patients. A recent expert review has announced the need for further validation of the R_2CHADS_2 in a real world cohort with full spectrum of estimated glomerular filtration rate (eGFR) [15].

We aimed to evaluate the ability of CHA_2DS_2-VASc, R_2CHADS_2 and ATRIA scores at predicting TE events in contemporary two different real world cohorts of non-anticoagulated and anticoagulated patients with non-valvular atrial fibrillation (NVAF) which have full spectrum of eGFR.

Methods

This retrospective study is composed of two separate and different cohorts: for the first cohort, we screened all the consultations which were registered in the emergency department of our tertiary hospital between January 2008 and June 2010, by this we were able to identify all consecutive patients ≥18 years of age with AF documented by electrocardiographic records ($n = 1873$). After excluding patients with prosthetic valve ($n = 473$), rheumatic heart disease ($n = 46$) and/or patients with active cancer ($n = 61$), there were 1293 patients with NVAF. We also excluded patients on anticoagulation ($n = 1135$) and those patients lost to follow up ($n = 4$). Thus, the non-anticoagulated cohort consisted of 154 consecutive patients with NVAF.

The second cohort of the present study was constituted by 911 patients with NVAF on vitamin K antagonists (VKAs), as was previously described [16].

For both cohorts, a detailed medical history was recorded for each patient, and the basal clinical characteristics at study entry together with information on follow up were carefully gathered by cardiologists.

The study was approved by the Clinical Research Ethics Committee of the University Clinical Hospital of Santiago de Compostela. The study protocol conforms to the ethical guidelines of the 1975 Declaration of Helsinki as reflected in a priori approval by the institution's human research committee.

TE risk calculation

CHA_2DS_2-VASc, R_2CHADS_2 and ATRIA scores for predicting TE complications were calculated in each patient from the original corresponding prognostic variables scores used in their derivation cohorts. CHA_2DS_2-VASc was calculated by adding 2 points for age ≥ 75 years; 2 points for prior stroke or transient ischemic attack (TIA); and 1 point for each of the following factors: congestive heart failure\left ventricular ejection fraction ≤40 %, hypertension, diabetes mellitus, vascular disease, age 65–74 and female sex, with a maximum score of 9 points.

R_2CHADS_2 was calculated by adding 2 points for renal dysfunction (i.e. estimated glomerular filtration rate [eGFR] <60 ml/min/1.73 m^2); 2 points for prior stroke or TIA; and one point for each of the following factors: congestive heart failure, hypertension, age ≥ 75 and diabetes mellitus with a maximum score of 8 points.

For CHA_2DS-VA_2Sc and R_2CHADS_2, patients with 0 point were defined as being in the low risk category and patients with 1 point were at intermediated risk, while patients with ≥2 points were in the high risk stratum.

The ATRIA TE risk score was calculated by adding 1 point for each of the following factors: female sex, diabetes mellitus, congestive heart failure, hypertension, proteinuria and renal dysfunction (i.e. eGFR < 45 ml/min/1.73 m^2 or end-stage renal disease) and by adding 0–9 points depending on the specific score weighting of patients age according to the presence or absence of prior ischemic stroke [14]. We did not have data about proteinuria, so the maximum score of the ATRIA risk score will be 14 points. Patients with ≤ 5 points were defined as low risk category and patients with 6 points were at intermediated risk, while patients with ≥7 points were in the high risk stratum.

eGFR was estimated at study entry for every patient in both cohorts using the 4 variable Modification of Diet in Renal Disease (MDRD-4) [17].

End point definition

The primary endpoint for the present study was the development of TE event during follow-up. A TE complication was defined as the occurrence of ischemic stroke, TIA or peripheral embolism (including fatal TE events). Diagnosis of stroke or transient ischemic attack required an acute neurological deficit lasting for more or less than 24 h, respectively, which could not be explained by other causes and with at least 1 image test (computed tomography or magnetic resonance) compatible with the diagnosis, as well as confirmation from a neurologist. A diagnosis of peripheral embolism was defined as non-central nervous system embolism leading to an abrupt vascular insufficiency associated with clinical or radiographic evidence of arterial occlusion in absence of another mechanism such as atherosclerosis, instrumentation or trauma.

For both cohorts, patients were followed up for 1-year after the enrolment or until TE event or death occurred. Data on TE event were gathered from the cardiology clinic visits and records, and through hospital files as well as through primary care centers reports. Data regarding death during the follow up period was also recorded.

Statistical analysis

Qualitative data were expressed as frequencies and percentages while quantitative data were summarized as mean and standard deviation. Each risk score was entered into separate Cox regression models to test their association with TE complication. Thereafter, we calculated the c-statistic as a measure of the predictive ability of the scores and tested the hypothesis that these schemes performed significantly better than chance (indicated by a c-statistic 0.50). We calculated and reported the p-values and hazard ratios (HR) with their 95 % confidence interval (95 % CI). P-value < 0.05 was considered statistically significant. The data was performed using the SPSS v.18 software.

Results

Baseline characteristics

Our study enrolled a total of 1065 patients, distributed in two different cohorts. The non-anticoagulated cohort had 154 patients with NVAF and the anticoagulated cohort consisted of 911 patients with NVAF on VKAs.

Table 1 summarizes the baseline characteristics of the patients in each cohort. For the non-anticoagulated cohort

Table 1 Baseline characteristics of patients with nonvalvular atrial fibrillation in the non-anticoagulated and the anticoagulated cohorts

	Non-anticoagulated cohort	Anticoagulated cohort
	$N = 154$	$N = 911$
Age (years)	74 ± 12	73 ± 11
Age ≥65 years, %	127 (82.5)	707 (77.6)
Age ≥75 years, %	75 (40.5)	445 (48.8)
Female sex, %	81 (52.6)	306 (33.6)
Systolic blood pressure at study entry (mmHg)	129 ± 15	139 ± 28
Current smoking, %	53 (30.4)	77 (8.5)
Hypertension, %	110 (71.4)	678 (74.4)
Diabetes mellitus, %	33 (21.4)	220 (24.1)
Peripheral arterial disease, %	20 (12.9)	92 (10.1)
Heart failure, %	10 (6.5)	343 (35.5)
History of stroke or TIA, %	9 (5.8)	103 (11.3)
Coronary artery disease, %	23 (14.9)	127 (13.9)
COPD, %	31 (20.1)	183 (20.1)
Hyperthyroidism, %	2 (1.3)	14 (1.5)
Anemia, %	27 (17.4)	178 (19.5)
Alcohol consumption ≥ 40 gr/daily, %	9 (5.8)	81 (8.9)
Antiplatelets, %	150 (97.4)	23 (2.5)
PINRR (%)	--	58 ± 18
eGFR < 60 ml/min/1.73 m^2, %	44 (28.6)	311 (34.1)
CHA$_2$DS$_2$-VASc		
0 point, %	5 (3.2)	62 (6.8)
1 point, %	18 (11.7)	77 (8.4)
≥ 2 points, %	131 (85.1)	772 (84.7)
R$_2$CHADS$_2$		
0 points, %	22 (14.3)	98 (10.8)
1 points, %	43 (27.9)	142 (15.6)
≥ 2 points, %	89 (57.8)	671 (73.7)
ATRIA		
≤ 5 points, %	79 (51.3)	389 (42.7)
6 points, %	14 (9.1)	115 (12.6)
≥ 7 points, %	61 (39.6)	407 (44.7)

ATRIA the anticoagulation and risk factors in atrial fibrillation score, *CHA2DS2-VASc* congestive heart failure, hypertension, age ≥75, diabetes mellitus, prior stroke or transient ischemic attack, vascular disease, age 65–74, female, *COPD* chronic obstructive pulmonary disease, *eGFR* estimated glomerular filtration rate, *PINNR* proportion of international normalized ratio within therapeutic range, *R$_2$CHADS$_2$* renal dysfunction, congestive heart failure, hypertension, age ≥75, diabetes mellitus, prior stroke or transient ischemic attack, *TIA* transient ischemic attack

the mean age was 74 ± 12 and 52.6 % were females. For the anticoagulated cohort, the mean age was 73 ± 11 and 33.6 % were females.

Outcomes during follow up

During follow up (11 ± 2.7 months) of the non-anticoagulated cohort, 8 (5.2 %) patients died and 9 (5.8 %) patients developed TE events, 8 of them were ischemic strokes and one event was a peripheral embolic event. For the anticoagulated cohort, 60 (6.6 %) patients died and 18 (2 %) patients developed TE events during the follow up (10 ± 3 months): 13 events were ischemic strokes, 2 events were TIAs and 3 were peripheral embolic events.

Risk scores performance

Risk scores performance in the non-anticoagulated cohort

CHA_2DS_2-VASc score classified 85.1 % of patients in the high risk category, while R_2CHADS_2 classified 57.8 % as high risk patients; ATRIA classified just 39.6 % of patients in the high risk category (Table 1).

The distribution of the TE events rates in the different risk categories of the three risk scores, demonstrated the absence of occurrence of TE event in the subgroups of patients classified as low risk (i.e. patients with 0 point) according to CHA_2DS_2-VASc and R_2CHADS_2. However, TE events occurred in 6.3 % of patients classified as at low risk according to ATRIA (Table 2).

CHA_2DS_2-VASc was the only score to show significant association with TE events: HR = 1.58 (95 % CI; 1.01–2.46). R_2CHADS_2 and ATRIA did not show significant association with TE event: HR = 1.23 (95 % CI; 0.86–1.77) and 1.20 (95 % CI; 0.93–1.56) for both scores, respectively (Table 3).

The discriminative capacity of the three risk scores at predicting TE event are shown in Table 4. CHA_2DS_2-

Table 2 Distribution of thromboembolic events according to the different risk category of each risk score

	Non-anticoagulated cohort N = 9	Anticoagulated cohort N = 18
CHA_2DS_2-VASc		
0 point, %	0 (0)	0 (0)
1 point, %	0 (0)	1 (1.3)
≥ 2 points, %	9 (6.9)	17 (2.2)
R_2CHADS_2		
0 point, %	0 (0)	0 (0)
1 point, %	1 (2.3)	0 (0)
≥ 2 points, %	8 (9)	18 (2.7)
ATRIA		
≤ 5 points, %	5 (6.3)	2 (0.5)
6 points, %	0 (0)	1 (0.9)
≥ 7 points, %	4 (6.6)	15 (3.7)

ATRIA the anticoagulation and risk factors in atrial fibrillation score, *CHA2DS2-VASc* congestive heart failure, hypertension, age ≥75, diabetes mellitus, prior stroke or transient ischemic attack, vascular disease, age 65–74, female, *R₂CHADS₂* renal dysfunction, congestive heart failure, hypertension, age ≥75, diabetes mellitus, prior stroke or transient ischemic attack

Table 3 Association between each risk score as continuous variables and thromboembolic event in both cohorts

	Non anticoagulated cohort HR (95 % CI)	Anticoagulated cohort HR (95 % CI)
CHA_2DS_2-VASc	1.58 (1.01–2.46)	1.49 (1.13–1.97)
	p = 0.044	p = 0.005
R_2CHADS_2	1.23 (0.86–1.77)	1.41 (1.13–1.77)
	p = 0.25	p = 0.03
ATRIA	1.20 (0.93–1.56)	1.37 (1.12–1.66)
	p = 0.17	p = 0.002

ATRIA the anticoagulation and risk factors in atrial fibrillation score, *CHA2DS2-VASc* congestive heart failure, hypertension, age ≥75, diabetes mellitus, prior stroke or transient ischemic attack, vascular disease, age 65–74, female, *CI* confidence interval, *HR* hazard ratio, *NVAF* nonvalvular atrial fibrillation, *p*; p value, *R₂CHADS₂* renal dysfunction, congestive heart failure, hypertension, age ≥75, diabetes mellitus, prior stroke or transient ischemic attack

VASc and R_2CHADS_2 had moderate discriminative capacity with c-statistics of 0.69 (95 % CI; 0.53–0.85) and 0.65 (95 % CI; 0.53–0.78), respectively. The ATRIA score showed a weaker discriminative ability at predicting TE events: c- statistics = 0.64 (95 % CI; 0.49–0.80).

Risk scores performance in the anticoagulated cohort

CHA_2DS_2-VASc score classified 84.7 % of patients in the high risk category, while R_2CHADS_2 classified 73.7 % and ATRIA classified just 44.7 % of patients in the high risk category (Table 1).

The distribution of the TE events rates in the different risk categories showed the absence of TE event in patients classified in the low risk category according to CHA_2DS_2-VASc and R_2CHADS_2. However, two TE events occurred among patients belonged to the low risk category by ATRIA (Table 2).

In terms of hazard ratios, as a measure of association between each risk score and TE events, all the studied scores demonstrated similar and significant association with TE events: HR = 1.49 (95 % CI; 1.13–1.97), 1.41 (95 % CI; 1.13–1.77) and 1.37 (95 % CI; 1.12–1.66) for CHA_2DS_2-VASc, R_2CHADS_2 and ATRIA, respectively (Table 3).

Table 4 Discriminatory capacity of risk scores as continuous variables at predicting thromboembolic event in both cohorts

	Non anticoagulated cohort c-statistics (95 % CI)	Anticoagulated cohort c-statistics (95 % CI)
CHA_2DS_2-VASc	0.69 (0.53–0.85)	0.72 (0.63–0.82)
R_2CHADS_2	0.65 (0.53–0.78)	0.70 (0.61–0.79)
ATRIA	0.64 (0.49–0.80)	0.72 (0.62–0.83)

ATRIA the anticoagulation and risk factors in atrial fibrillation score, *CHA2DS2-VASc* congestive heart failure, hypertension, age ≥75, diabetes mellitus, prior stroke or transient ischemic attack, vascular disease, age 65–74, female, *CI* confidence interval, *HR* hazard ratio, *R₂CHADS₂* renal dysfunction, congestive heart failure, hypertension, age ≥75, diabetes mellitus, prior stroke or transient ischemic attack

The three risk scores showed good discriminative ability at predicting TE event: c-statistics = 0.72 (95 % CI; 0.63–0.82) for CHA_2DS_2-VASc; 0.70 (95 % CI; 0.61–0.79) for R_2CHADS_2 and 0.72 (95 % CI; 0.62-0.83) for ATRIA (Table 4).

Discussion

In this study comparing three contemporary TE risk scores in non-anticoagulated and anticoagulated real world cohorts of patients with NVAF which have full spectrum of eGFR, CHA_2DS_2-VASc was the only score to show significant association in terms of hazard ratio at predicting TE events in the non-anticoagulated cohort.

In the anticoagulated cohort of this study, the three TE risk scores had similar and significant association and discrimination at predicting TE event. On note, only the CHA_2DS_2-VASc and R_2CHADS_2 were accurate at defining patients at truly low risk to develop TE event in both cohorts.

Oral anticoagulants are highly effective in preventing TE event in patients with AF. However, risk of major bleeding is the downside of oral anticoagulants therapy, so accurate risk estimation of TE event is of paramount importance to help decision making process regarding this issue [2]. Up to our knowledge, this is the first study to compare the most recommended CHA_2DS_2-VASc and the recently developed and more sophistically derived R_2CHADS_2 and ATRIA scores in real world non-anticoagulated and anticoagulated patients with NVAF.

It is clearly recognized that TE risk scores are best tested in a non-anticoagulated cohort from a real world [15]. In this regard, although R_2CHADS_2 and ATRIA contained new risk factors believed to have strong association with TE event like renal dysfunction [13, 14, 18]. However, CHA_2DS_2-VASc was the best score to have strong association with TE event in the non-anticoagulated cohort of our study, this may be explained by the fact that factors like renal dysfunction may coexist with advancing age, hypertension, diabetes, heart failure and vascular disease which are already individual components comprising the CHA_2DS_2-VASc score. Moreover, our results can be explained and supported if we take into account that R_2CHADS_2 score [13] was mainly derived and validated from the ROCKET AF trial of anticoagulated patients which excluded patients with creatinine clearance < 30 ml/min and this may limit its predictability in non-anticoagulated AF patients from the real world with full range of eGFR. Furthermore, similar to our findings in which CHA_2DS_2-VASc clearly outperformed ATRIA score in non-anticoagulated cohort of patients with AF, were found in a recent nationwide study [12].

The analysis of the anticoagulated cohort of the current study showed that the three TE risk scores have demonstrated similar association and discrimination at predicting thromboembolism. The improvement we have seen in the performance of the R_2CHADS_2 and ATRIA in the anticoagulated cohort may be explained by the fact that factors like renal dysfunction —which is involved in the R_2CHADS_2 and ATRIA— is a strong independent predictor of poor anticoagulation control and hence for more TE complications [16, 19]. Furthermore, these findings, in turn, may reflect that the non-anticoagulated and the anticoagulated cohorts of patients with NVAF are completely different groups of patients and re-emphasized the belief and strong hypothesis that TE risk scores are best tested in a non-anticoagulated cohort.

In our analysis, CHA_2DS_2-VASc and R_2CHADS_2 were accurate at identifying truly low risk patients in both cohorts. In previous studies, CHA_2DS_2-VASc had identified accurately patients at low risk in non-anticoagulated and anticoagulated patients with NVAF [7, 20]. Similar to our results regarding the reasonable ability of R_2CHADS_2 at identifying patients at low risk, were found in the external validation of R_2CHADS_2 in which the rates of TE event in the low risk patients at 3-years of follow up were as low as 0.36 % and 0.5 % in the non-anticoagulated and anticoagulated subgroups of the ATRIA study cohort, respectively [13].

In the two different cohorts of current study, ATRIA classified about half of patients in the low risk category, and this may limit its ability to correctly classify patients at truly low risk. Similar performance of the ATRIA risk score was found in a recent study enrolled large cohort of patients [12].

Similar to our findings in which CHA_2DS_2-VASc classified the greatest number of patients as being at high risk (85.1 %) and (84.7 %) in the non-anticoagulated and anticoagulated cohorts, respectively, were reported previously [12, 20]. This may aid and reflect the accuracy of CHA_2DS_2-VASc at classifying a small group of patients who are truly at low risk of TE event.

Finally, our analysis of the anticoagulated cohort showed that those patients in the high risk category according to CHA_2DS_2-VASc and the R_2CHADS_2 are still at high risk of developing TE event despite anticoagulation. Really, the identification of patients who remain at high risk of TE event despite anticoagulation could be of great importance in daily clinical practice as this high risk group of patients may need specific treatment strategy with close follow up and more efforts to improve the quality of anticoagulation control and to achieve the best management of their risk factors like hypertension, diabetes and heart failure.

Although this is the first study aimed to compare the CHA2DS2-VASc and the new R2CHADS2 and ATRIA scores in real world non-anticoagulated and anticoagulated cohorts of patients with NVAF. However, the relatively small number of patients enrolled in the current study - when compared with several previous studies [12–14] - might limit the validity of our results. This might reflect the need for future studies with large cohorts of patients for further validation of the interesting results obtained from our analysis.

Our overall results when taken together might indicate that the CHA_2DS_2-VASc still the best user friendly tool at predicting TE event as well as at identifying patients at truly low risk particularly in the non-anticoagulated patients who are actually need accurate TE risk stratification.

Limitations

The main limitation of our study is its retrospective design, but it has interesting strong points as it reflects real world practice by enrolment of two contemporary separate and different cohorts of non-anticoagulated and anticoagulated patients with NVAF consulted the emergency department or the outpatient cardiology clinics of a tertiary hospital with the advantage of careful follow-up and data collection by cardiologists. Nevertheless, in this regard prospective studies in the future may be needed for better assessment of the clinical validity of our results.

The sample size of the non-anticoagulated cohort of the current study might be another limitation of our study that could limit the likelihood of detecting small effects or significant relationships from the data. However, the availability of a contemporary large non-anticoagulated cohort of patients with NVAF is challenging and increasingly unlikely. Furthermore, the findings in our study might need to be enhanced by further studies with large real world cohorts of patients with NVAF. In the non-anticoagulated cohort, the vast majority of patients were taking antiplatelet therapy during follow up. However, antiplatelet therapy alone is not a substitute for thromboembolic prevention in AF and could not reduce significantly the TE risk [21], so patients in the non-anticoagulated cohorts continue to have high TE risk during the follow up.

Really, most patients in the non-anticoagulated cohort were at risk of TE event and despite this, the anticoagulation was underused in these patients. This may be mainly due to the effect of advance age, associated comorbidities and/or patient preference on the medical decisions taken by the emergency department doctors and the reluctance to change the medication regime.

Conclusions

CHA_2DS_2-VASc has better association with TE events than R_2CHADS_2 or ATRIA in non-anticoagulated patients with NVAF, and represents in this study the more accurate clinical tool for TE risk stratification in these patients. The CHA_2DS_2-VASc and the R_2CHADS_2

scores may accurately identify patients at truly low risk of developing future TE events regardless of the anticoagulation status.

Abbreviations

AF: atrial fibrillation; eGFR: estimated glomerular filtration; HR: hazard ratio; MDRD-4: 4 variable modification of diet in renal disease; NVAF: nonvalvular atrial fibrillation; TE: thromboembolic event; TIA: transient ischemic attack; VKAs: vitamin k antagonists.

Competing interests

The authors declare that they have no competing interest.

Authors' contributions

RRA is the principal investigator who participated substantially in the acquisition of data, design of the study, interpretation of data and drafting the manuscript. EAA participated significantly in the design of the study, statistical analysis and drafting the manuscript. ALL participated in the acquisition of data and drafting the manuscript. SRR participated in the interpretation of data and drafting the manuscript. MRM participated in the interpretation of data and critically revised the manuscript. JGS participated in the interpretation of data and drafting the manuscript. CPG participated in the design of the study and reviewed critically the manuscript. LMS participated in the interpretation of data and reviewed critically the manuscript. XFL participated in the interpretation of data and drafting the manuscript. JGJ participated in the design of the study and reviewed critically the manuscript. All authors read and approved the final manuscript.

Acknowledgements

None.

References

1. Wolf PA, Abbott RD, Kannel WB. Atrial fibrillation as an independent risk factor for stroke: the Framingham study. Stroke. 1991;22:983–8.
2. Hart RG, Benavente O, McBride R, Pearce LA. Antithrombotic therapy to prevent stroke in patients with atrial fibrillation: a meta-analysis. Ann Intern Med. 1999;131:492–501.
3. Wann LS, Curtis AB, January CT, Ellenbogen KA, Lowe JE, Estes NA3rd, et al. 2011 ACCF/AHA/HRS focused update on the management of patients with atrial fibrillation (updating the 2006 guideline): a report of the American College of Cardiology Foundation/ American Heart Association task force on practice guidelines. J Am Coll Cardiol. 2011;57:223–42.
4. You JJ, Singer DE, Howard PA, Lane DA, Eckman MH, Fang MC, et al. Antithrombotic therapy for atrial fibrillation: antithrombotic therapy and prevention of thrombosis, 9th ed: American College of Chest Physicians evidence-based clinical practice guidelines. Chest. 2012;141:e531S–75.
5. Camm AJ, Lip GY, De Caterina R, Atar D, Hohnloser SH, Hindricks G, et al. 2012 focused update of the ESC guidelines for the management of atrial fibrillation: an update of the 2010 ESC guidelines for the management of atrial fibrillation—developed with the special contribution of the European Heart Rhythm Association. Europace. 2012;14:1385–413.
6. Gage BF, Waterman AD, Shannon W, Boechler M, Rich MW, Radford MJ. Validation of clinical classification schemes for predicting stroke: results from the national registry of atrial fibrillation. JAMA. 2001;285:2864–70.
7. Lip GY, Nieuwlaat R, Pisters R, Lane DA, Crijns HJ. Refining clinical risk stratification for predicting stroke and thromboembolism in atrial fibrillation using a novel risk factor-based approach: the euro heart survey on atrial fibrillation. Chest. 2010;137:263–72.
8. Olesen JB, Torp-Pedersen C, Hansen ML, Lip GY. The value of the CHA_2DS_2-VASc score for refining stroke risk stratification in patients with atrial fibrillation with a $CHADS_2$ score 0–1: a nationwide cohort study. Thromb Haemost. 2012;107:1172–9.
9. Coppens M, Eikelboom JW, Hart RG, Yusuf S, Lip GY, Dorian P, et al. The CHA_2DS_2-VASC score identifies those patients with atrial fibrillation and a $CHADS_2$ of 1 who are unlikely to benefit from oral anticoagulant therapy. Eur Heart J. 2013;34:170–6.

10. Van Staa TP, Setakis E, Di Tanna GL, Lane DA, Lip GY. A comparison of risk stratification schemes for stroke in 79,884 atrial fibrillation patients in general practice. J Thromb Haemost. 2011;9:39–48.

11. Fang MC, Go AS, Chang Y, Borowsky L, Pomernacki NK, Singer DE, et al. Comparison of risk stratification schemes to predict thromboembolism in people with nonvalvular atrial fibrillation. J Am Coll Cardiol. 2008;51:810–5.

12. Chao TF, Liu CJ, Wang KL, Lin YJ, Chang SL, Lw L, et al. Using the CHA2DS2-VASc score for refining stroke risk stratification in 'low-risk' asian patients with atrial fibrillation. J Am Coll Cardiol. 2014;64:1658–65.

13. Piccini JP, Stevens SR, Chang Y, Singer DE, Lokhnygina Y, Go AS, et al. Renal dysfunction as a predictor of stroke and systemic embolism in patients with nonvalvular atrial fibrillation: validation of the R_2CHADS_2 index in the ROCKET AF (Rivaroxaban Once-Daily, Oral, Direct Factor Xa Inhibition Compared with Vitamin K Antagonism for Prevention of Stroke and Embolism Trial in Atrial Fibrillation) and ATRIA (Anticoagulation and Risk Factors in Atrial Fibrillation) study cohorts. Circulation. 2013;127:224–32.

14. Singer DE, Chang Y, Borowsky LH, Fang MC, Pomernacki NK, Udaltsova N, et al. A new risk scheme to predict ischemic stroke and other thromboembolism in atrial fibrillation: the ATRIA study stroke risk score. J Am Heart Assoc. 2013;2:e000250.

15. Dzeshka MS, Lane DA, Lip GY. Stroke and bleeding risk in atrial fibrillation: navigating the alphabet soup of risk-score acronyms (CHADS2, CHA2DS2-VASc, R2CHADS2, HAS-BLED, ATRIA, and More). Clin Cardiol. 2014;37:634–44.

16. Abumuaileq RR, Abu-Assi E, Raposeiras-Roubin S, Lopez-Lopez A, Redondo-Dieguez A, Alvarez-Iglesias D, et al. Evaluation of SAMe-TT2R2 risk score for predicting the quality of anticoagulation control in a real-world cohort of patients with non-valvular atrial fibrillation on vitamin-K antagonists. Europace. 2015;17:711–7.

17. Levey AS, Coresh J, Greene T, Marsh J, Stevens LA, Kusek JW, et al. Expressing the modification of diet in renal disease study equation for estimating glomerular filtration rate with standardized serum creatinine values. Clin Chem. 2007;53:766–72.

18. Baber U, Howard VJ, Halperin JL, Soliman EZ, Zhang X, McClellan W, et al. Association of chronic kidney disease with atrial fibrillation among adults in the united states. Reasons for Geographic and Racial Differences in Stroke (REGARDS) study. Circ Arrhythm Electrophysiol. 2011;4:26–32.

19. Rose AJ, Hylek EM, Ozonoff A, Ash AS, Reisman JI, Berlowitz DR. Patient characteristics associated with oral anticoagulation control: results of the Veterans AffaiRs Study to Improve Anticoagulation (VARIA). J Thromb Haemost. 2010;8:2182–91.

20. Lip GY, Frison L, Halperin JL, Lane DA. Identifying patients at high risk for stroke despite anticoagulation: a comparison of contemporary stroke risk stratification schemes in an anticoagulated atrial fibrillation cohort. Stroke. 2010;41:2731–8.

21. Hart RG, Pearce LA, Aguilar MI. Meta-analysis: antithrombotic therapy to prevent stroke in patients who have nonvalvular atrial fibrillation. Ann Intern Med. 2007;146:857–67.

17

Comparative effectiveness of rivaroxaban versus warfarin or dabigatran for the treatment of patients with non-valvular atrial fibrillation

Faye L. Norby[1][*], Lindsay G.S. Bengtson[2], Pamela L. Lutsey[1], Lin Y. Chen[3], Richard F. MacLehose[1], Alanna M. Chamberlain[4], Ian Rapson[1] and Alvaro Alonso[5]

Abstract

Background: Rivaroxaban is an oral anticoagulant approved in the US for prevention of stroke and systemic embolism in patients with non-valvular atrial fibrillation (NVAF). We determined the effectiveness and associated risks of rivaroxaban versus other oral anticoagulants in a large real-world population.

Methods: We selected NVAF patients initiating oral anticoagulant use in 2010–2014 enrolled in MarketScan databases. Rivaroxaban users were matched with warfarin and dabigatran users by age, sex, enrolment date, anticoagulant initiation date, and high-dimensional propensity score. Study endpoints, including ischemic stroke, intracranial bleeding (ICB), myocardial infarction (MI), and gastrointestinal (GI) bleeding, were identified from inpatient diagnostic codes. Multivariable Cox models were used to assess associations between type of anticoagulant and outcomes.

Results: The analysis included 44,340 rivaroxaban users matched to 89,400 warfarin and 16,957 dabigatran users (38% female, mean age 70) with 12 months of mean follow-up. Anticoagulant-naïve rivaroxaban initiators, but not those switching from warfarin, had lower risk of ischemic stroke [hazard ratio (HR) (95% confidence interval (CI)): 0.75 (0.62, 0.91)] and ICB [HR (95%CI): 0.55, (0.39, 0.78)] than warfarin users. In contrast, anticoagulant-experienced rivaroxaban initiators had higher risk of GI bleeding than warfarin users [HR (95%CI): 1.55 (1.32, 1.83)]. Endpoint rates were similar when comparing anticoagulant-naïve rivaroxaban and dabigatran initiators, with the exception of higher GI bleeding risk in rivaroxaban users [HR (95%CI) 1.28 (1.06, 1.54)]. There were no significant differences in the risk of MI among the comparison groups.

Conclusion: In this large real-world sample of NVAF patients, effectiveness and risks of rivaroxaban versus warfarin differed by prior anticoagulant status, while effectiveness of rivaroxaban versus dabigatran differed in GI bleeding risk.

Keywords: Non-valvular atrial fibrillation, Stroke, Warfarin, Dabigatran, Rivaroxaban

Background

Atrial fibrillation (AF) is the most common sustained cardiac arrhythmia, with a lifetime risk of 1 in 4 in the general population, and an increasing prevalence as the population ages [1]. The estimated prevalence of AF in the United States (US) is expected to rise to 12.1 million by 2030 [2, 3]. Patients with any type of AF, whether permanent, persistent, or paroxysmal, and whether they are symptomatic or asymptomatic, are at increased risk of thromboembolic ischemic stroke, [4–7] with nonvalvular AF (NVAF) associated with a 5 times greater risk compared to those without NVAF [4].

For patients with diagnosed NVAF, the current ACC/AHA/HRS Guideline for the Management of Patients with AF recommends oral anticoagulation in those with a prior stroke or transient ischemic attack, or those with a moderate or greater risk of stroke (CHA_2DS_2-VASc

* Correspondence: flopez@umn.edu
[1]Division of Epidemiology and Community Health, School of Public Health, University of Minnesota, 1300 S 2nd St, Suite 300, Minneapolis, MN 55454, USA
Full list of author information is available at the end of the article

score ≥ 1 in males or ≥2 in females) [8]. Vitamin K antagonist anticoagulants, with warfarin being the most common in the US, have been prescribed since the 1950's as an oral anticoagulant for stroke prevention in patients with NVAF. Over the last six years, several non-vitamin K antagonist oral anticoagulants (NOACs) have been approved by the US Food and Drug Administration (FDA) to reduce the risk of stroke and systemic embolism in patients with NVAF.

Rivaroxaban is a direct factor Xa inhibitor approved by the FDA in November, 2011 for the prevention of stroke and systemic embolism in patients with NVAF. Rivaroxaban is administered as a single daily dose of 20 mg for most patients or 15 mg for those with reduced kidney function. A dose of 10 mg may be prescribed for the prevention or treatment of deep venous thrombosis (approved in July 2011). In the large randomized controlled trial, ROCKET AF, NVAF patients randomized to rivaroxaban experienced lower rates of stroke, intracranial bleeds, and fatal bleeding than those assigned to warfarin [9]. However, concerns were raised regarding international normalized ratio (INR) measures in the warfarin (control) arm of the clinical trial data [10, 11]. Published real-world studies of rivaroxaban vs. warfarin in NVAF patients report similar results as the clinical trials, but have focused on limited outcomes and have not stratified on patient characteristics [12–14].

Dabigatran, a direct thrombin inhibitor, was the first NOAC to be FDA-approved (October, 2010) for the prevention of stroke and systemic embolism in patients with NVAF. Data indicate dabigatran is associated with a lower risk of stroke and intracranial bleeds compared to warfarin, however, dabigatran users may be more at risk of GI bleeds and myocardial infarctions (MI) compared to warfarin users [15, 16]. Head-to-head comparisons of the effectiveness of dabigatran vs. rivaroxaban in NVAF patients indicate rivaroxaban initiators have an increased risk of intracranial bleeding and major bleeding, including GI bleeds [12, 17].

In this real-world study, we determined the effectiveness and associated risks of rivaroxaban vs. warfarin and rivaroxaban vs. dabigatran use in anticoagulant-naïve NVAF patients. We also assessed the effectiveness of rivaroxaban in patients who switched from warfarin compared to those who use only warfarin.

Methods
Study population
A retrospective cohort study was conducted using healthcare claims data from January 1st, 2010 through December 31st, 2014 from the Truven Health MarketScan® Commercial Claims and Encounters Database and the Medicare Supplemental and Coordination of Benefits Database (Truven Health Analytics, Inc., Ann Arbor, MI) [18]. The MarketScan Commercial Database includes health insurance claims spanning all levels of care, as well as enrolment data from large employers and health plans across the United States, providing private healthcare coverage for employees, their spouses, and dependents. The MarketScan Medicare Supplemental Database includes claims from individuals and their dependents with employer-sponsored Medicare Supplemental plans. Both databases link medical and outpatient prescription drug claims and encounter data with patient enrolment data to provide individual-specific clinical utilization, expenditure, and outcomes information across inpatient and outpatient services and outpatient pharmacy services. Patients with AF enrolled in the MarketScan Medicare Supplemental Database have similar demographic characteristics to patients with AF in the general fee-for-service Medicare population [19, 20].

The initial sample included 1,021,079 patients age 22–99 with at least one inpatient or 2 outpatient claims for AF 7 to 365 days apart (International Classification of Diseases, Ninth Revision, Clinical Modification (ICD-9-CM) codes 427.3, 427.31, and 427.32 in any position). We excluded patients with ICD-9-CM codes for valvular disease or procedure codes for valvular repair or replacement because the NOACs have received FDA approval for NVAF only (n = 92,098). The analytic sample was 522,620 once we restricted to individuals with at least one prescription for warfarin, rivaroxaban or dabigatran after their first AF claim between January 1, 2010 and December 31st, 2014. The final available sample was 227,799 after requiring ≥90 days of continuous enrolment prior to the first oral anticoagulant prescription. If a patient discontinued enrolment and then re-enrolled, we analysed their first period of enrolment. A systematic review of studies using ICD-9-CM codes for AF identification reported a positive predicted value (PPV) of approximately 90% and a sensitivity of approximately 80% [21]. All patient information is Health Insurance Portability and Accountability Act compliant, de-identified, commercially available secondary data, and therefore the Institutional Review Board at the University of Minnesota deemed this analysis exempt from review.

Anticoagulant use and initial matching
Prescriptions for warfarin, rivaroxaban and dabigatran were identified following the first code for AF from 2010 to the end of 2014. Patients were initially categorized according to their first anticoagulant prescription during this period as a new warfarin user, a new rivaroxaban-only user, or a new dabigatran-only user. Warfarin users switching to rivaroxaban during follow-up were identified as switchers. Due to limited numbers, patients switching from dabigatran to rivaroxaban were not considered in this study, and neither were those taking other NOACS.

Each rivaroxaban-only initiator was matched with up to 3 warfarin-only initiators by age (± 3 years), sex, time since database enrolment (± 90 days) and drug initiation date (± 90 days). Computerized matching using a greedy matching algorithm was used to match rivaroxaban users to warfarin users [22]. New rivaroxaban users were matched 1:1 with new dabigatran users using the same matching criteria. Individuals switching from warfarin to rivaroxaban were matched with up to 5 warfarin-only users by age (± 3 years), sex, time since database enrolment (± 90 days) and warfarin initiation date (± 90 days). The date the individual switched to rivaroxaban (the index date) then became the index date for the matched warfarin-only user. Warfarin users must have had ≥90 days of warfarin use before the index date to be considered as a match. The validity of warfarin claims in administrative data has a PPV of 99% and a sensitivity of 94% [23]. Baseline characteristics after initial matching are provided in Additional file 1: Table S1.

Outcome ascertainment

The main outcomes of interest included ischemic stroke, intracranial bleeding, MI, and GI bleeding, and were identified from inpatient claims using validated algorithms described below. In addition, 3 control outcomes of hip/pelvic fracture, breast/prostate cancer, and asthma were also obtained from inpatient claims. Hip/pelvic fracture was included a priori as a control outcome where no association with anticoagulant type was expected. A similar risk of hip/pelvic fracture by anticoagulant type would provide indirect evidence of no confounding. The control outcomes of breast/prostate cancer and asthma were added post-hoc after unexpected associations were observed between hip/pelvic fracture and anticoagulant type. Codes for these variables are listed in the Additional file 1: Tables S1-S8.

Ischemic stroke was defined based on the presence of ICD-9-CM codes 434.xx (occlusion of cerebral arteries) and 436.xx (acute but ill-defined cerebrovascular disease) as the primary discharge diagnosis in any inpatient claim following the index date. A PPV of >80% has been reported in several validation studies that used this definition [24]. Intracranial bleeding was defined based on the presence of ICD-9-CM codes 430 (subarachnoid haemorrhage) and 431 (intracerebral haemorrhage) as the primary discharge diagnosis in an inpatient claim following the index date. The PPV has been reported as >90% in many different validation studies [24]. MI was defined as the presence of ICD-9-CM codes 410.xx in the 1st or 2nd position of an inpatient discharge diagnosis. This excluded code 410.x2, which is used to indicate follow-up of the initial episode. The PPV for this algorithm is between 88 and 94% in validation studies [25, 26]. GI bleeding was defined by an algorithm developed by Cunningham et al. [27] that

considers presence of bleeding-related ICD-9-CM codes in inpatient claims as primary and secondary diagnoses, presence of transfusion codes, and presence/absence of trauma codes to exclude trauma-related bleeding. The PPV of this algorithm is 86%, which is comparable to other peer-reviewed algorithms [26]. Hip/pelvic fracture, breast/prostate cancer and asthma were defined according to algorithms developed by the Centers for Medicare and Medicaid Chronic Condition Data Warehouse [28].

Assessment of covariates

Pre-determined covariates were defined based on inpatient, outpatient and pharmacy claims that took place prior to the index date using validated published algorithms [27, 29]. Demographic characteristics, comorbidities, procedures and pharmacy prescription fills were ascertained. Comorbidities of interest were ascertained with published algorithms from inpatient and outpatient claims and include prior stroke/transient ischemic attack, haemorrhagic stroke, heart failure, MI, hypertension, diabetes, peripheral arterial disease, liver disease, kidney disease, chronic pulmonary disease, malignancies (except malignant skin neoplasm), metastatic cancer, history of bleeding, haematological disorders (anaemia, coagulation defects), dementia, depression, and alcohol abuse [27, 29]. Cardiac, vascular, gastrointestinal, and neurologic procedures also were identified from inpatient and outpatient claims. Presence of prescription fills for the following medication groups were ascertained: digoxin, clopidogrel, other antiplatelets, angiotensin-converting enzyme inhibitors, angiotension receptor blockers, ß-blockers, calcium channel blockers, antiarrhythmics, statins, and antidiabetic medications. The CHA_2DS_2-VASc score [30] was calculated at index date to determine stroke risk. Codes for these variables are listed in the Additional file 1: Tables S1-S8.

Statistical analysis

High-dimensional propensity scores (HDPS) were calculated using methodology proposed by Schneeweiss et al., [31] and included the following pre-defined variables: age, age ≥ 75, calendar year, sex, the CHA_2DS_2-VASc score, any prevalent outcome before the start of the index date, and covariates listed above, which were obtained from inpatient and outpatient diagnostic codes and procedure codes, and outpatient pharmacy claims. HDPS were calculated with SAS macros developed by Rassen et al. and included the covariates described above and the most prioritized empirical covariates [32]. To define the empirical covariates, the data were categorized into 5 domains: inpatient diagnostic codes, inpatient procedure codes, outpatient diagnostic codes, outpatient procedure codes, and medications. Within each of the 5 domains, we selected the 200 most prevalent conditions. This resulted in 1000 covariates. All the covariates in the dimensions listed above were empirically rank ordered based on their potential for controlling confounding (i.e. strength of the covariate-outcome association and prevalence of the covariate) [33]. We selected the top 500 covariates based on this ordering. The 500 empirically-derived covariates, along with the pre-specified covariates mentioned above (also listed in Table 1), were included as covariates in a regression model to calculate the probability of receiving a DOAC versus warfarin. Separate HDPS were calculated for each of the anticoagulant comparison-outcome pairs (7 outcomes × 3 comparison groups = 21 total HDPS).

Separate models were used to compare 1) new rivaroxaban users to new warfarin-only users; 2) patients who switched to rivaroxaban from warfarin to warfarin-only users and 3) new rivaroxaban users to new dabigatran users. As noted above, anticoagulant users were initially matched by age, sex, enrolment date, and anticoagulant initiation date, for the purpose of defining an index date, and to collect covariate information at the time of drug initiation. To better compare the groups based on characteristics at the time of drug initiation, we then rematched patients according to each outcome-specific HDPS. A greedy matching technique with a calliper of 0.25 of a standard-deviation of each HDPS was used to improve exchangeability [22]. Using the calliper, new rivaroxaban users were matched with up to 2 warfarin-only users, rivaroxaban switchers were matched with up to 4 warfarin-only users, and new rivaroxaban users were matched 1:1 with new dabigatran users.

Cox proportional hazards models were used to estimate the association between anticoagulant type and the time to each outcome (ischemic stroke, intracranial bleeding, MI, GI bleeding, and the 3 control outcomes of hip/pelvic fracture, breast/prostate cancer, and asthma). The start of follow-up began at the drug index date. Time to event was considered as the time to each outcome event, health plan disenrollment, or the end of study follow-up, whichever occurred first. For each outcome, Cox proportional hazards models were adjusted for age (continuous), sex, CHA_2DS_2-VASc (categorical), HDPS (continuous), and prevalent outcome at the index date. We performed two sensitivity analyses. First, we required patients to have been enrolled in the database for at least 180 days (instead of 90 days) before the first oral anticoagulant prescription. Second, we limited the analysis to those who had AF after January 1st, 2011, to minimize selective prescribing.

Effect modification by sex, age (<75, ≥75), CHA_2DS_2-VASc score (<2, ≥2), early vs. late outcomes (<90 days ≥90 days), and rivaroxaban dose strength were explored using stratified analysis. A p-value for interaction was obtained by adding a multiplicative term in the model (i.e. sex*drug). All statistical analyses were performed with SAS v 9.3 (SAS Inc., Cary, NC).

Results

After exclusion criteria were applied, our study included 32,495 new rivaroxaban users matched to 45,496 warfarin-only users, 11,845 switchers to rivaroxaban matched to 43,904 warfarin-only users, and 16,957 new rivaroxaban users matched to 16,957 new dabigatran users. Numbers varied slightly across analyses due to endpoint-specific HDPS matching; therefore the total numbers listed in the tables are for the outcome of ischemic stroke. Characteristics of patients initiating rivaroxaban were comparable to their matched controls (Table 1). New rivaroxaban users were similar to new warfarin users, though slightly younger in age (mean age 69 vs. 71), and with a mean CHA_2DS_2-VASc score of 3.0 compared to 3.2 in warfarin-only users. Switchers to rivaroxaban from warfarin were comparable to their matched warfarin-only users, with a mean age of 71 and a mean CHA_2DS_2-VASc score of 4.0 vs. 3.9, respectively. New rivaroxaban users matched to new dabigatran users were similar, with the same mean age (67) and mean CHA_2DS_2-VASc score (2.6). Across comparison groups, the switchers (rivaroxaban switchers and their matched warfarin-only users) were older and had a higher prevalence of comorbidities (85% hypertensive, 35% diabetic, mean CHA_2DS_2-VASc score of 4.0) when compared to the new anticoagulant users. The new rivaroxaban and new dabigatran users tended to be younger (mean age 67) and had the fewest comorbidities among the comparison groups, with a mean CHA_2DS_2-VASc score of 2.6.

Overall, the characteristics of patients after the final matching (listed in Table 1) were similar to characteristics at the time of initial matching (listed in Additional file 1: Table S1). HDPS distributions for ischemic stroke by comparison group prior to HDPS matching are depicted in Additional file 1: Figure S1. The distributions are most similar between new rivaroxaban and new dabigatran users and least similar between new rivaroxaban users and new warfarin-only users. These distributions are prior to matching on HDPS; the extreme ends of each distribution were less likely to be included in analyses since it is less likely that there will be suitable matched patients.

New rivaroxaban users vs. new warfarin users

The hazard ratio (HR) and 95% confidence interval (CI) of each outcome for new rivaroxaban users compared to new warfarin users are reported in Table 2. During a mean follow-up of 12 months (median 10.5 months), new rivaroxaban users had a significantly lower rate of ischemic stroke and intracranial bleeds compared to warfarin users, HR (95% CI) = 0.75 (0.62–0.91) and 0.55 (0.39–0.78), respectively, in models adjusted for age, sex, CHA_2DS_2-VASc score, prevalent outcome and HDPS. Rates of MI and GI bleeding were comparable between the two groups. New users of rivaroxaban had a lower

Table 1 Characteristics of atrial fibrillation patients by anticoagulant use, MarketScan, 2010–2014

	New Users		Switchers		New Users	
	New Rivaroxaban (n = 32,495)	Matched Warfarin (n = 45,496)	Rivaroxaban Switcher (n = 11,845)	Matched Warfarin (n = 43,904)	New Rivaroxaban (n = 16,957)	Matched Dabigatran (n = 16,957)
Age, years	69.3 ± 12.2	71.1 ± 12.5	71.2 ± 12.1	71.4 ± 12.0	67.2 ± 12.1	67.2 ± 12.1
Age ≥ 75 years	37.1	43.5	44.3	44.9	29.9	29.8
Female, %	38.7	40.1	39.3	39.5	34.1	34.2
Comorbidities, %						
Hypertension	66.0	62.8	84.8	82.5	61.9	59.2
Diabetes	25.7	26.7	35.3	35.4	23.4	23.5
Myocardial infarction	7.1	8.1	11.1	11.0	5.5	5.2
Heart failure	23.1	26.0	38.7	38.3	19.5	19.3
Ischemic stroke/TIA	15.5	17.2	29.1	27.0	12.1	12.2
Hemorrhagic stroke	0.6	0.8	1.7	1.6	0.3	0.3
PAD	12.2	14.1	23.7	23.1	8.8	8.5
Dementia	1.1	1.5	2.9	2.6	0.6	0.7
Renal Disease	7.6	10.3	14.1	15.5	5.3	5.0
Chronic pulmonary disease	21.4	22.5	34.6	32.7	17.8	17.1
Liver disease	3.6	3.6	7.0	6.6	2.9	2.9
Malignancy	10.9	11.3	17.1	16.5	8.5	7.8
Depression	7.0	7.5	13.7	11.9	5.5	5.6
Hematological disorders	7.6	9.7	22.5	21.8	5.6	5.1
Metastatic cancer	1.6	1.9	2.6	2.5	1.0	0.9
Alcohol abuse	0.4	0.4	0.6	0.6	0.3	0.3
GI bleed	4.4	4.9	12.1	11.5	3.4	3.2
Other bleed	2.4	3.0	8.3	8.0	1.7	1.5
CHA$_2$DS$_2$-VASC score	3.0 ± 1.9	3.2 ± 2.0	4.0 ± 2.1	3.9 ± 2.1	2.6 ± 1.8	2.6 ± 1.8
CHA$_2$DS$_2$-VASC score ≥ 2	75.5	79.5	87.4	86.8	69.4	68.5
Prior procedures, %						
Cardiac	54.6	53.6	81.1	79.4	52.2	50.5
Vascular	4.5	6.3	9.7	9.2	2.8	2.7
Gastrointestinal	21.1	20.8	42.3	39.6	17.5	16.6
Neurological	12.7	12.0	23.7	19.7	9.7	8.5
Medications, %						
Digoxin	11.4	13.3	23.0	22.8	10.9	11.2
Clopidogrel	9.5	9.6	11.0	10.5	7.9	7.3
Antiplatelets	1.8	1.8	2.1	1.9	1.4	1.2
Angiotensin-converting enzyme inhibitors	30.0	30.7	41.7	41.4	27.5	28.2
Angiotensin receptor blockers	20.2	19.2	26.5	24.9	18.8	17.7
Beta-blockers	63.9	61.8	77.3	75.6	61.5	60.8
Calcium channel blockers	36.0	34.9	46.5	44.1	33.6	32.9
Anti-arrhythmias	20.2	17.9	32.9	28.2	21.9	21.5
Statins	46.6	47.4	62.2	62.0	42.7	42.5
Diabetes medications	19.6	20.7	25.4	25.4	18.2	19.2

Table 1 Characteristics of atrial fibrillation patients by anticoagulant use, MarketScan, 2010–2014 *(Continued)*

Initial dose of anticoagulant, %						
Rivaroxaban						
10 mg	6.2	–	5.4	–	4.8	–
15 mg	18.2	–	21.0	–	15.2	–
20 mg	75.6	–	73.7	–	80.0	–
Warfarin						
< 5 mg	–	33.2	30.2	31.8	–	–
5 mg	–	48.0	51.6	49.3	–	–
> 5 mg	–	18.9	18.3	18.9	–	–
Dabigatran						
75 mg	–	–	–	–	–	11.9
150 mg	–	–	–	–	–	88.1

Values correspond to mean ± standard deviation or percentage

risk of the control outcome hip/pelvic fractures compared to warfarin initiators; however, there was no association between anticoagulant type and the other 2 control outcomes. In stratified analysis, the reduction in stroke risk among new rivaroxaban users vs. warfarin was larger in women compared to men (HR (95% CI) = 0.61 (0.46, 0.81) vs. 0.90 (0.70, 1.17); p for interaction = 0.02) and in the first 90 days after initiation compared to the subsequent time period (HR (95% CI) = 0.52 (0.35, 0.76) vs. 0.86 (0.69, 1.07); p for interaction = 0.03), (Fig. 1, panel A). Rivaroxaban initiation (vs. warfarin) was associated with increased risk of GI bleeding in women but not in men (HR: 1.24 vs. 0.95, respectively; p for interaction = 0.02) and in those age ≥ 75 compared to those <75 (HR: 1.18 vs. 0.90, respectively; p for interaction = 0.01).

Rivaroxaban switchers vs. persistent warfarin users

Patients who switched to rivaroxaban from warfarin had a significantly higher rate of GI bleeding compared to warfarin-only users, HR (95% CI) = 1.55 (1.32–1.83) (Table 3). There was no significant difference in the rate of ischemic stroke, intracranial bleeding, or MI. Rivaroxaban switchers had a lower rate of hip/pelvic fractures compared to warfarin users while there was no association for the other 2 control outcomes. In stratified analysis, the increased risk of GI bleeding associated with switching to rivaroxaban was higher in the first 90 days after switching to rivaroxaban compared to the risk greater than 90 days after switching, HR (95% CI) = 2.31 (1.71–3.11) vs. 1.33 (1.10–1.62), p for interaction = 0.002 (Fig. 1, panel B). Rivaroxaban was associated with reduced risk of intracranial bleeding in those age < 75 but not in individuals 75 and older (HR: 0.43 vs. 1.45, respectively; p for interaction = 0.01). However, this interaction should be interpreted with caution due to the small numbers in the <75 age group (4 events in rivaroxaban users and 33 in warfarin users). The association of rivaroxaban use, compared to warfarin, was

Table 2 Adjusted hazard ratios (95% confidence intervals) of selected outcomes comparing new rivaroxaban users to new warfarin users for the treatment of non-valvular atrial fibrillation, MarketScan, 2010–2014

	Rivaroxaban User (*n* = 32,495)			Matched Warfarin User (*n* = 45,496)			Hazard Ratio (95% CI)[a]	*p*-value
Main outcomes	# Events	Person-years	IR (95% CI)	# Events	Person-years	IR (95% CI)		
Ischemic stroke	165	33,252	5.0 (4.3–5.8)	347	45,965	7.5 (6.8–8.4)	0.75 (0.62, 0.91)	0.003
Intracranial bleeding	46	33,309	1.4 (1.0–1.8)	124	45,958	2.7 (2.3–3.2)	0.55 (0.39, 0.78)	0.0008
Myocardial infarction	244	33,183	7.4 (6.5–8.3)	421	45,965	9.2 (8.3–10.1)	0.88 (0.75, 1.03)	0.11
Gastrointestinal bleeding	492	33,134	14.8 (13.6–16.2)	717	45,649	15.7 (14.6–16.9)	1.07 (0.95, 1.20)	0.29
Control outcomes								
Hip / pelvic fracture	194	33,214	5.8 (5.1–6.7)	408	45,866	8.9 (8.1–9.8)	0.83 (0.70, 0.99)	0.04
Breast / prostate cancer	272	33,236	8.2 (7.3–9.2)	419	45,941	9.1 (8.3–10.0)	0.92 (0.79, 1.08)	0.33
Asthma	443	33,157	13.4 (12.2–14.6)	606	45,769	13.2 (12.2–14.3)	0.99 (0.88, 1.13)	0.93

IR incidence rate, *CI* confidence interval
Incidence rate is per 1000 person-years
[a]Adjusted for age, sex, CHA$_2$DS$_2$-VASc score, prevalent outcome and high-dimensional propensity score

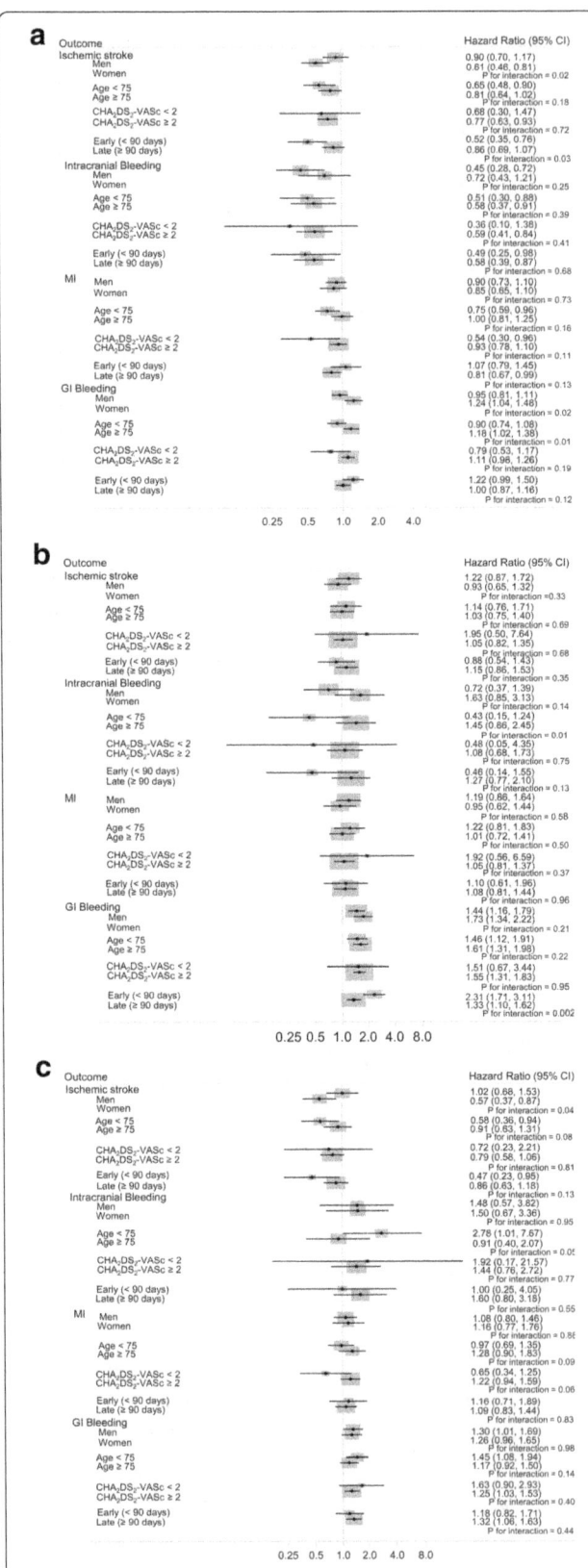

Fig. 1 Adjusted hazard ratios (95% confidence intervals) of outcomes among anticoagulant users, stratified by subgroups, MarketScan, 2010–2014. **Panel a:** New rivaroxaban users vs. new warfarin users. **Panel b:** Patients who switched from warfarin to rivaroxaban vs. persistent warfarin users. **Panel c:** New rivaroxaban users vs. new dabigatran users

significantly different between the anticoagulant-naïve and anticoagulant-experienced (switchers) groups for ischemic stroke [HR (95% CI) = 0.75 (0.62, 0.91) vs. 1.06 (0.83, 1.36); p for interaction 0.03] intracranial bleeding [HR (95% CI) = 0.55 (0.39, 0.78) vs. 1.04 (0.66, 1.65); p for interaction 0.03], and for GI bleeding [HR (95% CI) = 1.07 (0.95, 1.20) vs. 1.55 (1.32, 1.83); p for interaction <0.001].

New rivaroxaban users vs. new dabigatran users

Compared to new dabigatran users, those initiating rivaroxaban had a significantly higher risk of GI bleeding, HR (95% CI) = 1.28 (1.06–1.54) (Table 4). Rivaroxaban users had a non-significant lower risk of ischemic stroke compared to dabigatran users, HR (95% CI) = 0.77 (0.58–1.03), and this inverse association was present in women but not in men HR (95% CI) = 0.57 (0.37–0.87) vs. 1.02 (0.69–1.53), p for interaction = 0.04 (Fig. 1, panel C). There was no difference between rivaroxaban and dabigatran initiators in the risk of intracranial bleeds, MI, or any of the control outcomes, and no statistically significant interactions in the remaining stratified results.

Associations by rivaroxaban dose

Results stratified by initial rivaroxaban dose are listed in Additional file 1: Tables S2-S4. Most patients were taking the 20 mg dose (74–80% for each comparison group), while only around 5% were taking the 10 mg dose, and the remaining percentage taking the 15 mg dose. Because of low numbers in the 10 mg group, and since this dose is not FDA-approved for NVAF treatment, we focus only on the 15 mg and 20 mg groups. Overall, the associations were similar between the 15 mg and 20 mg groups when compared to their matched warfarin or dabigatran comparison groups. The exception was that for new rivaroxaban users, the 15 mg group had a higher risk of MI, HR (95% CI) = 1.19 (0.93–1.52), and GI bleeding = 1.40 (1.17–1.65) than the 20 mg group, 0.77 (0.63–0.93) and 0.97 (0.84–1.11), respectively, when compared to the matched warfarin-only users.

Sensitivity analyses

We performed a sensitivity analysis comparing new rivaroxaban users to new warfarin users, but restricted to patients with at least 180 days of enrolment before the first oral anticoagulation prescription. The results are listed in Additional file 1: Table S5, and indicate similar risks as our main results in Table 2, where we required

Table 3 Adjusted hazard ratios (95% confidence intervals) of selected outcomes comparing patients who switched to rivaroxaban from warfarin to warfarin-only users for the treatment of non-valvular atrial fibrillation, MarketScan, 2010–2014

	Rivaroxaban Switcher (n = 11,845)			Matched Warfarin User (n = 43,904)			Hazard Ratio (95% CI) [a]	p-value
Main outcomes	# Events	Person-years	IR (95% CI)	# Events	Person-years	IR (95% CI)		
Ischemic stroke	85	11,758	7.2 (5.8–8.9)	278	40,081	6.9 (6.2–7.8)	1.06 (0.83–1.36)	0.62
Intracranial bleeding	24	11,808	2.0 (1.3–3.0)	83	40,221	2.1 (1.7–2.5)	1.04 (0.66–1.65)	0.86
Myocardial infarction	77	11,776	6.5 (5.2–8.1)	252	40,283	6.3 (5.5–7.1)	1.08 (0.84–1.40)	0.55
Gastrointestinal bleeding	216	11,681	18.5 (16.1–21.1)	489	39,955	12.2 (11.2–13.4)	1.55 (1.32–1.83)	<0.0001
Control outcomes								
Hip / pelvic fracture	86	11,765	8.2 (6.6–9.9)	410	40,091	10.2 (9.3–11.3)	0.73 (0.58–0.92)	0.009
Breast / prostate cancer	107	11,749	9.1 (7.5–11.0)	297	40,164	7.4 (6.6–8.3)	1.21 (0.97–1.51)	0.10
Asthma	166	11,720	14.2 (12.1–16.4)	482	40,063	12.0 (11.0–13.1)	1.12 (0.94–1.34)	0.21

IR incidence rate, CI confidence interval
Incidence rate is per 1000 person-years
[a]Adjusted for age, sex, CHA_2DS_2-VASc score, prevalent outcome and high-dimensional propensity score

90 days of anticoagulation free enrolment. To account for selective prescribing based on FDA approval dates, we performed another sensitivity analysis in which restricted the analysis comparing new rivaroxaban users to new warfarin users to those with an enrolment date after January 1st, 2011. These results are listed in Additional file 1: Table S6 and are similar to our main results listed in Table 2.

Discussion

In this retrospective administrative claims analysis of NVAF patients, we found that anticoagulant-naïve rivaroxaban initiators had lower risks of ischemic stroke and intracranial bleeding compared to new warfarin users. These benefits of rivaroxaban were not observed for patients switching from warfarin to rivaroxaban compared to persistent warfarin users. However, among patients switching to rivaroxaban, risk of GI bleeding was higher, especially in the first 90 days after switching. New rivaroxaban users and new dabigatran users had comparable rates of ischemic stroke and intracranial bleeding, but the former had a higher risk of GI bleeding.

Results from our analysis are mostly consistent with efficacy and safety results from clinical trial data and results from real-world studies where rivaroxaban was non-inferior or superior to warfarin for the prevention of stroke or systemic embolism [9, 13, 14, 34, 35]. In the ROCKET AF trial, which included 14,264 patients with NVAF randomized to 20 mg rivaroxaban once daily or dose-adjusted warfarin, rates of ischemic stroke, intracranial bleeding, and fatal bleeding were lower among individuals assigned to rivaroxaban [9]. In a sub-analysis of the ROCKET AF trial comparing efficacy and risks separately in vitamin K antagonist-naïve and vitamin K antagonist-experienced patients, rivaroxaban was associated with decreased risk of ischemic stroke and bleeding

Table 4 Adjusted hazard ratios (95% confidence intervals) of selected outcomes comparing new rivaroxaban users to new dabigatran users for the treatment of non-valvular atrial fibrillation, MarketScan, 2010–2014

	Rivaroxaban User (n = 16,957)			Matched Dabigatran User (n = 16,957)			Hazard Ratio (95% CI) [a]	p-value
Main outcomes	# Events	Person-years	IR (95% CI)	# Events	Person-years	IR (95% CI)		
Ischemic stroke	82	21,721	3.8 (3.0–4.7)	107	21,723	4.9 (4.1–5.9)	0.77 (0.58–1.03)	0.08
Intracranial bleeding	26	21,787	1.2 (0.8–1.7)	17	21,774	0.8 (0.5–1.2)	1.47 (0.80–2.72)	0.22
Myocardial infarction	140	21,734	6.4 (5.4–7.6)	124	21,703	5.7 (4.8–6.8)	1.11 (0.87–1.41)	0.42
Gastrointestinal bleeding	255	21,633	11.8 (10.4–13.3)	198	21,641	9.1 (7.9–10.5)	1.28 (1.06–1.54)	0.01
Control outcomes								
Hip / pelvic fracture	101	21,770	4.6 (3.8–5.6)	116	21,706	5.3 (4.4–6.4)	0.88 (0.67–1.15)	0.34
Breast / prostate cancer	140	21,726	6.4 (5.4–7.6)	130	21,719	6.0 (5.0–7.1)	1.06 (0.84–1.35)	0.61
Asthma	245	21,645	11.3 (10.0–12.8)	203	21,629	9.4 (8.2–10.7)	1.18 (0.98–1.42)	0.09

IR incidence rate, CI confidence interval
Incidence rate is per 1000 person-years
[a]Adjusted for age, sex, CHA_2DS_2-VASc score, prevalent outcome and high-dimensional propensity score

only in the former group [36]. Our results follow a similar pattern, indicating that switching from warfarin to rivaroxaban may not provide any additional benefit for stroke prevention. In addition, we observed that the effectiveness of rivaroxaban for stroke prevention was more accentuated in women than men, and in the first 90 days after initiation compared to more than 90 days after initiation. The benefit of rivaroxaban versus warfarin in the first 90 days after initiation may be explained by the need of warfarin users to adjust their dose while they stabilize in the therapeutic range. Patients may be at increased risk for cardioembolic events during that critical period [37].

In the head-to-head NOAC analysis, we found rivaroxaban users had a non-significant lower risk of ischemic stroke compared to dabigatran users, similar to what has recently been reported, [17] however our results indicate this inverse association was significantly stronger in women compared to men. This protective association of rivaroxaban (vs. dabigatran) with stroke risk in women was of similar magnitude to that seen for new female rivaroxaban users compared to warfarin users. Future analysis may explore whether rivaroxaban use is more beneficial in women for stroke prevention, compared to warfarin or dabigatran use.

An elevated risk of GI bleeding in rivaroxaban patients has been reported in several studies, [9, 12, 17, 35, 38] with an increased risk in those age > 75 [39]. Our results partially corroborate these findings. New rivaroxaban users did not have a significantly increased risk of GI bleeds compared to warfarin users, however, in stratified analysis, women and patients age ≥ 75 were at an increased risk of GI bleeding. New rivaroxaban users had a higher risk of GI bleeding when compared to dabigatran users. Patients who switched to rivaroxaban also had a higher risk of GI bleeding, especially in the first 90 days after switching anticoagulants. This increased risk of GI bleeding in switchers could be confounded by clinical factors that made patients switch from warfarin to a NOAC, such as an adverse reaction to or complication from using warfarin, or the patient's inability to stabilize his/her warfarin dose. In our study, the switcher group was older and had more comorbidities compared to the new users, which are risk factors for GI bleeding. Further studies should examine patient characteristics in those who develop GI bleeding to identify in advance individuals most at risk of rivaroxaban-associated GI bleeding events, potentially using another oral anticoagulant in those patients.

Effectiveness and risks of rivaroxaban were similar by initial dose, except that new rivaroxaban users taking 15 mg had a higher risk of MI and GI bleeding compared to those prescribed the 20 mg dose. The 15 mg dose is indicated for patients with reduced kidney function, and that, along with other comorbidities associated with kidney disease, could be driving this association. The

comparative effectiveness of NOACs in patients with reduced kidney function should be addressed in future research.

We observed an unexpected association between rivaroxaban users and a lower risk of hip/pelvic fracture (a control outcome), when compared to warfarin use. In addition to its established effect of impairing synthesis of vitamin K-associated clotting factors, warfarin is believed to inhibit the activation of bone proteins and, therefore, warfarin users could be at a higher risk of osteoporotic fractures compared to users of other oral anticoagulants [40]. However, observational studies have reported conflicting results on whether this association exists, [41, 42] and chance or residual confounding may be responsible for the finding in the present analysis. Given uncertainty regarding whether warfarin may increase fracture risk, hip/pelvic fracture is likely not an ideal 'control' outcome. Nonetheless, for transparency we chose to report these results as they were pre-specified in our analysis plan. Importantly, we did not see any association of rivaroxaban with the other two control outcomes -breast/prostate cancer and asthma – for which no interrelations with warfarin are hypothesized.

This study has several limitations which should be considered. First, unmeasured confounding is a known limitation in observational studies using administrative claims data. To account for confounding, we matched and adjusted for HDPS, which utilizes pre-defined variables and a wide range of empirically-identified confounders and has shown to be an effective approach for control of confounding [31]. However, in order to make causal interference, the two treatment groups need to be similar- that means that the final matched sample based on HDPS may not be representative from the entire treated population. Therefore, our results only apply to the matched population, which may be different from the entire treated population. In addition, we included control outcomes in our analysis, which we would not expect to be associated with anticoagulant use, providing indirect evidence of no residual uncontrolled confounding. Second, outcomes and covariates are ascertained from administrative data, which has known limitations. However, validated algorithms were utilized to ascertain events of interest and it is likely that any misclassification is non-differential. Although administrative data may fail to capture all comorbidities, the mean CHA_2DS_2-VASc score and the prevalence of comorbidities is similar to the comorbidities in patients included in the NOAC clinical trials and in NVAF patient registries. In addition, the outcomes of interest are serious enough to require medical care and, therefore, unlikely to be missed in this administrative database. Third, these results may not be generalizable to the entire population. Lastly, we did not confirm medication adherence. We report only initial prescription fill and dose, and did not include information on whether patients adhered to medication for the duration of the study period. There is no information on time in therapeutic range for the warfarin group. These patients may or may not be well-controlled. Persistence of NOACs is higher than warfarin, with rivaroxaban users having a persistence of 75–80% at 1 year [34, 43].

Despite these limitations, our study has numerous key strengths. This is a large, real-world population, with enough power to detect adverse outcomes over time. This study reports in-depth, stratified results (by sex, age, CHA_2DS_2-VASc score, and early vs. late outcomes) in patients who switched from warfarin to rivaroxaban, and also reports these stratified results for head-to-head comparisons between rivaroxaban and dabigatran users. In addition, we report associations for each outcome by initial rivaroxaban dose strength. These results provide information on the safety profile of rivaroxaban and may help clinicians make informed decisions when selecting an oral anticoagulant for thromboembolic prevention in NVAF patients.

Conclusion

In conclusion, in this large real-world sample of NVAF patients, effectiveness and risks of rivaroxaban versus warfarin differed by prior anticoagulant status, while effectiveness of rivaroxaban versus dabigatran differed in GI bleeding risk. These results bolster prior clinical trials and observational studies, and provide more in-depth information on effectiveness and adverse events across patient subgroups, including those defined by prior use of warfarin.

Additional file

Additional file 1: Supplemental Materials. Table S1. Characteristics of atrial fibrillation patients by anticoagulant use prior to final matching based on high-dimensional propensity score, MarketScan, 2010–2014. **Table S2.** Adjusted hazard ratios (95% confidence intervals) of selected outcomes comparing new rivaroxaban users (categorized by initial dose) to new warfarin users for the treatment of non-valvular atrial fibrillation, MarketScan, 2010–2014. **Table S3.** Adjusted hazard ratios (95% confidence intervals) of selected outcomes comparing patients who switched to rivaroxaban (categorized by initial dose) from warfarin to warfarin-only users for the treatment of non-valvular atrial fibrillation, MarketScan, 2010–2014. **Table S4.** Adjusted hazard ratios (95% confidence intervals) comparing new rivaroxaban users (categorized by initial dose) to new dabigatran users for the treatment of non-valvular atrial fibrillation, MarketScan, 2010–2014. **Table S5.** Adjusted hazard ratios (95% confidence intervals) of selected outcomes comparing new rivaroxaban users to new warfarin users for the treatment of non-valvular atrial fibrillation, MarketScan, 2010–2014. Restricted to 36,623 patients with at least 180 days of enrolment before first oral anticoagulation prescription. **Table S6.** Adjusted hazard ratios (95% confidence intervals) of selected outcomes comparing new rivaroxaban users to new warfarin users for the treatment of non-valvular atrial fibrillation, MarketScan, 2010–2014. Restricted to 68,927 patients with an enrolment date later than January 1st, 2011. **Table S7.** ICD-9-CM codes for outcomes. **Table S8.** ICD-9-CM codes used to define comorbidities. **Figure S1.** High-dimensional propensity score distribution by oral anticoagulant status for the outcome of stroke. These are the

distributions prior to final matching based on high-dimensional propensity score. (DOCX 356 kb)

Abbreviations
AF: Atrial fibrillation; CI: Confidence interval; FDA: Food and Drug Administration; GI: Gastrointestinal; HDPS: High-dimensional propensity score; HR: Hazard ratio; ICB: Intracranial bleeding; ICD-9-CM: International Classification of Diseases, Ninth Revision, Clinical Modification; INR: International normalized ratio; MI: Myocardial infarction; NOACs: Non-vitamin K antagonist oral anticoagulants; NVAF: Non-valvular atrial fibrillation; PPV: Positive predicted value; US: United States

Acknowledgements
None.

Funding
Research reported in this publication was supported by grant R01-HL122200 from the National Heart, Lung, and Blood Institute and grant 16EIA26410001 from the American Heart Association.

Authors' contributions
FN and AA have designed this study in whole. FN, LB, AA, RM have contributed to statistical analyses in this study. FN, LB, PL, LC, AC, AA have contributed to writing this manuscript. LB, PL, LC, AC, IR, AA have revised this manuscript. All authors read and approved the final manuscript.

Competing interests
Dr. Bengtson is an employee of Optum. All other authors have no competing interests.

Author details
[1]Division of Epidemiology and Community Health, School of Public Health, University of Minnesota, 1300 S 2nd St, Suite 300, Minneapolis, MN 55454, USA. [2]Health Economics and Outcomes Research, Life Sciences, Optum, Eden Prairie, MN, USA. [3]Cardiac Arrhythmia Center, Cardiovascular Division, Department of Medicine, University of Minnesota Medical School, Minneapolis, MN, USA. [4]Department of Health Sciences Research, Mayo Clinic, Rochester, MN, USA. [5]Department of Epidemiology, Rollins School of Public Health, Emory University, Atlanta, GA, USA.

References
1. Lloyd-Jones DM, Wang TJ, Leip EP, Larson MG, Levy D, Vasan RS, D'Agostino RB, Massaro JM, Beiser A, Wolf PA, et al. Lifetime risk for development of atrial fibrillation: the Framingham heart study. Circulation. 2004;110(9):1042–6.
2. Mozaffarian D, Benjamin EJ, Go AS, Arnett DK, Blaha MJ, Cushman M, Das SR, de Ferranti S, Despres JP, Fullerton HJ, et al. Heart disease and stroke statistics-2016 update: a report from the American Heart Association. Circulation. 2016;133(4):e38–e360.
3. Colilla S, Crow A, Petkun W, Singer DE, Simon T, Liu X. Estimates of current and future incidence and prevalence of atrial fibrillation in the U.S. adult population. Am J Cardiol. 2013;112(8):1142–7.
4. Wolf PA, Abbott RD, Kannel WB. Atrial fibrillation as an independent risk factor for stroke: the Framingham study. Stroke. 1991;22(8):983–8.
5. Glotzer TV, Daoud EG, Wyse DG, Singer DE, Ezekowitz MD, Hilker C, Miller C, Qi D, Ziegler PD. The relationship between daily atrial tachyarrhythmia burden from implantable device diagnostics and stroke risk: the TRENDS study. Circ Arrhythm Electrophysiol. 2009;2(5):474–80.
6. Ziegler PD, Glotzer TV, Daoud EG, Singer DE, Ezekowitz MD, Hoyt RH, Koehler JL, Coles J Jr, Wyse DG. Detection of previously undiagnosed atrial fibrillation in patients with stroke risk factors and usefulness of continuous monitoring in primary stroke prevention. Am J Cardiol. 2012;110(9):1309–14.
7. Ziegler PD, Glotzer TV, Daoud EG, Wyse DG, Singer DE, Ezekowitz MD, Koehler JL, Hilker CE. Incidence of newly detected atrial arrhythmias via implantable devices in patients with a history of thromboembolic events. Stroke. 2010;41(2):256–60.

8.   January CT, Wann LS, Alpert JS, Calkins H, Cigarroa JE, Cleveland JC Jr, Conti JB, Ellinor PT, Ezekowitz MD, Field ME, et al. 2014 AHA/ACC/HRS guideline for the management of patients with atrial fibrillation: a report of the American College of Cardiology/American Heart Association task force on practice guidelines and the Heart Rhythm Society. Circulation. 2014;130(23):e199–267.

9.   Patel MR, Mahaffey KW, Garg J, Pan G, Singer DE, Hacke W, Breithardt G, Halperin JL, Hankey GJ, Piccini JP, et al. Rivaroxaban versus warfarin in nonvalvular atrial fibrillation. N Engl J Med. 2011;365(10):883–91.

10. Cohen D. Rivaroxaban: can we trust the evidence? BMJ. 2016;352:i575.

11. Patel MR, Hellkamp AS, Fox KA. Point-of-care Warfarin monitoring in the ROCKET AF trial. N Engl J Med. 2016;374(8):785–8.

12. Lip GY, Keshishian A, Kamble S, Pan X, Mardekian J, Horblyuk R, Hamilton M: Real-world comparison of major bleeding risk among non-valvular atrial fibrillation patients initiated on apixaban, dabigatran, rivaroxaban, or warfarin. A propensity score matched analysis. Thromb Haemost. 2016;116(5):975–86.

13. Coleman CI, Antz M, Ehlken B, Evers T. REal-LIfe evidence of stroke prevention in patients with atrial fibrillation - the RELIEF study. Int J Cardiol. 2015;203:882–4.

14. Laliberte F, Cloutier M, Nelson WW, Coleman CI, Pilon D, Olson WH, Damaraju CV, Schein JR, Lefebvre P. Real-world comparative effectiveness and safety of rivaroxaban and warfarin in nonvalvular atrial fibrillation patients. Curr Med Res Opin. 2014;30(7):1317–25.

15. Connolly SJ, Ezekowitz MD, Yusuf S, Eikelboom J, Oldgren J, Parekh A, Pogue J, Reilly PA, Themeles E, Varrone J, et al. Dabigatran versus warfarin in patients with atrial fibrillation. N Engl J Med. 2009;361(12):1139–51.

16. Holster IL, Valkhoff VE, Kuipers EJ, Tjwa ET. New oral anticoagulants increase risk for gastrointestinal bleeding: a systematic review and meta-analysis. Gastroenterology. 2013;145(1):105–12. e115

17. Graham DJ, Reichman ME, Wernecke M, Hsueh YH, Izem R, Southworth MR, Wei Y, Liao J, Goulding MR, Mott K, et al: Stroke, Bleeding, and Mortality Risks in Elderly Medicare Beneficiaries Treated With Dabigatran or Rivaroxaban for Nonvalvular Atrial Fibrillation. JAMA Intern Med. 2016;176(11):1662–71.

18. Hansen LG, Chang S. White paper. Health research data for the real world: the MarketScan databases. http://truvenhealth.com/Portals/0/assets/2012_Truven_MarketScan_white_paper.pdf. 2012.

19. Naccarelli GV, Johnston SS, Dalal M, Lin J, Patel PP. Rates and implications for hospitalization of patients >/=65 years of age with atrial fibrillation/flutter. Am J Cardiol. 2012;109(4):543–9.

20. Piccini JP, Hammill BG, Sinner MF, Jensen PN, Hernandez AF, Heckbert SR, Benjamin EJ, Curtis LH. Incidence and prevalence of atrial fibrillation and associated mortality among Medicare beneficiaries, 1993-2007. Circ Cardiovasc Qual Outcomes. 2012;5(1):85–93.

21. Jensen PN, Johnson K, Floyd J, Heckbert SR, Carnahan R, Dublin S. A systematic review of validated methods for identifying atrial fibrillation using administrative data. Pharmacoepidemiol Drug Saf. 2012;21(Suppl 1):141–7.

22. GMATCH macro http://www.mayo.edu/research/departments-divisions/department-health-sciences-research/division-biomedical-statistics-informatics/software/locally-written-sas-macros.

23. Garg RK, Glazer NL, Wiggins KL, Newton KM, Thacker EL, Smith NL, Siscovick DS, Psaty BM, Heckbert SR. Ascertainment of warfarin and aspirin use by medical record review compared with automated pharmacy data. Pharmacoepidemiol Drug Saf. 2011;20(3):313–6.

24. Andrade SE, Harrold LR, Tjia J, Cutrona SL, Saczynski JS, Dodd KS, Goldberg RJ, Gurwitz JH. A systematic review of validated methods for identifying cerebrovascular accident or transient ischemic attack using administrative data. Pharmacoepidemiol Drug Saf. 2012;21(Suppl 1):100–28.

25. Kiyota Y, Schneeweiss S, Glynn RJ, Cannuscio CC, Avorn J, Solomon DH. Accuracy of Medicare claims-based diagnosis of acute myocardial infarction: estimating positive predictive value on the basis of review of hospital records. Am Heart J. 2004;148(1):99–104.

26. Wahl PM, Rodgers K, Schneeweiss S, Gage BF, Butler J, Wilmer C, Nash M, Esper G, Gitlin N, Osborn N, et al. Validation of claims-based diagnostic and procedure codes for cardiovascular and gastrointestinal serious adverse events in a commercially-insured population. Pharmacoepidemiol Drug Saf. 2010;19(6):596–603.

27. Cunningham A, Stein CM, Chung CP, Daugherty JR, Smalley WE, Ray WA. An automated database case definition for serious bleeding related to oral anticoagulant use. Pharmacoepidemiol Drug Saf. 2011;20(6):560–6.

28. Chronic Disease Warehouse. Chronic Conditions https://www.ccwdata.org/web/guest/condition-categories.

29. Quan H, Sundararajan V, Halfon P, Fong A, Burnand B, Luthi JC, Saunders LD, Beck CA, Feasby TE, Ghali WA. Coding algorithms for defining comorbidities in ICD-9-CM and ICD-10 administrative data. Med Care. 2005; 43(11):1130–9.

30. Lip GY, Nieuwlaat R, Pisters R, Lane DA, Crijns HJ. Refining clinical risk stratification for predicting stroke and thromboembolism in atrial fibrillation using a novel risk factor-based approach: the euro heart survey on atrial fibrillation. Chest. 2010;137(2):263–72.

31. Schneeweiss S, Rassen JA, Glynn RJ, Avorn J, Mogun H, Brookhart MA. High-dimensional propensity score adjustment in studies of treatment effects using health care claims data. Epidemiology. 2009;20(4):512–22.

32. Rassen JA, Doherty, M., Huang, W., Schneeweiss, S. : Pharmacoepidemiology Toolbox. http://www.drugepi.org/dope-downloads/#Pharmacoepidemiology%20Toolbox.

33. Bross ID. Spurious effects from an extraneous variable. J Chronic Dis. 1966;19:637–47.

34. Camm AJ, Amarenco P, Haas S, Hess S, Kirchhof P, Kuhls S, van Eickels M, Turpie AG: XANTUS: a real-world, prospective, observational study of patients treated with rivaroxaban for stroke prevention in atrial fibrillation. Eur Heart J. 2016;37(14):1145–53.

35. Gorst-Rasmussen A, Lip GY, Bjerregaard Larsen T. Rivaroxaban versus warfarin and dabigatran in atrial fibrillation: comparative effectiveness and safety in Danish routine care. Pharmacoepidemiol Drug Saf. 2016;25(11):1236–44.

36. Mahaffey KW, Wojdyla D, Hankey GJ, White HD, Nessel CC, Piccini JP, Patel MR, Berkowitz SD, Becker RC, Halperin JL, et al. Clinical outcomes with rivaroxaban in patients transitioned from vitamin K antagonist therapy: a subgroup analysis of a randomized trial. Ann Intern Med. 2013;158(12):861–8.

37. Nelson WW, Desai S, Damaraju CV, Lu L, Fields LE, Wildgoose P, Schein JR. International normalized ratio stabilization in newly initiated warfarin patients with nonvalvular atrial fibrillation. Curr Med Res Opin. 2014;30(12):2437–42.

38. Sherwood MW, Nessel CC, Hellkamp AS, Mahaffey KW, Piccini JP, Suh EY, Becker RC, Singer DE, Halperin JL, Hankey GJ, et al. Gastrointestinal bleeding in patients with Atrial fibrillation treated with rivaroxaban or Warfarin: ROCKET AF trial. J Am Coll Cardiol. 2015;66(21):2271–81.

39. Abraham NS, Singh S, Alexander GC, Heien H, Haas LR, Crown W, Shah ND. Comparative risk of gastrointestinal bleeding with dabigatran, rivaroxaban, and warfarin: population based cohort study. BMJ. 2015;350:h1857.

40. Booth SL, Mayer J. Warfarin use and fracture risk. Nutr Rev. 2000;58(1):20–2.

41. Gage BF, Birman-Deych E, Radford MJ, Nilasena DS, Binder EF. Risk of osteoporotic fracture in elderly patients taking warfarin: results from the National Registry of Atrial fibrillation 2. Arch Intern Med. 2006;166(2):241–6.

42. Mamdani M, Upshur RE, Anderson G, Bartle BR, Laupacis A. Warfarin therapy and risk of hip fracture among elderly patients. Pharmacotherapy. 2003;23(1):1–4.

43. Nelson WW, Song X, Coleman CI, Thomson E, Smith DM, Damaraju CV, Schein JR. Medication persistence and discontinuation of rivaroxaban versus warfarin among patients with non-valvular atrial fibrillation. Curr Med Res Opin. 2014;30(12):2461–9.

The study protocol for PREDICT AF RECURRENCE: a PRospEctive cohort stuDy of survelllanCe for perioperaTive Atrial Fibrillation RECURRENCE in major non-cardiac surgery for malignancy

Satoshi Higuchi[1,10]*[iD], Yusuke Kabeya[2,3], Kenichi Matsushita[1], Keisei Tachibana[4], Riken Kawachi[5], Hidefumi Takei[4], Yutaka Suzuki[6], Nobutsugu Abe[6], Yorihisa Imanishi[7], Kiyoshi Moriyama[8], Tomoko Yorozu[8], Koichiro Saito[9], Masanori Sugiyama[6], Haruhiko Kondo[4] and Hideaki Yoshino[1]

Abstract

Background: A previous retrospective cohort study established the relationship between perioperative atrial fibrillation (POAF) and subsequent mortality and stroke. However, the details regarding the cause of death and etiology of stroke remain unclear.

Methods: The prospective cohort study of surveillance for perioperative atrial fibrillation recurrence in major non-cardiac surgery for malignancy (PREDICT AF RECURRENCE) registry is an ongoing prospective cohort study to elucidate the long-term recurrence rate and the clinical impact of new-onset POAF in the setting of head and neck, non-cardiac thoracic, and abdominal surgery for malignancy. In this study, cardiologists collaborate with a surgical team during the perioperative period, carefully observe the electrocardiogram (ECG) monitor, and treat arrhythmia as required. Furthermore, patients who develop new-onset POAF are followed up using a long-term Holter ECG monitor, SPIDER FLASH-t AFib®, to assess POAF recurrence.

Discussion: Even if patients with malignancy survive by overcoming the disease, they may die from any preventable cardiovascular diseases. In particular, those with POAF may develop cardiogenic stroke in the future. Because details of the natural history of patients with POAF remain unclear, investigating the need to continue anticoagulation therapy for such patients is necessary. This study will provide essential information on the recurrence rate of POAF and new insights into the prediction and treatment of POAF.

Keywords: Perioperative atrial fibrillation (POAF), Non-cardiac surgery, Oncology, Stroke

* Correspondence: sahiguchi-circ@umin.ac.jp
[1]Division of Cardiology, Department of Internal Medicine II, Kyorin University School of Medicine, Tokyo, Japan
[10]Division of Cardiology, Department of Internal Medicine II, Kyorin University School of Medicine, 6-20-2 Shinkawa, Mitaka City, Tokyo 181-8611, Japan
Full list of author information is available at the end of the article

Background

Atrial fibrillation (AF) is one of the most common types of arrhythmia and a common health-related problem, with increasing incidence and prevalence worldwide [1, 2]. AF is associated with increased mortality and incidence of thromboembolic events, such as stroke [3–5], and is most likely induced by clinical conditions, such as hypertension, diabetes mellitus, and heart failure [6–8]. Furthermore, AF often occurs after both cardiac and non-cardiac surgeries, usually on the second or third postoperative day [9], with an incidence rate of 10–65% and 1–9%, respectively [9–11]. The massive differences in the reported incidence rate could be attributed to the possible overlooking of short-duration AF and the variable impact of each surgical procedure on the incidence. Although perioperative AF (POAF) seems to be a temporary cardiac event that does not affect the subsequent clinical course, POAF is reported to be associated with long-term mortality and stroke, even in the setting of non-cardiac surgery and general clinical situations [10]. Furthermore, some recent studies demonstrated that malignancy was related to a higher prevalence of AF [12–14]. Notably, Conen et al. demonstrated that the multi-variate adjusted hazard ratio of AF after diagnosis of breast cancer was as high as 4.67 (95% CI, 2.85–7.64) in the first 3 months, regardless of treatment assignments [14].

Despite recognizing AF as an independent risk factor for mortality, the evidence to determine AF as a causal factor is insufficient [15]. Hence, determining whether AF is the direct and decisive cause of death in the general population without any cardiac disease remains doubtful. In cardiac surgery, the frequent occurrence of POAF with impaired cardiac function might induce cardiac events, such as heart failure and cardiac death. However, in non-cardiac surgery, wherein patients do not usually present with such impairment whether AF directly correlates with mortality or only a surrogate marker remains undetermined.

The recent advancements in the treatment of malignancies have enhanced the prognosis of such patients, increasing the subsequent survivor population at the risk of cardiovascular events [16]. Patients with AF recurrence after the perioperative period are susceptible to subsequent embolic events; therefore, both long- and short-term POAF management to prevent adverse clinical events should be considered. Although a previous study [10] suggested that anticoagulation therapy could be beneficial for patients with POAF, it did not identify patients who were at high risk for subsequent stroke and who should start anticoagulation therapy after discharge. If most factors causing stroke are related to atherosclerosis, antiplatelet therapy along with appropriate risk management regimen should be provided. Particularly, patients with malignancy sometimes face complicated treatment choices because of elevated thrombotic and bleeding risks [17]. In such cases, a survey detailing the short- and long-term clinical course of those with POAF might be helpful for subsequent daily clinical management.

Hypothesis

The present study has been conducted to investigate our primary hypothesis that the patients with new-onset POAF will develop AF recurrence in the future.

Methods/design

Study design and population

The PRospEctive cohort stuDy of surveIllanCe for perioperaTive Atrial Fibrillation RECURRENCE (PREDICT AF RECURRENCE) in major non-cardiac surgery for malignancy is an ongoing prospective, single-center, observational study that is designed to illustrate the clinical impact of POAF on mortality and morbidity as cardiologists collaborate with a surgical team during the perioperative period and investigate the frequency of AF recurrence after discharge in patients with malignancy. In this study, we examined consecutive patients who underwent non-cardiac surgery under general anesthesia due to definitive or suspected malignancy. We followed patients who developed new-onset AF by using a cardiac event recorder. Figure 1 shows the flowchart of the study. The present study enrolled from July 2014 and the registered patients will be followed up until December 2022.

Inclusion criteria

In this study, we enrolled patients (age: ≥20 and ≤90 years) who planned to undergo surgery in Kyorin University Hospital (Tokyo, Japan) from July 2014. The malignancies registered were as follows: head and neck (e.g., pharyngeal, laryngeal, tongue, mandible, buccal mucosal, gingival, and glottic), chest (e.g., esophageal, lung, and lung metastases), or abdomen (gallbladder, extra- and intrahepatic bile duct, pancreatic, duodenal, Vater papillary, hepatic cell, and liver metastases) cancers. Some previous studies have demonstrated that the prevalence of POAF was frequently associated with the surgery site and, thus, could be infrequent in less-invasive surgical treatments [10, 18]. Hence, we did not include patients with gastric and colon cancers in this study because a majority of them were treated with less-invasive laparoscopic surgery in our institute.

Exclusion criteria

In this study, we excluded patients with persistent or chronic AF and atrial flutter. Although those with known paroxysmal AF before surgery were included for in-hospital analysis, they were excluded in the analysis of long-term AF recurrence.

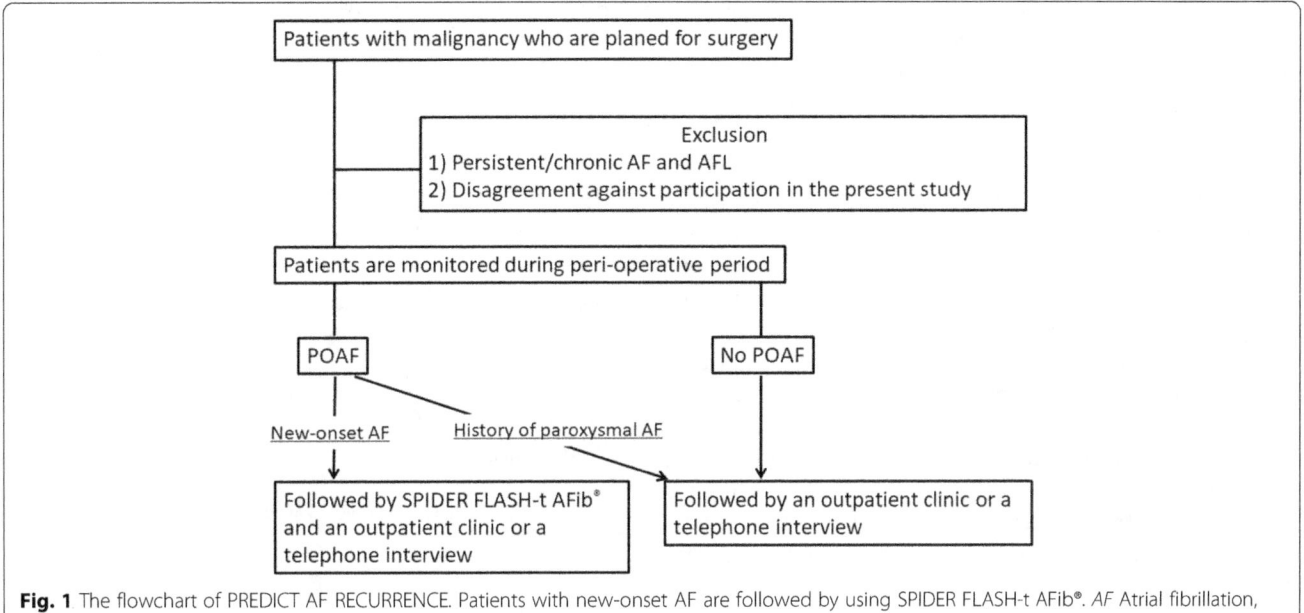

Fig. 1 The flowchart of PREDICT AF RECURRENCE. Patients with new-onset AF are followed by using SPIDER FLASH-t AFib®. *AF* Atrial fibrillation, *AFL* Atrial flutter, *POAF* Perioperative atrial fibrillation

Baseline assessment

The baseline survey was conducted 1–3 days preoperatively by using a study-specific questionnaire for collecting information, including age, sex, current medications, alcohol consumption, smoking status, past histories of thoracotomy and cardiogenic stroke, and complications, such as heart failure, coronary artery disease, peripheral artery diseases, and chronic obstructive pulmonary disease. Table 1 shows the definition of each complication. We performed blood examination within 3 months preoperatively, which included blood cell counts, C-reactive protein (CRP), D-dimer, liver enzyme, electrolytes, serum creatinine, thyroid hormone, and B-type natriuretic peptide (BNP). In addition, we performed a respiratory function test (including forced expiratory volume and forced vital capacity) and 12-lead electrocardiography (ECG) at the same time with blood examination. As a routine clinical practice in the institute, Doppler ultrasonography was performed on patients with D-dimer level of ≥0.5 µg/mL to assess superficial and deep venous thromboses of the lower extremities.

Data collection during general anesthesia

During the surgery, anesthesiologists provided general care to patients. In addition, heart rate, rhythm, and ST-T changes were continuously monitored by an ECG and appropriately recorded. The final diagnosis of each arrhythmia was confirmed by cardiologists.

Operation record

We recorded the stage of malignancy, type of surgery, extent of tumor resection and lymph node dissection,

Table 1 Definition of complications

Heart Failure	Fulfills any of the following:
	1) Any symptoms such as orthopnea, paroxysmal nocturnal dyspnea, or dyspnea on effort and BNP≥100 pg/mL
	2) A history of admission because of congestive heart failure.
Hypertension	Systolic blood pressure ≥140 mmHg and/or diastolic blood pressure ≥90 mmHg
Diabetes Mellitus	Fulfills 1) and 2)
	1) Fasting plasma glucose ≥126 mg/dL or casual plasma glucose ≥200 mg/dL
	2) HbA1c ≥6.5%
Coronary Artery Disease	Patients with any of the following: LAD, LCx, or RCA with stenosis ≥75%, or LMT with stenosis ≥50% if a patient has undergone coronary angiography or computed tomography.
Peripheral Artery Disease	The term includes carotid artery stenosis/occlusion, intracranial middle- and large-artery stenosis/occlusion, renal stenosis, arteriosclerosis obliterans, and aortic aneurysm, all of which are diagnosed by any imaging modality.
Chronic Obstructive Pulmonary Disease	fulfills 1) and 2)
	1) FEV$_1$/FVC ratio <0.7
	2) Predicted to be irreversible after the administration of an inhaled bronchodilator

BNP, B-type natriuretic peptide; LAD, left anterior descending artery; LCx, left circumflex artery; RCA, right coronary artery; LMT, left main trunk; FEV$_1$, forced expiratory volume in 1 second; FVC, forced vital capacity

and pathological findings in the patients. The stage and extent of lymph node dissection in each surgery were determined based on the Union of International Cancer Control (UICC) TNM classification seventh edition.

Postoperative data collection

In this study, all patients were observed with an ECG monitor device for a minimum of 24 h up to 30 days postoperatively; the monitoring duration was based on each surgeon's discretion. In addition, duration of monitoring and surgical intensive care unit stay were recorded. Patients with any type of arrhythmia requiring an intervention were treated by cardiologists in accordance with the current guideline. Furthermore, anticoagulation therapy was provided for those who developed AF if CHA2DS2 VASc score [19] was ≥1 and ≥2 in men and women, respectively, after surgeons assessed the bleeding risk and permitted the prescription. Subsequently, the presence of symptoms, onset time/day, and total duration of AF during hospitalization were recorded, and blood examination, such as white blood cell, hemoglobin, serum creatinine, CRP, and electrolytes, was planned on the following and the fourth postoperative day. We examined the presence of postoperative complications, including myocardial infarction; congestive heart failure; bleeding; thrombosis, such as stroke, transient ischemic attack, ischemic bowel disease, and pulmonary embolism; any infections; acute kidney injury; and desaturation necessary for home oxygen therapy. Finally, echocardiography was immediately performed for patients with new-onset AF.

Follow-up after discharge

In this ongoing study, the follow-up data would be collected from a face-to-face interview in an outpatient clinic, a telephone interview, or a medical record. The follow-up flow chart is shown in Table 2. Regardless of the presence of POAF, the patients in this study would be followed up for all-cause, cardiac, non-cardiac, and malignancy-related mortality; AF occurrence or recurrence; and stroke. The diagnosis and etiology of stroke in this study were determined by two or more neurologists and radiologists independent from the investigators. The patients who developed new-onset AF were continuously followed up using SPIDER FLASH-t AFib* (LivaNova, London, UK) for approximately 2 weeks after 1 and 12 months postoperatively. The device can record heart rhythm non-invasively for the longest duration in Japan. The dynamic memory in the device allows for rhythm episodes to be accurately identified regardless of their duration. Any arrhythmia, including AF, is recorded automatically (Additional file 1: Table S1). In addition, follow-up was performed after 6 months if required.

Table 2 Follow-up in chronological order

	1	3	6	12	24	36	48	60	(month)
New-onset POAF									
clinic visit	✓	✓	✓	✓	✓	✓	✓	✓	
blood examination	✓		✓	✓					
event recorder	✓		✓ᵃ	✓					
12-lead ECG	✓	✓	✓	✓	✓	✓	✓	✓	
No POAF									
clinic visit	✓		✓	✓	✓	✓	✓	✓	
blood examination	✓		✓	✓					
Known PAF prior to surgery									
clinic visit	✓		✓	✓	✓	✓	✓	✓	
blood examination	✓		✓	✓					

ᵃ: if required
ECG: electrocardiogram; PAF: paroxysmal atrial fibrillation; POAF: perioperative atrial fibrillation

Follow-up was recorded throughout the day except during the time when patients were taking a bath. Patients who were unable to handle SPIDER FLASH-t AFib* were examined using 24-h Holter ECG for 2 to 4 times. If AF recurrence was documented 1 month postoperatively, the following event monitoring was not planned. The patients who developed a rash because of an electrode seal at the first record could stop the following examination. If the patients were hospitalized at 1, 6, or 12 months postoperatively, they could be evaluated using an ECG monitor device of the residing ward instead of SPIDER FLASH-t AFib*. The records acquired by SPIDER FLASH-t AFib* were assessed by an external expert organization, and the final decision was confirmed by two cardiologists. With regard to the 24-h Holter ECG and ECG monitor device in the ward, two cardiologists analyzed and diagnosed the recorded ECG. In the case of differential diagnosis, they attain consensus after sufficient discussion to conclude the final diagnosis. Information on anticoagulation, such as type, dose, duration, and adherence, are collected by cardiologists. Of note, patients without AF recurrence for a year can discontinue anticoagulation treatment.

Outcome definition

Detailed outcomes defined in Additional file 2.

Short-term outcome

In this study, short-term outcomes comprise new-onset POAF; any arrhythmia; embolic events, such as stroke; and mortality until the thirtieth day after surgery. We defined POAF as AF during and/or after surgery until the thirtieth postoperative day. In addition, we also evaluated the type of arrhythmia, etiology of stroke, and cause of death.

The study protocol for PREDICT AF RECURRENCE: a PRospEctive cohort stuDy of surveIllanCe...

149

Long-term outcome

We followed up all patients with and without POAF in this study. Long-term outcomes included AF recurrence (evaluated only in those with new-onset POAF); embolic events, such as stroke; recurrent or de novo malignancy; and mortality on and after the thirty-first postoperative day. New-onset AF occurring on and after the thirty-first day was not considered as POAF, but as "conventional" paroxysmal AF. We defined AF recurrence as repetitive AF lasting ≥30 s on and after the thirty-first day, which was documented by SPIDER FLASH-t AFib*, 24-h Holter ECG, or hospital ECG monitor [20]. Notably, patient's self-assessment and symptoms did not contribute to the definitive diagnosis. Furthermore, the cause of death included cardiac, non-cardiac, and cancer-related mortalities.

Sub-analysis

We will conduct sub-analyses investigating the predictor of POAF in each malignancy, and the incidence and the characteristics of other arrhythmias.

Statistical analysis

No preceding study evaluated the incidence of AF recurrence in patients with POAF. Therefore, we assumed the incidence in reference to the first 200 patietns in our study, which indicated a 25% recurrence rate. We assumed a 0.97% incidence of AF in patients without POAF based on a previous study [6]. Based on 80% power and a significance level of 0.05, 38 patients with new-onset POAF were required. Assuming a 15% dropout rate and a 9% incidence rate of POAF, 497 (new-onset POAF, $n = 45$; non-POAF, $n = 452$) were required at least. In this study, the relationship between exposure variables and in-hospital outcomes was assessed using logistic regression analyses and expressed as odds ratio, 95% confidential interval, and P value. Variables with $P < 0.10$ in the univariate logistic regression analysis were included in the multivariate logistic regression analysis. In addition, we assessed the long-term outcomes using the survival analysis methods. The cumulative incidence of long-term outcomes was assessed using the Kaplan–Meier statistics. Furthermore, the hazard ratios of long-term outcomes were calculated using the Cox regression analysis.

Discussion

To the best of our knowledge, this study is the first research to prospectively investigate the long-term recurrence and the clinical impact of POAF using an event recorder in patients with malignancy.

Early documentation of POAF could be essential to prevent potential embolic events. In addition, underdiagnoses are often possible because AF lasts for a very short period, and an ECG monitor is the only means to provide a definitive diagnosis. To date, several risk scores and equations for the prediction of AF in the general population have been developed and validated. In this study, we will validate the efficacy of such risk scores in the setting of the perioperative period by assessing our dataset.

Even if patients with malignancy survive by overcoming the disease, they might die from any preventable cardiovascular diseases. In particular, those with POAF might develop cardiogenic stroke in the future. Because details of the natural history of patients with POAF remain unclear, investigating the need to continue anticoagulation therapy for such patients is necessary.

The apparent correlation between POAF and stroke can be explained by other atherosclerotic factors, such as age, hypertension, and diabetes mellitus [6, 7, 21]. Therefore, whether AF causes subsequent stroke remains unclear. Physicians in this study follow up patients in real time and record the incidence of POAF and any complications, which might be helpful for assuming the causal relationship between AF and morbidities, chronologically. Furthermore, the instrumental variable method, if appropriate, could reinforce the supposed correlation.

Although POAF post-non-cardiac surgery is an increasingly common problem and attracts clinicians' attention, both short- and long-term characteristics and management have remained unclear because of limited evidence [22].

This study has some limitations. First, the present cohort incudes limited subsets of non-cardiac surgery. The results acquired from the present study may not be adapted for the other subsets, such as non-malignancy. Second, the incidence of AF in the patietns without POAF may be underestimated because they do not wear the event recorder. However, the most important question is whether we should prescribe anticoagulation for patients with POAF in future. We believe that the results of this cohort will provide several indications for the management of patients with malignancy who developed POAF.

Abbreviations

AF: Atrial fibrillation; ECG: Electrocardiogram; POAF: Perioperative atrial fibrillation

Funding

This study is funded by JSPS KAKENHI Grant Number 17 K18085.

Authors' contributions

SH designed the study and drafted manuscript. YK, KM, KT, RK, HT, YS, NA, YI, KM, TY, KS, MS, HK, and HY designed the study and revised the manuscript critically for important intellectual content. Final approval of the manuscript submitted was done by SH.

Competing interests

The authors declare that they have no competing interests.

Author details

[1]Division of Cardiology, Department of Internal Medicine II, Kyorin University School of Medicine, Tokyo, Japan. [2]Division of General Internal Medicine, Department of Internal Medicine, Tokai University, Isehara, Kanagawa, Japan. [3]Department of Home Care Medicine, Saiyu Clinic, Saitama, Japan. [4]Department of General Thoracic Surgery, Kyorin University School of Medicine, Tokyo, Japan. [5]Department of General Thoracic Surgery, Nihon University School of Medicine, Tokyo, Japan. [6]Department of Surgery, Kyorin University School of Medicine, Tokyo, Japan. [7]Department of Otorhinolaryngology, Head and Neck Surgery, Kawasaki Municipal Kawasaki Hospital, Kawasaki, Kanagawa, Japan. [8]Department of Anesthesiology, Kyorin University School of Medicine, Tokyo, Japan. [9]Department of Otolaryngology-Head and Neck Surgery, Kyorin University School of Medicine, Tokyo, Japan. [10]Division of Cardiology, Department of Internal Medicine II, Kyorin University School of Medicine, 6-20-2 Shinkawa, Mitaka City, Tokyo 181-8611, Japan.

References

1. Lip GYH, Brechin CM, Lane DA. The global burden of atrial fibrillation and stroke: a systematic review of the epidemiology of atrial fibrillation in regions outside North America and Europe. Chest. 2012;142(6):1489–98.

2. Chugh SS, Havmoeller R, Narayanan K, Singh D, Rienstra M, Benjamin EJ, Gillum RF, Kim YH, McAnulty JH Jr, Zheng ZJ, et al. Worldwide epidemiology of atrial fibrillation: a global burden of disease 2010 study. Circulation. 2014;129(8):837–47.

3. Benjamin EJ, Wolf PA, D'Agostino RB, Silbershatz H, Kannel WB, Levy D. Impact of atrial fibrillation on the risk of death: the Framingham heart study. Circulation. 1998;98(10):946–52.

4. Chugh SS, Blackshear JL, Shen WK, Hammill SC, Gersh BJ. Epidemiology and natural history of atrial fibrillation: clinical implications. J Am Coll Cardiol. 2001;37(2):371–8.

5. Patel NJ, Deshmukh A, Pant S, Singh V, Patel N, Arora S, Shah N, Chothani A, Savani GT, Mehta K, et al. Contemporary trends of hospitalization for atrial fibrillation in the United States, 2000 through 2010: implications for healthcare planning. Circulation. 2014;129(23):2371–9.

6. Krahn AD, Manfreda J, Tate RB, Mathewson FA, Cuddy TE. The natural history of atrial fibrillation: incidence, risk factors, and prognosis in the Manitoba follow-up study. Am J Med. 1995;98(5):476–84.

7. Benjamin EJ, Levy D, Vaziri SM, D'Agostino RB, Belanger AJ, Wolf PA. Independent risk factors for atrial fibrillation in a population-based cohort. The Framingham Heart Study. JAMA. 1994;271(11):840–4.

8. Santhanakrishnan R, Wang N, Larson MG, Magnani JW, McManus DD, Lubitz SA, Ellinor PT, Cheng S, Vasan RS, Lee DS, et al. Atrial fibrillation begets heart failure and vice versa: temporal associations and differences in preserved versus reduced ejection fraction. Circulation. 2016;133(5):484–92.

9. Maisel WH, Rawn JD, Stevenson WG. Atrial fibrillation after cardiac surgery. Ann Intern Med. 2001;135(12):1061–73.

10. Gialdini G, Nearing K, Bhave PD, Bonuccelli U, Iadecola C, Healey JS, Kamel H. Perioperative atrial fibrillation and the long-term risk of ischemic stroke. JAMA. 2014;312(6):616–22.

11. Batra GS, Molyneux J, Scott NA. Colorectal patients and cardiac arrhythmias detected on the surgical high dependency unit. Ann R Coll Surg Engl. 2001; 83(3):174–6.

12. O'Neal WT, Lakoski SG, Qureshi W, Judd SE, Howard G, Howard VJ, Cushman M, Soliman EZ. Relation between cancer and atrial fibrillation (from the REasons for geographic and racial differences in stroke study). Am J Cardiol. 2015;115(8):1090–4.

13. Erichsen R, Christiansen CF, Mehnert F, Weiss NS, Baron JA, Sorensen HT. Colorectal cancer and risk of atrial fibrillation and flutter: a population-based case-control study. Intern Emerg Med. 2012;7(5):431–8.

14. Conen D, Wong JA, Sandhu RK, Cook NR, Lee IM, Buring JE, Albert CM. Risk of malignant Cancer among women with new-onset atrial fibrillation. JAMA Cardiol. 2016;1(4):389–96.

15. Leong DP, Eikelboom JW, Healey JS, Connolly SJ. Atrial fibrillation is associated with increased mortality: causation or association? Eur Heart J. 2013;34(14):1027–30.

16. Chung R, Maulik A, Hamarneh A, Hochhauser D, Hausenloy DJ, Walker JM, Yellon DM. Effect of remote Ischaemic conditioning in oncology patients undergoing chemotherapy: rationale and design of the ERIC-ONC study–a single-center, blinded, randomized controlled trial. Clin Cardiol. 2016;39(2): 72–82.

17. Melloni C, Shrader P, Carver J, Piccini JP, Thomas L, Fonarow GC, Ansell J, Gersh B, Go AS, Hylek E, et al. Management and outcomes of patients with atrial fibrillation and a history of cancer: the ORBIT-AF registry. Eur Heart J Qual Care Clin Outcomes. 2017;3(3):192–7.

18. Bhave PD, Goldman LE, Vittinghoff E, Maselli J, Auerbach A. Incidence, predictors, and outcomes associated with postoperative atrial fibrillation after major noncardiac surgery. Am Heart J. 2012;164(6):918–24.

19. Lip GY, Nieuwlaat R, Pisters R, Lane DA, Crijns HJ. Refining clinical risk stratification for predicting stroke and thromboembolism in atrial fibrillation using a novel risk factor-based approach: the euro heart survey on atrial fibrillation. Chest. 2010;137(2):263–72.

20. Barthelemy JC, Feasson-Gerard S, Garnier P, Gaspoz JM, Da Costa A, Michel D, Roche F. Automatic cardiac event recorders reveal paroxysmal atrial fibrillation after unexplained strokes or transient ischemic attacks. Ann Noninvasive Electrocardiol. 2003;8(3):194–9.

21. Majeed A, Moser K, Carroll K. Trends in the prevalence and management of atrial fibrillation in general practice in England and Wales, 1994-1998: analysis of data from the general practice research database. Heart. 2001; 86(3):284–8.

22. Vallurupalli S, Shanbhag A, Mehta JL. Controversies in postoperative atrial fibrillation after noncardiothoracic surgery: clinical and research implications. Clin Cardiol. 2017;40(5):329–32.

19

Analysis of cardiovascular mortality, bleeding, vascular and cerebrovascular events in patients with atrial fibrillation vs. sinus rhythm undergoing transfemoral Transcatheter Aortic Valve Implantation (TAVR)

Joerg Herold[1]* (iD), Vasiliki Herold-Vlanti[1], Mohammad Sherif[2], Blerim Luani[1], Christin Breyer[1], Klaus Bonaventura[3] and Ruediger Braun-Dullaeus[1]

Abstract

Background: Transcatheter aortic valve replacement (TAVR) has been demonstrated to be an established therapy for high-risk, inoperable patients with severe symptomatic aortic valve stenosis. For patients with moderate surgical risk, TAVR is equivalent to conventional aortic valve surgery. However, atrial fibrillation (AF) is also present in many of these patients, thus requiring post-implantation oral anticoagulation therapy in addition to the inhibition of thrombocyte aggregation, which poses the risk of bleeding complications. The aim of our work was to investigate the influence of AF on mortality and the occurrence of bleeding, vascular and cerebrovascular complications related to TAVR according to the VARC-2 criteria.

Methods: Two hundred eighty-three patients who underwent TAVR between March 2010 and April 2016 were retrospectively examined. In total, 257 patients who underwent transfemoral access were included in this study. The mean patient age was 81 ± 6 years, 54.1% of the patients were women, and 42.4% had pre-interventional AF.

Results: Compared to patients with sinus rhythm (SR, $n = 148$), patients with AF ($n = 109$) had an almost three-fold higher incidence of major vascular complications (AF 14.7% vs. SR 5.4%, $p = 0.016$) and life-threatening bleeding (AF 11.9% vs. SR 4.1%, $p = 0.028$) during the first 30 post-procedural days. However, the rate of cerebrovascular complications (AF 3.7% vs. SR 2.7%, $p = 0.726$) did not significantly differ between the two groups. Overall mortality was significantly higher in patients with AF during the first month (AF 8.3% vs. SR 2.0%, $p = 0.032$) and the first year (AF 28.4% vs. SR 15.3%; $p = 0.020$) following TAVR.

Conclusion: Patients with AF had significantly more severe bleeding complications after TAVR, which were significantly related to mortality. Future prospective randomized studies must clarify the optimal anticoagulation therapy for patients with AF after TAVR.

Keywords: TAVR, VARC-2, Sinus rhythm, NOAC, Bleeding, Atrial fibrillation, Antiplatelet therapy

* Correspondence: joerg_herold@hotmail.com
[1]Department of Internal Medicine/Cardiology and Angiology,
Otto-von-Guericke University of Magdeburg, Leipziger Str. 44, 39120
Magdeburg, Germany
Full list of author information is available at the end of the article

Background

Degenerative aortic stenosis is the most common form of heart valve disease affecting the elderly population [1]. Transcatheter aortic valve implantation (TAVR) has been shown to be superior to medical therapy for inoperable patients and is not inferior to surgical aortic valve replacement (SAVR) in terms of all-cause mortality [2–5]. Five-year data from the PARTNER study recently confirmed the long-term success of the TAVR strategy [4, 6, 7].

However, patients undergoing TAVR are also at high risk for both bleeding and stroke complications. The mechanisms of peri-procedural bleeding complications appear to be mainly related to vascular/access site complications, whereas the pathophysiology of cerebrovascular events remains largely unknown. Life-threatening bleeding complications may also dramatically increase mortality [8, 9].

Nevertheless, among elderly patients for whom TAVR is indicated, prescreening often reveals other comorbidities. Both aortic valve stenosis and atrial fibrillation (AF) are particularly common among patients in the 8th decade of life [10, 11]. Managing these patients, who require oral anticoagulation to address AF-associated increased thromboembolic risk and who undergo TAVR due to severe aortic valve stenosis, presents a challenge in clinical practice. In particular, the question arises regarding whether to administer anticoagulant therapy after TAVR to prevent vascular complications or bleeding and cerebrovascular events. No consistent evidence-based anticoagulant therapy recommendations are currently available for patients with AF after TAVR. The aim of this retrospective study was to examine the influence of AF in a "real world" TAVR cohort.

Methods

Study design and patients

A total of 283 patients underwent TAVR between March 2010 and April 2016 at the University Hospital of Cardiology and Angiology of Otto-von-Guericke-University Magdeburg. The trial was registered at German Clinical Trials Register (DRKS) (DRKS00011798). The access route to the aortic valve was through the femoral artery and the subclavian artery. Patients whose implantation procedures were discontinued (frustrated TAVR, $n = 4$; 1.4%) and those requiring immediate cardiac surgery due to acute life-threatening intraprocedural complications ($n = 3$; 1.1%) were excluded from further analysis. Patients with transsubclavian TAVR ($n = 19$; 6.7%) were not included in the evaluation because this subgroup was too small for statistical calculations (Fig. 1). Thus,

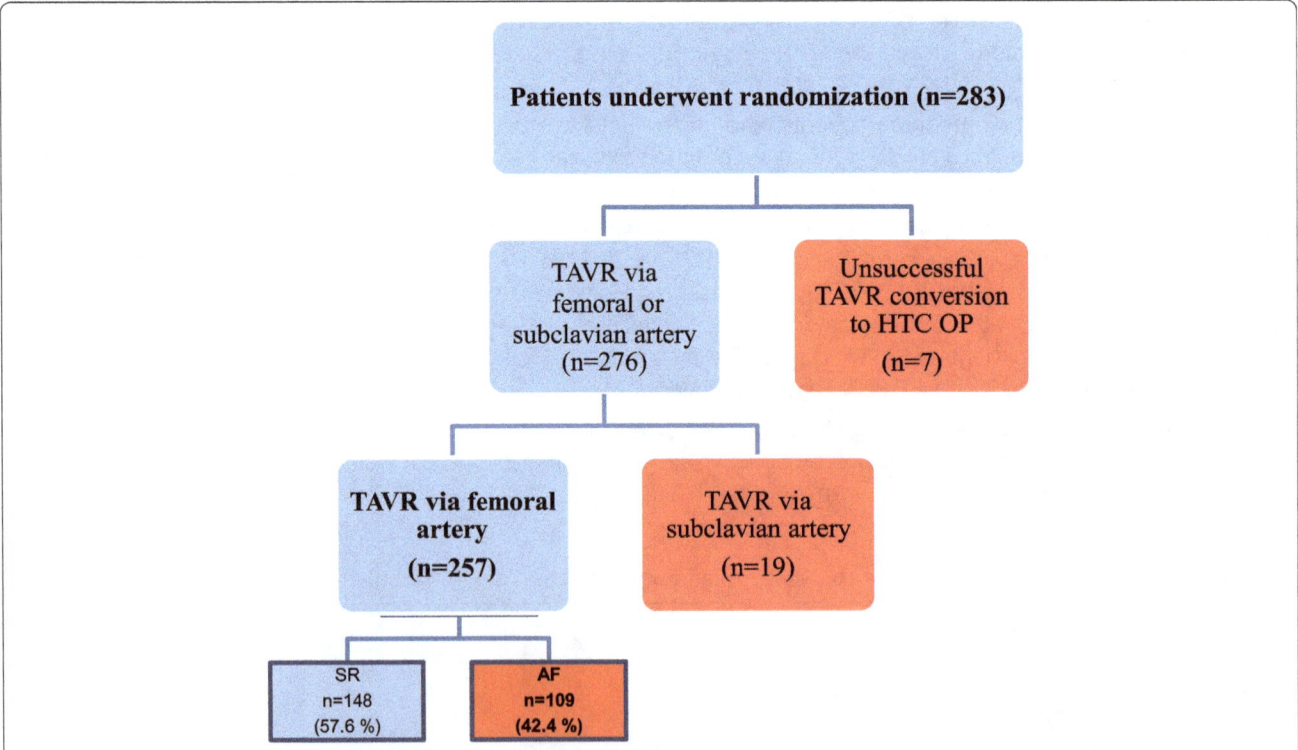

Fig. 1 Trial enrollment showing the total population of patients who received a TAVR procedure from 03/2010 to 04/2016. Patients without a successfully implanted TAVR ($n = 4$, 1.4%) or patients who had to be converted to open cardiac surgery (HTC-OP; $n = 3$; 1.1%) were excluded. Due to the small group size, the patients who received a TAVR over the subclavian artery ($n = 19$; 6.7%) were not included in the study. Thus, 257 patients with transfemoral access were included in the further analysis. Visualization of the classification of the patient collective according to the preprocedural cardiac rhythm: Almost half of the total patient population (42.4%) suffered from AF

257 patients were retrospectively divided into SR and AF groups according to pre-procedural cardiac rhythm. The presence of AF prior to TAVR was determined electro-cardiographically and/or on the basis of outpatient or in-patient records. The two groups were compared for baseline characteristics, post-procedural mortality and complications, and vascular and cerebrovascular compli-cations within 30 days, 3 months, 6 months, and 1 year after TAVR. The complications following TAVR were documented using the VARC-2 criteria [12]. To evaluate the use of coagulation inhibitors in patients with AF after TAVR, patients with AF were divided post-procedurally into subgroups. Because most patients with AF were treated with either vitamin K antagonist (VKA) plus clopidogrel or with a NOAC plus clopidogrel for 3 months, these two subgroups were compared for mortal-ity and complication rates.

Medication

The patients with AF and TAVR received triple therapy (phenprocoumon/clopidogrel (75 mg o.d./aspirin 100 mg o.d.)), phenprocoumon/clopidogrel (75 mg o.d.) or a com-bination of a NOAC and clopidogrel (75 mg o.d.) for 3 months. Bleeding complications were defined by the VARC- 2 criteria.

Endpoints

Clinical follow-up, including echocardiography, electro-cardiography, and laboratory testing for creatinine, transaminases, red blood cells and thrombocytes was performed before and after valve implantation prior to discharge and at 1, 3, 6, 9 and 12 months following the procedure.

Statistical analyses

The statistical data analyses were performed using SPSS 24.0 (SPSS Inc., Chicago, USA). The results were pre-sented both descriptively and graphically. Continuous values were presented as mean values with standard de-viations and are represented by box plots for the individ-ual groups being examined. Categorical variables were presented as absolute and relative frequencies of the overall study population and by using bar graphs. A comparison of the groups (AF vs. SR) for statistically sig-nificant differences was performed using the unpaired t-test (Satterthwaite) for continuous variables and Fisher's exact test for categorical variables. In the case of strong deviations from a normal distribution, a natural loga-rithm transformation was used to facilitate use of the t-test. Survival curves were calculated using the Kaplan-Meier method, and the groups were compared using the log-rank test, taking censored data into account. Add-itionally, cumulative mortality was analyzed in the same manner as other complications without regard for

censored data. Using the multivariate COX regression model, different baseline characteristics were examined for their prognostic significance in relation to survival probability and one-year overall mortality. In this process, influential variables were selected using step-wise conditional forward selection. The results were pre-sented in the form of odds or hazard ratios, 95% confidence intervals and/or p values. The p values were calculated as exact two-tailed values. The significance level was set to 0.05, such that p values ≤ 0.05 indicated statistically significant results. All analyses were deliber-ately performed to the full level of significance. No cor-rections were performed for multiple comparisons due to the exploratory nature of this investigation.

Results
Patient characteristics

Overall, 283 patients were screened. According to the in-clusion and exclusion criteria, 257 patients were eventu-ally included. Nineteen screened patients were excluded because of subclavian access. TAVR was not successful in 7 of the 257 patients (2.4%). After these exclusions, 148 patients with SR vs. One hundred and nine with AF who underwent TAVR via transfemoral access were in-cluded for further analysis (Fig. 1).

The average age of the entire study group was 80.8 ± 6.0 years on the day of implantation, with 45.9% male patients ($n = 118$). The baseline characteristics of the en-tire patient group and the two groups classified accord-ing to preprocedural cardiac rhythm are summarized in Table 1. With regard to comorbidities, significantly more patients in the AF group than in the SR group had PAD (21.1% vs. 11.5%, respectively, $p = 0.038$). Furthermore, significantly more patients in the AF group had already received a pacemaker (SR 7.4% vs. AF 19.3%, $p = 0.007$). The remaining features were not significantly different between the two groups.

Laboratory parameters, echocardiographic characteristics and risk scores

Table 2 lists the laboratory parameters of the samples col-lected 2 days before valve implantation and the echocar-diographic characteristics. These are listed as the mean values for the entire patient population and for the two groups in direct comparison. There were no statistically significant differences between the two groups. Concern-ing the baseline risk assessment, patients with AF did not significantly differ from those with SR (Fig. 2).

DAPT vs. triple therapy

Patients with AF received postoperative therapeutic heparinization (AF 51.4% vs. SR 4.1%, $p < 0.001$) and combination therapy consisting of either OAC and APT (AF 67.9% vs. SR 6.1%, $p < 0.001$) or triple therapy (AF

Table 1 Characteristics of the patients at baseline

Characteristics of the Patients at Baseline	Total population ($n = 257$)	SR-group ($n = 148$)	AF-group ($n = 109$)	p Value
Age — yr	80.8 ± 6.0	80.6 ± 6.0	80.9 ± 6.0	0.736
Male sex — no. (%)	118 (45.9%)	62 (41.9%)	56 (51.4%)	0.163
Body-mass index (kg/m^2)	28.2 ± 5.5	28.3 ± 5.6	28.1 ± 5.3	0.724
Diabetes mellitus (n. %)	110 (42.8%)	57 (38.5%)	53 (48.6%)	0.126
Diabetes treated with insulin	68 (26.5%)	33 (22.3%)	35 (32.1%)	0.087
Hypertension	223 (86.8%)	126 (85.1%)	97 (89.0%)	0.457
Dyslipidemia (n. %)	179 (69.6%)	102 (68.9%)	77 (70.6%)	0.785
PAD	40 (15.6%)	17 (11.5%)	23 (21.1%)	0.038
Chronic obstructive pulmonary disease (n %)	50 (19.5%)	33 (22.3%)	17 (15.6%)	0.204
Medical history — no. (%)				
Chronic kidney disease on dialysis	8 (3.1%)	7 (4.7%)	1 (0.9%)	0.143
History of cancer	64 (24.9%)	40 (27.0%)	24 (22.0%)	0.384
Active cancer	20 (7.8%)	10 (6.8%)	10 (9.2%)	0.489
Coronary heart disease	210 (81.7%)	120 (81.1%)	90 (82.6%)	0.871
Coronary-artery bypass surgery	36 (14.0%)	18 (12.2%)	18 (16.5%)	0.365
Myocardial infarction	30 (11.7%)	15 (10.1%)	15 (13.8%)	0.433
PCI	67 (26.1%)	42 (28.4%)	25 (22.9%)	0.389
Pacemaker	32 (12.5%)	11 (7.4%)	21 (19.3%)	0.007
Stroke	40 (15.6%)	22 (14.9%)	18 (16.5%)	0.731
NYHA III	164 (63.8%)	96 (64.9%)	68 (62.4%)	0.695
NYHA IV	61 (23.7%)	31 (20.9%)	30 (27.5%)	0.238

All values correspond to the mean ± standard deviation or the number n (proportion in %). PAD was defined as claudication intermittens or any symptom corresponding to ≥ Fontaine stage II and / or as amputation in the context of an arterial occlusion and/or present or planned endovascular intervention for the revascularization of the peripheral vessels

9.2% vs. SR 0.7%, $p = 0.001$). Conversely, DAPT was administered significantly more frequently to patients with SR (SR 93.2% vs. AF 16.5%, $p < 0.001$).

Vascular complications
The incidence of major vascular complications was 9.3% overall during the first 30 days and differed significantly between the two groups. Specifically, almost three times as many major vascular complications occurred in patients with AF than in patients with SR (AF 14.7% vs. SR 5.4%, $p = 0.016$) (Table 3).

Regarding minor vascular complications, a similar, non-significant difference was found between the two groups (Table 4). The temporal distribution of minor

Table 2 Summary of the main parameters of the baseline laboratory and echocardiographic findings. There was no significant difference between the two groups regarding the laboratory and echocardiographic parameters

Baseline laboratory	Total population (n = 257)	SR-group(n = 148)	AF-group(n = 109)	p Value
Hemoglobin (mmol/l)	7.5 ± 1.1	7.5 ± 1.1	7.4 ± 1.1	0.227
Creatinin (umol/l[1])	108.1 ± 44.1	103.5 ± 37.1	114.2 ± 51.3	0.121*
Glomerular filtration rate CKD-EPI (ml/min[1])	54.5 ± 19.2	54.9 ± 17.9	54.0 ± 20.9	0.718
Thrombocyte (Gpt/l)	222.5 ± 75.6	225.3 ± 77.5	218.6 ± 73.2	0.479
Echocardiographic parameters	Total population (n = 257)	SR-group (n = 148)	AF-group (n = 109)	p Value
Aortic valve area (cm2)	0.72 ± 0.17	0.72 ± 0.17	0.71 ± 0.16	0.799
Pulmonary hypertension (PaSP >55 mmHg)	23 (8.9%)	11 (7.4%)	12 (11.0%)	0.379
Ejection fraction (%)	46.1 ± 13.8	47.2 ± 13.7	44.5 ± 13.9	0.113
Ejection fraction <40%	59 (23.0%)	30 (20.3%)	29 (26.6%)	0.293

[1]Patients not requiring dialysis ($n = 8$; 3.1% or SR: $n = 7$; 4.7% AF: $n = 1$, 0.9%). * Test using log-transformed values
All values correspond to the mean ± standard deviation or the number n (proportion in %)

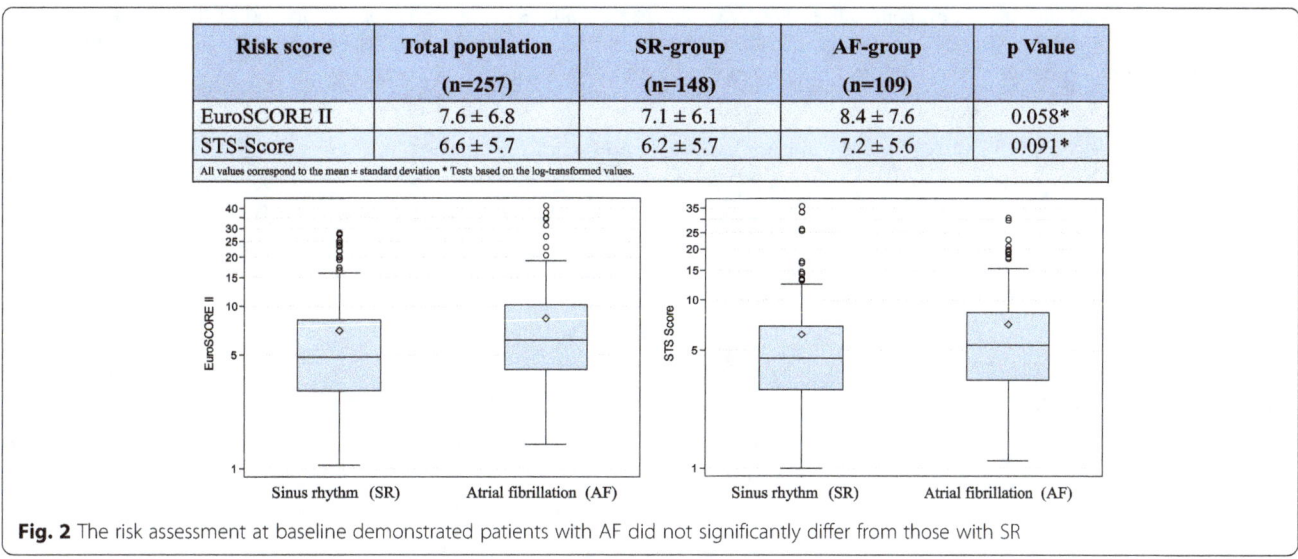

Risk score	Total population (n=257)	SR-group (n=148)	AF-group (n=109)	p Value
EuroSCORE II	7.6 ± 6.8	7.1 ± 6.1	8.4 ± 7.6	0.058*
STS-Score	6.6 ± 5.7	6.2 ± 5.7	7.2 ± 5.6	0.091*

All values correspond to the mean ± standard deviation * Tests based on the log-transformed values.

Fig. 2 The risk assessment at baseline demonstrated patients with AF did not significantly differ from those with SR

vascular complications was also correlated with the occurrence of major vascular complications (Table 4).

Major and minor bleeding

With regard to the occurrence of major and minor bleeding, no significant differences between the two groups could be demonstrated. However, patients with SR had more severe major and minor bleeding (Table 4).

Life-threating bleeding

During the first 30 days, a total of 19 life-threatening secondary bleeding events were recorded in the overall patient group (7.4%). Patients with pre-interventional AF had nearly three times as many events as patients with SR (AF 11.9% vs. SR 4.1%, p = 0.028). This result corresponds to the rates and the temporal development of major vascular complications. Thus, most life-threatening bleeding occurred around the time of implantation and the changeover to OAC (NOAC or VKA) and DAPT. Once the patients became accustomed to the medication, there were no further significant changes (increases or decreases in bleeding) between the two groups (Table 5).

Transfusion of erythrocyte concentrates

During the first 30 days, a blood transfusion with at least one erythrocyte concentrate (RBC) unit was required for approximately one of every five (21.0%) patients. The need for RBC transfusion was significantly different between the two groups, as significantly more patients with AF required RBC administration (AF 27.5% vs. SR 16.2%, p = 0.031, OR 1.96, 95% CI 1.07–3.60). The difference in RBC requirements between the two groups is shown schematically in Fig. 3.

Stroke

The incidence of stroke within the first 30 days was 3.1% in the overall patient group. There was no significant difference between the two groups in stroke incidence during the first 30 days after TAVR (SR 2.7% vs. AF 3.7%, p = 0.726) or during the complete follow-up period (Table 6). There was also no significant difference in the incidence of transient ischemic attacks (TIAs) between the two groups (SR 0.0% vs. AF 1.8%, p = 0.179) within the first 30 days after TAVR.

Table 3 Major vascular complications

Follow-up	Total population (n = 257)	SR-group(n = 148)	AF-group(n = 109)	p Value	OR (95% CI)
30 days	9.3% (24/257)	5.4% (8/148)	14.7% (16/109)	0.016	3.01 (1.24–7.32)
3 months	9.3% (24/257)	5.4% (8/148)	14.7% (16/109)	0.016	3.01 (1.24–7.32)
6 months	9.9% (24/241)	5.8% (8/137)	15.4% (16/104)	0.016	2.98 (1.22–7.26)
12 months	10.8% (24/219)	6.3% (8/124)	16.7% (16/95)	0.017	2.95 (1.20–7.22)

The table shows the major vascular complications of the total patient group and of the two groups over the course of the follow-up period. The parentheses list the number of major vascular complications and the number of patients available for analysis

In patients with AF, almost three times as many major vascular complications occurred during the first 30-day post-procedural complications than in patients with SR. No further increase in major vascular complications after the first 30 days were noted, as these complications mainly occurred around the intervention

Table 4 The upper part (lite blue) summarizes the minor vascular complications of the total population and of the two groups. The parentheses list the number of minor vascular complications and the number of patients available for analysis. No significant difference was observed between the two groups with respect to minor vascular complications

	Total population (n = 257)	SR-group(n = 148)	AF-group (n = 109)	p Value	OR (95% CI)
Follow-up Minor vascular complication					
30 days	22.6% (58/257)	22.3% (33/148)	22.9% (25/109)	1.00	1.09 (0.61–1.96)
3 months	23.0% (59/257)	22.3% (33/148)	23.9% (26/109)	0.767	1.09 (0.61–1.96)
6 months	24.8% (60/241)	23.9% (33/137)	26.0% (27/104)	0.764	1.12 (0.62–2.01)
12 months	27.3% (60/219)	26.4% (33/124)	28.4% (27/95)	0.762	1.11 (0.61–2.01)
Follow-up Major bleeding					
30 days	3.5% (9/257)	4.1% (6/148)	2.8% (3/109)	0.737	0.67 (0.16–2.74)
3 months	3.9% (10/257)	4.7% (7/148)	2.8% (3/109)	0.525	0.57 (0.14–2.26)
6 months	4.5% (11/241)	5.8% (8/137)	2.9% (3/104)	0.360	0.48 (1.13–1.87)
12 months	5.5% (12/219)	7.2% (9/124)	3.2% (3/95)	0.240	0.42 (0.11–1.60)
Follow-up Minor bleeding					
30 days	19.8% (51/257)	21.6% (32/148)	17.4% (19/109)	1.00	1.09 (0.61–1.96)
3 months	19.8% (51/257)	21.6% (32/148)	17.4% (19/109)	0.767	1.09 (0.61–1.96)
6 months	21.0% (51/241)	23.0% (32/137)	18.3% (19/104)	0.764	1.12 (0.62–2.01)
12 months	23.1% (51/219)	25.4% (32/124)	20.0% (19/95)	0.762	1.11 (0.61–2.01)

The middle part of the table (blue) shows the major bleeding events of the total collective and of the two groups during the course of the follow-up period. The lower part of the table (deep blue) lists the minor bleeding events. The parentheses list the number of bleeding events and the number of patients available for analysis. With regard to the occurrences of major and minor bleeding, no significant accumulation was found in one of the two groups

Overall mortality and cardiovascular mortality associated with TAVR

The total patient population showed cumulative 30-day, 3-month, 6-month and one-year overall mortality rates of 4.7, 9.3, 14.9 and 21.0%, respectively. With respect to pre-interventional heart rhythms, patients with pre-existing AF had markedly higher cumulative mortality than patients in the SR group at 30 days (AF 8.3% vs. SR 2.0%, $p = 0.032$), 3 months (AF 14.7% vs. SR 5.4%, $p = 0.016$), 6 months (AF 22.1% vs. SR 9.5%, $p = 0.010$) and 1 year (AF 28.4% vs. SR 15.3%, $p = 0.020$). A statistically significant ($p = 0.012$) difference was found in AF patient mortality over the entire first year according to the Kaplan-Meier survival analysis (Fig. 4). Concerning cardiovascular mortality, the total patient population had cumulative 30-day, 3-month, 6-month and one-year cardiovascular mortality rates of 3.9, 8.2, 12.0 and 17.4%,

respectively. Patients with pre-existing AF clearly had consistently higher cardiovascular mortality than patients in the SR group at 30 days (AF 7.3% vs. SR 1.4%, $p = 0.020$), 3 months (AF 12.8% vs SR 4.7%, $p = 0.022$), 6 months (AF 18.3% vs. SR 7.3%, $p = 0.015$) and 1 year (AF 24.2% vs. SR 12.1%, $p = 0.030$) (Fig. 5).

Days of hospitalization

The average duration of hospitalization was 17.3 ± 10.2 days overall. Patients with AF had a significantly longer hospital stay than patients with SR (SR 16.2 ± 9.2 vs. AF 18.9 ± 11.3; $p = 0.043$) (Fig. 6).

Predictors of one-year overall mortality after TAVR

Multivariate analysis revealed that pre-existing AF was an independent predictor of increased mortality at 1 year

Table 5 Life-threatening bleeding

Follow-up	Total population (n = 257)	SR-group(n = 148)	AF-group(n = 109)	p Value	OR (95% CI)
30 days	7.4% (19/257)	4.1% (6/148)	11.9% (13/109)	0.028	3.21 (1.18–8.72)
3 months	7.8% (20/257)	4.7% (7/148)	11.9% (13/109)	0.057	2.73 (1.05–7.09)
6 months	8.2% (20/241)	5.0% (7/137)	12.5% (13/104)	0.057	2.69 (1.04–7.01)
12 months	9.0% (20/219)	5.6% (7/124)	13.5% (13/95)	0.057	2.66 (1.02–6.96)

Shows the life-threatening bleeding events of all patients and of the two groups during the course of the follow-up period. The parentheses list the number of life-threatening bleeding events and the number of patients available for analysis
Patients with AF showed nearly three times more life-threatening bleeding events than patients with SR. This result corresponds to the rates and the temporal development of major vascular complications. Most of the life-threatening bleeding occurred peri-precidually and during initiation of oral anticoagulation or dual anti-platelet therapy. Thereafter, no significant differences were determined

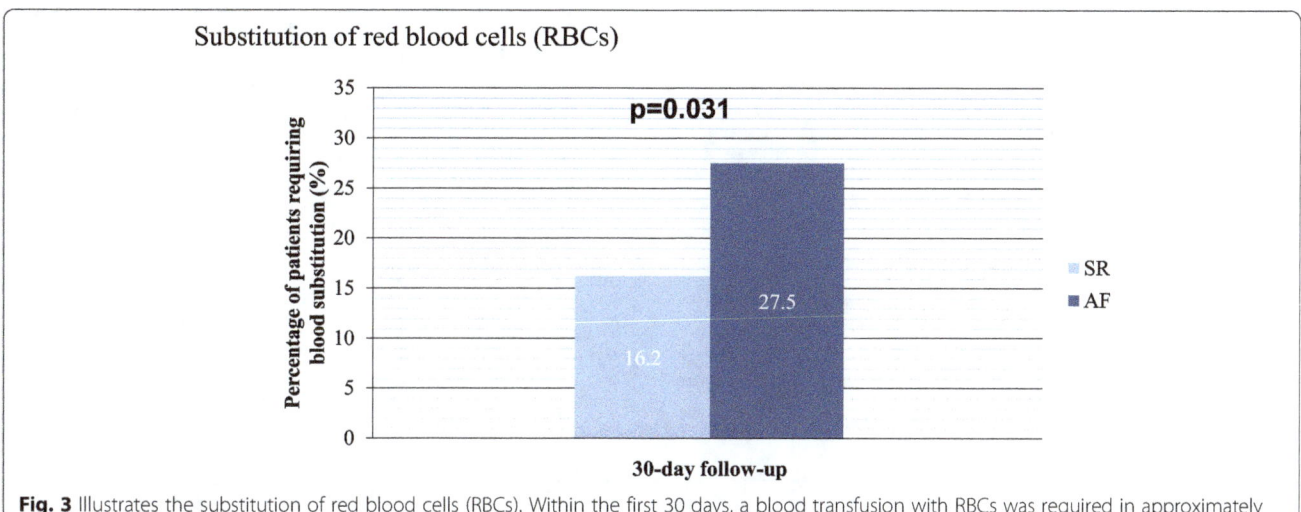

Fig. 3 Illustrates the substitution of red blood cells (RBCs). Within the first 30 days, a blood transfusion with RBCs was required in approximately one of every five (21.0%) patients. Significantly more RBCs had to be administered to patients with AF

(HR: 2.10). All significant predictors for 1-year mortality are reported in Table 7.

Discussion

Following the first aortic value implantation in 2002, TAVR was characterized by Cribier et al. [13] as an established therapy for high-grade, symptomatic aortic valve stenosis [14]. Furthermore, recently published data from the PARTNER-2 and SURTAVI studies show that TAVR is equivalent to conventional aortic valve replacement surgery for patients who present with intermediate surgical risk [7, 15]. In addition to other comorbidities, pre-existing AF is present in a significant proportion of elderly patients with high-grade degenerative aortic valve stenosis, with a rapidly increasing prevalence with increasing age [16, 17]. Because of the multi-morbidity of patients who often exhibit elevated bleeding risk, medical treatment after TAVR remains challenging. In practice, the limited dual platelet inhibition with aspirin and clopidogrel as an antithrombotic therapy has been most widely accepted according to TAVR and SR. The European Society of Cardiology (ESC) recommendations for IIa C indicate that dual antiplatelet therapy should be considered for the first 3–6 months after TAVR, followed by lifelong single antiplatelet

therapy in patients who do not need oral anticoagulation for other reasons, whereas single antiplatelet therapy may be considered after TAVR in patients with high bleeding risk (III B) [18]. Nevertheless, there are clinical challenges in the management of patients with AF and TAVR. According the ESC guidelines, triple therapy for longer than 1 month should be considered for patients with a high risk of ischemia, which outweighs bleeding risk (IIa B); on the contrary, dual therapy comprising VKA and clopidogrel should be considered as an alternative to 1-month triple antithrombotic therapy (IIa A) in patients with high bleeding risk [18].

However, there are still uncertainties in both the clinical implementation and in the duration of triple-therapy or use of NOAC for patients with AF. The combination of anticoagulation with an antiplatelet therapy is used to prevent stroke and valve thrombosis but likely increases bleeding complications.

Therefore, 257 patients were included in this study between March 2010 and April 2016. Regarding pre-procedural cardiac rhythm, nearly half of the patients ($n = 109$; 42.4%) had AF. Therefore, the question arose as to whether the patients were randomly distributed into the SR and AF groups in this study. As

Table 6 Cerebrovascular complications

Follow-upStroke	Total population (n = 257)	SR-group(n = 148)	AF-group(n = 109)	p Value	OR (95% CI)
30 days	3.1% (8/257)	2.7% (4/148)	3.7% (4/109)	0.726	1.37 (0.34–5.61)
3 months	3.1% (8/257)	2.7% (4/148)	3.7% (4/109)	0.726	1.37 (0.34–5.61)
6 months	3.3% (8/241)	2.9% (4/137)	3.8% (4/104)	0.728	1.34 (0.33–5.49)
12 months	5.0% (11*/219)	4.0% (5/124)	6.3% (6/95)	0.537	1.62 (0.48–5.47)

Lists the cerebrovascular complications up to the one-year follow-up. The strokes are shown for the entire patient population and for the two groups during the follow-up period. The parentheses list the number of strokes and the number of patients available for analysis. * Ten ischemic strokes and one hemorrhagic stroke. The occurrence of stroke in the two groups showed no significant difference

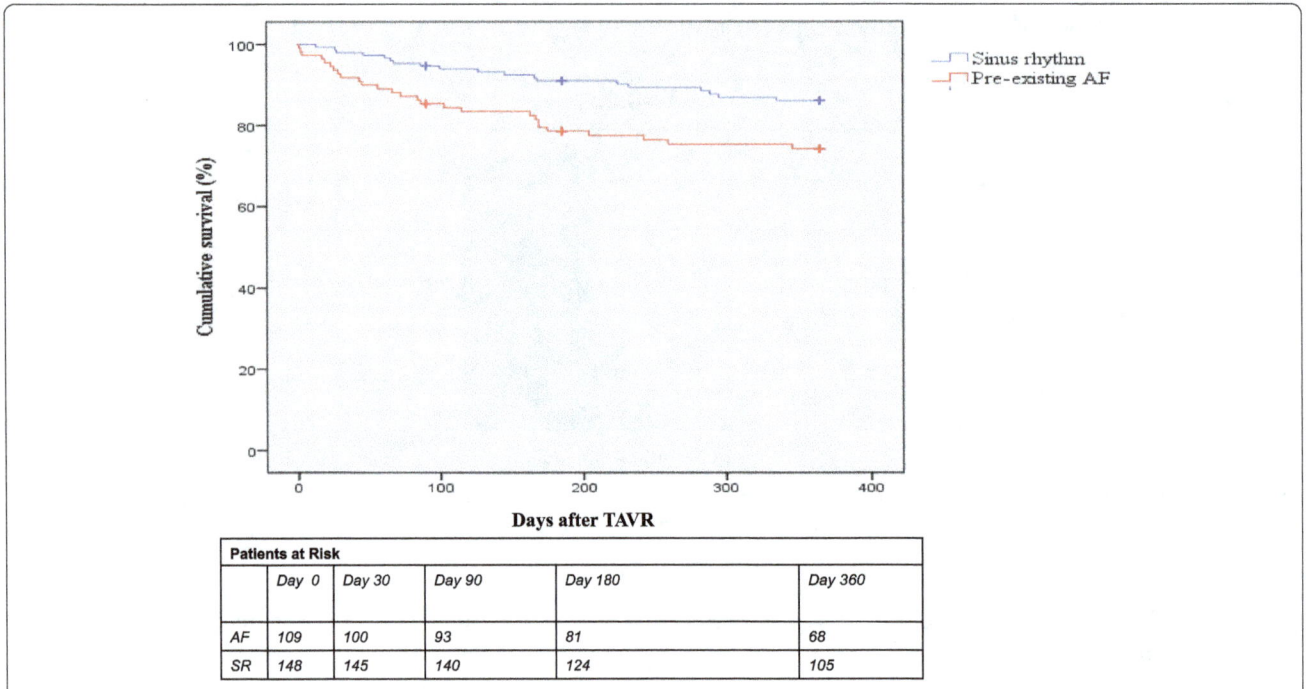

Fig. 4 Kaplan-Meier curves of the one-year cumulative survival of patients with and without pre-existing atrial fibrillation (AF). Event rates were also calculated with the use of the log-rank test. Deaths from unknown causes were assumed to be deaths from cardiovascular cause. AF caused a higher overall mortality according to TAVR

previously mentioned, AF is the most frequent cardiac arrhythmia. Based on its age-dependent prevalence, the average age of those affected is between 75 and 85 years [16]. Additionally, the occurrence of AF is likely due to a high number of pre-valvular cardiac diseases, such as arterial hypertension, coronary heart disease and cardiac valve disease [17]. The increased incidence of AF in this patient population is therefore predictable given the mean study population age of 80.8 ± 6.0 years, comorbidity rates of 81.7% for

coronary heart disease and 86.8% for arterial hypertension, and above all, the fact that all patients had high-grade aortic valve stenosis.

Although this was a retrospective survey rather than a prospective study, the baseline characteristics differed in only two parameters. Specifically, previous pacemaker implantation was significantly more common among patients with AF. In one sense, this might confer a prophylactic effect against AF in these patients. For the entire patient population, the EuroSCORE II was 7.6 ± 6.8 and

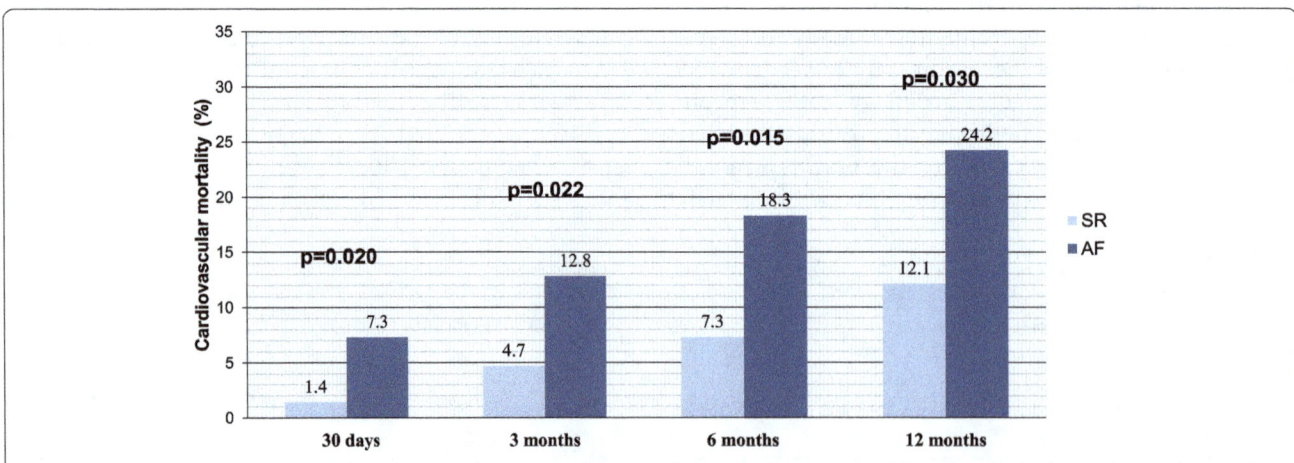

Fig. 5 Shows the cardiovascular mortality rates up to the one-year follow-up. Patients with pre-existing AF presented a higher cardiovascular mortality after 30 days. This difference persisted for 12 months

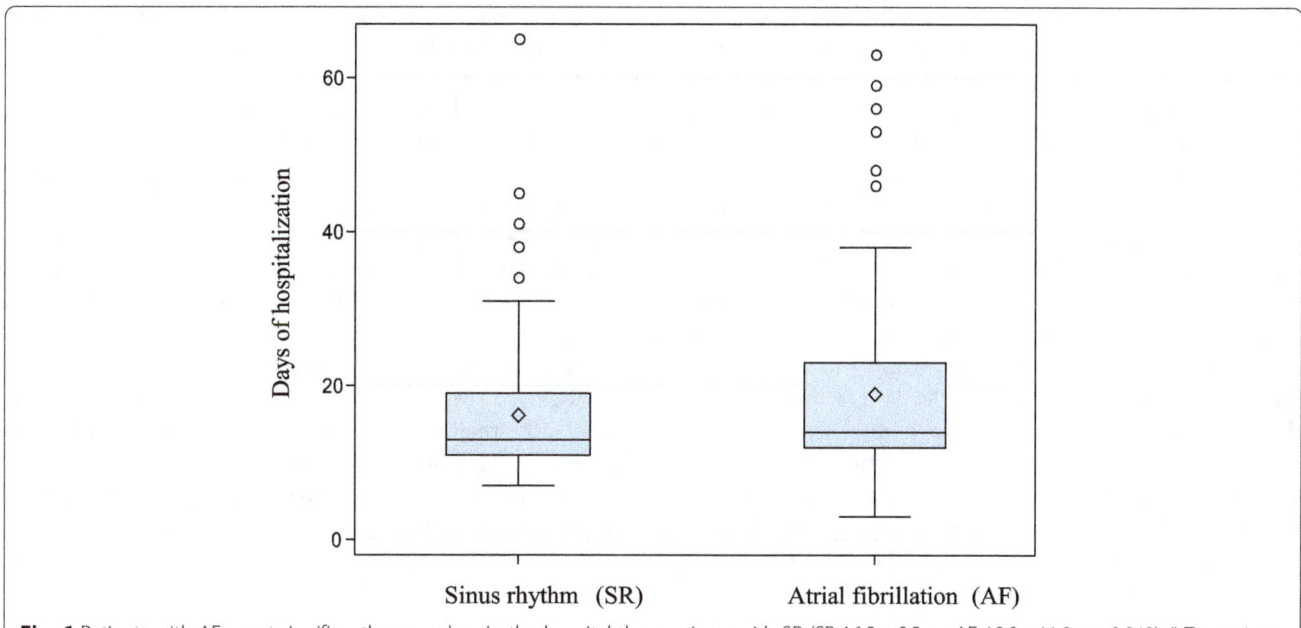

Fig. 6 Patients with AF spent significantly more days in the hospital than patients with SR (SR 16.2 ± 9.2 vs. AF 18.9 ± 11.3 p = 0.043). * Test using log-transformed values

the STS score was 6.6 ± 5.7, similar to the scores in the largest German registry (German Aortic Valve Registry, GARY). Current data from the GARY registry also show that more patients with low-risk scores underwent TAVR in recent years (the mean STS score according to the GARY registry was 5.0) [19].

Vascular complications during transfemoral TAVR cover a wide range of vascular injuries, such as perforations, ruptures, dissections and their sequelae involving access vessels or the aorta [20, 21]. Vascular complications were subdivided into major and minor complications according to VARC-2 criteria [22] and were compared between the AF and SR groups. The overall incidence of major vascular complications during the first 30 postoperative days was 9.3%. However, it is important to note that no further increase in vascular complications was observed after the first 30 days, as these events were mainly peri-procedural.

Due to the different recruitment periods of the patients included in the study, the use of different valve

generations and valve implantation systems, and the different definitions of vascular complications depending on the study situation, existing published data on vascular complications differ considerably among large TAVR studies and registries. For example, in the PARTNER study, the rate of major vascular complications during the first 30 post-interventional days was as high as 16.2% using the modified VARC criteria [3, 5]. In the PARTNER-2 study, the rate of vascular complications according to the advanced VARC-2 criteria decreased to only 7.9% and to 8.5% for the transsubclavian and transfemoral cohorts, respectively [15]. The FRANCE-2 trial and SOURCE-XT registries showed major vascular complication rates (according to VARC-2 criteria) of 5.5% and 7.9%, respectively, for transfemoral access [23, 24]. A major vascular complication rate (according to VARC criteria) of 10.9% was reported in the ADVANCE study, predominantly with transfemoral implanted valve prostheses [25]. In the GARY registry, however, a low incidence of major vascular complications (4.1%) was

Table 7 Shows the significant independent predictors for mortality by the 1-year follow-up according to the multivariate logistic regression

Significant predictors	Multivariate data analysis at baseline	
	Hazard Ratio (95% Confidence Interval)	p Value
Pre-existing AF	2.10 (1.17–3.78)	0.013
Anemia (Hb < 10.5 g/dL)	2.39 (1.28–4.47)	0.007
STS-score	1.08 (1.04–1.12)	< 0.001
Previous coronary artery bypass graft surgery (CABG)	0.25 (0.08–0.83)	0.024
Previous coronary artery disease (CAD)	3.27 (1.00–10.72)	0.050

observed. This can be explained by the fact that in the GARY registry, as in other studies, vascular complications are classified using different classification criteria than the VARC criteria. The GARY registry detects and divides complications into three categories. For example, aortic dissection and annular rupture after TAVR are classified as severe vital complications rather than as vascular complications [19]. Furthermore, the VARC-2 criteria significantly differ from the VARC-1 criteria in the definition of major vascular complications. These differences must be accounted for when interpreting the study results. For example, when using the VARC-2 criteria, any vascular injury that leads not only to life-threatening bleeding but also to major hemorrhage is recorded as a major vascular complication. Additionally, any unplanned endovascular or surgical intervention associated with a severe event such as death, life-threatening or major hemorrhage, visceral ischemia, or neurological impairment is defined as a major vascular complication according to the VARC-2 criteria [22, 26]. In an analysis of 403 consecutive TAVR patients, Steinvil et al. 0reported that use of the VARC-2 criteria led to a higher reported rate of major vascular complications than use of the VARC-1 criteria due to the detection of major bleeding [8]. Therefore, directly comparing the major vascular complication rate in our study population with the rates from previous large studies is difficult.

This study clearly shows that patients with AF have nearly three times more major vascular complications within the first 30 days after TAVR than patients with SR. Therefore, special attention should be paid to patients with AF during pre-procedural consultation and during the peri-procedural period in consideration of the significantly higher rates of major vascular complications and life-threatening bleeding.

Another relevant point is that there were more patients with PAD in the AF group. The association of PAD with significantly more frequent major vascular complications may be associated with the poorer vascular access in this patient group. Sinning et al. [27] observed that patients with PAD had a two-fold higher rate of major vascular complications after TAVR compared to patients without PAD.

Because most peri-procedural vascular injuries lead to bleeding, it can be assumed that these events are more pronounced in patients with AF than in patients with SR. To date, few studies have investigated vascular complications or bleeding after TAVR in connection with AF. Seeger et al. recently published a clinical follow-up study, reporting a promising anticoagulation regime using apixaban in patients with AF after TAVR [28]. This strategy suggests that an early safety endpoint in patients with AF receiving apixaban was significantly less frequent compared with patients receiving a VKA [28].

Nonetheless, some analyses have revealed contradictory results. The BRAVO-3 trial revealed similar early outcomes across groups regardless of anticoagulant strategy (AF and SR) and demonstrated that AF was not associated with significantly higher risk of adjusted 30-day outcomes [29]. A possible reason could be that 29.5% of AF patients were treated with DAPT without OAC, while only 16.5% of patients were treated without OAC in our study. Therefore, an increased number of left atrial occlusions could be responsible for this discrepancy.

In a recently published subgroup analysis from the SOURCE-XT registry [30], a significantly higher incidence of major vascular complications and life-threatening bleeding was reported among patients with pre-existing AF. However, the anticoagulation strategy was not investigated in this study. Maan et al. [31] found no statistically significant differences in major vascular complications between SR and AF patients in a retrospective study of 137 patients. Although bleeding after TAVR was not considered. Chopard et al. [32] did not show any significant difference in the occurrence of major vascular complications within 30 days after TAVR between patients with pre-existing AF and those with SR based on their analysis of data from the FRANCE-2 registries. However, there was a noticeably lower overall rate of major vascular complications. Furthermore, the rate of life-threatening bleeding was not explicitly stated in this study.

Bleeding complications

Overall, 7.4% of the patients experienced life-threatening bleeding, 3.5% had major bleeding and 19.8% had minor bleeding during the first 30 post-procedural days.

In the large TAVR studies and registry data already published, the rates of life-threatening bleeding have differed among transfemoral (or mainly transfemoral) cohorts based on the VARC/VARC-2 criteria. The reported bleeding rates have ranged from 1.2% in the FRANCE-2 registry [23] to 13.6% in the CoreValve High Risk study [33], with rates of 6.7% in the PARTNER-2 study [15], 4.0% in the ADVANCE study [25] and 3.8% in the SOURCE-XT registry [24].

In the PARTNER study, hemorrhages were classified as major or minor using the modified VARC-2 criteria rather than classifying as major life-threatening bleeding. This resulted in major bleeding rates of 10.9% in cohort A and 16.8% in cohort B [3, 5]. Recent data from the GARY registry showed a decrease in the incidence of major bleeding (bleeding requiring transfusion of $\geq$ two RBC units) of 30.6% in 2011, 27.6% in 2012 and 23.0% in 2013 [19]. The SURTAVI study concluded an incidence of life-threatening or major bleeding of 12.2% [7] due to both technical advancements and increased user knowledge regarding TAVR. Accordingly, the year data were acquired in published studies must also be considered when interpreting the results and also applies to nearly all complication rates.

Concerning the distribution of bleeding complications between the two groups within the first 30 post-procedural days, patients with AF had life-threatening bleeding three times more frequently than patients with SR. A similar difference was evident in the rates and temporal development of major vascular complications. Although this difference remained constant throughout the follow-up period, further bleeding complications were unlikely in all successful TAVR procedures not complicated by bleeding or vascular complications during the first 30 post-procedural days. Concerning the occurrence of major or minor bleeding, no significant difference between the two groups was demonstrated either within 30 days after TAVR or during the complete follow-up period. Considering that 93.2% of SR patients were treated with DAPT, these results may indicate that the bleeding incidence of 3.7% per year already described in the literature for DAPT therapy may also be applicable to TAVR patients [34]. The propensity matched analysis from the ITER registry indicated aspirin alone does not increase the risk of prosthetic valve dysfunction and reduces the risk of peri-procedural complications and the risk of 30-day all-cause death compared to DAPT therapy after TAVI in patients with SR [35]. Supporting results were shown by Ichibori et al., who suggested that treatment with aspirin alone is an acceptable regimen for TAVR patients with SR [36]. Although the risk of bleeding is lowered by a single antiplatelet therapy, valve thrombosis and dysfunction are frequently observed. Indeed, observational studies found subclinical leaflet thrombosis rates up to 13% [37]. Subclinical leaflet thrombosis occurred frequently in bioprosthetic aortic valves, more commonly in TAVR than in surgical valves [38]. Anticoagulation therapy (both NOACs and VKA), but not DAPT, was effective in preventing or treating subclinical leaflet thrombosis. Subclinical leaflet thrombosis was associated with increased rates of TIAs and strokes [37].

These collective findings indicate that there remains a great need for further clarification. Ongoing large prospective, randomized, multicenter studies such as the GALILEO Trial [39] are needed to analyze the combination of rivaroxaban and aspirin compared to aspirin and clopidogrel.

To date, few studies have specifically investigated the influence of AF on the occurrence of bleeding after TAVR. Stortecky et al. [40] demonstrated a comparable incidence of life-threatening and major bleeding among patients with AF and SR in a collective study of 389 patients, 131 of whom (33.7%) had AF. Interestingly, in this study, only 39% of AF patients received combined VKA and APT post-procedural therapy (the remainder of patients received aspirin or clopidogrel therapy). Of the patients in the present study, 67.9% of those with AF were treated with OAC plus APT for 3 months, which may explain the different occurrence rate of life-threatening bleeding. Tarantini et al. [30] similarly reported significantly more life-threatening bleeding in a group of AF patients within the first year after TAVR. Although the incidence of major bleeding was similar between the two groups in their study, minor bleeding was significantly more frequently observed among the patients with AF. Chopard et al. [32] considered life-threatening bleeding only as part of a 30-day combined safety endpoint (total mortality, stroke, major vascular complications, acute renal failure, coronary artery obstruction, and flap dysfunction requiring re-intervention) in a comparison between patients with AF or SR. However, it should be noted that the overall anticoagulant therapy regimen was not recorded in Chopard et al. [32] or Tarantini et al. [30]. Vavuranakis et al. [41] also observed no significant difference in the occurrence of major bleeding between patients with AF and SR in their small analysis of 80 patients (20 patients with AF and 20 with SR after propensity scoring). However, this result is likely due to the small number of patients. Furthermore, in contrast to the present study, Vavuranakis et al. did not analyze life-threatening or minor bleeding [41]. While anticoagulation strategies suggest a reduction in antiplatelet agents with SR [35], the optimal regime for patients with AF after TAVR remains to be addressed. Ongoing studies with apixaban (Atlantis) and edoxaban, such as the ENVISAGE-TAVI AF study, have been initiated to shed light on this gray area.

Seeger et al. evaluated the impact of AF on outcomes in TAVR and evaluated the safety and efficacy of apixaban compared with VKA in patients with AF [28]. In agreement with our results, they showed a significantly higher rate of all-cause mortality throughout the 12-month follow-up in patients suffering from AF undergoing TAVR. Moreover, the study of Seeger et al. included more patients treated with the Xa inhibitor apixaban than our study (data not shown). While Seeger et al. found more life-threatening bleeding events but no difference in major vascular complications in patients with AF, the number of major vascular bleeding events was not separately shown. Seeger et al. evaluated after 4 weeks of treatment with a combination of APT and either NOAC or VKA the single use of an anticoagulation regime without platelet inhibitors. Single or double antiplatelet regimes were prescribed according to the valve type.

For the first time, pre- and post-procedural (within 48 h after TAVR) hemoglobin levels (Hb) were compared in this study for a more precise analysis and better under-standing of the cause and extent of bleeding. A post-procedural Hb drop of $14.4 \pm 11.7\%$ was observed in the entire patient population. Interestingly, patients with SR had relatively greater post-procedural Hb level reductions than those with AF. This finding could be explained by the fact that the AF group received more RBC transfu-sions due to more life-threatening bleeding.

Cerebrovascular events

Since the first TAVR, neurological complications have been a primary concern, with particular care dedicated to prevention. Notably, in the PARTNER study, the over-all rate of neurological events after TAVR was twice that of conventional aortic valve repair [5]. Furthermore, cerebral magnetic resonance tomography revealed new, although usually asymptomatic, cerebral lesions in the majority of patients after TAVR [42, 43].

The stroke rates within 30 days and 1 year after TAVR in this study were 3.1 and 5.0%, respectively, comparable to reported rates of 1.5–4.2 and 4.1–6.9%, respectively, in previously published TAVR studies and registries [15, 19, 23–25, 44]. Furthermore, post-procedural transient ischemic attacks were observed in only 0.8% of our total patient population, consist-ent with the rates of below 1.0% reported in the lit-erature [15, 25, 40]. The strategy of Seeger et al. using an Xa inhibitor instead of VKA was related to a significantly lower rate of early safety endpoint in patients with AF compared with patients treated with a VKA (13.5% vs. 30.5%; $p < 0.01$), with a lower stroke rate (2.1% vs. 5.3%; $p = 0.17$) at the 30-day and 12-month (1.2% vs. 2.0%; $p = 0.73$) follow-ups [28].

A limitation of the international data and of the present patient cohort is that only patients with symp-tomatic neurological deficits underwent MR or CT in-vestigations. Accordingly, subclinical strokes may not have been detected.

Although AF is the most common cause of embolic stroke [16], no significant differences in the incidence of stroke were detected within 30 days or within 1 year after TAVR between the AF and SR study groups. Add-itionally, the number of patients who suffered a TIA did not differ significantly between the two groups. This re-sult may be attributable to the good post-procedural anti-coagulant therapy for patients with AF. Fortunately, no elevated rates of cerebral bleeding were observed during the observation period.

Mortality associated with TAVR

The overall 30-day and one-year mortality rates in this study were 4.7% and 21.0%, respectively, with most deaths attributable to cardiovascular events. Accordingly, the corresponding cumulative 30-day and one-year

cardiovascular mortality rates after TAVR were 3.9% and 17.4%, respectively. Considering pre-existing cardiac rhythm, patients with AF in this study experienced sig-nificantly higher cardiovascular and overall mortality than patients with SR. These findings can be explained mainly by the more frequent occurrence of severe com-plications (life-threatening bleeding, major vascular complications) among patients with AF. The results of the present study and the subgroup analyses to date underscore the need to include AF in future risk scores, particularly for TAVR, and to optimize the post-procedural management of these patients, including anticoagulant therapy as appropriate, to avoid the com-plications of TAVR.

No prospective, randomized study has been con-ducted thus far to evaluate antithrombotic therapy after TAVR among patients with AF. Until now, guidelines have been derived from retrospective stud-ies and meta-analyses [14, 18, 28, 45–47]. As a re-sult, anticoagulation regimens associated with TAVR are primarily either empirical or are administered at the discretion of the attending physician [48, 49]. The observed diversity of treatment regimens con-firms the clinical challenge of selecting post-procedural medications, even among the patients in this study. The two anticoagulation regimens for pa-tients with AF in our study included VKA plus clopi-dogrel or NOAC plus clopidogrel for 3 months. These two treatment subgroups were studied for mortality and complications after TAVR. Subgroup analyses were not conducted for other treatment reg-imens due to the small group sizes in this study. Considering the analysis of this retrospective data, the selection criteria for treatment with either VKA or a NOAC must be questioned. According to the statistical analysis of the baseline characteristics, pa-tients in the NOAC group were significantly older than patients in the VKA group. Additionally, they had a higher bleeding risk based on their HASBLED scores. This observation could reflect the fact that older patients with increased bleeding risk have com-monly been treated with an NOAC due to the diffi-cultly of regular INR monitoring necessary for therapeutic VKA anticoagulation. Regarding the com-plication and mortality rates after TAVR during the follow-up period, no significant differences between the two groups were found in this analysis. These re-sults support the future use of NOAC after TAVR. However, it is also important to note that the pa-tients in the NOAC and VKA groups underwent im-plantation during different time periods. Specifically, the earliest patients with AF (2010) were treated with VKA, whereas NOACs, although not recommended in standard guidelines, were preferred after 2014.

To recommend the findings of Seeger et al. [14] and the results from this study for patients with SR, we anticipate the results of future randomized, prospective, large studies, such as the GALILEO trial [16]. Furthermore, this topic of interest is currently being investigated in multicenter, phase IIIb, prospective, open-label, randomized trial studies (ClinicalTrials.gov Identifier: NCT02664649) using apixaban or lixiana (Edoxaban Compared to Standard Care After Heart Valve Replacement Using a Catheter in Patients With Atrial Fibrillation (ENVISAGE-TAVI AF); ClinicalTrials.gov Identifier: NCT02943785) to determine the advantages of the current standard of care for patients with AF undergoing a successful TAVR procedure.

We believe that the unidentified risk for valve thrombosis and subclinical stroke might be adequately addressed with oral anticoagulation agents. In the future, patients undergoing TAVR might benefit from post-intervention anticoagulation therapy in combination with an NOAC, and possibly at a reduced dose in patients with concomitant disease in other vascular beds according to the results of the COMPASS trial [17]. However, the optimal dose and duration of therapy still need to be clarified. Thus, it is recommended to adhere to current guidelines, with routine DAPT and recourse to OAC when specifically indicated, while tailoring therapy based on bleeding and thromboembolic risk in individual patients [50].

Conclusion

The presence of AF was associated with markedly increased risk for life-threating bleeding and major vascular complications in patients with aortic valve stenosis treated with TAVR. AF had an independent detrimental effect on one-year overall mortality after TAVR. More data are needed to define the role of AF prevention and treatment on outcomes in these patients. Additionally, optimization of the anticoagulation strategy is warranted. Finally, the implementation of more comprehensive TAVR risk scores, taking into account AF, remains a relevant clinical need. Prospective studies may further clarify this phenomenon.

Abbreviations

AF: Atrial fibrillation; APT: Anti-platelet therapy; CI: Confidence interval; DAPT: Dual anti-platelet therapy; HR: Hazard ratio; NOAF: New-onset atrial fibrillation; OAC: Oral anticoagulation; OR: Odds ratio; PAD: Peripheral arterial disease; PCI: Percutaneous coronary intervention.; RBC: Red blood cell; SR: Sinus rhythm; TAVR: Transcatheter aortic valve replacement; TIA: Transient ischemic attack; VKA: Vitamin K antagonist

Acknowledgements

F.W. Röhl Institute for Biometry and Medical Informatics, Otto-von-Guericke University of Magdeburg, Germany and Antje Weniger Controlling Otto-von-Guericke University of Magdeburg, Germany.

Funding

This research received no grants from any funding agencies in the public and commercial or not-for-profit sectors.

Authors' contributions

JH: Concept, data collection, statistics and drafting. VHV: Analysis and interpretation of data, statistics, drafted the manuscript. RBD: Analysis and interpretation of data, revising the manuscript critically and final approval. KB: Concept and drafting, revising the manuscript critically. MS: Statistics, revising the manuscript critically, concept. CB: Acquisition of data and draft the manuscript. BL: Acquisition of data and draft the manuscript. All authors read and approved the final manuscript.

Competing interests

The authors declare that they have no competing interests.

Author details

[1]Department of Internal Medicine/Cardiology and Angiology, Otto-von-Guericke University of Magdeburg, Leipziger Str. 44, 39120 Magdeburg, Germany. [2]Department of Internal Medicine/Cardiology and Angiology, University of Rostock, Ernst-Heydemann-Straße 6, 18057 Rostock, Germany. [3]Department of Internal Medicine/Cardiology and Angiology, Ernst-von-Bergmannstrost Clinic, Charlottenstraße 72, 14467 Potsdam, Germany.

References

1. Iung B, Baron G, Butchart EG, Delahaye F, Gohlke-Barwolf C, Levang OW, Tornos P, Vanoverschelde JL, Vermeer F, Boersma E, et al. A prospective survey of patients with valvular heart disease in Europe: the euro heart survey on Valvular heart disease. Eur Heart J. 2003;24(13):1231–43.
2. Thourani VH, Kodali S, Makkar RR, Herrmann HC, Williams M, Babaliaros V, Smalling R, Lim S, Malaisrie SC, Kapadia S, et al. Transcatheter aortic valve replacement versus surgical valve replacement in intermediate-risk patients: a propensity score analysis. Lancet. 2016;387(10034):2218–25.
3. Leon MB, Smith CR, Mack M, Miller DC, Moses JW, Svensson LG, Tuzcu EM, Webb JG, Fontana GP, Makkar RR, et al. Transcatheter aortic-valve implantation for aortic stenosis in patients who cannot undergo surgery. N Engl J Med. 2010;363(17):1597–607.
4. Mack MJ, Leon MB, Smith CR, Miller DC, Moses JW, Tuzcu EM, Webb JG, Douglas PS, Anderson WN, Blackstone EH, et al. 5-year outcomes of transcatheter aortic valve replacement or surgical aortic valve replacement for high surgical risk patients with aortic stenosis (PARTNER 1): a randomised controlled trial. Lancet. 2015;385(9986):2477–84.
5. Smith CR, Leon MB, Mack MJ, Miller DC, Moses JW, Svensson LG, Tuzcu EM, Webb JG, Fontana GP, Makkar RR, et al. Transcatheter versus surgical aortic-valve replacement in high-risk patients. N Engl J Med. 2011;364(23):2187–98.
6. Kapadia SR, Leon MB, Makkar RR, Tuzcu EM, Svensson LG, Kodali S, Webb JG, Mack MJ, Douglas PS, Thourani VH, et al. 5-year outcomes of transcatheter aortic valve replacement compared with standard treatment for patients with inoperable aortic stenosis (PARTNER 1): a randomised controlled trial. Lancet. 2015;385(9986):2485–91.
7. Reardon MJ, Van Mieghem NM, Popma JJ, Kleiman NS, Sondergaard L, Mumtaz M, Adams DH, Deeb GM, Maini B, Gada H, et al. Surgical or Transcatheter aortic-valve replacement in intermediate-risk patients. N Engl J Med. 2017;376(14):1321–31.
8. Steinvil A, Leshem-Rubinow E, Halkin A, Abramowitz Y, Ben-Assa E, Shacham Y, Bar-Dayan A, Keren G, Banai S, Finkelstein A. Vascular complications after transcatheter aortic valve implantation and their association with mortality reevaluated by the valve academic research consortium definitions. Am J Cardiol. 2015;115(1):100–6.
9. Herold J, Friedl A, Huth C, Braun-Dullaeus RC. Unusual aortic perforation after transcutaneous aortic valve implantation. Eur Heart J. 2013;34(14):1049.
10. Levy S, Breithardt G, Campbell RW, Camm AJ, Daubert JC, Allessie M, Aliot E, Capucci A, Cosio F, Crijns H, et al. Atrial fibrillation: current knowledge and recommendations for management. Working group on arrhythmias of the European society of cardiology. Eur Heart J. 1998;19(9):1294–320.
11. Go AS, Hylek EM, Phillips KA, Chang Y, Henault LE, Selby JV, Singer DE. Prevalence of diagnosed atrial fibrillation in adults: national implications for

rhythm management and stroke prevention: the AnTicoagulation and risk factors in Atrial fibrillation (ATRIA) study. JAMA. 2001;285(18):2370–5.

12. Kappetein AP, Head SJ, Genereux P, Piazza N, van Mieghem NM, Blackstone EH, Brott TG, Cohen DJ, Cutlip DE, van Es GA, et al. Updated standardized endpoint definitions for transcatheter aortic valve implantation: the valve academic research Consortium-2 consensus document (VARC-2). Eur J Cardiothorac Surg. 2012;42(5):S45–60.

13. Cribier A, Eltchaninoff H, Bash A, Borenstein N, Tron C, Bauer F, Derumeaux G, Anselme F, Laborde F, Leon MB. Percutaneous transcatheter implantation of an aortic valve prosthesis for calcific aortic stenosis: first human case description. Circulation. 2002;106(24):3006–8.

14. Vahanian A, Alfieri O, Andreotti F, Antunes MJ, Baron-Esquivias G, Baumgartner H, Borger MA, Carrel TP, De Bonis M, Evangelista A, et al. Guidelines on the Management of Valvular Heart Disease (version 2012): the joint task force on the management of Valvular heart disease of the European Society of Cardiology (ESC) and the European Association for Cardio-Thoracic Surgery (EACTS). Eur J Cardiothorac Surg. 2012;42(4):S1–44.

15. Leon MB, Smith CR, Mack MJ, Makkar RR, Svensson LG, Kodali SK, Thourani VH, Tuzcu EM, Miller DC, Herrmann HC, et al. Transcatheter or surgical aortic-valve replacement in intermediate-risk patients. N Engl J Med. 2016; 374(17):1609–20.

16. Camm AJ, Lip GY, De Caterina R, Savelieva I, Atar D, Hohnloser SH, Hindricks G, Kirchhof P, Guidelines ESCCfP. 2012 Focused update of the ESC guidelines for the management of atrial fibrillation: an update of the 2010 ESC guidelines for the management of atrial fibrillation. Developed with the special contribution of the European heart rhythm association. Eur Heart J. 2012;33(21):2719–47.

17. European Heart Rhythm A, European Association for Cardio-Thoracic S, Camm AJ, Kirchhof P, Lip GY, Schotten U, Savelieva I, Ernst S, Van Gelder IC, Al-Attar N, et al. Guidelines for the Management of Atrial Fibrillation: the task force for the management of Atrial fibrillation of the European Society of Cardiology (ESC). Eur Heart J. 2010;31(19):2369–429.

18. Baumgartner H, Falk V, Bax JJ, De Bonis M, Hamm C, Holm PJ, Iung B, Lancellotti P, Lansac E, Munoz DR, et al. 2017 ESC/EACTS guidelines for the management of valvular heart disease. Eur Heart J. 2017;38(36):2739–91.

19. Walther T, Hamm CW, Schuler G, Berkowitsch A, Kotting J, Mangner N, Mudra H, Beckmann A, Cremer J, Welz A, et al. Perioperative results and complications in 15,964 Transcatheter aortic valve replacements: prospective data from the GARY registry. J Am Coll Cardiol. 2015;65(20):2173–80.

20. Khatri PJ, Webb JG, Rodes-Cabau J, Fremes SE, Ruel M, Lau K, Guo H, Wijeysundera HC, Ko DT. Adverse effects associated with transcatheter aortic valve implantation: a meta-analysis of contemporary studies. Ann Intern Med. 2013;158(1):35–46.

21. Neragi-Miandoab S, Michler RE. A review of most relevant complications of transcatheter aortic valve implantation. ISRN cardiology. 2013;2013:956252.

22. Kappetein AP, Head SJ, Genereux P, Piazza N, van Mieghem NM, Blackstone EH, Brott TG, Cohen DJ, Cutlip DE, van Es GA, et al. Updated standardized endpoint definitions for transcatheter aortic valve implantation: the valve academic research Consortium-2 consensus document. Eur Heart J. 2012; 33(19):2403–18.

23. Gilard M, Eltchaninoff H, Iung B, Donzeau-Gouge P, Chevreul K, Fajadet J, Leprince P, Leguerrier A, Lievre M, Prat A, et al. Registry of transcatheter aortic-valve implantation in high-risk patients. N Engl J Med. 2012;366(18):1705–15.

24. Schymik G, Lefevre T, Bartorelli AL, Rubino P, Treede H, Walther T, Baumgartner H, Windecker S, Wendler O, Urban P, et al. European experience with the second-generation Edwards SAPIEN XT transcatheter heart valve in patients with severe aortic stenosis: 1-year outcomes from the SOURCE XT registry. JACC Cardiovasc Interv. 2015;8(5):657–69.

25. Linke A, Wenaweser P, Gerckens U, Tamburino C, Bosmans J, Bleiziffer S, Blackman D, Schafer U, Muller R, Sievert H, et al. Treatment of aortic stenosis with a self-expanding transcatheter valve: the international multi-centre ADVANCE study. Eur Heart J. 2014;35(38):2672–84.

26. Leon MB, Piazza N, Nikolsky E, Blackstone EH, Cutlip DE, Kappetein AP, Krucoff MW, Mack M, Mehran R, Miller C, et al. Standardized endpoint definitions for transcatheter aortic valve implantation clinical trials: a consensus report from the valve academic research consortium. Eur Heart J. 2011;32(2):205–17.

27. Sinning JM, Horack M, Grube E, Gerckens U, Erbel R, Eggebrecht H, Zahn R, Linke A, Sievert H, Figulla HR, et al. The impact of peripheral arterial disease on early outcome after transcatheter aortic valve implantation: results from the German Transcatheter aortic valve interventions registry. Am Heart J. 2012;164(1):102–10. e101

28. Seeger J, Gonska B, Rodewald C, Rottbauer W, Wohrle J. Apixaban in patients with Atrial fibrillation after Transfemoral aortic valve replacement. JACC Cardiovasc Interv. 2017;10(1):66–74.

29. Hengstenberg C, Chandrasekhar J, Sartori S, Lefevre T, Mikhail G, Meneveau N, Tron C, Jeger R, Kupatt C, Vogel B, et al. Impact of pre-existing or new-onset atrial fibrillation on 30-day clinical outcomes following transcatheter aortic valve replacement: results from the BRAVO 3 randomized trial. Catheter Cardiovasc Interv. 2017;90(6):1027-37. doi:10.1002/ccd.27155.

30. Tarantini G, Mojoli M, Windecker S, Wendler O, Lefevre T, Saia F, Walther T, Rubino P, Bartorelli AL, Napodano M, et al. Prevalence and impact of Atrial fibrillation in patients with severe aortic Stenosis undergoing Transcatheter aortic valve replacement: an analysis from the SOURCE XT prospective multicenter registry. JACC Cardiovasc Interv. 2016;9(9):937–46.

31. Maan A, Heist EK, Passeri J, Inglessis I, Baker J, Ptaszek L, Vlahakes G, Ruskin JN, Palacios I, Sundt T, et al. Impact of atrial fibrillation on outcomes in patients who underwent transcatheter aortic valve replacement. Am J Cardiol. 2015;115(2):220–6.

32. Chopard R, Teiger E, Meneveau N, Chocron S, Gilard M, Laskar M, Eltchaninoff H, Iung B, Leprince P, Chevreul K, et al. Baseline characteristics and prognostic implications of pre-existing and new-onset Atrial fibrillation after Transcatheter aortic valve implantation: results from the FRANCE-2 registry. JACC Cardiovasc Interv. 2015;8(10):1346–55.

33. Adams DH, Popma JJ, Reardon MJ, Yakubov SJ, Coselli JS, Deeb GM, Gleason TG, Buchbinder M, Hermiller J Jr, Kleiman NS, et al. Transcatheter aortic-valve replacement with a self-expanding prosthesis. N Engl J Med. 2014;370(19):1790–8.

34. Sorensen R, Hansen ML, Abildstrom SZ, Hvelplund A, Andersson C, Jorgensen C, Madsen JK, Hansen PR, Kober L, Torp-Pedersen C, et al. Risk of bleeding in patients with acute myocardial infarction treated with different combinations of aspirin, clopidogrel, and vitamin K antagonists in Denmark: a retrospective analysis of nationwide registry data. Lancet. 2009;374(9706):1967–74.

35. D'Ascenzo F, Benedetto U, Bianco M, Conrotto F, Moretti C, D'Onofrio A, Agrifoglio M, Colombo A, Ribichini F, Tarantini G, et al. Which is the best anti-aggregant or anti-coagulant therapy after TAVI? A propensity matched analysis from the ITER registry. The management of DAPT after TAVI. EuroIntervention. 2017;13(12):e1392-400. doi:10.4244/EIJ-D-17-00198.

36. Ichibori Y, Mizote I, Maeda K, Onishi T, Ohtani T, Yamaguchi O, Torikai K, Kuratani T, Sawa Y, Nakatani S, et al. Clinical outcomes and bioprosthetic valve function after Transcatheter aortic valve implantation under dual Antiplatelet therapy vs. aspirin alone. Circ J. 2017;81(3):397–404.

37. Chakravarty T, Sondergaard L, Friedman J, De Backer O, Berman D, Kofoed KF, Jilaihawi H, Shiota T, Abramowitz Y, Jorgensen TH, et al. Subclinical leaflet thrombosis in surgical and transcatheter bioprosthetic aortic valves: an observational study. Lancet. 2017;389(10087):2383–92.

38. Ruile P, Jander N, Blanke P, Schoechlin S, Reinohl J, Gick M, Rothe J, Langer M, Leipsic J, Buettner HJ, et al. Course of early subclinical leaflet thrombosis after transcatheter aortic valve implantation with or without oral anticoagulation. Clin Res Cardiol. 2017;106(2):85–95.

39. Windecker S, Tijssen J, Giustino G, Guimaraes AH, Mehran R, Valgimigli M, Vranckx P, Welsh RC, Baber U, van Es GA, et al. Trial design: rivaroxaban for the prevention of major cardiovascular events after Transcatheter aortic valve replacement: rationale and design of the GALILEO study. Am Heart J. 2017;184:81–7.

40. Stortecky S, Buellesfeld L, Wenaweser P, Heg D, Pilgrim T, Khattab AA, Gloekler S, Huber C, Nietlispach F, Meier B, et al. Atrial fibrillation and aortic stenosis: impact on clinical outcomes among patients undergoing transcatheter aortic valve implantation. Circ Cardiovasc Interv. 2013;6(1):77–84.

41. Vavuranakis M, Kalogeras K, Vrachatis D, Kariori M, Moldovan C, Mpei E, Lavda M, Kolokathis AM, Siasos G, Tousoulis D. Antithrombotic therapy in patients undergoing TAVI with concurrent atrial fibrillation. One center experience. J Thromb Thrombolysis. 2015;40(2):193–7.

42. Ghanem A, Muller A, Nahle CP, Kocurek J, Werner N, Hammerstingl C, Schild HH, Schwab JO, Mellert F, Fimmers R, et al. Risk and fate of cerebral embolism after transfemoral aortic valve implantation: a prospective pilot study with diffusion-weighted magnetic resonance imaging. J Am Coll Cardiol. 2010;55(14):1427–32.

43. Kahlert P, Knipp SC, Schlamann M, Thielmann M, Al-Rashid F, Weber M, Johansson U, Wendt D, Jakob HG, Forsting M, et al. Silent and apparent cerebral ischemia after percutaneous transfemoral aortic valve implantation: a diffusion-weighted magnetic resonance imaging study. Circulation. 2010; 121(7):870–8.

44. Eltchaninoff H, Prat A, Gilard M, Leguerrier A, Blanchard D, Fournial G, Iung B, Donzeau-Gouge P, Tribouilloy C, Debrux JL, et al. Transcatheter aortic valve implantation: early results of the FRANCE (FRench aortic national CoreValve and Edwards) registry. Eur Heart J. 2011;32(2):191–7.

45. Webb J, Rodes-Cabau J, Fremes S, Pibarot P, Ruel M, Ibrahim R, Welsh R, Feindel C, Lichtenstein S. Transcatheter aortic valve implantation: a Canadian cardiovascular society position statement. Can J Cardiol. 2012; 28(5):520–8.

46. Holmes DR Jr, Mack MJ, Kaul S, Agnihotri A, Alexander KP, Bailey SR, Calhoon JH, Carabello BA, Desai MY, Edwards FH, et al. 2012 ACCF/AATS/ SCAI/STS expert consensus document on transcatheter aortic valve replacement: developed in collaboration with the American Heart Association, American Society of Echocardiography, European Association for Cardio-Thoracic Surgery, Heart Failure Society of America, mended hearts, Society of Cardiovascular Anesthesiologists, Society of Cardiovascular Computed Tomography, and Society for Cardiovascular Magnetic Resonance. Catheter Cardiovasc Interv. 2012;79(7):1023–82.

47. Nishimura RA, Otto CM, Bonow RO, Carabello BA, Erwin JP 3rd, Guyton RA, O'Gara PT, Ruiz CE, Skubas NJ, Sorajja P, et al. 2014 AHA/ACC guideline for the Management of Patients with Valvular Heart Disease: a report of the American College of Cardiology/American Heart Association task force on practice guidelines. Circulation. 2014;129(23):e521–643.

48. Rodes-Cabau J, Dauerman HL, Cohen MG, Mehran R, Small EM, Smyth SS, Costa MA, Mega JL, O'Donoghue ML, Ohman EM, et al. Antithrombotic treatment in transcatheter aortic valve implantation: insights for cerebrovascular and bleeding events. J Am Coll Cardiol. 2013;62(25):2349–59.

49. Vavuranakis M, Kolokathis AM, Vrachatis DA, Kalogeras K, Magkoutis NA, Fradi S, Ghostine S, Karamanou M, Tousoulis D. Atrial fibrillation during or after TAVI: incidence, implications and Therapeutical considerations. Curr Pharm Des. 2016;22(13):1896–903.

50. Gargiulo G, Collet JP, Valgimigli M. Antithrombotic therapy in TAVI patients: changing concepts. EuroIntervention. 2015;11 Suppl W:W92–5.

20

Long-term clinical outcomes of catheter ablation in patients with atrial fibrillation predisposing to tachycardia-bradycardia syndrome: a long pause predicts implantation of a permanent pacemaker

Dong-Hyeok Kim, Jong-Il Choi[*] ⓘ, Kwang No Lee, Jinhee Ahn, Seung Young Roh, Dae In Lee, Jaemin Shim, Jin Seok Kim, Hong Euy Lim, Sang Weon Park and Young-Hoon Kim

Abstract

Background: There is a controversy as to whether catheter ablation should be the first-line therapy for tachycardia-bradycardia syndrome (TBS) in patients with atrial fibrillation (AF).

Methods: We aimed to investigate long-term clinical outcomes of catheter ablation in patients with TBS and AF. Among 145 consecutive patients who underwent catheter ablation of AF with TBS, 121 patients were studied.

Results: Among 121 patients, 11 (9.1%) received implantation of a permanent pacemaker during a mean 21 months after ablation. Length of pause on termination of AF was significantly greater in patients who received pacemaker implantation after ablation than those who underwent ablation only (7.9 ± 3.5 vs. 5.1 ± 2.1 s, $p < 0.001$). Using a multivariate model, a long pause of 6.3 s or longer after termination of AF was associated with the requirement to implant a permanent pacemaker after ablation (HR 1.332, 95% CI 1.115-1.591, $p = 0.002$).

Conclusion: This study suggests that, in patients with AF predisposing to TBS, long pause on termination of AF predicts the need to implant a permanent pacemaker after catheter ablation.

Keywords: Atrial fibrillation, Tachycardia, Bradycardia, Catheter ablation, Pacemaker

Background

Tachycardia-bradycardia syndrome (TBS) is literally a two-fold disease that is characterized by prolonged sinus pause on termination of atrial tachyarrhythmias, including atrial fibrillation (AF). Implantation of a permanent pacemaker plus antiarrhythmic drug (AAD) prescription is the mainstay therapy for patients with TBS due to sinus pause or its aggravation on AAD [1]. However, AF-related problems (e.g. AF symptoms, progression to persistent AF [2], tachycardia-mediated cardiomyopathy [3, 4], AAD use, anticoagulation) may remain even after implantation of a permanent pacemaker. Furthermore,

* Correspondence: jongilchoi@korea.ac.kr
Division of Cardiology, Department of Internal Medicine, Korea University College of Medicine and Korea University Medical Center, 73, Inchon-ro, Seongbuk-gu, Seoul 02841, Republic of Korea

device-related complications (e.g. infection, endocarditis, vascular complications, need for generator change) may also occur.

Catheter ablation has been widely performed in patients with AF, and its clinical benefits and safety in patients with AF have been well documented. Catheter ablation is also known to be curative for TBS, especially in PV-triggered AF [5], through elimination of triggers for tachycardia. Recent studies demonstrated that ablation, compared to pacemaker implantation, decreased tachycardia-related hospitalization and was effective at controlling AF and prolonged sinus pause [6]. However, long term follow-up data are needed because some populations of patients are likely to have intrinsic sinus node dysfunction (SND) even in the clinical setting of TBS, and SND can gradually progress in those patients who require a pacemaker after catheter ablation of AF [7, 8]. Thus, whether catheter ablation should be considered the first line therapy for TBS in AF remains debated. In this study, we investigated the long-term clinical outcomes of catheter ablation in patients with TBS on termination of AF. Furthermore, we determined predictors for triage of patients in whom catheter ablation is expected to be more beneficial than implantation of a permanent pacemaker.

Methods

Patient population

Figure 1 shows the study populations. Patients who visited Korea University Medical Center and underwent catheter ablation of AF or pacemaker implantation during June 2004-June 2015 were retrospectively examined. Definitions of AF type and catheter ablation of AF followed the Guidelines for the management of atrial fibrillation and the 2014 consensus documents of the American Heart Association/American College of Cardiology/Heart Rhythm Society [9, 10]. TBS was defined as in previous studies, namely a ventricular pause following termination of atrial tachyarrhythmia (e.g. AF) [11, 12]. TBS was defined when more than 3 s of sinus pause was documented on ECG immediately after termination of AF leading to related symptoms, such as dizziness and syncope. If long sinus pause more than 3 s after termination of tachyarrhythmia could not be documented, we checked Holter ECG or event ECG recorder repeatedly. Although ECG with long pause more than 3 s was documented, TBS was not diagnosed if there were no symptoms related to the ECG documentation. Catheter ablation of AF in patients with AF and TBS

was determined at the physicians' discretion based on symptoms of palpitations, dizziness, syncope, and history of stroke.

Among the 145 patients, 24 patients were excluded; 20 with a pause of less than three seconds, 3 because of no documented electrocardiography (ECG) of pause, and 1 due to follow-up loss. Finally, 121 patients with catheter ablation were studied. A permanent pacemaker was implanted in 11 patients who were highly symptomatic due to a long pause after ablation. This study was approved by the institutional review board in Korea University Medical Center.

Procedures for catheter ablation

After written informed consent was obtained, all the patients underwent electrophysiology study and catheter ablation. Prior to the procedure, all antiarrhythmic drugs were discontinued, and more than 5 half-lives were allowed to pass before the study was performed. Amiodarone was discontinued at least 1 month before the ablation procedure. All catheters were inserted via the femoral vein. A duodecapolar catheter (St. Jude Medical Inc., Lowell, MA, USA) was placed in the coronary sinus (CS) to record both the low right atrium (RA) and CS electrograms, and a decapolar catheter (Bard Electrophysiology Inc., Lowell, MA, USA) was positioned at the high RA. A quadripolar catheter was placed at either the His bundle or superior vena cava (SVC). Intracardiac electrograms were recorded using a Prucka CardioLab™ electrophysiology system (General Electric Health Care System Inc., Milwaukee, WI, USA) or EP Workmate system (EP MedSystem, Inc./St. Jude Medical Inc., St. Paul, MN, USA). After double transseptal puncture, the

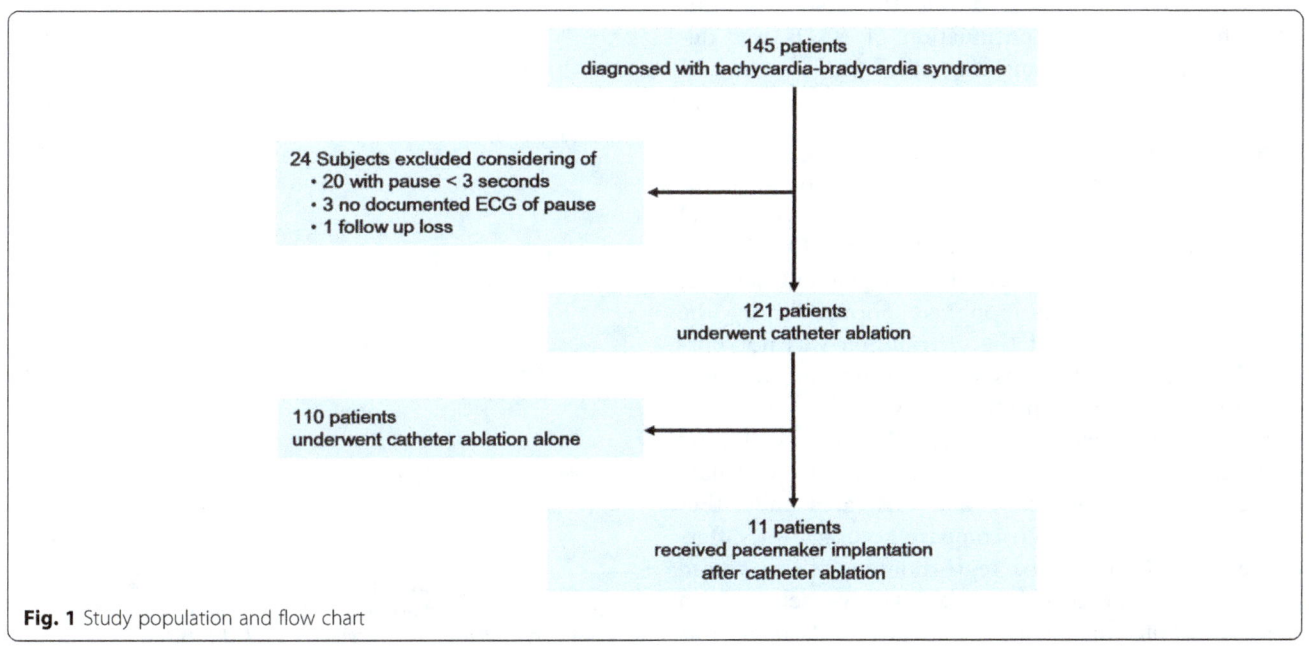

Fig. 1 Study population and flow chart

patients were administered anticoagulants such as intravenous heparin to maintain an activated clotting time of between 300 and 400 s. Three-dimensional geometries of the LA and PVs were reconstructed using Ensite-NavX mapping system (St. Jude Medical Inc., St. Paul, MN, USA). Trigger was defined as initiation of AF before PV isolation. When non-PV trigger was detected, and then was also ablated [13, 14]. Circumferential pulmonary vein isolation (CPVI) with electrical PV isolation was performed. When AF followed CPVI, either linear ablation or complex fractionated atrial electrogram-guided ablation was performed additionally. When AF converted into atrial tachycardia (AT), AT was ablated according to the mechanisms of AT. For focal AT, RF energy was delivered at the focus; for macroreentrant AT, a line of block was created at the critical isthmus. The endpoints of the ablation were AF or AT termination. Each radiofrequency energy application was performed using an open-irrigated ablation catheter with a maximum temperature of 48 °C and a power of 25-35 W.

Outcome measurements and patient follow-up

Primary outcome measurement was freedom from atrial tachyarrhythmia(s), AF or AT, after the procedures. After ablation, patients were asked to visit the outpatient clinic at 1, 3, 6, 9, and 12 months and then every 6 months thereafter or whenever they experienced tachycardia-related symptoms. ECG was performed at every visit. Holter monitor recording was performed in patients who were thought to have arrhythmia-related intermittent symptoms. Recurrence of atrial tachyarrhythmia was defined as an event lasting more than 30 s after a 3-month blanking period. Antiarrhythmic drugs (AADs) were taken during the first 3 months after the ablation. Discontinuation of AADs was determined at the physicians' discretion.

Statistical analysis

All values are expressed as means ± SD or as numbers and percentages where appropriate. Categorical data were compared by the χ^2 test. Continuous variable data were compared by independent samples t-test when the distribution was normal or by the Mann-Whitney test if it the distribution was not normal. Kaplan-Meier analysis with the log-rank test was used to determine the probability of freedom from recurrent atrial tachyarrhythmia. Receiver operating characteristic (ROC) analysis was used to calculate sensitivity and specificity, and the area-under-the-curve (AUC) was used to compare accuracy for different lengths of pause. Cox regression analysis was used for the predictor model. Variables were selected on the basis of univariate significance. $P < 0.05$ was considered statistically significant. Statistical analyses were performed using SPSS Statistics 19.0 software (SPSS Inc., Armonk, NY, USA).

Results

Clinical characteristics

Total 121 patients underwent catheter ablation and clinical characteristics at baseline are summarized in Table 1. Mean longest pause following termination of AF were 5.4 s. After ablation, anticoagulant and antiplatelet therapy was continued according to CHADS$_2$ score or CHA$_2$DS$_2$-VASc score: warfarin 37.2%, anti-platelet drug 49.6%, and NOAC 3.3% (Table 1).

Complications after ablation and clinical outcomes

After AF ablation, 9 complications were noted: cardiac tamponade ($n = 6$, 4.9%), groin hematoma ($n = 2$, 1.6%), and atrial esophageal fistula ($n = 1$, 0.8%). One patient (0.8%) died among total 121 patients. Four patients (3.3%) experienced stroke.

Table 1 Demographics and clinical characteristics of the study participants

Factors	$n = 121$
Age, years old	61.1 ± 10.4
Male, n (%)	64 (52.9)
Longest pause, seconds	5.4 ± 2.4
Time of AF symptom onset, months	36.5 ± 32.3
Type of persistent AF, n (%)	17 (14.0)
AAD before procedure, n (%)	77 (63.6)
Class I drug	66 (54.5)
Class III drug	11 (9.1)
Antithrombotic drug, n (%)	109 (90.1)
Warfarin	45 (37.2)
Anti-platelet drug	60 (49.6)
NOAC	4 (3.3)
LVEF	57.8 ± 7.9
LA size, mm	41.0 ± 5.6
E/e'	9.6 ± 5.2
Hypertension, n (%)	66 (54.5)
Diabetes mellitus, n (%)	16 (13.2)
CHAS$_2$DS$_2$-VASc score	1.9 ± 1.3
0, n (%)	15 (12.4)
1, n (%)	39 (32.2)
≥ 2, n (%)	67 (55.4)
HAS-BLED score	1.6 ± 1.1

Values are expressed as means±SDs and numbers (percentages). *AF* atrial fibrillation, *AAD* anti-arrhythmic drug, *NOAC* non-vitamin K antagonist anticoagulant, *LVEF* left ventricular ejection fraction, *LA* left atrium

Recurrence of atrial tachyarrhythmia after catheter ablation

After catheter ablation, the rate of any atrial tachyarrhythmia (AF or AT) recurrence is 19.0% (23 of 121) during mean 29.3 months of follow up. We investigate factors affecting recurrence according to age and trigger sites. Thirty-one patients (25.6%) were 70-year-old or more. Atrial tachyarrhythmia recurrence was not significantly different between patients with 70-year-old or more and those with younger than 70-year-old (18.9% vs. 19.4%, log-rank test $p = 0.732$). During the ablation procedures, triggers were identified in 73 patients (60. 3%) and no trigger was identified in 48 patients (39.7%). There was no significant difference of atrial tachyarrhythmia recurrence between patients with triggers and those with no trigger (17.8% vs. 20.8%, log-rank test $p = 0.559$, Additional file 1: Figure S1). Among total patients, sixty-three patients (52.1%) had a pulmonary vein (PV) trigger; left superior PVs, left inferior PVs, right superior PVs, right middle PV, right inferior PV, and multiple PVs accounted for 27 (22.3%), 7 (5.8%), 13 (10.7%), 1 (0.8%), 2 (1.7%), and 13 (10.7%) trigger sites, respectively. Ten patients (8.3%) had non-PV triggers; eight (6.6%) at SVC and two (1.7%) at the high RA septum. There was no significant difference of atrial tachyarrhythmia recurrence between patients with PV trigger and those with non-PV trigger (18.6% vs. 14.3%, log-rank test $p = 0.817$, Additional file 2: Figure S2).

Pacemaker implantation after catheter ablation

Following catheter ablation of AF, eleven patients (9.1%) received implantation of permanent pacemaker. Mean time interval from catheter ablation to pacemaker implantation was 21 months. The patients' characteristics are shown in Table 2. Mean longest pause on termination of AF prior to catheter ablation was significantly longer in patients who underwent pacemaker implantation after catheter ablation compared to those who underwent catheter ablation alone (7.9 ± 3.5 vs. 5.1 ± 2.1 s, $p < 0.001$) (Fig. 2). ROC curve analysis showed that the optimal cutoff point for predicting implantation of a permanent pacemaker following catheter ablation was 6.3 s (sensitivity 72.7%, specificity 79.1%, AUC = 0.75). The longest pause was associated with a need for implantation of a permanent pacemaker using both univariate analyses (HR 1.287, 95% CI 1.101-1.506, $p = 0.002$) and a multivariate model (HR 1.576, 95% CI 1.060-2.343, $p = 0.025$) adjusted by age, sex, time of AF symptom onset, HTN, DM, use of post-procedural AAD, LVEF, LA diameter, and trigger (Table 3). Antiplatelet therapy (aspirin, $n = 1$) was continued during pacemaker implantation. Anticoagulation therapy with warfarin ($n = 9$) was continued without heparin bridge during pacemaker implantation. One patient did not receive any antithrombotic therapy before the procedure. Among total 11 patients with pacemaker implantation after ablation, there was no pocket hematoma.

Discussion
Main findings

This study demonstrated that recurrence rate after catheter ablation were 19% in patients with AF predisposing to TBS during mean 29 months of follow up, 9.1% of patients were required implantation of a permanent pacemaker after catheter ablation, and they had a longer pause on termination of AF compared to those with catheter ablation alone. Multivariate analysis showed that a pause of 6.3 s or longer at baseline was associated with the need to implant a permanent pacemaker after catheter ablation.

Table 2 Patients who underwent implantation of permanent pacemaker after RFCA

No.	Age (years)	Sex	Longest pause (seconds)	LA size (mm)	CHA$_2$DS$_2$-VASc score	Trigger	AAD or NB after ablation	AF recur	Symptom after ablation	PM indication	Pause after ablation (seconds)	Time interval from RFCA to PM (days)	PM mode
1	71	M	10.1	39.5	1	None	None	recur	dizziness	SP	4.2	2422	DDD
2	60	F	5.2	49.5	1	None	None	SR	dizziness	SP	5.1	14	DDDR
3	67	M	12.8	37.8	1	LSPV	None	SR	syncope	SP	5.2	7	DDDR
4	49	F	13.6	47.9	1	SVC	None	SR	syncope	SP	8.5	70	DDDR
5	59	M	6.3	40.7	1	LSPV	None	SR	dizziness	SP	7.2	566	DDDR
6	52	F	6.9	36.0	2	SVC	None	recur	dizziness	SP	5.3	1504	DDDR
7	58	F	3.4	43.3	2	LSPV	None	SR	dizziness	SP	7.0	1269	DDDR
8	70	M	8.2	43.1	2	LSPV	None	SR	dizziness	SP	6.8	27	DDDR
9	61	F	7.2	60.8	2	None	None	SR	dizziness	SP	6.8	1126	DDDR
10	70	F	9.8	32.2	3	SVC	None	SR	dizziness	SP	5.2	51	DDDR
11	69	F	3.1	39.7	3	None	None	SR	dizziness	SP	4.7	250	DDDR

No. patients number, *M* male, *F* female, *RFCA* radiofrequency catheter ablation, *PM* pacemaker, *AAD* anti-arrhythmic drug, *NB* nodal blocker, *SR* sinus rhythm, *AF* atrial fibrillation, *SP* sinus pause

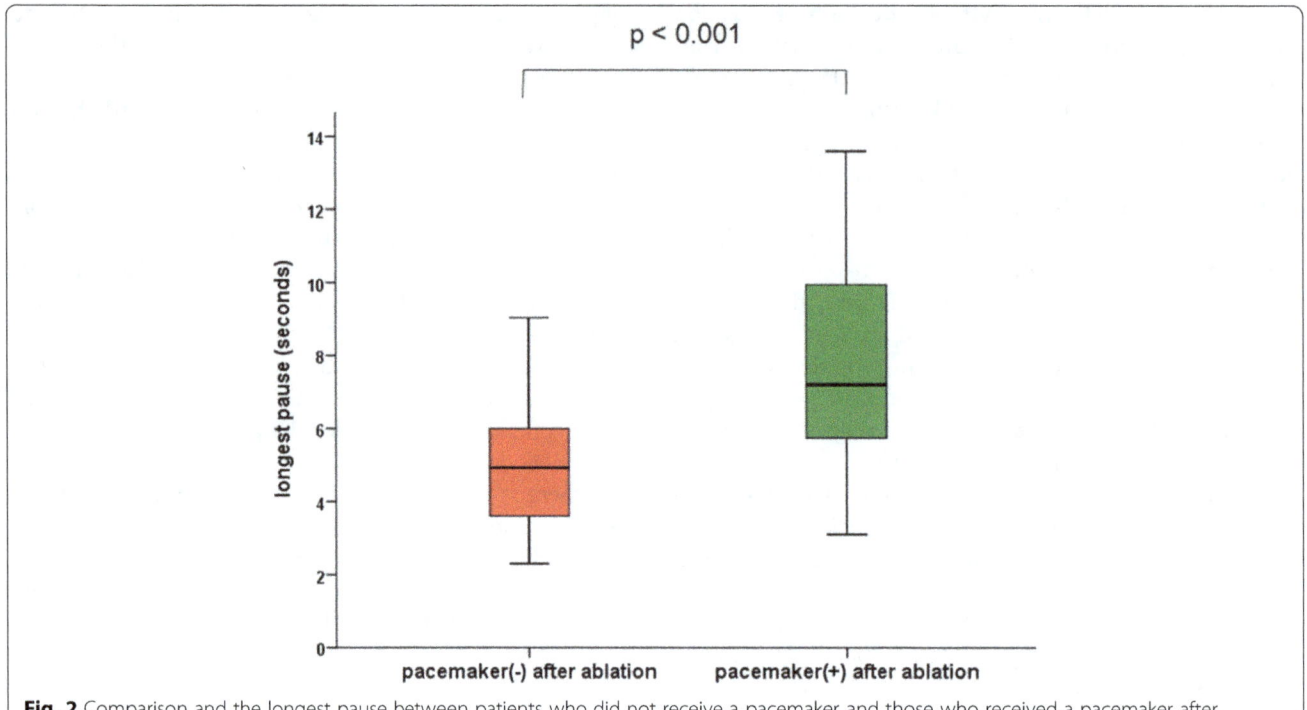

Fig. 2 Comparison and the longest pause between patients who did not receive a pacemaker and those who received a pacemaker after catheter ablation

Mechanisms of TBS with AF

SND is frequently associated with AF [11], and is caused by inhomogeneous refractoriness [15]. A study in a chronic pacing-induced AF dog model demonstrated sinus node remodeling as a result of AF that was characterized by prolongation of corrected sinus node recovery time and P-wave duration and a decrease in maximal and intrinsic heart rate [2]. Sick sinus syndrome can be regarded as an atrial disease rather than as sinus node disease per se [16–18]. The mechanism of TBS, where the pause is manifested just after AF terminates, remains to be determined. Yeh et al. suggested that funny current (I_f) down-regulation may contribute to the clinically significant association between SND and supraventricular tachyarrhythmias [19]. Recently, Duhme et al.

demonstrated that altered C-linker interaction in hyperpolarized-activated ion channel HCN4 is associated with familial TBS and AF, indicating that funny channel dysfunction contributes to the development of atrial tachyarrhythmias [20]. Ectopic activities that elicit triggers for initiation of AF may also be induced in HCN4-K530 N by the switch from enforced inhibition of gating to stimulation of gating due to binding of cAMP under adrenergic stress. Furthermore, slow heart rates may increase susceptibility to ectopic beats. Therefore, molecular and structural remodeling of the sinus node increases arrhythmogenesis, promoting the vicious cycle of "AF begets AF" [21]. Thus, early ablation for TBS likely decreases the rate of implantation of permanent pacemakers before predisposition to SND by AF burden.

Table 3 Factors associated with pacemaker implantation after ablation

Factors	HR (univariate analysis)	P value	HR (multivariate analysis)	P value
Age, years	1.014 (0.954-1.078)	0.657		
Female sex	0.488 (0.142-1.676)	0.254		
Longest pause, seconds	1.287 (1.101-1.506)	0.002	1.576 (1.060-1.343)	0.025
Time of AF symptom onset, months	0.978 (0.933-1.025)	0.357		
AAD after ablation	1.459 (0.308-6.904)	0.634		
LVEF, %	1.024 (0.952-1.102)	0.525		
LA diameter, mm	1.086 (0.990-1.191)	0.080	1.230 (0.860-1.757)	0.257
Trigger (vs. no-trigger)	0.753 (0.217-2.614)	0.655		

Values are expressed as hazard ratios (HRs) with CI 95%. *AAD* anti-arrhythmic drug, *LVEF* left ventricular ejection fraction, *LA* left atrium

Catheter ablation for TBS with AF

Catheter ablation has been used to treat patients with AF for several decades. Clinical outcome is better in paroxysmal AF than in persistent AF. The reasons for this include the lower severity of the remodeling process in paroxysmal AF than persistent AF, and the main cause of AF onset being ectopic beats that can be eliminated by catheter ablation. Catheter ablation may also improve sinus node function in patients with TBS and AF by inducing reverse remodeling. Hocini et al. demonstrated that successful ablation of AF was followed by marked recovery in sinus atrial node function when AF patients showed prolonged sinus pauses on AF termination [7]. These concepts suggest that TBS that manifests as trigger-AF may be cured by catheter ablation. Premature beat or activity originating from the PV is well-known and is the most common trigger in patients with AF [22, 23]. Miyazaki et al. demonstrated that SVC plays a role in AF not only as a trigger, but also as a perpetuator [24]. We identified triggers in 60.3% of patients. PV trigger activity was 86% and the most common non-PV trigger originated from the SVC (8 of 10). However, there was no significant difference in the rate of freedom from atrial tachyarrhythmia between PV trigger and non-PV trigger patients.

Permanent pacemaker or catheter ablation?

Whether catheter ablation or implantation of a permanent pacemaker should be the first-line treatment remains debated. Prior to the AF-ablation era, pacing was the only option for treatment of TBS because tachycardia therapy using AAD aggravated bradycardia. Patients with drug-resistant tachycardia were considered to be candidates for catheter ablation even at that time [25]. However, the treatment strategy of pacemaker plus AAD has many weaknesses, including pacemaker- and AF-related problems. In patients who receive a pacemaker, various device-related complications may occur, such as infection, endocarditis, vascular injury, lead extraction, and pocket hematoma. In our study, there was no pocket hematoma in 11 patients who underwent pacemaker implantation. Recently, Malagù M et al. demonstrated that uninterrupted antiplatelet therapy or continued anticoagulation therapy without heparin bridge based on thromboembolic risk stratification was associated with a reduced incidence of clinically significant pocket hematoma [26]. The incidence of pocket hematoma was 1.6% in no-bridge protocol group and 6.5% in conventional management group. Pacing-induced heart failure may be a potential comorbidity. Need for generator change will increase as average life expectancy increases compared to device longevity. Because the risk of stroke increases in elderly patients with AF, use of certain diagnostic tools, such as magnetic resonance imaging, becomes problematic. Furthermore, AF still remains as a comorbidity in patients who undergo implantation of pacemaker. Moreover, AF itself may lead to medical problems (e.g. progression to persistent AF, tachycardia-mediated cardiomyopathy, proarrhythmic events due to uses of AAD, bleeding due to maintenance of antithrombotic therapy), and the management for AF is also needed indefinitely. In contrast to pacemaker implantation, catheter ablation of AF has several strengths in patients with TBS including eradication of AF and no need for a device. However, it was not clear whether catheter ablation or pacemaker implantation was better for treating paroxysmal AF-related TBS. Furthermore, recent studies demonstrated that maintenance of sinus rhythm following catheter ablation might reduce the risk of stroke compared with AAD therapy alone [27–29]. In our study, two patients were hospitalized due to stroke after catheter ablation. Further study is required to address whether ablation is more beneficial than implantation of permanent pacemaker for preventing stroke.

Prediction for implantation of a pacemaker in TBS: TBS or intrinsic SND?

Miyanaga et al. reported that mean heart rate did not increase in TBS patients, probably due to pre-existing SND, although parasympathetic modulation was significantly attenuated after CPVI [30]. Inada et al. reported that a pacemaker was required in 8% of patients with paroxysmal AF and prolonged sinus pauses following catheter ablation, but gradual progression of SND occurred after long-term follow-up of over 3 years [8]. In our study, a pacemaker had to be implanted in 9.1% of patients who underwent catheter ablation due to bradycardia-related symptoms, such as syncope. Mean time interval from catheter ablation to implantation of a permanent pacemaker was 21 months, which suggests that intrinsic SND was progressive. Nevertheless, it is difficult to differentiate between patients who have AF with TBS or intrinsic SND because the characteristics of intrinsic SND are similar to those of TBS. We found that implantation of a permanent pacemaker after catheter ablation was required in patients with a long pause (≥ 6.3 s). This finding suggests that a pacemaker should primarily be considered in patients with a long pause on AF termination. Of course, SND might be caused or accelerated by the ageing process [31, 32]. However, this still remains unclear [33]. The ages of patients who received pacemaker implantation and those who did not after catheter ablation were similar. In addition, the rates of freedom from atrial tachyarrhythmia following catheter ablation were similar between patients who were 70 years or older versus those younger than 70 years. Recently, Nademanee et al. demonstrated that elderly patients with AF benefited from AF ablation, which was safe and effective at maintaining sinus rhythm and was associated with lower mortality and stroke risk [34]. Thus, the ageing process may not be the sole mechanism affecting the pathophysiology of TBS and AF.

Study limitations

This was not a randomized trial that was designed to determine whether ablation was superior to pacemaker implantation. In this retrospective study, the decision of whether to perform catheter ablation or to implant a permanent pacemaker as the first-line treatment was at the physicians' discretion based on clinical manifestations. Rates of recurrence of atrial tachyarrhythmias might also have been underestimated because we did not use a continuous rhythm monitoring device, such as an implantable loop recorder, for detection of AF [35].

Conclusions

This long-term follow-up study of patients with TBS and AF showed that implantation of a permanent pacemaker after catheter ablation of AF may be required in patients who have a long pause on AF termination. Individualized treatment considering the length of pause when AF terminates is recommended in patients with TBS due to AF.

Abbreviations

AAD: Antiarrhythmic drug; AF: Atrial fibrillation; AT: Atrial tachycardia; AUC: Area-under-the-curve; CI: Confidential interval; CPVI: Circumferential pulmonary vein isolation; CS: Coronary sinus; ECG: Electrocardiography; LA: Left atrium; LVEF: Left ventricular ejection fraction; NOAC: Non-vitamin K antagonist anticoagulant; RA: Right atrium; ROC: Receiver operating characteristic; SND: Sinus node dysfunction; SVC: Superior vena cava; TBS: Tachycardia-bradycardia syndrome

Acknowledgements

We are grateful to the entire staff of the electrophysiology laboratory of the Korea University Medical Center for their technical assistance.

Funding

This work was supported by a Korea University Grant (J-IC) and in part by a grant from Basic Science Research Program through the National Research Foundation of Korea funded by the Ministry of Education (NRF-2015R1D1A1A02061859 to J-IC) and the Ministry of Science, ICT & Future Planning (NRF-2012R1A1A1013260 to J-IC).

Authors' contributions

DHK and JIC contribute concept, design, data collection, analysis, interpretation, drafting manuscript, and critical review of the manuscript. YHK contribute concept, data collection, interpretation, and critical review of the manuscript. KNL, JHA, SYR, DIL, JMS, JSK, HEL, and SWP contribute data collection, analysis, and interpretation. All authors read and approved the final manuscript.

Competing interests

The authors declare that they have no competing interests.

References

1. Epstein AE, DiMarco JP, Ellenbogen KA, Estes NA 3rd, Freedman RA, Gettes LS, Gillinov AM, Gregoratos G, Hammill SC, Hayes DL, et al. 2012 ACCF/AHA/HRS focused update incorporated into the ACCF/AHA/HRS 2008 guidelines for device-based therapy of cardiac rhythm abnormalities: a report of the American College of Cardiology Foundation/American Heart Association task force on practice guidelines and the Heart Rhythm Society. J Am Coll Cardiol. 2013;61(3):e6–75.
2. Elvan A, Wylie K, Zipes DP. Pacing-induced chronic atrial fibrillation impairs sinus node function in dogs. Electrophysiological remodeling. Circulation. 1996;94(11):2953–60.
3. Sanders P, Morton JB, Kistler PM, Vohra JK, Kalman JM, Sparks PB. Reversal of atrial mechanical dysfunction after cardioversion of atrial fibrillation: implications for the mechanisms of tachycardia-mediated atrial cardiomyopathy. Circulation. 2003;108(16):1976–84.
4. Shinbane JS, Wood MA, Jensen DN, Ellenbogen KA, Fitzpatrick AP, Scheinman MM. Tachycardia-induced cardiomyopathy: a review of animal models and clinical studies. J Am Coll Cardiol. 1997;29(4):709–15.
5. Haissaguerre M, Jais P, Shah DC, Takahashi A, Hocini M, Quiniou G, Garrigue S, Le Mouroux A, Le Metayer P, Clementy J. Spontaneous initiation of atrial fibrillation by ectopic beats originating in the pulmonary veins. N Engl J Med. 1998;339(10):659–66.
6. Chen YW, Bai R, Lin T, Salim M, Sang CH, Long DY, Yu RH, Tang RB, Guo XY, Yan XL, et al. Pacing or ablation: which is better for paroxysmal atrial fibrillation-related tachycardia-bradycardia syndrome? Pacing and clinical electrophysiology: PACE. 2014;37(4):403–11.
7. Hocini M, Sanders P, Deisenhofer I, Jais P, Hsu LF, Scavee C, Weerasooriya R, Raybaud F, Macle L, Shah DC, et al. Reverse remodeling of sinus node function after catheter ablation of atrial fibrillation in patients with prolonged sinus pauses. Circulation. 2003;108(10):1172–5.
8. Inada K, Yamane T, Tokutake K, Yokoyama K, Mishima T, Hioki M, Narui R, Ito K, Tanigawa S, Yamashita S, et al. The role of successful catheter ablation in patients with paroxysmal atrial fibrillation and prolonged sinus pauses: outcome during a 5-year follow-up. Europace: European pacing, arrhythmias, and cardiac electrophysiology: journal of the working groups on cardiac pacing, arrhythmias, and cardiac cellular electrophysiology of the European Society of Cardiology. 2014;16(2):208–13.
9. Camm AJ, Kirchhof P, Lip GY, Schotten U, Savelieva I, Ernst S, Van Gelder IC, Al-Attar N, Hindricks G, Prendergast B, et al. Guidelines for the management of atrial fibrillation: the task force for the management of atrial fibrillation of the European Society of Cardiology (ESC). Eur Heart J. 2010;31(19):2369–429.
10. January CT, Wann LS, Alpert JS, Calkins H, Cigarroa JE, Cleveland JC Jr, Conti JB, Ellinor PT, Ezekowitz MD, Field ME, et al. 2014 AHA/ACC/HRS guideline for the management of patients with atrial fibrillation: a report of the American College of Cardiology/American Heart Association task force on practice guidelines and the Heart Rhythm Society. J Am Coll Cardiol. 2014; 64(21):e1–76.
11. Ferrer MI. The sick sinus syndrome in atrial disease. JAMA. 1968;206(3):645–6.
12. Kaplan BM. The tachycardia-bradycardia syndrome. The Medical clinics of North America. 1976;60(1):81–99.
13. Markowitz SM. Ablation of atrial fibrillation: patient selection, technique, and outcome. Current cardiology reports. 2008;10(5):360–6.
14. Calkins H, Hindricks G, Cappato R, Kim YH, Saad EB, Aguinaga L, Akar JG, Badhwar V, Brugada J, Camm J, et al. 2017 HRS/EHRA/ECAS/APHRS/SOLAECE expert consensus statement on catheter and surgical ablation of atrial fibrillation. Heart rhythm: the official journal of the Heart Rhythm Society. 2017;14(10):e275–444.
15. Luck JC, Engel TR. Dispersion of atrial refractoriness in patients with sinus node dysfunction. Circulation. 1979;60(2):404–12.
16. Kaplan BM, Langendorf R, Lev M, Pick A. Tachycardia-bradycardia syndrome (so-called "sick sinus syndrome"). Pathology, mechanisms and treatment. Am J Cardiol. 1973;31(4):497–508.
17. Evans R, Shaw DB. Pathological studies in sinoatrial disorder (sick sinus syndrome). Br Heart J. 1977;39(7):778–86.
18. Dobrzynski H, Boyett MR, Anderson RH. New insights into pacemaker activity: promoting understanding of sick sinus syndrome. Circulation. 2007;115(14): 1921–32.
19. Yeh YH, Burstein B, Qi XY, Sakabe M, Chartier D, Comtois P, Wang Z, Kuo CT, Nattel S. Funny current downregulation and sinus node dysfunction associated with atrial tachyarrhythmia: a molecular basis for tachycardia-bradycardia syndrome. Circulation. 2009;119(12):1576–85.

Long-term clinical outcomes of catheter ablation in patients with atrial fibrillation predisposing...

173

20. Duhme N, Schweizer PA, Thomas D, Becker R, Schroter J, Barends TR, Schlichting I, Draguhn A, Bruehl C, Katus HA, et al. Altered HCN4 channel C-linker interaction is associated with familial tachycardia-bradycardia syndrome and atrial fibrillation. Eur Heart J. 2013;34(35):2768–75.

21. Wijffels MC, Kirchhof CJ, Dorland R, Allessie MA. Atrial fibrillation begets atrial fibrillation. A study in awake chronically instrumented goats. Circulation. 1995;92(7):1954–68.

22. Haissaguerre M, Jais P, Shah DC, Arentz T, Kalusche D, Takahashi A, Garrigue S, Hocini M, Peng JT, Clementy J. Catheter ablation of chronic atrial fibrillation targeting the reinitiating triggers. J Cardiovasc Electrophysiol. 2000;11(1):2–10.

23. Pappone C, Oreto G, Rosanio S, Vicedomini G, Tocchi M, Gugliotta F, Salvati A, Dicandia C, Calabro MP, Mazzone P, et al. Atrial electroanatomic remodeling after circumferential radiofrequency pulmonary vein ablation: efficacy of an anatomic approach in a large cohort of patients with atrial fibrillation. Circulation. 2001;104(21):2539–44.

24. Miyazaki S, Takigawa M, Kusa S, Kuwahara T, Taniguchi H, Okubo K, Nakamura H, Hachiya H, Hirao K, Takahashi A, et al. Role of arrhythmogenic superior vena cava on atrial fibrillation. J Cardiovasc Electrophysiol. 2014;25(4):380–6.

25. Yadav A, Scheinman M. Current management of the tachybrady syndrome. ACC Curr J Rev. 2002;11(1):68–72.

26. Malagu M, Trevisan F, Scalone A, Marcantoni L, Sammarco G, Bertini M. Frequency of "pocket" hematoma in patients receiving vitamin K antagonist and antiplatelet therapy at the time of pacemaker or cardioverter defibrillator implantation (from the POCKET study). Am J Cardiol. 2017; 119(7):1036–40.

27. Friberg L, Tabrizi F, Englund A. Catheter ablation for atrial fibrillation is associated with lower incidence of stroke and death: data from Swedish health registries. Eur Heart J. 2016;37(31):2478–87.

28. Kochhauser S, Alipour P, Haig-Carter T, Trought K, Hache P, Khaykin Y, Wulffhart Z, Pantano A, Tsang B, Birnie D, et al. Risk of stroke and recurrence after AF ablation in patients with an initial event-free period of 12 months. J Cardiovasc Electrophysiol. 2017;28(3):273–9.

29. Saliba W, Schliamser JE, Lavi I, Barnett-Griness O, Gronich N, Rennert G. Catheter ablation of atrial fibrillation is associated with reduced risk of stroke and mortality: a propensity score-matched analysis. Heart rhythm: the official journal of the Heart Rhythm Society. 2017;14(5):635–42.

30. Miyanaga S, Yamane T, Date T, Tokuda M, Aramaki Y, Inada K, Shibayama K, Matsuo S, Miyazaki H, Abe K, et al. Impact of pulmonary vein isolation on the autonomic modulation in patients with paroxysmal atrial fibrillation and prolonged sinus pauses. Europace: European pacing, arrhythmias, and cardiac electrophysiology: journal of the working groups on cardiac pacing, arrhythmias, and cardiac cellular electrophysiology of the European Society of Cardiology. 2009;11(5):576–81.

31. Alings AM, Bouman LN. Electrophysiology of the ageing rabbit and cat sinoatrial node–a comparative study. Eur Heart J. 1993;14(9):1278–88.

32. Haqqani HM, Kalman JM. Aging and sinoatrial node dysfunction: musings on the not-so-funny side. Circulation. 2007;115(10):1178–9.

33. Monfredi O, Boyett MR. Sick sinus syndrome and atrial fibrillation in older persons - a view from the sinoatrial nodal myocyte. J Mol Cell Cardiol. 2015;83:88–100.

34. Nademanee K, Amnueypol M, Lee F, Drew CM, Suwannasri W, Schwab MC, Veerakul G. Benefits and risks of catheter ablation in elderly patients with atrial fibrillation. Heart rhythm: the official journal of the Heart Rhythm Society. 2015;12(1):44–51.

35. Verma A, Champagne J, Sapp J, Essebag V, Novak P, Skanes A, Morillo CA, Khaykin Y, Birnie D. Discerning the incidence of symptomatic and asymptomatic episodes of atrial fibrillation before and after catheter ablation (DISCERN AF): a prospective, multicenter study. JAMA Intern Med. 2013;173(2):149–56.

Evaluating the effect of magnesium supplementation and cardiac arrhythmias after acute coronary syndrome

Shirvan Salaminia[1], Fatemeh Sayehmiri[2], Parvin Angha[3], Koroush Sayehmiri[4] and Morteza Motedayen[5]* (iD)

Abstract

Background: Atrial and ventricular cardiac arrhythmias are one of the most common early complications after cardiac surgery and these serve as a major cause of mortality and morbidity after cardiac revascularization. We want to evaluate the effect of magnesium sulfate administration on the incidence of cardiac arrhythmias after cardiac revascularization by doing this systematic review and meta-analysis.

Methods: The search performed in several databases (SID, Magiran, IranDoc, IranMedex, MedLib, PubMed, EmBase, Web of Science, Scopus, the Cochrane Library and Google Scholar) for published Randomized controlled trials before December 2017 that have reported the association between Magnesium consumption and the incidence of cardiac arrhythmias. This relationship measured using odds ratios (ORs) with a confidence interval of 95% (CIs). Funnel plots and Egger test used to examine publication bias. STATA (version 11.1) used for all analyses.

Results: Twenty-two studies selected as eligible for this research and included in the final analysis. The total rate of ventricular arrhythmia was lower in the group receiving magnesium sulfate than placebo (11.88% versus 24.24%). The same trend obtained for the total incidence of supraventricular arrhythmia (10.36% in the magnesium versus 23.91% in the placebo group). In general the present meta-analysis showed that magnesium could decrease ventricular and supraventricular arrhythmias compared with placebo (OR = 0.32, 95% CI 0.16–0.49; $p < 0.001$ and OR = 0.42, 95% CI 0.22–0.65; $p < 0.001$, respectively). Subgroup analysis showed that the effect of magnesium on the incidence of cardiac arrhythmias was not affected by clinical settings and dosage of magnesium. Meta-regression analysis also showed that there was no significant association between the reduction of ventricular arrhythmias and sample size.

Conclusion: The results of this meta-analysis study suggest that magnesium sulfate can be used safely and effectively and is a cost-effective way in the prevention of many of ventricular and supraventricular arrhythmias.

Keywords: Serum magnesium level, Arrhythmias, Atrial, Ventricular, Meta-analysis

* Correspondence: mor.mot2@gmail.com
[5]Department of Cardiology, Faculty of Medicine, Zanjan University of Medical Sciences, Zanjan, Iran
Full list of author information is available at the end of the article

Background

Coronary artery disease is one of the major causes of death in most industrialized and also other countries. Despite newer medical treatments as well as interventional and surgical techniques, mortality is still significant. In addition to medical treatments for this disease, many patients with the coronary artery disease need surgical treatment. Coronary artery bypass graft is an effective procedure to reduce or eliminate symptoms of angina. However, despite being effective, it also has special complications during and following surgery. One of the most common early complications after open heart surgery is atrial and ventricular arrhythmias, which leads to increased mortality and morbidity in the postoperative period. This complication by increasing hospital stay, it also raises the involved economic costs [1]. The use of cardiopulmonary bypass, as one of the essentials for coronary bypass graft, results in decreased serum magnesium level. Hypomagnesemia is a relatively common electrolyte disorder in hospitalized patients[2] with associated arrhythmias. The arrhythmias which caused by magnesium deficiency are resistant to both antiarrhythmic drugs and cardioversion[3]. As a result, the addition of magnesium sulfate to compensate for Hypomagnesemia could be a method for preventing arrhythmias. During cardiopulmonary bypass, total Magnesium concentration reduces due to the ultrafiltration and also hydration with Albumin and other blood products. However, increasing renal excretion of magnesium does not occur during bypass[4].

Magnesium deficiency presents among about 71% of patients who underwent Cardiopulmonary bypass (CPB) [5]. In many studies intraoperative addition of the magnesium sulfate was beneficial. These benefits were decreasing postoperative arrhythmia rate; lowering the rate of postoperative hypertension and reducing postoperative electrocardiographic changes [6]; increasing coronary blood flow and increased cardiac indexes [7], reduced inflammatory response [8], decreased platelet function [9], and reduced mortality [10].

There is evidence to suggest that low magnesium level could relate to the incidence of ventricular arrhythmias after cardiac surgery and may reduce postoperative ventricular arrhythmia. However, there are different opinions about the relationship between magnesium level and the Arrhythmia in patients with acute coronary syndromes [11]. Many studies performed in this regard and some of them showed relation.

In this systematic review and meta-analysis study, it has been tried to integrate the results of studies that investigate the effect of magnesium sulfate on cardiac arrhythmias. The fundamental aim is to provide a safe and effective way for prevention of cardiac arrhythmias and its complications.

Methods

Data sources and search strategy

The present study is a meta-analysis of all data resources about the effect of magnesium sulfate on cardiovascular events after coronary revascularization. The study conducted by the review and meta-analysis of existing electronic sources between 1986 and 2017, including SID, Magiran, IranDoc, IranMedex, MedLib, PubMed, ISI, Web of Science, Scopus, and Google Scholar. The selected studies must evaluate the effect of magnesium sulfate on cardiac arrhythmias and mortality after cardiac revascularization and in both Farsi and English languages. Our keywords were magnesium sulfate, bypass, coronary artery, arrhythmia, atrial, ventricular and their Persian equivalents and with all their possible combinations. Also, all titles and references of the selected articles used as additional search tools for relevant studies.

Study selection) inclusion and exclusion criteria)

This review considered all randomized controlled trials which evaluated the relationship between magnesium sulfate with cardiac arrhythmias. Inclusion criteria were as follow: any study carried out in the patients with acute coronary syndromes (all patients undergoing CABG or PCI and also medically treated subjects); evaluated the correlation of the arrhythmias and serum magnesium sulfate; compared the administration of magnesium to a placebo group, and reported clinical events such as incidence and type of arrhythmias (supraventricular arrhythmias / ventricular arrhythmias) and or mortality. Any study excluded if was in conjunction with another heart disease; not reported the incidence of arrhythmias, were case studies, and those not compared magnesium with placebo. Also, studies excluded if published in languages other than English or Persian, those that were meta-analyses or systematic reviews, and those that presented insufficient data or were duplicate publications.

Data extraction

Data extracted after study appraisal. Quality assessment was assayed by NOS scale (New Ottawa Scale). For this purpose, a form designed with multiple pieces of information and the fundamental data needed for analysis (participants, interventions, outcomes, and study quality). The following information extracted and recorded: the first author, the year of publication, study location, number of patients in the treatment and control groups, average group age, group gender, the systemic magnesium dose, mortality, the incidence and types of arrhythmias (supraventricular and ventricular arrhythmias) and mortality. Two authors evaluated independently all included trials and extracted data on the basis of a standard protocol extraction. In cases which needed more information, the articles' writers contacted for supplementary data or further elucidation.

Disagreements about study eligibility resolved by group discussion. The data entered into Microsoft Excel.

Statistical analysis

One of the main objectives of this study was to evaluate the incidence of arrhythmia; therefore, the binomial distribution used to calculate the variance in each study and Weighted Average used to combine arrhythmia rate in different studies. Each study weight was proportional to its inverse of the variance. The odds ratio (OR) with a confidence interval of 95% computed as the effect measure for both individual trials and pooled estimates. For dichotomous data (adverse effects), the Peto odds ratio (to account for the potential of 0 counts in the cells for low-frequency outcomes) and 95% CI reported.

Statistical heterogeneity evaluated in studies using Q and I^2 Cochran statistics. When the results of studies were heterogeneous, the analysis performed using a random-effects model. Also, wherever there was no heterogeneity for the outcome, the fix effects model used to pool analysis and verses. Thus, in this meta-analysis, two main approaches used: the fix effects model and the random-effects model.

Subgroup analyses carried out to investigate the dosage effect of magnesium used (< 10 g, > 10 g) and clinical settings (surgery and not surgery) on the evaluated outcomes. We conducted a meta-regression analysis with sample size, mean age and magnesium dose as independent variables and log OR as the dependent variable to assess sources of heterogeneity. Integrated estimations and the related confidence interval of 95% evaluated using forest plots as visuals. Funnel plots and Egger test used to examine publication bias. Values of $p < 0/05$ considered as valid for heterogeneity tests. The analysis conducted with software R (version 3.2.1) and STATA (version 11.1). All statistical tests were two-sided.

Results

Selected articles

In this meta-analysis, we first identified 253 clinical trials. By manual search of the bibliographies and reference lists of these articles, we identified another 61 additional articles. Altogether, 314 articles identified through the literature search and 43 of them eliminated because of being repetitive. Article selection completed considering three steps: title, abstract and the full text. After the initial screening of clinical trials, 31 papers excluded with unrelated titles. In a secondary screening of the abstracts, 190 papers excluded with unrelated abstracts. In the next step and after a full-text review, another 28 article excluded; finally, twenty-two published articles from 1986 to 2017 [12–33] selected to be appropriate for the final analysis (Fig. 1). Collected number of participants were 6061 individuals, which contained 2987 in Magnesium and 3074 in the placebo group respectively. Table 1 summarizes the characteristics of the eligible studies.

Ventricular arrhythmias (ventricular tachycardia or ventricular fibrillation)

Table 2 represents the total rate of arrhythmias after meta-analysis of the extracted data. As seen in this table, thirteen studies [12–14, 16–20, 23, 27, 29, 31, 32] included for evaluating the prevalence of the ventricular arrhythmia. The prevalence of ventricular tachycardia in the group receiving magnesium sulfate and placebo was 5.67% (95% CI, 1.38–11.97) and 15.04% (95% CI, 6.47–26.06) respectively.

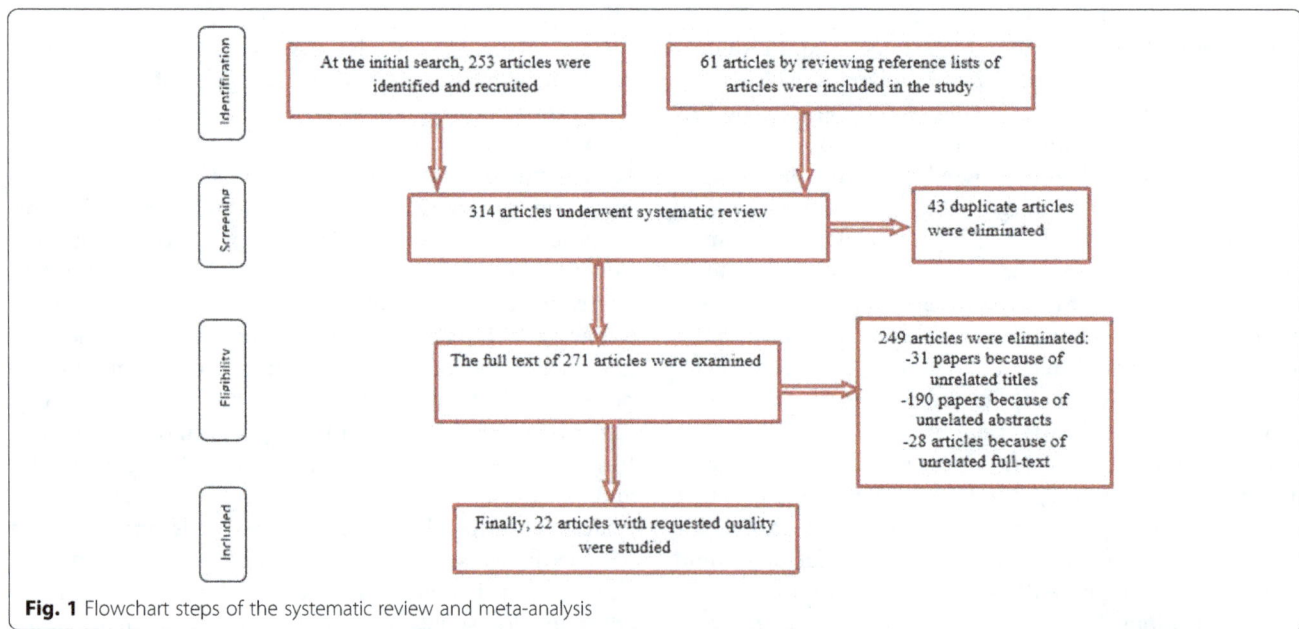

Fig. 1 Flowchart steps of the systematic review and meta-analysis

Table 1 General characters of studies entered meta-analysis

Authors	Year of Publication	Country	Clinical settings	number		Mean Age		Treatment
				Mg	P	Mg	p	
L.F. Smith[12]	1986	U.K.	Not surgery	92	93	59.7 ± 0.9	58.4 ± 1.1	65 mmol MgSO4 over 24 h
Rasmussen HS[13]	1987	Denmark	Not surgery	55	75	64.6	67.6	12 mmol MgSO4 over 24 h
Shechter.M[14]	1990	Israel	Not surgery	50	53	64 ± 10	63 ± 11	22 g MgSO4 over 24 h
M.Thiigersen.A[15]	1993	Sweden	Not surgery	54	55	67 ± 10	67 ± 11	50 mmol MgSO4 over 20 h
Roffe.C[16]	1994	U.K.	Not surgery	22	26	65.7 ± 12.7	60.2 ± 9.7	73 mmol MgSO4 over 24 h
Bhargava.B[17]	1995	India	Not surgery	40	38	58 ± 10	56 ± 8	65 mmol MgSO4 over 24 h
Karmy-Jones.R[18]	1995	Canada	CABG	46	54	64.5 ± 7.9	60.2 ± 11.9	2.4 g MgSO4 over 24 h
Shakerinia.T[19]	1996	Iran	CABG	25	25	67.2 ± 8.3	64.9 ± 6.7	15 mmol/L MgSO4 over 24 h
Raghu.C[20]	1999	India	Not surgery	169	181	52.9 ± 11	53.1 ± 10.8	18 g MgSO4 over 24 h
Parikka.H[21]	1999	Finland	Not surgery	31	26	60 ± 6	59 ± 6	70 mmol MgSO4 over 24 h
Treggiari-Venzi MM[22]	2000	Switzerland	CABG	47	51	65	65	4 g MgSO4 over 24 h
M. Santoro.G[23]	2000	Italy	Angioplasty	75	75	60 ± 11	60 ± 12	7 g MgSO4 over 5 h
Toraman F[24]	2001	Turkey	CABG	100	100	62 ± 6.7	61.4 ± 8.7	0.8 g MgSO4 over 24 h
Nakashima H[25]	2004	Japan	Angioplasty	89	91	67 ± 11	69 ± 11	20 g MgSO4 over 24 h
Ebadi.A[26]	2008	Iran	CABG	81	81	61.6 ± 5.5	61.7 ± 8.5	2 g MgSO4 over 24 h
Tiryakioglu.O[27]	2009	Turkey	CABG	64	64	58 ± 8	57.6 ± 8.8	3 g MgSO4 over 24 h
Cook RC[28]	2009	Canada	CABG	462	465	–	–	5 g MgSO4 over 24 h
MoeenVaziri MT[29]	2009	Iran	CABG	25	26	60.1 ± 8.9	60.8 ± 10.5	30 mg/kg MgSO4 in 5 min
Tabari.M[30]	2009	Iran	CABG	60	60	61.3 ± 0.6	58.4 ± 10.3	4.5 g MgSO4 over 24 h
Mhaskar DM[31]	2013	India	Not surgery	50	50	59.1 ± 13.4	59.5 ± 15.03	20 g MgSO4 over 24 h
Abbas SH[32]	2015	Pakistan	CABG	130	130	51.7 ± 10.2	51.7 ± 10.2	1 g MgSO4 over 24 h
Mohammadzadeh A[33]	2017	Iran	CABG	125	125	60.8 ± 7.6	61.3 ± 6.6	30 mg/kg MgSO4 in 5 min

Notes: Mg, magnesium; P, placebo; CABG, coronary artery bypass grafting

Moreover, the prevalence of ventricular fibrillation in the magnesium sulfate group was 2.13% (95% CI, 0.00–6.59) compared to 4.43% (95% CI, 0.31–11.69) in the placebo group. The total rate of ventricular arrhythmia was 11.88% (95% CI, 6.71–11.17) and 24.24% (95% CI, 14.52–35.43) within the magnesium and placebo groups respectively.

We also compared patients with and without arrhythmia in magnesium and placebo groups to determine the association between magnesium and the incidence of ventricular arrhythmias (Table 3).

The present meta-analysis with a fixed-effect model showed no difference in ventricular fibrillation within the magnesium group compared with placebo (OR = 0.69, 95%CI, 0.47–1.01; $I^2 = 48.9\%$, $p = 0.098$); however a significant decrease observed in ventricular tachycardia between magnesium and placebo groups (OR = 0.65, 95% CI, 0.50–0.85; $I^2 = 55.6\%$, $p = 0.035$). By using random effects model this meta-analysis showed that magnesium could decrease ventricular arrhythmias compared with placebo (OR = 0.32, 95% CI 0.16–0.49; $p < 0.001$, Fig. 2). There was heterogeneity among trials ($I^2 = 69.7\%$; $p = 0.000$).

Supraventricular arrhythmias (atrial fibrillation or supraventricular tachycardia)

As shown in Table 2, fourteen studies [13, 15–19, 22, 24, 26–28, 30–32] reported the prevalence of supraventricular arrhythmia. The incidence of arrhythmias was as follows: atrial fibrillation was 9.72% (95% CI, 3.31–18.63) within the magnesium sulfate group and 22.37% (95% CI, 15.86–29.59) within the placebo group. Supraventricular tachycardia was 4.90% in the magnesium group (95% CI, 0.84–11.28) and 14.62% in the placebo group(95% CI, 7.26–23.82). The total rate of supraventricular arrhythmia was 10.36% (95% CI, 5.55–16.32) and 23.91% (95% CI, 18.82–29.38) within the magnesium and placebo groups respectively.

Random effects analysis showed a significant decrease in atrial fibrillation comparing magnesium with placebo (OR = 0.46, 95%CI, 0.28–0.76; $I^2 = 76.9\%$, $p = 0.000$); also a reduction in supraventricular tachycardia observed via fixed-effect model (OR = 0.65, 95% CI, 0.50–0.85; $I^2 = 48.5\%$; $p = 0.035$). Overall, meta-analysis with random effects model showed that magnesium could decrease supraventricular arrhythmia compared with placebo (OR = 0.42, 95% CI

Table 2. Arrhythmias prevalence using Random Effect Meta-Analysis

Type of arrhythmia	Treatment	Number of studies	Prevalence%	Confidence interval 95% (CI%95)	Heterogeneity index I^2 (%)	P value
Ventricular tachycardia	Magnesium	7	5.67	1.38–11.97	71.81	0.003
	placebo	7	15.04	6.47–26.06	88.9	0.00
Ventricular fibrillation	Magnesium	7	2.13	0.00–6.59	76.81	0.00
	Placebo	7	4.43	0.31–11.69	86.09	0.00
Total of Ventricular arrhythmia	Magnesium	13	11.88	6.71–18.17	82.99	0.00
	Placebo	13	24.24	14.52–35.43	92.11	0.00
Atrial fibrillation	Magnesium	9	9.72	3.31–18.63	92.15	0.00
	Placebo	9	22.37	15.86–29.59	85.3	0.00
Supraventricular tachycardia	Magnesium	6	4.90	0.84–11.28	75.36	0.00
	Placebo	6	14.62	7.26–23.82	78.76	0.00
	Magnesium	14	10.36	5.55–16.32	87.16	0.00
Total of supraventricular arrhythmia	Placebo	14	23.91	18.82–29.38	75.10	0.00
Bradycardia	Magnesium	4	6.46	0.71–12.21	78.9	0.00
	Placebo	4	7.2	1.03–1.37	79.8	0.00
Total Arrhythmia	Magnesium	22	41	11.44–21.0	85.89	0.00
	Placebo	22	30.85	25.07–39.63	86.21	0.00

0.22–0.65; $p < 0.001$, Fig. 3). There was significant heterogeneity among trials ($I^2 = 77.6\%$; $p = 0.000$), (Table 3).

Bradycardia

Among reviewed studies, four articles reported the prevalence of bradycardia. The rate of bradycardia in the magnesium sulfate and placebo groups was 6.46% (95% CI, 0.71–12.21) and 7.2% (95% CI, 1.03–1.37) respectively (Table 2). Random effects meta-analysis did not show a beneficial effect of magnesium on the reduction of bradycardia (OR = 1.29, 95% CI 0.99–1.69; $p = 0.329$). The reviewed studies showed limited evidence of heterogeneity ($I^2 = 12.7\%$; $p > 0.001$), (Table 3).

Subgroup analyses

It was clear that some factors might influence the associations between magnesium and the incidence of cardiac arrhythmias. Therefore, we conducted subgroup analyses to minimize heterogeneity among various studies. In the current study, the effect of magnesium consumption versus placebo on the reduction of cardiac arrhythmias examined by the dosage of magnesium (< 10 g, > 10 g); fourteen trials used magnesium less than 10 g and eight used magnesium 10 g or more within the first 24 h. We found a significant decrease in cardiac arrhythmias comparing magnesium with placebo in both groups (magnesium< 10 g OR = 0.42, 95% CI: 0.24–0.59; I2 = 71.0%, $p = 0.000$ and magnesium ≥10 g OR = 0.34, 95% CI: 0.08–0.60; I2 = 90.1%, p = 0.000).

We also performed subgroup meta-analysis based on the clinical settings; surgery or not surgery. Nine trials evaluated the effect of magnesium consumption on the incidence of arrhythmias in nonsurgical patients. The results of the meta-analysis showed a significant decrease comparing magnesium with placebo (OR = 0.33, 95%CI,

Table 3 Magnesium administration and the incidence and type of arrhythmias compared to placebo

Type of fractures	Summary odds ratio (OR)	95% confidence interval	Between studies	
			I^2	p for heterogeneity
Ventricular tachycardia	0.65	0.50–0.85	55.6%	0.035
Ventricular fibrillation	0.69	0.47–1.01	48.9%	0.098
Total of Ventricular arrhythmia	0.38	0.23–0.64	79.0%	0.000
Atrial Fibrillation	0.46	0.28–0.76	76.9%	0.000
Supraventricular tachycardia	0.48	0.33–0.70	48.5%	0.084
Total of Supraventricular arrhythmia	0.43	0.28–0.65	73.4%	0.000
Bradycardia	1.29	0.99–1.69	12.7	0.329
Total Arrhythmia	0.41	0.29–0.58	82.1	0.000

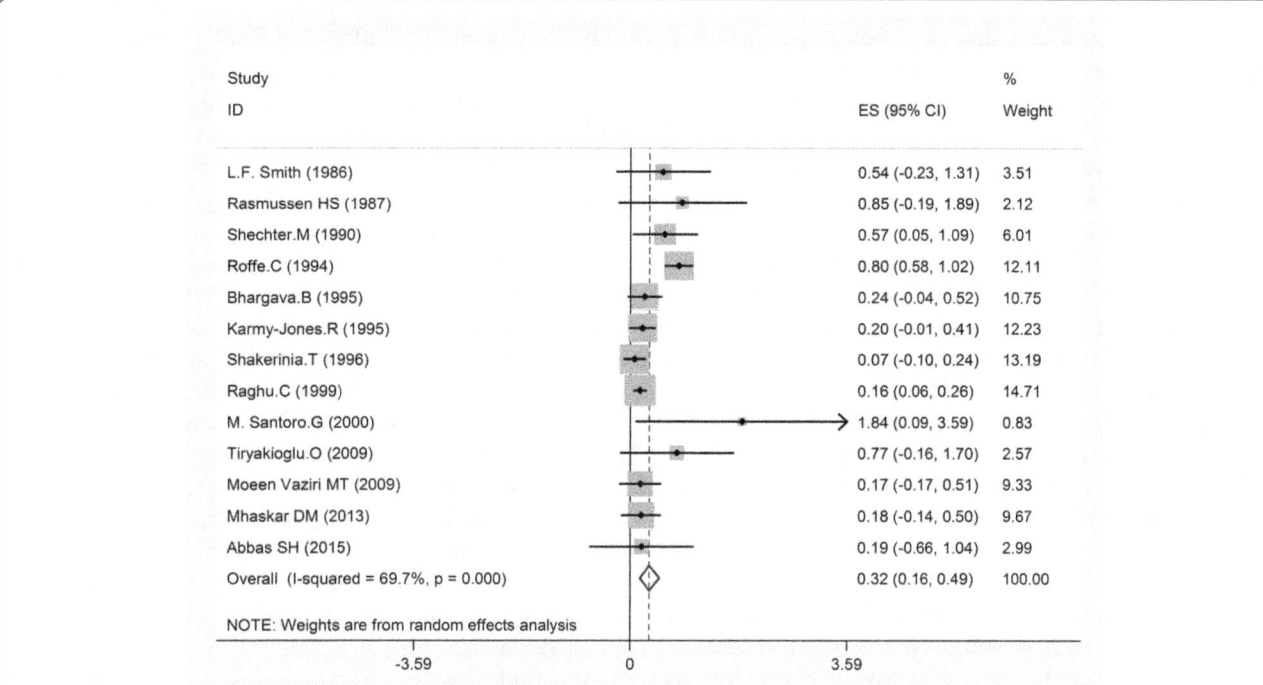

Fig. 2 Forest plot and the rate of ventricular arrhythmias (left: magnesium, right: placebo).Square represents effect estimate of individual studies with their 95% confidence intervals with size of squares proportional to the weight assigned to the study in the meta-analysis. In this chart, studies are stored in order of the year of publication and author's names, based on a random effects model

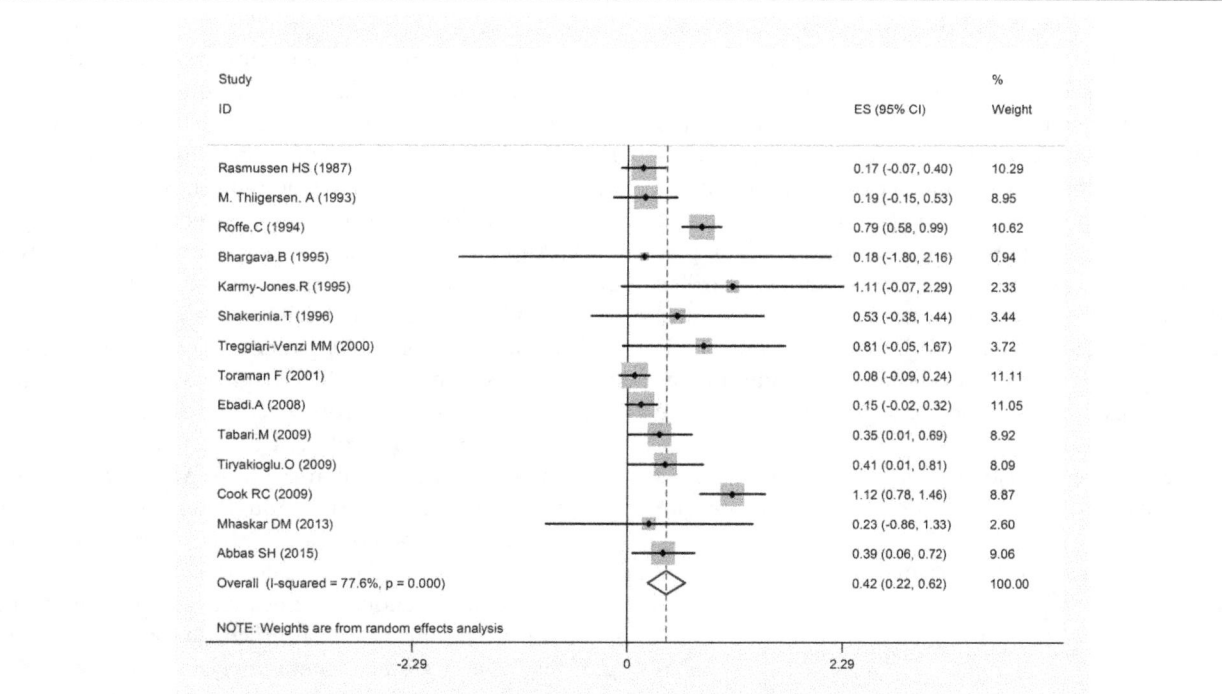

Fig. 3 Forest plot and the rate of supraventricular arrhythmias (left: magnesium, right: placebo). Square represents effect estimate of individual studies with their 95% confidence intervals with size of squares proportional to the weight assigned to the study in the meta-analysis. In this chart, studies are stored in order of the year of publication and author's names, based on a random effects model

0.10–0.57; I2 = 88.7%, p = 0.000). Also, thirteen trials performed in surgical patients and showed that magnesium consumption could have a positive effect in reducing cardiac arrhythmias (OR = 0.43, 95%CI 0.24–0.62; I2 = 73.3%, p = 0.000).

The results of subgroup analyses showed that the dose of magnesium used or the clinical settings did not affect the reduction of arrhythmias.

To find the source of heterogeneity a meta-regression performed. As seen in Table 4, the association between sample size, mean age, published year, the consumed dose of magnesium and the effect size of the outcomes evaluated. Our results showed that there was no significant association between the reduction of ventricular arrhythmias and sample size (p = 573), mean age (p = 553), published year (p = 283), and the consumed dose of the magnesium (p = 410).

Publication Bias

Figure 4 presents the Begg's funnel plot for publication bias in the risk difference analysis of the effect of magnesium in reducing ventricular arrhythmias. According to the publication bias figure, the effect of bias was not significant when Begg's funnel plot evaluated (p = 0.204, Fig. 4); P-values for Egger's regression asymmetry test were 0.008; thus, the Egger tests revealed the evidence of publication bias in this study.

Discussion

Cardiac arrhythmia is caused by a wrong rate or rhythm of the heartbeat, which are under the control of the cardiac conduction system [34]. Magnesium sulfate is frequently used to reduce cardiac arrhythmias in patients with the acute coronary syndrome [35]. Numerous attempts are in action to diminish cardiac arrhythmias. This study is a meta-analysis of previously conducted studies comparing magnesium consumption versus placebo control in reducing the incidence of cardiac arrhythmia; the current systematic review and meta-analysis of these twenty-two randomize control trials found a positive correlation between the administrations of magnesium sulfate and the reduction of cardiac arrhythmias.

Our results were consistent with those of the previous meta-analyses which evaluated the effect of magnesium

Table 4 Source of heterogeneity by multivariate meta-regression analysis

Factors	Coefficient	Standard error	P
Published year	−.0121418	.010758	0.283
Sample size	−.0010426	.0017948	0.573
Mean age	.0118355	.0192186	0.553
Dose of Magnesium	.2159504	.0109332	0.410

on the incidence of arrhythmias. A meta-analysis of eight trials included 930 patients with acute myocardial infarction, showed the beneficial effect of magnesium to prevent arrhythmias. Horner's study showed that the administration of magnesium in acute myocardial infarction associated with 49% reduction in ventricular arrhythmias and 54% reduction in supraventricular tachycardia [36]. A meta-analysis of seventeen trials with 2069 patients reported that magnesium administration could reduce the risk of supraventricular arrhythmias by 23% (atrial fibrillation by 29%) and of ventricular arrhythmias by 48% after cardiac surgery [37]. Our meta-analysis showed that magnesium could decrease the risk of ventricular arrhythmias about 32% and supraventricular arrhythmias about 42% respectively.

One of our results was that magnesium sulfate could reduce the incidence of supraventricular arrhythmias more than ventricular arrhythmias. However, the effect of magnesium in reducing the incidence of ventricular arrhythmias has not investigated as widely as the same for supraventricular arrhythmias. A meta-analysis of twenty studies with 3696 patients who underwent coronary artery bypass did not find any effect of magnesium on the incidence of ventricular arrhythmias; the authors identified the effect of magnesium sulfate in reducing postoperative supraventricular arrhythmias when examined by lower-quality studies [38].

This study suggests that magnesium sulfate administration reduces supraventricular arrhythmia. Moreover, the observed effects were greater for atrial fibrillation. The most common arrhythmia after coronary artery bypass graft is atrial fibrillation. Alghamdi and colleagues in a meta-analysis of eight randomized controlled trials revealed that the use of intravenous magnesium associated with a significant reduction in the incidence of atrial fibrillation after coronary artery bypass surgery [39]. Another meta-analysis of twenty-two trials with 2896 patients showed that there was an overall reduction in atrial fibrillation after magnesium administration [40]. A meta-analysis of 2490 patients from twenty randomized trials concluded that magnesium administration could be an effective prophylactic measure for prevention of the postoperative atrial fibrillation [41]. Another meta-analysis of seven clinical trials with 1028 participants revealed that intravenous magnesium reduced the incidence of postoperative atrial fibrillation about 36% [42]. Many of the conducted studies encouraged the use of intravenous magnesium to prevent postoperative atrial fibrillation after coronary artery bypass grafting. The present meta-analysis was consistent with previous studies; we confirmed the previous results and concluded that magnesium administrating could be useful in prevention and treatment of various cardiac arrhythmias.

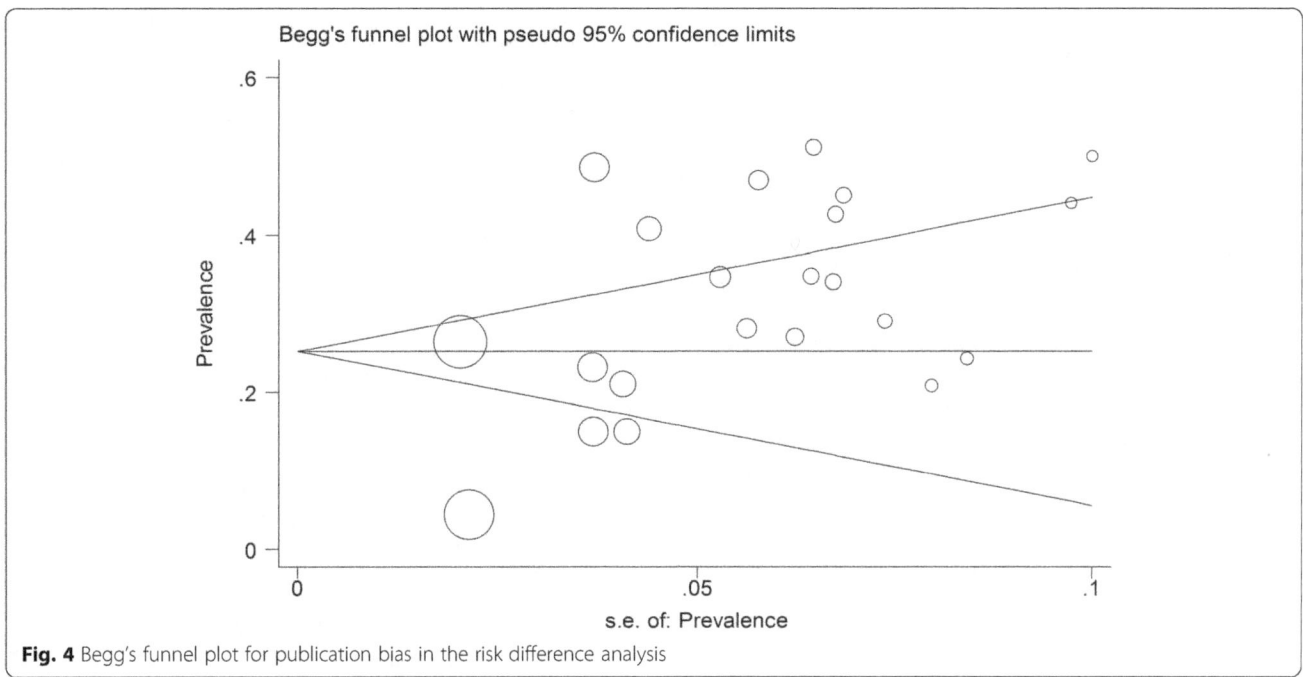

Fig. 4 Begg's funnel plot for publication bias in the risk difference analysis

As discussed above, several meta-analyses have explored the effects of magnesium administration and cardiac arrhythmias, but there was also data not included. Furthermore, there have been further developments and newer trials since the publication of previous meta-analyses, which did not include these trials. In fact, this study is also the largest one which examined the effect of magnesium on the incidence of cardiac arrhythmias.

Magnesium plays an essential role in many fundamental biological processes, for example, it participates in many enzymatic reactions and many ion channels functions [34]. Magnesium also is a cofactor of the membrane Na-K pump; it regulates the outward K+ movement and potassium is transported equally in both directions when Mg2+ is absent [43, 44]. Magnesium deficiency can reduce the amount of intracellular K+ and the pump's activity, which leads to partial depolarization and changes in the activity of many potential-dependent membrane channels [43, 44]. So, its deficiency also disturbs the resting membrane potential of the cardiac cells and results in cardiac arrhythmias [44].

Hypomagnesaemia is common among patients with cardiovascular diseases [45]. Therefore, measurement of the serum magnesium level of patients with cardiovascular disease before surgery is necessary and indicate injection of magnesium sulfate to prevent these complications. Hypomagnesaemia in cardiovascular disease may occur due to various reasons such as treatment of hypertension with diuretics, diabetic patients, and patients with cardiomyopathy [46].

Magnesium deficiency is an important factor responsible for supraventricular and ventricular arrhythmias

[34]. Beluri and colleagues found that the risk of ventricular arrhythmias in magnesium deficiency increased dramatically and suggested that hypomagnesemia could be considered one of the most important causes of ventricular arrhythmias [47]. Hypomagnesemia in patients with congestive heart failure causes arrhythmia. Fall Solomon and colleagues found that 55% of patients with congestive heart failure suffer hypomagnesemia, which results in ventricular premature beats and atrial fibrillation [48].

All these findings indicate the importance of serum magnesium monitoring level in cardiac patients. Therefore, by checking and correcting serum magnesium level, it is possible to prevent many cardiac arrhythmias and improve the care of cardiac patients.

This meta-analysis had several limitations. First, there was a lack of uniformity in the reviewed trials regarding the clinical settings and the amount of magnesium administered. For example, some study was among revascularized patients (CABG or angioplasty) while others in non-surgical patients; however, we performed a meta-analysis and concluded that the effect of magnesium on the incidence of arrhythmias not affected by either clinical settings or the amount of magnesium administered. Secondly, we were unable to conduct a subgroup analysis regarding the concurrent use of other antiarrhythmic medications. Insufficient available data about the concurrent use of other antiarrhythmic agents, which could modify effect size, prevented us from the evaluation of such cases. Third, in a meta-analysis sample size and standard deviation are very important in combining the results of studies and may be influenced the evaluated outcomes. Fourth, the possible effects of publication bias inherent in any meta-analysis could not be ruled out. Finally, some identified studies presented defective quantitative data and could not be included in this meta-analysis.

Conclusion

The present meta-analysis showed that the total rate of cardiac arrhythmia was significantly lower in the group receiving magnesium sulfate than placebo The current finding also showed that magnesium consumption would decrease ventricular and supraventricular arrhythmias compared with placebo. In conclusion, our study suggested that administration of magnesium sulfate could be safe, effective and cost-effective in the prevention of many cardiac arrhythmias. Therefore, by checking and correcting serum magnesium level, it may be possible to prevent a large proportion of cardiac arrhythmias and improve cardiac patient's health. However, other studies should be done about the dose and the time of adding magnesium sulfate until proved that this method is effective in the prevention of cardiac arrhythmias.

Abbreviations
CABG: Coronary Artery Bypass Grafting; PCI: Percutaneous Coronary Intervention

Acknowledgements
The authors extend their gratitude to the Social Determinants of Health Research Center, Yasoj University of Medical Sciences.

Authors' contributions
ShS and MM designed the conception of the study; KS and FS focus of the statically analysis; PA, technical support and conceptual advise. All authors contributed to the drafted the manuscript, revised it critically and approved the final version.

Competing interests
The authors declare that they have no competing interests.

Author details
[1]Department of Cardiac Surgery, Yasuj University of Medical Science, Yasuj, Iran. [2]Proteomics Research Center, Shahid Beheshti University of Medical Sciences, Tehran, Iran. [3]Social Determinants of Health Research Center, Yasuj University of Medical Sciences, Yasuj, Iran. [4]Department of Social Medicine, School of Medicine, Ilam University of Medical Sciences, Ilam, Iran. [5]Department of Cardiology, Faculty of Medicine, Zanjan University of Medical Sciences, Zanjan, Iran.

References
1. Chung M, Asher R, Yamada D, Eagle K. Arrhythmias after cardiac and non-cardiac Surgery. In: Podrid P, Kowey P, editors. Cardiac arrhythmia. 2nded. Philadelphia: Lippincott Williams Wilkins; 2001. p. 631–8.
2. Dipiro JT, Al. Talbea R, Yee g C, et al. Pharmacotherapy, vol. 976. 6th ed. New York: McGraw-Hill; 2005.
3. Kaplan JA, Reich DL, Lake CL, et al. Kaplan's cardiac anesthesia, vol. 268. 5th ed. Philadelphia: Saunders; 2006.
4. Butterworth J, Prielipp R. Endocrin, metabolic and electrolyte responses. In: Gravlec G, Davis R, Kurusz M, Utley J, editors. Cardiopulmonary Bypass. 2nded. Philadelphia: Lippincott Williams Wilkins; 2000. p. 358–60.

5. Shirey T. Monitoring magnesium to guid magnesium therapy for heart surgery. J Anesth. 2004;18:118–28.
6. Fanning WJ, et al. Prophylaxis of atrial fibrillation with magnesium sulfate after coronary artery bypass grafting. Ann Thorac Surg. 1991;52:529–33.
7. Kaplan M, Kut MS, Demirtas MM. Intravenous magnesium sulfate prophylaxis for artery bypass surgery. J Thorac Cardiavasc Surg. 2003;125:344–52.
8. Pinrad A, Donati F. Magnesium potentiates neuromuscular block with cisatracurium during cardiac surgery. Can J Anaesth. 2003;50:72–8.
9. Yeatman M, Angelini GD, Shnaider H. Magnesium in cardiac arrhythmias digoxin-induced nonparoxysmal atrioventricular junctional tachycardia responsive to parenteral magnesium sulfate. Br J Anaesth. 1988;24:230–40.
10. Wistbacka JO, Koistinen J. Magnasium substitution in elective artery surgery. J Cardiothorac Vasc Anesth. 1995;9:140–6.
11. Antman EM. Early administration of intravenous magnesium to high-risk patients with acute myocardial infarction in the magnesium in coronaries (MAGIC) trial: a randomized controlled trial. Lancet. 2002;360:1189–96.
12. Smith LF, Heagerty AM, Bing RF, Barnett DB. Intravenous infusion of magnesium sulfate after acute myocardial infarction: effects on arrhythmias and mortality. Int J Cardiol. 1986;12:175–80.
13. Rusmussen HS, Suenson M, Mcnairm P, Nbrregard P, Balslevm S. Magnesium infusion reduces the incidence of arrhythmias in acute myocardial infarction. A double-blind placebo-controlled study. Clin Cardiol. 1987;10:351–6.
14. Shechter M, Hod H, Marks N, Behar S, Kaplinsky E, Rabinowitz B. Beneficial effect of magnesium sulfate in acute myocardial infarction. Am J Cardiol. 1990;66:271–4.
15. M. Thiigersen A, Johnson O. O, Wester P. Effects of magnesium infusion on thrombolytic and non-thrombolytic treated patients with acute myocardial infarction. Int J Cardiol 1993;39:13–22.
16. Roffe C, Fletcher S, Woods KL. Investigation of the effects of intravenous magnesium sulfates on cardiac rhythm in acute myocardial infarction. Br Heart. 1994;71:141–5.
17. Bhargava B, Chandra S, .Agarwal VV, Kaul U, Vashishth S, Wasir HS. Adjunctive magnesium infusion therapy in acute myocardial infarction. Int J Cardiol 1995; 52: 95–99.
18. Karmy Jones R, Hamilton A, Dzavik V, Allegreto M, Finegan BA, Koshal A. Magnesium sulfate prophylaxis after cardiac operations. Ann Thorac Surg. 1995;59:502–7.
19. Shakerinia T, Ali IM, And Sullivan JA. magnesium in cardioplegia: is it necessary. CJS 1996; 39(5): 397–400.
20. Raghu C, Peddeswara P, Seshagiri Rao D. Protective effect of intravenous magnesium in acute myocardial infarction following thrombolytic therapy. Int J Cardiol. 1999;71:209–15.
21. Parikka H, Toivonen L, Naukkarinen V, Tierala I, Pohjola-Sintonen S, Heikkila¨ J, Nieminen MS. Decreases by magnesium of QT dispersion and ventricular arrhythmias in patients with acute myocardial infarction. Eur Heart J. 1999; 20:111–20.
22. Treggiari-Venzi MM, Waeber JL, Perneger TV, Suter PM, Adamec R, Romand JA. Intravenous amiodarone or magnesium sulfate is not cost-beneficial prophylaxis for atrial fibrillation after coronary artery bypass surgery. Br J Anaesth. 2000;85(5):690–5.
23. Santoro GM, Antoniucci D, Bolognese L, Valenti R, Buonamici P, Trapani M, Santini A, Filippo Fazzini P. A randomized study of intravenous magnesium in acute myocardial infarction treated with direct coronary angioplasty. Am Heart J. 2000;140:891–7.
24. Toraman F, Karabulut EH, Alhan C, Dagdelen S, Tarcan S. Magnesium infusion dramatically decreases the incidence of atrial fibrillation after coronary artery bypass grafting. Ann Thorac Surg. 2001;72:1256–62.
25. Nakashima H, Katayama T, Honda Y, Suzuki S, Yano K. Cardioprotective effects of magnesium sulfate in patients undergoing primary coronary angioplasty for acute myocardial infarction. Circ J. 2004;68:23–8.
26. Ebadi A, Mohammad Hosseini F, Tabatabai SK, Rostaminejad A. Evaluation of using IV magnesium sulfate for prevention of postoperative atrial fibrillation arrhythmia in patients undergoing coronary artery bypass grafting. Journal of Armaghan Danesh. 2008;13(2):1–10.
27. Tiryakioglu O, Demirtas S, Ari H, Tiryakioglu SK, Huysal K, Selimoglu O, Ozyazicioglu A. Magnesium sulfate and amiodarone prophylaxis for prevention of postoperative arrhythmia in coronary by-pass operations. J Cardiothorac Surg. 2009;4(8):2–7.
28. Cook RC, Humphries KH, Gin K, Janusz MT, Slavik RS, Pharm D, Bernstein V, Tholin M, Lee MK. Prophylactic Intravenous Magnesium Sulphate in addition

Evaluating the effect of magnesium supplementation and cardiac arrhythmias after acute coronary...

183

to oral blockade does not prevent atrial arrhythmias after coronary artery or Valvular heart surgery a randomized. Controlled Trial Circulation. 2009; 120(15):163–9.

29. Moeen Vaziri MT, Jouibar R, Akhlagh SHA, Janati M. The effect of lidocaine and magnesium sulfate on prevention of ventricular fibrillation in coronary artery bypass grafting surgery. Iran Red Crescent Med J. 2010;12(3):298–301.

30. Tabari M, Soltani Gh, Zirak N, Ghoshayeshi L. the effect of magnesium sulfate on cardiac arrhythmias after open heart surgery. J Med Sci 2009;88.[article in persian].

31. Mhaskar MM, Mahajan SK, Pawar KC. Significance of serum magnesium levels in reference to acute myocardial infarction and role of intravenous magnesium therapy in prevention of cardiac arrhythmias following myocardial infarction. International Journal of Medicine and Public Health. 2013;3(3):187–91.

32. Abbas S, Khan FJ, Abbas A, Sharif Nassery S, RiaZz W, Iqbal M. Waheed. Prophylactic magnesium and rhythm disorders after open cardiac surgery. Journal of Cardiology & Current Research. 2015;2(6):00081.

33. Mohammadzadeh A, Towfighi F, Jafari N. Effect of magnesium on arrhythmia incidence in patients undergoing coronary artery bypass grafting. ANZ J Surg. 2017; https://doi.org/10.1111/ans.14056.

34. Cieoelewicz A, Jankowski J, Korzeniowska K, Balcer-Dymel N, Jabecka A. The role of magnesium in cardiac arrhythmias. J Elem s. 2013; https://doi.org/10.5601/jelem.2013.18.2.11.

35. Shechter M, Hod H, Marks N, Behar S, Kaplinsky E, Rabinowitz B. Beneficial effect of Magnessium sulfate in acute myocardial infarction. Am J Cardiol. 1990;66:271–4.

36. Horner SM. Efficacy of intravenous magnesium in acute myocardial infarction in reducing arrhythmias and mortality: meta-analysis of magnesium in acute myocardial infarction. Circulation. 1992;86:774–9.

37. Shiga T, Wajima Z, Inoue T, et al. Magnesium prophylaxis for arrhythmias after cardiac surgery: a meta-analysis of randomized controlled trials. Am J Med. 2004;117:325–33.

38. De Oliveira GS Jr, Knautz JS, Sherwani S, McCarthy RJ. Systemic magnesium to reduce postoperative arrhythmias after coronary artery bypass graft surgery: a meta-analysis of randomized controlled trials. J Cardiothorac Vasc Anesth. 2012;26(4):643–50.

39. Alghamdi AA, Al-Radi OO, Latter DA. Intravenous magnesium for prevention of atrial fibrillation after coronary artery bypass surgery: a systematic review and meta-analysis. J Cardiovasc Surg. 2005;20:293–9.

40. Burgess DC, Kilborn MJ, Keech AC. Interventions for prevention of post-operative atrial fibrillation and its complications after cardiac surgery: a meta-analysis. Eur Heart J. 2006;27:2846–57.

41. Miller S, Crystal E, Garfinkle M, et al. Effects of magnesium on atrial fibrillation after cardiac surgery: a meta-analysis. Heart. 2005;91:618–23.

42. Gu WJ, WU ZJ, WANG PF, AUNG LH, YIN RX. Intravenous magnesium prevents atrial fibrillation after coronary artery bypass grafting: a meta-analysis of 7 double-blind, placebo-controlled, randomized clinical trials. Trials. 2012;13:41.

43. ANGUS M, ANGUS Z. Cardiovascular actions of magnesium. Crit Care Clin. 2001;53:299–307.

44. Rude r, Shils ME. Magnesium. In: Modern Nutrition in health and disease, Shils ME, Shike M, Ross AC, Caballero B, Cousins RJ, editors. 10th edition: Lippincott Williams & Wilkins; 2006.

45. Big RP, Chia R. Magnesium deficiency. Role in arrhythmias complicating acute myocardial infarction? Med J Aust. 1981;1(7):346–8.

46. Al-Ghamdi SM, Cameron EC, Sutton RA. Magnesium deficiency: pathophysiologic and clinical overview. Am J Kidney Dis. 1994;24(5):737–52.

47. Bolouri A, Mehrabi GHA, Salehi M. Evaluation of the prevalence of ventricular tachyarrhythmia in patients with acute myocardial infarction and serum magnesium in Khatam-Al-Anbia hospital, Zahedan, Iran. Zahedan J Res Med Sci, Tabib-e-Shaegh. 2006; 8(2): 93–100.[article in Persian].

48. Fal Soleiman H, Kazemi T. The serum magnesium level in patients with congestive heart failure. Med J Mashad Univ Med Sci. 2006;90(48):399–404.

22

Uncertainty on the effectiveness and safety of rivaroxaban in premenopausal women with atrial fibrillation: empirical evidence needed

Herbert J. A. Rolden[1,2]*, Angela H. E. M. Maas[3], Gert Jan van der Wilt[2] and Janneke P. C. Grutters[2]

Abstract

Background: Novel anticoagulations (NOACs) are increasingly prescribed for the prevention of stroke in premenopausal women with atrial fibrillation. Small studies suggest NOACs are associated with a higher risk of abnormal uterine bleeds than vitamin K antagonists (VKAs). Because there is no direct empirical evidence on the benefit/risk profile of rivaroxaban compared to VKAs in this subgroup, we synthesize available indirect evidence, estimate decision uncertainty on the treatments, and assess whether further research in premenopausal women is warranted.

Methods: A Markov model with annual cycles and a lifetime horizon was developed comparing rivaroxaban (the most frequently prescribed NOAC in this population) and VKAs. Clinical event rates, associated quality adjusted life years, and health care costs were obtained from different sources and adjusted for gender, age, and history of stroke. A Monte Carlo simulation with 10,000 iterations was then performed for a hypothetical cohort of premenopausal women, estimated to be reflective of the population of premenopausal women with AF in The Netherlands.

Results: In the simulation, rivaroxaban is the better treatment option for the prevention of ischemic strokes in premenopausal women in 61% of the iterations. Similarly, this is 98% for intracranial hemorrhages, 24% for major abnormal uterine bleeds, 1% for minor abnormal uterine bleeds, 9% for other major extracranial hemorrhages, and 23% for other minor extracranial hemorrhages. There is a 78% chance that rivaroxaban offers the most quality-adjusted life years. The expected value of perfect information in The Netherlands equals 122 quality-adjusted life years and 22 million Euros.

Conclusions: There is a 22% risk that rivaroxaban offers a worse rather than a better benefit/risk profile than vitamin K antagonists in premenopausal women. Although rivaroxaban is preferred over VKAs in this population, further research is warranted, and should preferably take the shape of an internationally coordinated registry study including other NOACs.

Keywords: Abnormal uterine bleeding, Atrial fibrillation, Premenopausal women, Rivaroxaban, Value of information, Vitamin K antagonists

* Correspondence: herbert.rolden@gmail.com
[1]Council for Public Health and Society, The Hague, The Netherlands
[2]Department for Health Evidence, Radboud University Medical Center, Nijmegen, The Netherlands
Full list of author information is available at the end of the article

Background

Atrial fibrillation (AF) is the most common cardiac arrhythmia and is a chronic or recurrent illness that greatly affects patients' quality of life. It is estimated that over 2% of people suffer from AF and its prevalence is expected to increase, in part due to population ageing in combination with a deterioration of lifestyle factors such as overweight, leading to more diabetes, hypertension and ischemic heart disease at a young age [1–3]. AF drastically increases the risk of ischemic stroke, and Vitamin K Antagonists (VKAs) have been prescribed for decades to prevent such stroke events in patients with AF. Unfortunately, VKAs are associated with serious side-effects, of which intracranial hemorrhage is the most severe, causing extremely high rates of emergency hospital admissions [4], requiring regular monitoring for dose titration [5].

Since 2010, four different pharmaceutical agents have entered the market as an alternative to VKAs: dabigatran, rivaroxaban, apixaban and edoxaban. Their phase III trials suggest that these novel oral anticoagulants (NOACs) are at least non-inferior to VKAs in terms of effectiveness, and are associated with a lower risk of intracranial hemorrhages [6–10]. Another important benefit of NOACs is that they are provided in a standard dose and do not require frequent monitoring. Results from observational studies suggest that rivaroxaban (Rvx) is the most prescribed NOAC, at least in Canada and the UK [11, 12]. A plausible reason for its popularity is that RVX is taken once daily, where other NOACs have a twice daily dose regimen [13].

Regardless of the advantages that RVX provides, some researchers and clinicians still have reservations in clinical practice. A main problem with RVX is that - as for other NOACs - there is a lack of empirical evidence on its benefit/risk profile in certain patient subgroups, and premenopausal women form a marked example, for whom an important neglected factor is that RVX is associated with a higher risk of abnormal uterine bleeds (AUBs) than VKAs [14, 15]. It is therefore possible that RVX might be the "wrong" treatment choice for premenopausal women, and that its widespread use in this subgroup may cause more harm than benefit, especially considering that heavy and irregular menstrual bleeding is common in women in their forties and requires specific attention [16].

As premenopausal women have not been separately investigated, we aim to assess the impact of RVX prescription in this subgroup by synthesizing and modeling all relevant indirect empirical evidence that is currently available. We have done this by simulating clinical event rates from the phase III trial on RVX, and the different subgroup analyses performed on this trial (sometimes adjusted using additional empirical evidence), and the consequences of these events in a hypothetical cohort of premenopausal women in a specific model. An adjoining value-of-information analysis shows whether further research in this subgroup is warranted.

Methods

Model description

A decision-analytic Markov model with annual cycles and a lifetime horizon was developed in which VKAs and RVX were compared as treatments for the prevention of stroke in premenopausal women with AF. VKAs were provided in adjusted doses (target INR between 2.0 and 3.0) and RVX in a dose of 20 mg. The model included five different health states – "no history of stroke", "previous stroke or TIA", "previous stroke and minor disability", "previous stroke and major disability", and "death" – and nine clinical events: ischemic stroke, TIA, systemic embolism, myocardial infarction, intracranial hemorrhage, major and minor abnormal uterine bleeds (AUBs), and other major and minor extracranial hemorrhages. In each cycle, women from the hypothetical cohort remained in their health state or moved from one health state to another when a TIA, ischemic stroke, intracranial hemorrhage, or death occurred. See Fig. 1 for an overview of the model.

Population

At baseline, the cohort of women in our analysis was 20 years of age and 0.5% had a history of stroke. This estimate was based on consultation of clinical experts. Menopause was assumed to set in at age 51 years. After this age, the occurrence of abnormal uterine bleeds is less common in women, although they do occur. In the model we conservatively assumed that after 51 years of age, women were no longer at risk for abnormal uterine bleeds. Based on the age distribution of premenopausal women in the Netherlands in 2015 and different studies on the prevalence of AF in age subgroups, [1, 2, 17, 18] we estimated that 10,000 premenopausal women had AF in The Netherlands in 2015, of which 10.5% were aged 20–29 years, 20% were 30–39, 49% were 40–49, and 20.5% were 50–51 years. We assumed that around 40% of these women were eligible for oral anticoagulation due to their co-morbidities [2]. See Additional file 1 (including Table S1) for more details.

This study focuses on a simulation model of a hypothetical cohort of premenopausal women with AF. Data on this cohort was based solely on publicly available data. This study was therefore not submitted to an institutional ethics committee. Approval from an ethics committee is required in The Netherlands only when scientific research subjects persons to at least one intervention or imposes on them a form of behavior, as stated in the Medical Research Involving Human Subjects Act.

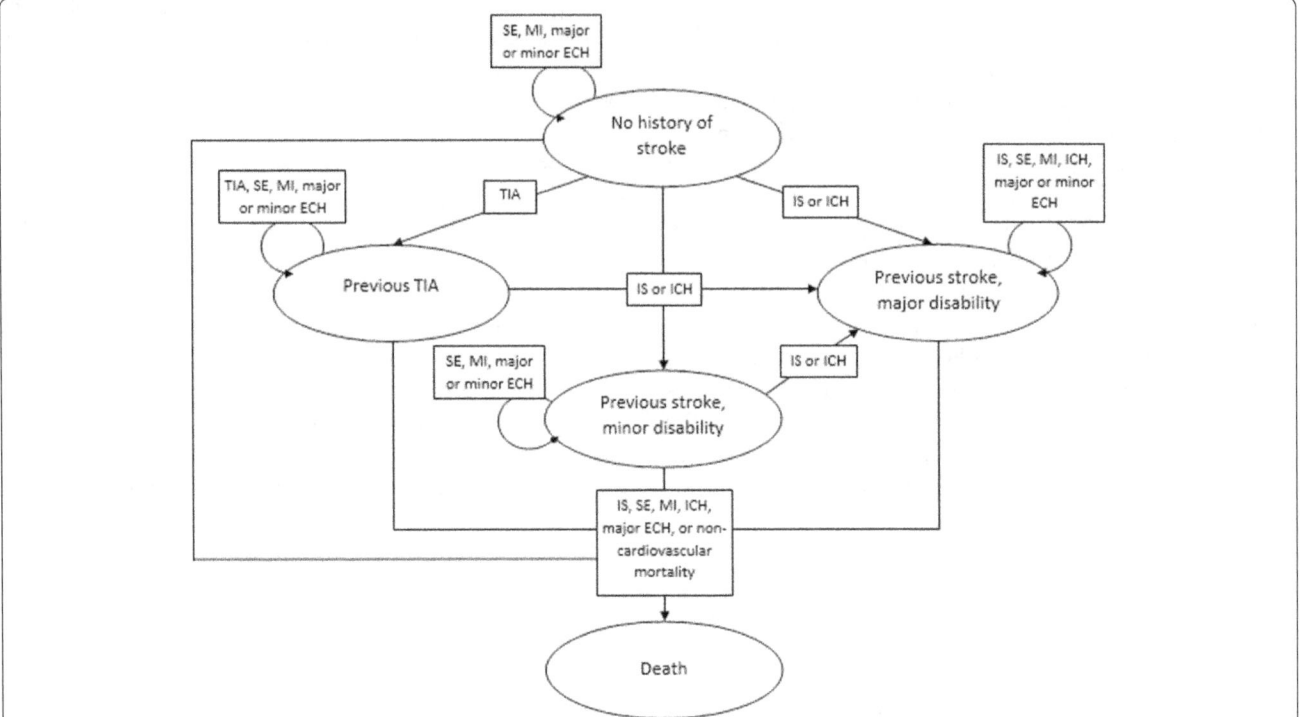

Fig. 1 Illustration of the Markov model with health states (circles), clinical events (rectangles), and transition possibilities (arrows). Abbreviations: *IS* ischemic stroke, *TIA* transient ischemic attack, *SE* systemic embolism, *MI* myocardial infarction, *ICH* intracranial hemorrhage, *ECH* extracranial hemorrhage (either abnormal uterine bleed or other form of extracranial hemorrhage)

Probabilities

Clinical event rates were retrieved from different studies on the phase III trial on RVX [8, 19, 20] as well as a post approval study on RVX and VKAs for the prevention of venous thromboembolism in premenopausal women [8, 15]. The study population from the ROCKET-AF trial differed from the hypothetical cohort of premenopausal women in terms of gender, age, and history of stroke. This was important to consider as these variables influence the risk of different clinical events with VKAs as well as the relative risks with RVX. Adjustments were made for different clinical events on the basis of gender, age and history of stroke using different sources [8, 19–23]. The clinical event rates and risk adjustments that were used are listed in Additional file 1: Table S2.

Utility

To assess whether RVX or VKAs form the preferred option, we needed to compare the benefit/risk profiles of both treatments. This is difficult because many different clinical events and health states are important to consider. However, these events and states can be transformed into a single utility measure – quality adjusted life years (QALYs) – and this measure was used to reflect the overall benefit/risk profiles. Quality of life was considered as a single index utility, on a scale from 0 (representing death) to 1 (representing perfect health).

The decrement in utility caused by clinical events as well as the utility scores of health events were retrieved from different sources [24–26]. An overview of (dis)utilities is provided in Additional file 1: Table S3. QALYs were discounted at an annual rate of 1.5% [27].

Costs

Health care costs were also used as input in the model. Costs and frequency of treatment/monitoring were collected from the websites of Dutch institutions [28, 29], and advise from clinical experts. Costs for clinical events and health states were obtained from health economic literature [30–33]. Price indices were used to convert costs to the 2015 price level [34]. Future costs were discounted to their present value by an annual rate of 4% [27]. An overview of the health care costs associated with treatment, monitoring, clinical events and health states can be found in the Additional file 1.

Monte Carlo simulation

We performed a Monte Carlo simulation to obtain insight into how the uncertainty on the model parameters impact utility and cost-effectiveness. In the simulation, we ran the Markov model 10,000 times for a hypothetical cohort of 10,000 women aged 20 years, whereby – for every iteration – parameter values for clinical event rates, utilities and costs were randomly selected from their uncertainty distributions. The averages, and the 95% confidence intervals of these averages, were calculated over the 10,000 iterations, as well as the average increments of RVX compared to VKAs. We also calculated in how many iterations RVX performed better than VKAs with regard to clinical events and QALYs.

Cost-effectiveness of RVX was expressed as the "incremental cost-effectiveness ratio" (ICER) and the "net monetary benefit" (NMB). The ICER is a standard cost-effectiveness measure that expresses the healthcare costs associated with gaining one QALY. It is calculated here by dividing the incremental costs of RVX by its incremental effects. The NMB is the monetary value assigned to the total amount of QALYs that is associated with a treatment, subtracted by the costs of the treatment. The monetary value that is assigned to QALYs differs per context; the unofficial value of €50,000 per QALY in the Netherlands was used in our analysis [27]. The treatment with the highest NMB is considered cost-effective.

Value of information analysis

Through a value of information (VOI) analysis, one can assess what the impact is of making more informed decisions because uncertainty on what is the best treatment option is reduced. For this purpose, we estimated the "expected value of perfect information" (EVPI). The EVPI is the expected value of eliminating all parameter uncertainty, here expressed as the maximum in QALYs that can be gained. The EVPI is estimated by calculating for each of the 10,000 iterations in the Monte Carlo simulation the difference between QALYs with the treatment that is chosen under uncertainty and QALYs with the treatment that would be chosen if "true" parameter values were known [35].

Not all women who initiate treatment before their menopause are 20 years old (the baseline age in the base case analysis). Therefore, the EVPI was calculated for different baseline ages before menopause, namely 20, 30, 40 and 50 years. To estimate the population EVPI, we multiplied these age-dependent EVPIs with the estimated number of women in each age group in The Netherlands.

If the VOI analysis would reveal that further research is warranted, we further investigated which variables mainly contribute to the decision uncertainty. A Tornado plot is useful for this purpose, which shows for the most important model parameters how their uncertainty influences the results in terms of incremental QALYs.

Results
Monte Carlo simulation

On average, RVX provides better protection against thromboembolic events and intracranial hemorrhages than VKAs do, but is associated with a higher risk of all forms of extracranial hemorrhages (Table 1). However,

for many clinical events there is a large uncertainty on which treatment provides better protection. For example, the risk of ischemic stroke is found to be, on average, lower with RVX than VKAs – i.e. 0.44 less ischemic strokes per 10 patients over their lifetime. However, according to the 95% uncertainty range, this incremental effect may be even bigger (down to 3.18 less ischemic strokes) but RVX may also be harmful, leading up to 2.22 *more* ischemic strokes.

The last column shows that, in the 10,000 iterations of the Monte Carlo simulation, RVX prevents more ischemic strokes than VKAs (around 61% of the time). Notable from Table 1 is that there is little uncertainty on which treatment is associated with less intracranial hemorrhages (RVX in 98% of the iterations), and less major non-AUB extracranial hemorrhages and minor AUBs (VKAs in 91% and 99% of the iterations respectively).

For each iteration in the simulation, the clinical events associated with each treatment were translated into a single health-related utility measure, namely QALYs. Treatment with RVX results, on average, in more QALYs than treatment with VKAs (30.48 vs. 29.91 per subject respectively). There is, however, a 22% chance that VKAs outperform RVX in this respect. This is also made visible in Fig. 2, which shows all the iterations from the Monte Carlo simulation, designating for each iteration the incremental QALYs (x-axis) and incremental costs (y-axis) with RVX as compared to VKAs.

RVX is associated with higher costs than VKAs in 92% of the iterations (Table 1). The mean increment of 0.57 QALYs with RVX comes at an average expense of €16,251. This implies that for every QALY gained with RVX, an additional expense of €28,506 is required. Assuming that within Dutch health care policy-makers are willing to pay €50,000 for each QALY gained, RVX has a 60% probability of being cost-effective.

Value of information analysis

Table 2 shows for each 10-year age group before the age of 51 the estimated number of women in the Netherlands in 2015, as well the results from the VOI analysis. Visible from the table is that the VOI lowers with rising age. For each woman with a baseline age of 20, perfect information on effectiveness and safety yields 0.0849 QALY and has a net monetary benefit of €12,795 when compared with the current status of uncertainty. However, these values are 0.0076 and €1710 with a baseline age of 50. In the total group of premenopausal women in the Netherlands (2015), perfect information would improve women's health with around 122 QALYs and would yield over 22 million Euros. The net monetary benefit represents the value of gaining QALYs and preventing healthcare costs because better decisions are being made.

Table 1 Outcomes of the Monte Carlo simulation in which rivaroxaban (RVX) is compared to vitamin K antagonists (VKAs) for the prevention of stroke in a hypothetical cohort of premenopausal women with atrial fibrillation over their lifetime

	Rivaroxaban (RVX)		Vitamin K antagonists (VKAs)		Increment of RVX vs. VKAs		Chance RVX performs better
	Mean	95% CI[a]	Mean	95% CI[a]	Mean	95% CI[a]	
Benefit/Risk profile							
Clinical events, per 1000 subjects over the lifetime							
Ischemic stroke or TIA	567	408 to 759	611	428 to 832	−44	−318 to +222	61%
Systemic embolism	87	36 to 169	102	47 to 182	−15	−110 to +84	63%
Myocardial infarction	319	190 to 496	362	228 to 533	−43	−141 to +49	84%
Intracranial hemorrhage	136	74 to 226	210	146 to 290	−74	−140 to −8	98%
Extracranial hemorrhage (ECH)							
Major AUB	928	57 to 1990	429	21 to 894	499	−5.83 to +1690	24%
Major other ECH	1023	685 to 1458	832	639 to 1060	191	−65 to +536	9%
Minor AUB	3872	2194 to 5739	1868	1442 to 2314	2004	227 to +3929	1%
Minor other ECH	3763	2670 to 5137	3401	2716 to 4188	362	−513 to +1436	23%
QALYs, per subject	30.48	26.89 to 33.86	29.91	26.31 to 33.34	0.57	−0.80 to 2.15	78%
Cost-effectiveness (×€1000, per subject)							
Healthcare costs	63.7	45.2 to 91.4	47.5	32.5 to 66.7	16.3	−6.1 to 43.1	8%
Costs per QALY gained[b]	–	–	–	–	28.5	–	60%[c]
Net monetary benefit[c]	1460	1276 to 1637	1448	1265 to 1625	12	−75 to 109	60%

[a]The lower bound of the range equals the 2.5th percentile, and the upper bound equals the 97.5th percentile
[b]Otherwise defined as the incremental cost-effectiveness ratio (ICER)
[c]The net monetary benefit (NMB) is the monetary value assigned to the total amount of QALYs that is associated with a treatment, subtracted by the costs of the treatment. We assumed that one QALY was valued with €50,000. The treatment with the highest NMB is considered cost-effective

The tornado plot in Fig. 3 shows what the impact is of the uncertainty concerning the relative risks of RVX versus VKAs on incremental QALYs with RVX as compared to VKAs with regard to specific parameters. Uncertainty on the relative risk of ischemic stroke and major abnormal uterine bleeding has the most prominent impact on incremental QALYs with RVX. For example, under current uncertainty, the relative risk of ischemic stroke with RVX vs. VKAs in premenopausal women ranges from 0.66 to 1.37. If the relative risk would be 1.37, treatment with RVX will lead to a loss of −0.32 QALYs. If, on the other side of the spectrum, the relative risk equals 0.66, treatment with RVX will lead to a gain of 1.69 QALYs. Uncertainty on the relative risk of major non-AUB extracranial hemorrhages has the least impact of the parameters shown here; other parameters like the relative risk of minor hemorrhage, disutilities of clinical events, and utility scores of health states are not shown because the impact of their uncertainty is even smaller.

Discussion

We set out to assess the decision uncertainty on whether RVX or VKAs should be prescribed in premenopausal women with AF. Although RVX is widely prescribed in this subgroup [11–13], first results suggested that the risk of AUB is higher with RVX than with VKAs whereas

it may even be less effective in preventing ischemic strokes [19]. Using a model-based approach, we estimated that there is a 22% chance that the wrong decision is being made by prescribing RVX, implicating worse health outcomes than treatment with VKAs. This does not imply that there is sufficient reason to withhold RVX from premenopausal women – after all, RVX seems to have a 78% probability to have a better benefit/risk profile than VKAs. However, our study suggests that more research needs to be done for this subgroup because of the decision uncertainty.

Further research on the benefit/risk profile of RVX and VKAs in premenopausal women may add to decision-making by clinicians and policy-makers. We estimate that eliminating uncertainty will yield around 122 QALYs and has a value of over 22 million Euros in the Netherlands. The risks of ischemic stroke and major AUB provide the largest contribution to decision uncertainty, and should therefore be of primary concern in further research. As the number of premenopausal women with (paroxysmal) AF is relatively low and a large study population is required to gain enough statistical power to effectively investigate the risk of ischemic stroke, a large registry study is presumably the best option for further research, preferably on an international basis. Another reason to perform a registry study rather

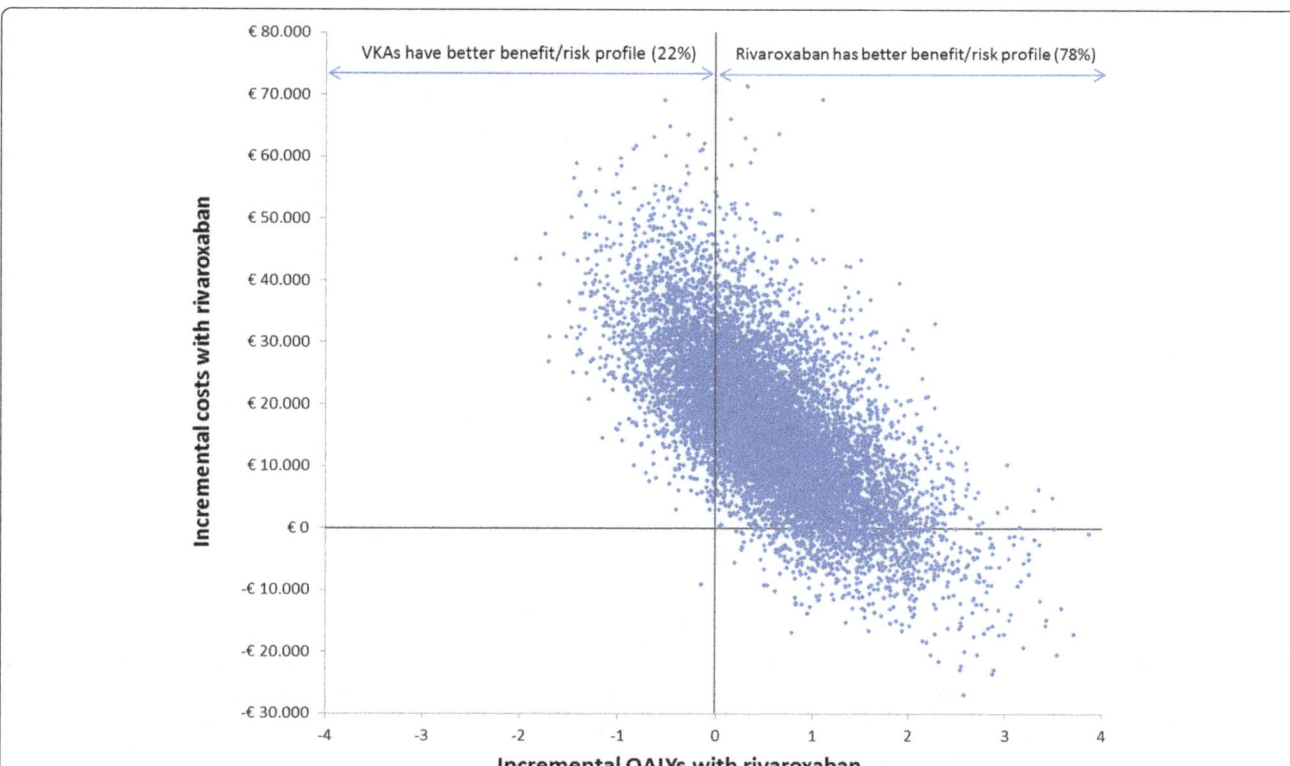

Fig. 2 The probabilities that rivaroxaban leads to better or worse health (x-axis) than vitamin K antagonists (VKAs) in terms of Quality Adjusted Life Years (QALYs) and is more or less costly (y-axis). The figure is the result of the Monte Carlo simulation, in which the Markov model was iterated 10,000 times, whereby clinical event rates, utility scores and health care costs were randomly selected from their uncertainty distributions in each iteration

Table 2 The value of reducing the decision uncertainty surrounding the choice between either rivaroxaban (RVX) or vitamin K antagonists (VKAs) in premenopausal women with atrial fibrillation in the Netherlands

	Per person			Total population		
	Estimated chance[a]	EVPI[b]		Estimated number	Population EVPI[b]	
		QALYs	NMB		QALYs	NMB
Baseline age[c]						
20 yrs	10.5%	0.0849	€12,795	420	35.7	€5,373,900
30 yrs	20%	0.0467	€8311	800	37.4	€6,648,800
40 yrs	49%	0.0219	€4430	1960	42.9	€8,682,800
50 yrs	20.5%	0.0076	€1710	820	6.2	€1,402,200
Total	100%	0.0305	€5527	4000	122.2	€22,107,700

[a]Represents the chance that the female patient with atrial fibrillation belongs to the respective age category

[b]Expected value of perfect information, which equals the outcomes (in terms of QALYs or NMB) when making treatment decisions under perfect information, subtracted with the outcomes when making decisions under current uncertainty. The EVPI consequently also equals the maximum value of information that can be gained with further research

[c]We assumed that the probability of having suffered a previous stroke increases with age: 0.5% in women aged 20; 1% in women aged 30; 2% in women aged 40; and 5% in women aged 50 years

than a randomized controlled trial, is that there is currently no classical equipoise with regard to the right treatment. If other NOACs are prescribed in this population, these should also be included in the registry study.

The empirical evidence used in our model stems from various countries and clinical settings, therefore we believe that the results on the benefit/risk profile per individual are largely expandable to other countries and settings – although possible discrepancies in time in therapeutic with VKAs need to be considered. Our simulation model has several limitations. First, we could not include all currently available NOACs in our analysis. Although dabigatran, apixaban and edoxaban are also likely candidates for the prevention of stroke in premenopausal women with AF, we decided to restrict our analysis to RVX because this is the most prescribed NOAC. However, the bleeding risks that are specific for these women also hold for other NOACs. Therefore, if other NOACs are prescribed to premenopausal women, the events should also be registered in order to perform a comprehensive analysis in the future on which - if any - NOAC is preferred in these specific patients. Second, in general, results of modeling studies greatly depend on the choices made by the researchers, and results might therefore differ between various studies. For example, we assumed that treatment decisions were not associated with

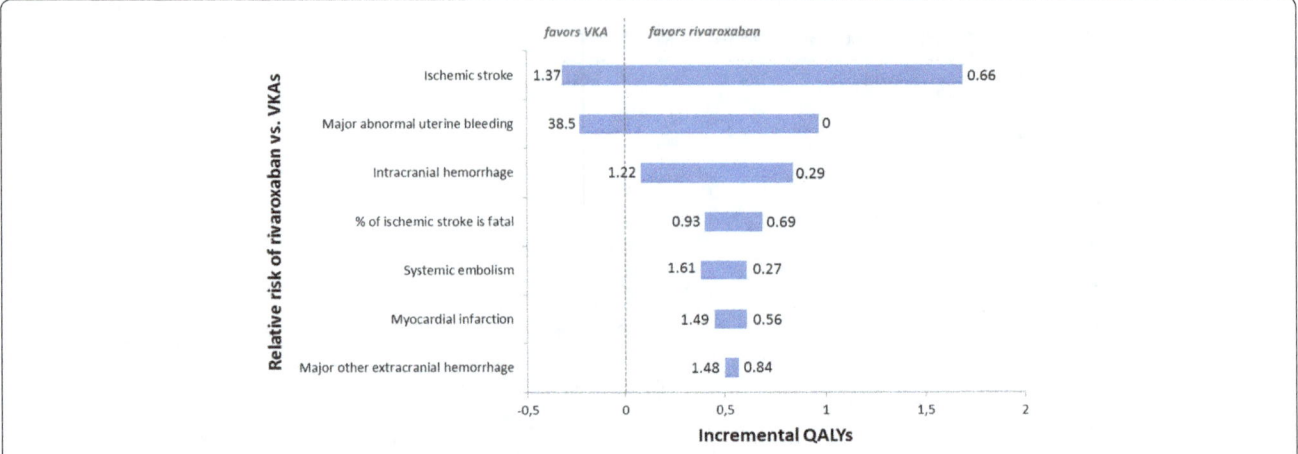

Fig. 3 Tornado plot: Overview of the impact of the main health outcomes on decision uncertainty. The figure shows the impact of the current uncertainty on the relative risks (RRs) of rivaroxaban vs. Vitamin K Antagonists (VKAs) in premenopausal women with atrial fibrillation on Quality Adjusted Life Years (QALYs). For example, the RR of ischemic stroke with rivaroxaban vs. VKAs in premenopausal women currently ranges from 0.66 to 1.37. When the RR is 1.37, treatment with rivaroxaban leads to a loss of −0.32 QALYs. If the RR is 0.66, treatment with rivaroxaban leads to a gain of 1.69 QALYs

a decrement in quality of life. In contrast, several previous cost-effectiveness studies on NOACs did include such decrements [36–38]. We acknowledge that treatment with VKAs are potentially associated with more inconvenience, but do not consider this to have an impact on health-related quality of life. Also, self-measurement of INR may be very common under younger AF patients, and may be less costly than visits to thrombotic clinics. Because we did not include self-measurement in our analysis, the costs associated with treatment with VKAs may be overestimated, which means cost-effectiveness of RVX may also be overestimated.

Our study shows that the limited inclusion of premenopausal women in the phase III trial on RVX, and the omission of a subgroup analysis on them, has provoked decision uncertainty in clinical practice which may be potential harmful for them. This is related to the recurring fact that women are underrepresented in clinical trials, often leading to a false extrapolation of general results [39–41]. Of course, it is important to consider that specific subgroups may need to be excluded from phase III trials for ethical reasons, but the choice for patient exclusion is often not made explicit, raising questions on whether exclusion was justifiable [42, 43].

We propose a more frequent use of model-based studies to aid clinicians in decision making for optimal treatment when clinical study data are missing. Results from such an analyses may also be helpful for funding agencies or governmental bodies in prioritizing research [44, 45], also with the purpose of preventing wasteful studies [46].

Conclusions

As AF often affects patients for the remainder of their life, it is important that the justified weighing of benefits and risks of long-term treatment are being made. We set out to assess the decision uncertainty surrounding a promising new treatment for AF in premenopausal women, a growing subgroup that has been overlooked in previous trials. Our study shows that although RVX seems promising, there is still uncertainty on whether RVX or VKAs should be prescribed in premenopausal women, mainly because of the uncertainty on the risk of AUBs and ischemic strokes. Further research on the use of NOACs in premenopausal women is warranted, and should preferably take the form of an internationally co-ordinated registry study. Estimating and reducing uncertainty on treatment decisions will benefit public health, and estimating the value of additional research may prevent additional wasteful research.

Additional file

Additional file 1: Table S1. Overview of the number of women according to different age groups in the Netherlands in 2015, based on data from Statistics Netherlands, and used as input for the hypothetical cohort in the Markov model. **Table S2.** Relevant clinical event rates in patients with atrial fibrillation treated with rivaroxaban or vitamin K antagonists, as well as possible risk adjustments of these rates (for example based on gender and age), used as input in the Markov model. **Table S3.** Disutility scores associated with the clinical events associated with atrial fibrillation (such as stroke or myocardial infarction), as well as the utility scores associated with health states, used as input in the Markov model. **Table S4.** Costs associated with the treatment of patients with atrial fibrillation with rivaroxaban and vitamin K antagonists, clinical events, as well as health states, used as input in the Markov model. **Table S5.** Costs associated with the monitoring of treatment with rivaroxaban as well as with vitamin K antagonists, used as input in the Markov model. (DOCX 57 kb)

Abbreviations
AF: Atrial fibrillation; AUB: Abnormal uterine bleed; ICER: Incremental cost-effectiveness ratio; NMB: Net monetary benefit; QALY: Quality adjusted life year; Rvx: Rivaroxaban; VKAs: Vitamin K antagonists

Acknowledgements
We would like to thank Anouck Kluytmans for reviewing the Markov model.

Funding
This study was funded by The Netherlands Organisation for Health Research and Development (ZonMw), Project number: 113,105,004; project title: The value of reducing uncertainty: merging ethics and economics; programme: Priority Medicines Elderly.

Authors' contributions
HR, AM, GW, and JG participated in generation of the study idea and aims. HR collected the data for the Markov model from pre-existing empirical studies, and built the model. AM, GW, and JG reviewed and approved the model. HR, AM, GW, and JG participated in the interpretation of study findings, the writing of the manuscript, and the review and approval of the manuscript before submitting it for peer-review.

Competing interests
The authors declare that they have no competing interests.

Author details
[1]Council for Public Health and Society, The Hague, The Netherlands. [2]Department for Health Evidence, Radboud University Medical Center, Nijmegen, The Netherlands. [3]Department of Cardiology, Radboud University Medical Center, Nijmegen, The Netherlands.

References
1. Ball J, Carrington MJ, McMurray JJ, Stewart S. Atrial fibrillation: profile and burden of an evolving epidemic in the 21st century. Int J Cardiol. 2013;167:1807–24.
2. Friberg L, Bergfeldt L. Atrial fibrillation prevalence revisited. J Intern Med. 2013;275:461–8.
3. Chugh SS, Havmoeller R, Narayanan K, Singh D, Rienstra M, Benjamin EJ, et al. Worldwide epidemiology of atrial fibrillation: a global burden of disease 2010 study. Circulation. 2014;129:837–47.
4. Budnitz DS, Lovegrove MC, Shebab N, Richards CL. Emergency hospitalizations for adverse drug events in older Americans. N Engl J Med. 2011;365:2002–12.
5. Yang E. A clinician's perspective: novel oral anticoagulants to reduce the risk of stroke in nonvalvular atrial fibrillation–full speed ahead or proceed with caution? Vasc Health Risk Manag. 2014;10:507–22.
6. Connolly SJ, Ezekowitz MD, Yusuf S, Eikelboom J, Oldgren J, Parekh A, et al. Dabigatran versus warfarin in patients with atrial fibrillation. N Engl J Med. 2009;361:1139–51.
7. Granger CB, Alexander JH, McMurray JJ, Lopes RD, Hylek EM, Hanna M, et al. Apixaban versus warfarin in patients with atrial fibrillation. N Engl J Med. 2011;365:981–92.
8. Patel MR, Mahaffey KW, Garg J, Pan G, Singer DE, Hacke W, et al. Rivaroxaban versus warfarin in nonvalvular atrial fibrillation. N Engl J Med. 2011;365:883–91.
9. Giugliano RP, Ruff CT, Braunwald E, Murphy SA, Wiviott SD, Halperin JL, et al. Edoxaban versus warfarin in patients with atrial fibrillation. N Engl J Med. 2013;369:2093–104.
10. Kirchhof P, Benussi S, Kotecha D, Ahlsson A, Atar D, Casadei B, et al. 2016 ESC guidelines for the management of atrial fibrillation developed in collaboration with EACTS. Eur Heart J. 2016;37:2893–962.
11. Andrade JG, Krahn AD, Skanes AC, Ciaccia A, Connors S. Values and preferences of physicians and patients with nonvalvular atrial fibrillation who receive oral anticoagulation therapy for stroke prevention. Can J Cardiol. 2016;32:747–53.
12. Lee SI, Sayers M, Lip GY, Lane DA. Use of non-vitamin K antagonist oral anticoagulants in atrial fibrillation patients: insights from a specialist atrial fibrillation clinic. Int J Clin Pract. 2015;69:1341–8.
13. Böttger B, Thate-Waschke IM, Bauersachs R, Kohlmann T, Wilke T. Preferences for anticoagulation therapy in atrial fibrillation: the patients' view. J Thromb Thrombolysis. 2015;40:406–15.
14. Ferreira M, Barsam S, Patel JP, Czuprynska J, Roberts LN, Patel RK, et al. Heavy menstrual bleeding on rivaroxaban. Br J Haematol. 2016;173:314–5.
15. Martinelli I, Lensing AW, Middeldorp S, Levi M, Beyer-Westendorf J, van Bellen B, et al. Recurrent venous thromboembolism and abnormal uterine bleeding with anticoagulant and hormone therapy use. Blood. 2016;127:1417–25.
16. Maas AH, Mv E, Bongers MY, Rolden HJ, Grutters JP, Ulrich L, et al. Practice points in gynecardiology: abnormal uterine bleeding in premenopausal women taking oral anticoagulant or antiplatelet therapy. Maturitas. 2015;82:355–9.
17. Statistics Netherlands. CBS Statline: http://statline.cbs.nl/statweb. Accessed 16 Sept 2016.
18. Renoux C, Patenaude V, Suissa S. Incidence, mortality, and sex differences of non-valvular atrial fibrillation: a population-based study. J Am Heart Assoc. 2014;3:e001402.
19. Johnson & Johnson Pharmaceutical Research & Development. Advisory committee briefing document. Rivaroxaban for the prevention of stroke and non-central nervous system (CNS) systemic embolism in patients with atrial fibrillation. 2011. http://www.fda.gov/downloads/AdvisoryCommittees/CommitteesMeetingMaterials/Drugs/CardiovascularandRenalDrugsAdvisoryCommittee/UCM270797.pdf. Accessed 20 Dec 2016. [10 Oct 2017: Link is no longer working, document is no longer available.].
20. Hankey GJ, Patel MR, Stevens SR, Becker RC, Breithardt G, Carolei A, et al. Rivaroxaban compared with warfarin in patients with atrial fibrillation and previous stroke or transient ischaemic attack: a subgroup analysis of ROCKET AF. Lancet Neurol. 2012;11:315–22.
21. Van Walraven C, Hart RG, Connolly S, Austin PC, Mant J, Hobbs FD, et al. Effect of age on stroke prevention therapy in patients with atrial fibrillation: the atrial fibrillation investigators. Stroke. 2009;40:1410–6.
22. Fang MC, Go AS, Chang Y, Hylek EM, Henault LE, Jensvold NG, et al. Death and disability from warfarin-associated intracranial and extracranial hemorrhages. Am J Med. 2007;120:700–5.
23. Leurent G, Garlantézec R, Auffret V, Hacot JP, Coudert I, Filippi E, et al. Gender differences in presentation, management and inhospital outcome in patients with ST-segment elevation myocardial infarction: data from 5000 patients included in the ORBI prospective French regional registry. Arch Cardiovasc Dis. 2014;107:291–8.
24. Sullivan PW, Arant TW, Ellis SL, Ulrich H. The cost effectiveness of anticoagulation management services for patients with atrial fibrillation and at high risk of stroke in the US. PharmacoEconomics. 2006;24:1021–33.
25. O'Brien CL, Gage BF. Costs and effectiveness of ximelagatran for stroke prophylaxis in chronic atrial fibrillation. JAMA. 2005;293:699–706.
26. Tengs TO, Lin TH. A meta-analysis of quality-of-life estimates for stroke. PharmacoEconomics. 2003;21:191–200.
27. The National Health Care Institute [Zorginstituut Nederland]. Kostenhandleiding: Methodologie van kostenonderzoek en referentieprijzen voor economische evaluaties in de gezondheidszorg. https://www.zorginstituutnederland.nl/binaries/content/documents/zinl-www/documenten/publicaties/overige-publicaties/1602-richtlijn-voor-het-uitvoeren-van-economische-evaluaties-in-de-gezondheidszorg-bijlagen/1602-richtlijn-voor-het-uitvoeren-van-economische-evaluaties-in-de-gezondheidszorg-bijlagen/Richtlijn+voor+het+uitvoeren+van+economische+evaluaties+in+de+gezondheidszorg+(verdiepings-modules).pdf. Accessed 16 Sept 2016.
28. Dutch drug costs. Available from: http://www.medicijnkosten.nl.
29. Federation of Dutch Anticoagulant clinics. Samenvatting medische jaarverslagen 2014. http://www.fnt.nl/media/docs/FNT_Samenvatting_Medisch_JV_2014.pdf. Accessed 16 Sept 2016.
30. Struijs JN, van Genugten ML, Evers SM, Ament AJ, Baan CA, van den Bos GA. Future costs of stroke in The Netherlands: the impact of stroke services. Int J Technol Assess Health Care. 2006;22:518–24.
31. Greving JP, Visseren FLJ, De Wit GA, Algra A. Statin treatment for primary prevention of vascular disease: whom to treat? Cost-effectiveness analysis. BMJ. 2011;342:d1672.
32. De Leest HT, Van Dieten HE, Van Tulder MW, Lems WF, Dijkman BA, Boers M. Costs of treating bleeding and perforated peptic ulcers in The Netherlands. J Rheumatol. 2004;31:788–91.
33. Mensch A, Stock S, Stollenwerk B, Müller D. Cost effectiveness of

rivaroxaban for stroke prevention in German patients with atrial fibrillation. PharmacoEconomics. 2015;33:271–83.

34. Statistics Netherlands. CBS Statline: http://statline.cbs.nl/statweb. Accessed 20 Dec 2016.

35. Briggs A, Sculpher M, Claxton K. Decision modelling for health economic evaluation. Oxford: Oxford University Press; 2006.

36. Gage BF, Cardinalli AB, Owens DK. Cost-effectiveness of preference-based antithrombotic therapy for patients with nonvalvular atrial fibrillation. Stroke. 1998;29:1083–91.

37. Rognoni C, Marchetti M, Quaglini S, Liberato NL. Apixaban, dabigatran, and rivaroxaban versus warfarin for stroke prevention in non-valvular atrial fibrillation: a cost-effectiveness analysis. Clin Drug Investig. 2014;34:9–17.

38. Verhoef TI, Redekop WK, Hasrat F, de Boer A, Maitland-van der Zee AH. Cost effectiveness of new oral anticoagulants for stroke prevention in patients with atrial fibrillation in two different European healthcare settings. Am J Cardiovasc Drugs. 2014;14:451–62.

39. Rosano GM, Lewis B, Agewall S, Wassmann S, Vitale C, Schmidt H, et al. Gender differences in the effect of cardiovascular drugs: a position document of the working group on pharmacology and drug therapy of the ESC. Eur Heart J. 2015;36:2677–80.

40. Kim AM, Tingen CM, Woodruff TK. Sex bias in trials and treatment must end. Nature. 2010;465:688–9.

41. Pilote L, Humphries KH. Incorporating sex and gender in cardiovascular research: the time has come. Can J Cardiol. 2014;30:699–702.

42. Van Spall HG, Toren A, Kiss A, Fowler RA. Eligibility criteria of randomized controlled trials published in high-impact general medical journals: a systematic sampling review. JAMA. 2007;297:1233–40.

43. Rolden HJ, Grutters JP, van der Wilt GJ, Maas AH. Closing the information gap between clinical and postmarketing trials: the case of dabigatran. Eur Heart J Cardiovasc Pharmacother. 2015;1:153–6.

44. Claxton KP, Sculpher MJ. Using value of information analysis to prioritise health research: some lessons from recent UK experience. PharmacoEconomics. 2006;24:1055–68.

45. Minelli C, Baio G. Value of information: a tool to improve research prioritization and reduce waste. PLoS Med. 2015;12:e1001882.

46. Chalmers I, Bracken MB, Djulbegovic B, Garattini S, Grant J, Gülmezoglu AM, et al. How to increase value and reduce waste when research priorities are set. Lancet. 2014;383:156–65.

23

Risk profiles and pattern of antithrombotic use in patients with non-valvular atrial fibrillation in Thailand

Rungroj Krittayaphong[1]*[iD], Arjbordin Winijkul[1], Komsing Methavigul[2], Wattana Wongtheptien[3], Chaiyasith Wongvipaporn[4], Treechada Wisaratapong[5], Rapeephon Kunjara-Na-Ayudhya[6], Smonporn Boonyaratvej[7], Chulalak Komoltri[8], Pontawee Kaewcomdee[1], Ahthit Yindeengam[1] and Piyamitr Sritara[9] for the COOL-AF Investigators

Abstract

Background: Anticoagulation therapy is a standard treatment for stroke prevention in patients with non-valvular atrial fibrillation (NVAF) that have risk factors for stroke. However, anticoagulant increases the risk of bleeding, especially in Asians. We aimed to investigate the risk profiles and pattern of antithrombotic use in patients with NVAF in Thailand, and to study the reasons for not using warfarin in this patient population.

Methods: A nationwide multicenter registry of patients with NVAF was created that included data from 24 hospitals located across Thailand. Demographic data, atrial fibrillation-related data, comorbid conditions, use of antithrombotic drugs, and reasons for not using warfarin were collected. Data were recorded in a case record form and then transferred into a web-based system.

Results: A total of 3218 patients were included. Average age was 67.3 ± 11.3 years, and 58.2% were male. Average $CHADS_2$, CHA_2DS_2-VASc, and HAS-BLED score was 1.8 ± 1.3, 3.0 ± 1.7, and 1.5 ± 1.0, respectively. Antiplatelet was used in 26.5% of patients, whereas anticoagulant was used in 75.3%. The main reasons for not using warfarin in those with CHA_2DS_2-VASc ≥ 2 included already taking antiplatelet (26.6%), patient preference (23.1%), and using non-vitamin K antagonist oral anticoagulants (NOACs) (22.7%). Anticoagulant was used in 32.3% of CHA_2DS_2-VASc 0, 56.8% of CHA_2DS_2-VASc 1, and 81.6% of CHA_2DS_2-VASc ≥ 2. The use of NOACs increased from 1.9% in 2014 to 25.6% in 2017.

Conclusions: Anticoagulation therapy was prescribed in 75.3% of patients with NVAF. Among those receiving anticoagulant, 90.9% used warfarin and 9.1% used NOACs. The use of NOACs increased over time.

Keywords: Risk profiles, Antithrombotics, Non-valvular atrial fibrillation, Thailand

Background

Non-valvular atrial fibrillation (NVAF) is a common cardiac arrhythmia in clinical practice with a prevalence of approximately 1–2% [1, 2] which may be higher in patients with structural disease [3]. NVAF create a slow-flow situation within the atrium especially left atrial appendage leading to thrombus formation and thromboembolic event [1]. Current practice guidelines recommend the use of anticoagulant in patients with NVAF that have additional risk factor(s) for stroke [4, 5]. CHA_2DS_2VASc score has been recommended as a risk stratification tool for predicting stroke in this group [4]. The annual risk of ischemic stroke in patients with non-valvular atrial fibrillation (NVAF) may be higher than 5% in patients with a high CHA_2DS_2-VASc score [1]. Warfarin is associated with many types of food- and drug-related interactions, so international normalized ratio (INR) monitoring is needed [6, 7]. Although there are many non-vitamin K antagonist oral anticoagulants (NOAC), such as direct thrombin inhibitor and factor Xa inhibitors, warfarin is still widely used in Asian, and in low and middle income countries [8, 9]. Although anticoagulation therapy can reduce ischemic stroke, it can also cause or contribute to major bleeding or intracerebral

* Correspondence: rungroj.kri@mahidol.ac.th
[1]Division of Cardiology, Department of Medicine, Faculty of Medicine Siriraj Hospital, Mahidol University, 2 Wanglang Road, Bangkoknoi, Bangkok 10700, Thailand
Full list of author information is available at the end of the article

hemorrhage. Asian population was reported to have a higher risk of intracerebral hemorrhage, as a proportion of subtype of stroke, compared to Western population [2, 10]. Asian population also demonstrated a higher risk of warfarin-related intracerebral hemorrhage and bleeding-related complications [11, 12]. For a variety of reasons, anticoagulant is prescribed in less than half of patients with AF, including those in the intermediate- and high-risk groups [13, 14]. It is, therefore, important to study and understand the pattern of use of anti-thrombotic medication via the analysis of real-world data in this era.

Accordingly, the aim of this study was to investigate the risk profiles and pattern of antithrombotic use in patients with NVAF in Thailand, and to study the reasons for not using warfarin in this patient population.

Methods

Study population and data

NVAF patients were consecutively enrolled from 24 hospitals located all across Thailand. Thirteen of those centers are university hospitals, and ten are regional or general hospitals. The protocol for this study was approved by the institutional review boards (IRBs) of the Thailand Ministry of Public Health and IRB of each participating hospital namely Buddhachinaraj Hospital, Central Chest Institute of Thailand, Charoen Krung Pracha Rak Hospital, Chiangrai Prachanukroh Hospital, Chonburi Hospital, Chiang Mai Hospital, King Chulalongkorn Memorial Hospital, Naresuan University Hospital, Songklanakarind Hospital, Ramathibodi Hospital, Siriraj Hospital, Thammasat Hospital, Golden Jubilee Medical Center, Srinakarind Hospital, Lampang Hospital, Maharat Nakorn Ratchasima Hospital, Nakornping Hospital, Phramongkutklao Hospital, Police General Hospital, Prapokklao Hospital (Chanthaburi), Ratchaburi Hospital, Surat Thani Hospital, Surin Hospital, and Udonthani Hospital. All patients provided written informed consent prior to participation in this study. Patients aged ≥18 years with atrial fibrillation diagnosed by standard ECG or ambulatory monitoring were eligible for inclusion. Patients having one or more of the following were excluded: 1) ischemic stroke within 3 months; 2) thrombocytopenia (< 100,000/mm3), myeloproliferative disorders, hyperviscosity syndrome, or antiphospholipid syndrome; 3) prosthetic valve or valve repair; 4) rheumatic valve disease or significant valve disease; 5) atrial fibrillation from transient reversible cause (e.g., during respiratory tract infection or bronchospasm); 6) ongoing participation in a clinical trial; 7) life expectancy less than 3 years; 8) pregnancy; 9) inability to attend scheduled follow-up appointments; 10) refusal to join the study; and/or, 11) current hospitalization or hospitalization within 1 month prior to inclusion in the study.

Baseline demographic and clinical data were collected and recorded. Patients were followed-up at 6, 12, 18, 24, 30, and 36 months. Data relating to cardiovascular events, blood pressure, heart rate, and medications were collected at each follow-up visit. Data from each patient was written on a case record form and keyed into a web-based data collection and management system. The following data were collected: 1) demographic information; 2) history of stroke and bleeding; 3) type and duration of atrial fibrillation; 4) component parameters of CHADS2 score, CHA2DS2VASc score for stroke risk, and HAS-BLED score for risk of bleeding; 5) history of medical and cardiovascular disease; 6) antithrombotic medication; 7) reason for not using warfarin in those not taking warfarin; 8) concomitant medications; 9) twelve-lead ECG; and, 10) current INR. Protocols were established and followed by the data management team and statisticians to ensure the integrity and quality of the data before final analysis. Random site monitoring was also regularly performed. Approximately 70% of sites were audited. Data were collected during the 2014 to 2017 study period.

Statistical analysis

Demographic and clinical data were interpreted using descriptive statistics. Continuous data are presented as mean ± standard deviation, and categorical data are shown as number and percentage. All statistical analyses were performed using SPSS Statistics version 20 (SPSS, Inc., Chicago, IL, USA).

Results

A total of 3218 patients from 24 hospitals were included. Average age was 67.3 ± 11.3 years, and 1873 (58.2%) were male. Baseline demographic data, clinical characteristics, and use of antithrombotic medications are shown in Table 1. Average $CHADS_2$, CHA_2DS_2-VASc, and HAS-BLED score was 1.8 ± 1.3, 3.0 ± 1.7, and 1.5 ± 1.0, respectively. One-hundred and three patients (3.2%) had history of radiofrequency ablation for atrial fibrillation. Among patients with coronary artery disease (CAD), 60 patients (1.9%) had history of percutaneous coronary intervention (PCI) within 12 months.

Antiplatelet and anticoagulant was used in 854 (26.5%) and 2422 (75.3%) patients, respectively. Anticoagulant alone was used in 2125 (66.0%) patients. Antiplatelet alone was prescribed in 557 (17.3%) patients, and used in combination with anticoagulant in 297 (9.2%) patients. Two hundred and thirty-nine (9.2%) patients were taking no antithrombotic medications. Figure 1 describes the rate of use of antithrombotic agents in patients with different CHA_2DS_2-VASc and HAS-BLED scores. The rate of anticoagulant use increased in patients with a higher CHA_2DS_2-VASc score. Anticoagulant was used in 67 (32.3%) patients with a CHA_2DS_2-VASc of 0, in 238 (56.8%) patients with a

Table 1 Baseline characteristics of the study population and reasons for not using warfarin for those with CHA2DS2-VASc score ≥ 2

Variables	$N = 3218$
Age (years), mean ± SD	67.3 ± 11.3
Male gender, n (%)	1873 (58.2%)
Time after diagnosis of atrial fibrillation (years), mean ± SD	3.4 ± 4.4
Type of atrial fibrillation, n (%)	
- New	74 (2.3%)
- Paroxysmal	1001 (31.1%)
- Persistent	623 (19.4%)
- Permanent	1520 (47.2%)
History of heart failure, n (%)	875 (27.2%)
History of coronary artery disease, n (%)	505 (15.7%)
Devices, n (%)	330 (10.3%)
History of transient ischemic attack, n (%)	121 (3.8%)
History of ischemic stroke, n (%)	451 (14.0%)
Hypertension, n (%)	2183 (67.8%)
Diabetes mellitus, n (%)	777 (24.1%)
History of bleeding, n (%)	308 (9.6%)
Antithrombotic medications, n (%)	
Antiplatelet	854 (26.5%)
- Aspirin	761 (88.0%)
- ADP/P2Y12 inhibitors	191 (22.2%)
Anticoagulant	2422 (75.3%)
- Warfarin	2202 (90.9%)
- Direct thrombin inhibitor	80 (3.3%)
- Factor Xa inhibitors	140 (5.8%)
CHADS$_2$ score, n (%)	
- 0	479 (14.9%)
- 1	955 (29.7%)
- 2	977 (30.4%)
- 3	480 (14.9%)
- 4	237 (7.4%)
- 5	79 (2.5%)
- 6	11 (0.3)
CHA2DS2-VASc score, n (%)	
- 0	207 (6.4%)
- 1	419 (13.0%)
- 2	674 (20.9%)
- 3	736 (22.9%)
- 4	589 (18.3%)
- 5	365 (11.3%)

Table 1 Baseline characteristics of the study population and reasons for not using warfarin for those with CHA2DS2-VASc score ≥ 2 (Continued)

Variables	$N = 3218$
- 6	163 (5.1%)
- 7	51 (1.6%)
- 8	13 (0.4%)
- 9	1 (0%)
HAS-BLED score, n (%)	
- 0	458 (14.2%)
- 1	1190 (37.0%)
- 2	1067 (33.2%)
- 3	403 (12.5%)
- 4	84 (2.6%)
- 5	15 (0.5%)
- 6	1 (0%)
Main reasons for not using warfarin, n (%)	653 (20.3%)
- Already taking anti-platelet drugs	174 (26.6%)
- Patient preference	151 (23.1%)
- Using NOACS	148 (22.7%)
- Bleeding risk	90 (13.8%)
- Physician preference	89 (13.6%)
- Fall risk	27 (4.1%)
- Warfarin compliance concern	22 (3.4%)
- Taking medication contra-indicated or cautioned for use with Warfarin	6 (0.9%)
- Allergy	1 (0.2%)

CHA$_2$DS$_2$-VASc score of 1, and in 2117 (81.6%) patients with a CHA$_2$DS$_2$-VASc score of ≥2 (Fig. 1a). Increased risk of bleeding, as reflected by a higher HAS-BLED score, did not influence a reduction in the use of anticoagulant (Fig. 1b). Among those who received anticoagulant, 2202 (90.9%) used warfarin and 220 (9.1%) used NOACs. When we analyzed the rate of NOAC use stratified by year of recruitment, an increase in the rate of NOAC use from 1.9% in 2014 to 25.6% in 2017 was observed (Additional file 1).

The reasons for not using warfarin in patients with a CHA$_2$DS$_2$-VASc score ≥ 2 that were not taking warfarin are shown in Table 1. The main reasons included already taking antiplatelet in 174 (26.6%) patients, patient preference not to take warfarin in 151 (23.1%), and current use of NOACs in 148 (22.7%).

Discussion

In this study of 2014–2017 data from a multicenter registry in Thailand for patients with NVAF, we found a rate of anticoagulant use of 75.3%. However, only 41.8%

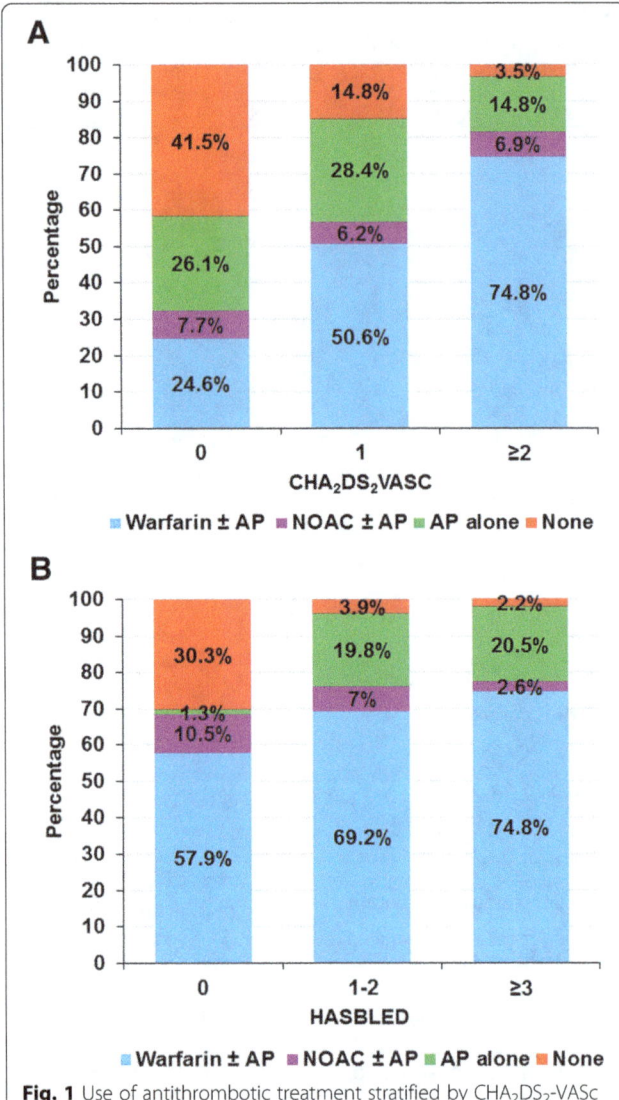

Fig. 1 Use of antithrombotic treatment stratified by CHA$_2$DS$_2$-VASc score (**a**) and HAS-BLED (**b**) score. (Abbreviations: AP, antiplatelet; NOAC, non-vitamin K antagonist oral anticoagulant)

Data from the initial phase of GLORIA AF during 2011 to 2013 indicated that the rate of anticoagulant use was only 33% [26]. Anticoagulant use increased to 80% during phase 2, which enrolled patients until 2014. There was a difference in the rate of anticoagulant use (90% vs. 52%) and NOAC use (52% vs. 28%) between Western and Asian populations in GLORIA phase 2 [27]. Anticoagulant use in the present study was greater than the rate among Asian population in GLORIA phase 2, but the use of NOACs in our study was lower. In addition to China – Japan, Korea, Taiwan, and Singapore participated in GLORIA – all of which are high income Asian countries. In many other low to middle income countries like Thailand, governments limit the use of and reimbursement for new and expensive drugs. Regardless, our data shows an increase in the use of NOACs over time by year of enrollment.

Other registries in Western population include the ORBIT AF registry [16], which was conducted in the US during 2010 to 2011, and EORP AF, which was conducted in European countries [18]. Both studies confirmed a high rate of anticoagulant use (76% and 80%, respectively). However, among very low-risk patients (i.e., CHA$_2$DS$_2$-VASc 0), the rate of anticoagulant use from previous reports is 38–56% [16, 18, 22], which is close to consistent with the 32% rate of use found in the present study. Some patients may be on anticoagulation for reasons that include pre-cardioversion and/or post-cardioversion anticoagulation therapy, or they might have some degree of left ventricular systolic dysfunction, but they did not fit the criteria for CHA$_2$DS$_2$-VASc scor. This data also suggests that physicians fear stroke, even in patients at very low risk. In very low-risk patients, especially when young, an anatomical approach should be considered to delay relapse and to maintain sinus rhythm in order to reduce the need for OAC [28].

We herewith propose some possible explanations regarding why we observed a relatively high rate of anticoagulant use in this study. First, our registry is more recent. Second, almost all of the patients included in this study were managed by cardiologists, which may provide better care for patients with NVAF than non-cardiologists [29]. Third, most of the centers that participated in this registry are tertiary care hospitals.

Reasons for not using warfarin in this study included taking antiplatelet in 26.6%, patient preference (or patient prefers not to take anticoagulants) in 23.1%, and current use of NOACs in 22.7%. The main reason for not using warfarin from the GARFIELD registry [22] was physician's choice (48.3%). Already taking antiplatelet is the reason for not using warfarin in only 7.2% of patients in the GARFIELD registry. This rate is much lower than the rate from our study, which indicates that the use of antiplatelet remains more common among Asian population.

of NVAF patients on warfarin had an INR within the 2–3 therapeutic range.

The baseline profiles of our study population are similar to the profiles described in previous reports [15–18]. The higher rate of anticoagulant use of 75.3% in this study compared to previous publications [13, 19] may be due to the implementation of clinical practice guidelines for the management of patients with NVAF [5, 20, 21].

GARFIELD AF enrolled patients with newly diagnosed NVAF starting with Cohort 1 in 2010–2011 [22, 23]. Only 56% of patients in Cohort 1 received anticoagulant. The rate of anticoagulant use markedly increased in 2015 [24]. Asian population in the GARFIELD registry had a lower percentage of anticoagulant use when compared to other regions of the world (38% vs. 53%) [25].

This study has some mentionable limitations. First, our study population was enrolled mainly from university hospitals or large regional hospitals, which limits the generalizability. Second, we were unable to correlate the findings of this study with clinical outcomes since the 3-year follow-up data acquisition process is not yet completed.

Conclusion

Antithrombotic drugs were prescribed in 75.3% of patients with NVAF. Among those who received anticoagulant, 90.9% used warfarin and 9.1% used NOACs.

Abbreviations

INR: International normalized ratio; IRB: Institutional review board; NOAC: Non-vitamin K antagonist oral anticoagulant; NVAF: Non-valvular atrial fibrillation; TIA: Transient ischemic attack

Acknowledgements

The authors gratefully acknowledge Wipaporn Wangworatrakul, Olaree Chaiphet, and Wilasinee Phromawan for data management, and all investigators and nurse coordinators for their assistance with patient enrollment and their commitment to maintaining a high level of data quality. The authors would also like to thank all of the patients that agreed to participate in this study.

Investigators list

Buddhachinaraj Hospital: Tomorn Thongsri, MD; Central Chest Institute of Thailand: Kriengkrai Hengrussamee, MD; Charoen Krung Pracha Rak Hospital: Pattraporn Srirattana, MD; Chiangrai Prachanukroh Hospital: Wattana Wongtheptien, MD; Chonburi Hospital: Pornchai Ngamjanyaporn, MD; Faculty of Medicine, Chiang Mai University: Arintaya Phrommintikul, MD; Faculty of Medicine, Chulalongkorn University: Smonporn Boonyaratavej, MD; Faculty of Medicine, Naresuan University: Pongpun Jittham, MD; Faculty of Medicine, Prince of Songkla University: Treechada Wisaratapong, MD; Faculty of Medicine Ramathibodi Hospital, Mahidol University: Sirin Apiyasawat, MD; Faculty of Medicine Siriraj Hospital, Mahidol University: Arjbordin Winijkul, MD, Rungroj Krittayaphong, MD; Faculty of Medicine, Thammasat University (Rangsit Campus): Roj Rojjarekampai, MD; Faculty of Medicine Vajira Hospital, Navamindradhiraj University: Kulyot Jongpiputvanich, MD; Golden Jubilee Medical Center: Somchai Dutsadeevettakul, MD; Srinakarind Hospital, Faculty of Medicine, Khon Kaen University: Chaiyasith Wongvipaporn, MD; Lampang Hospital: Thanita Boonyapiphat, MD; Maharat Nakorn Ratchasima Hospital: Weerapan Wiwatworapan, MD; Nakornping Hospital: Khanchai Siriwattana, MD; Pattani Hospital: Eakarnantha Arnanththanitha, MD; Photharam Hospital: Watchara Konkaew, MD; Phramongkutklao College of Medicine: Thoranis Chantrarat, MD; Police General Hospital: Kasem Ratanasumawong, MD; Prapokklao Hospital (Chanthaburi): Wiwat Kanjanarutjawiwat, MD; Queen Savang Vadhana Memorial Hospital: Sakaorat Kornbongkotmas; MD; Ratchaburi Hospital: Thanasak Patmuk, MD; Sapphasitthiprasong Hospital: Praprut Thanakitcharu, MD; Surat Thani Hospital: Suchart Arunsiriwattana, MD; Surin Hospital: Thaworn Choochunklin; MD; Udonthani Hospital: Sumon Tangsuntornwiwat, MD.

Funding

This study was funded by the Health System Research Institute (HSRI) (59–053), the Heart Association of Thailand under the Royal Patronage of H.M. the King, and the Royal College of Physicians of Thailand. None of the aforementioned funding sources influenced any aspect of this study or the authors' decision to submit this manuscript for publication.

Authors' contributions

RK - concept and design, data acquisition, interpretation of data, manuscript preparation, manuscript revision, and manuscript review; AW, KM, RKN, SB, PS - concept and design, data acquisition, interpretation of data, manuscript revision, and manuscript review; WW, CW, TW - data acquisition, manuscript revision, and manuscript review; CK - data interpretation, manuscript revision, and manuscript review; PK, AY - concept and design, data acquisition, manuscript revision, and manuscript review. All authors read and approved the final manuscript, and approved the submission of this manuscript for journal publication.

Competing interests

The authors declare that they have no competing interest.

Author details

[1]Division of Cardiology, Department of Medicine, Faculty of Medicine Siriraj Hospital, Mahidol University, 2 Wanglang Road, Bangkoknoi, Bangkok 10700, Thailand. [2]Department of Cardiology, Central Chest Institute of Thailand, Nonthaburi, Thailand. [3]Chiangrai Prachanukroh Hospital, Chiang Rai, Thailand. [4]Srinakarind Hospital, Faculty of Medicine, Khon Kaen University, Khon Kaen, Thailand. [5]Faculty of Medicine, Prince of Songkla University, Songkla, Thailand. [6]Vichaiyut Hospital and Medical Center, Bangkok, Thailand. [7]Faculty of Medicine, Chulalongkorn University, Bangkok, Thailand. [8]Department of Research Promotion, Faculty of Medicine Siriraj Hospital, Mahidol University, Bangkok, Thailand. [9]Faculty of Medicine Ramathibodi Hospital, Mahidol University, Bangkok, Thailand.

References

1. Lip GYH, Brechin CM, Lane DA. The global burden of atrial fibrillation and stroke: a systematic review of the epidemiology of atrial fibrillation in regions outside North America and Europe. Chest. 2012;142(6):1489–98.
2. Tse HF, Wang YJ, Ahmed Ai-Abdullah M, Pizarro-Borromeo AB, Chiang CE, Krittayaphong R, Singh B, Vora A, Wang CX, Zubaid M, et al. Stroke prevention in atrial fibrillation--an Asian stroke perspective. Heart Rhythm. 2013;10(7):1082–8.
3. Anselmino M, Ferraris F, Cerrato N, Barbero U, Scaglione M, Gaita F. Left persistent superior vena cava and paroxysmal atrial fibrillation: the role of selective radio-frequency transcatheter ablation. J Cardiovasc Med (Hagerstown). 2014;15(8):647–52.
4. Kirchhof P, Benussi S, Kotecha D, Ahlsson A, Atar D, Casadei B, Castella M, Diener HC, Heidbuchel H, Hendriks J, et al. 2016 ESC guidelines for the management of atrial fibrillation developed in collaboration with EACTS. Eur Heart J. 2016;37(38):2893–962.
5. Chiang CE, Okumura K, Zhang S, Chao TF, Siu CW, Wei Lim T, Saxena A, Takahashi Y, Siong Teo W. 2017 consensus of the Asia Pacific Heart Rhythm Society on stroke prevention in atrial fibrillation. J Arrhythm. 2017;33(4):345–67.
6. Holbrook AM, Pereira JA, Labiris R, McDonald H, Douketis JD, Crowther M, Wells PS. Systematic overview of warfarin and its drug and food interactions. Arch Intern Med. 2005;165(10):1095–106.
7. Connolly SJ, Pogue J, Eikelboom J, Flaker G, Commerford P, Franzosi MG, Healey JS, Yusuf S, Investigators AW. Benefit of oral anticoagulant over antiplatelet therapy in atrial fibrillation depends on the quality of international normalized ratio control achieved by centers and countries as measured by time in therapeutic range. Circulation. 2008;118(20):2029–37.
8. Guo Y, Wang H, Tian Y, Wang Y, Lip GYH. Time trends of aspirin and warfarin use on stroke and bleeding events in Chinese patients with new-onset atrial fibrillation. Chest. 2015;148(1):62–72.
9. Jedsadayanmata A. Patterns and adherence to guidelines of antithrombotic therapy in Thai patients with nonvalvular atrial fibrillation. J Med Assoc Thail. 2013;96(1):91–8.
10. Chau PH, Woo J, Goggins WB, Tse YK, Chan KC, Lo SV, Ho SC. Trends in stroke incidence in Hong Kong differ by stroke subtype. Cerebrovasc Dis. 2011;31(2):138–46.
11. Shen AY, Yao JF, Brar SS, Jorgensen MB, Chen W. Racial/ethnic differences in the risk of intracranial hemorrhage among patients with atrial fibrillation. J Am Coll Cardiol. 2007;50(4):309–15.
12. Chiang CE, Wang KL, Lip GYH. Stroke prevention in atrial fibrillation: an Asian perspective. Thromb Haemost. 2014;111(5):789–97.
13. Waldo AL, Becker RC, Tapson VF, Colgan KJ, Committee NS. Hospitalized patients with atrial fibrillation and a high risk of stroke are not being provided with adequate anticoagulation. J Am Coll Cardiol. 2005;46(9):1729–36.

14. Yang X, Li Z, Zhao X, Wang C, Liu L, Wang C, Pan Y, Li H, Wang D, Hart RG, et al. Use of warfarin at discharge among acute ischemic stroke patients with Nonvalvular atrial fibrillation in China. Stroke. 2016;47(2):464–70.

15. Chiang CE, Wang KL, Lin SJ. Asian strategy for stroke prevention in atrial fibrillation. Europace. 2015;17(Suppl 2):ii31–9.

16. Cullen MW, Kim S, Piccini JP Sr, Ansell JE, Fonarow GC, Hylek EM, Singer DE, Mahaffey KW, Kowey PR, Thomas L, et al. Risks and benefits of anticoagulation in atrial fibrillation: insights from the outcomes registry for better informed treatment of atrial fibrillation (ORBIT-AF) registry. Circ Cardiovasc Qual Outcomes. 2013;6(4):461–9.

17. Oldgren J, Healey JS, Ezekowitz M, Commerford P, Avezum A, Pais P, Zhu J, Jansky P, Sigamani A, Morillo CA, et al. Variations in cause and management of atrial fibrillation in a prospective registry of 15,400 emergency department patients in 46 countries: the RE-LY atrial fibrillation registry. Circulation. 2014;129(15):1568–76.

18. Lip GY, Laroche C, Dan GA, Santini M, Kalarus Z, Rasmussen LH, Oliveira MM, Mairesse G, Crijns HJ, Simantirakis E, et al. A prospective survey in European Society of Cardiology member countries of atrial fibrillation management: baseline results of EUObservational research Programme atrial fibrillation (EORP-AF) pilot general registry. Europace. 2014;16(3):308–19.

19. Gage BF, Boechler M, Doggette AL, Fortune G, Flaker GC, Rich MW, Radford MJ. Adverse outcomes and predictors of underuse of antithrombotic therapy in medicare beneficiaries with chronic atrial fibrillation. Stroke. 2000; 31(4):822–7.

20. Guidelines for Pharmacotherapy of Atrial Fibrillation (JCS 2013). Circ J 2014, 78(8):1997–2021.

21. Chiang CE, Wu TJ, Ueng KC, Chao TF, Chang KC, Wang CC, Lin YJ, Yin WH, Kuo JY, Lin WS, et al. 2016 guidelines of the Taiwan Heart Rhythm Society and the Taiwan Society of Cardiology for the management of atrial fibrillation. J Formos Med Assoc. 2016;115(11):893–952.

22. Kakkar AK, Mueller I, Bassand JP, Fitzmaurice DA, Goldhaber SZ, Goto S, Haas S, Hacke W, Lip GY, Mantovani LG, et al. Risk profiles and antithrombotic treatment of patients newly diagnosed with atrial fibrillation at risk of stroke: perspectives from the international, observational, prospective GARFIELD registry. PLoS One. 2013;8(5):e63479.

23. Fox KAA, Gersh BJ, Traore S, John Camm A, Kayani G, Krogh A, Shweta S, Kakkar AK, Investigators G-A. Evolving quality standards for large-scale registries: the GARFIELD-AF experience. Eur Heart J Qual Care Clin Outcomes. 2017;3(2):114–22.

24. Camm AJ, Accetta G, Ambrosio G, Atar D, Bassand JP, Berge E, Cools F, Fitzmaurice DA, Goldhaber SZ, Goto S, et al. Evolving antithrombotic treatment patterns for patients with newly diagnosed atrial fibrillation. Heart. 2017;103(4):307–14.

25. Oh S, Goto S, Accetta G, Angchaisuksiri P, Camm AJ, Cools F, Haas S, Kayani G, Koretsune Y, Lim TW, et al. Vitamin K antagonist control in patients with atrial fibrillation in Asia compared with other regions of the world: real-world data from the GARFIELD-AF registry. Int J Cardiol. 2016;223:543–7.

26. Huisman MV, Ma CS, Diener HC, Dubner SJ, Halperin JL, Rothman KJ, Teutsch C, Schoof N, Kleine E, Bartels DB, et al. Antithrombotic therapy use in patients with atrial fibrillation before the era of non-vitamin K antagonist oral anticoagulants: the global registry on long-term oral antithrombotic treatment in patients with atrial fibrillation (GLORIA-AF) phase I cohort. Europace. 2016;18(9):1308–18.

27. Huisman MV, Rothman KJ, Paquette M, Teutsch C, Diener HC, Dubner SJ, Halperin JL, Ma CS, Zint K, Elsaesser A, et al. The changing landscape for stroke prevention in AF: findings from the GLORIA-AF registry phase 2. J Am Coll Cardiol. 2017;69(7):777–85.

28. Barbero U, Ho SY. Anatomy of the atria : A road map to the left atrial appendage. *Herzschrittmacherther Elektrophysiol*. 2017;28(4):347–54.

29. Turakhia MP, Hoang DD, Xu X, Frayne S, Schmitt S, Yang F, Phibbs CS, Than CT, Wang PJ, Heidenreich PA. Differences and trends in stroke prevention anticoagulation in primary care vs cardiology specialty management of new atrial fibrillation: the retrospective evaluation and assessment of therapies in AF (TREAT-AF) study. Am Heart J. 2013;165(1):93–101. e101

24

Vasodilator-stimulated phosphoprotein-guided Clopidogrel maintenance therapy reduces cardiovascular events in atrial fibrillation patients requiring anticoagulation therapy and scheduled for percutaneous coronary intervention

Chaoyue Hu[1†], Xumin Zhang[2†], Yonghua Liu[3], Yang Gao[2], Xiaohong Zhao[2], Hua Zhou[2], Yu Luo[2], Yaling Liu[4*] and Xiaodong Wang[2*] ⓘ

Abstract

Background: In a previous study, we found that titrating clopidogrel maintenance doses (MDs) according to vasodilator-stimulated phosphoprotein (VASP) monitoring minimised the rate of major adverse cardiovascular and cerebral events (MACCE) after percutaneous coronary intervention (PCI) without increasing bleeding in patients with high on-treatment platelet reaction to clopidogrel. This study aimed to investigate whether VASP-guided clopidogrel MD could reduce thromboembolism and bleeding in atrial fibrillation (AF) patients requiring anticoagulation and scheduled for PCI.

Methods: AF patients scheduled for PCI were recruited between July 2014 and July 2016. These patients were allocated into VASP-guided ($n = 250$) and control ($n = 253$) groups depending on the clopidogrel MD profile. In the VASP-guided group, clopidogrel MD was titrated by the platelet reactivity index (PRI), whereas in the control group, clopidogrel MD was fixed at 75 mg per day. The primary endpoint was MACCE and secondary endpoints were thrombolysis in myocardial infarction (TIMI) major and minor bleeding 1 year after PCI.

Results: Five hundred and three patients were included in the present study, with 1-year data available for 95.6% patients. The average CHA_2DS_2-VASc score of the whole population was 3.7 ± 0.7 and the average HAS-BLED score was 3.2 ± 0.4. MACCE was less in the VASP-guided group than in the control group (2.5% vs. 5.0%, $P = 0.02$). The incidence of major bleeding was comparable between both groups (3.0% vs. 2.8%, $P = 0.72$) and minor bleeding was higher in the VASP-guided group than in the control group (15.3% vs. 9.7%, $P = 0.03$). Kaplan-Meier analysis indicated that there was no difference in survival between both groups (log-rank test, $P = 0.68$).

(Continued on next page)

* Correspondence: liuyaling198003@126.com; 1978wangxiaodong@163.com
†Chaoyue Hu and Xumin Zhang contributed equally to this work.
⁴Department of Anesthesiology, Renji Hospital, Shanghai Jiaotong University School of Medicine, 160 Pujian Road, Shanghai 200127, China
²Department of Cardiology, Shanghai East Hospital, Tongji University School of Medicine, 150 Jimo Road, Shanghai 200120, China
Full list of author information is available at the end of the article

(Continued from previous page)

Conclusions: In AF patients requiring anticoagulation and scheduled for PCI, VASP-guided antiplatelet therapy reduced major cardiovascular and cerebral adverse events, accompanied by increased minor bleeding events.

Keywords: Atrial fibrillation, Anticoagulation, Vasodilator-stimulated phosphoprotein, Clopidogrel, Percutaneous coronary intervention

Background

Atrial fibrillation (AF) is the most common abnormal cardiac rhythm, having a high risk of thromboembolism and causing detrimental clinical outcomes. About 5 to 10% of AF patients requiring oral anticoagulation undergo coronary stent implantation [1]. This spectrum of patients requires combined therapy with oral anticoagulation, aspirin, and P2Y12 receptor blocker, which is known as triple therapy (TT). The most common combination currently consists of the vitamin K antagonist warfarin, and aspirin and clopidogrel.

Although TT has a potentially beneficial antithrombotic effect, prolonged TT therapy may increase bleeding risk. Current guidelines recommend the concomitant administration of TT for short consecutive periods [2]. Clopidogrel, preferred to other novel P2Y12 receptor blockers (prasugrel and ticagrelor), is the only thienopyridine recommended in guidelines. In our previous study, we found that titrating clopidogrel maintenance doses (MDs) according to vasodilator-stimulated phosphoprotein (VASP) monitoring minimised the rate of major adverse cardiovascular and cerebral events (MACCE) after percutaneous coronary intervention (PCI) without increasing bleeding in patients with high on-treatment platelet reaction (HTPR) to clopidogrel at 1-year follow-up [3].

Methods

Aim

In the present study, we aimed to clarify whether VASP-guided clopidogrel MD could decrease adverse clinical events in AF patients requiring anticoagulation and scheduled for PCI.

Study design and patients

This was a prospective cohort study that included consecutive patients with stable coronary artery disease who had AF requiring anticoagulation and were scheduled for PCI. Patients were included if they 1) were older than 18 years and no more than 80 years, 2) had a preexisting diagnosis of paroxysmal, persistent, or permanent AF with anticoagulation therapy warfarin, 3) had effort angina pectoris despite optimal medical therapy, and 4) had silent ischaemia on radionuclide imaging. Exclusion criteria included cardiac

arrest, New York Heart Association III/IV function, platelet count $< 100 \times 10^9$/L, creatinine clearance rate < 25 mL/min.

We included patients from Shanghai East Hospital, a teaching hospital of Tongji University serving a population of approximately 5,500,000, with 12 intervention specialists and 2000 PCI procedures each year. Five hundred patients were randomly allocated to the VASP-guided and control groups. A statistician performed the allocation. Blinding was used for the participants and/or researchers. We collected data on demographic and clinical characteristics, prothrombotic risk factors, and antithrombotic therapy strategies before and after PCI. Patients' thromboembolism risk was evaluated by the CHA_2DS_2-VASc (Congestive heart failure, 1 point; Hypertension, 1 point; Age $\geq$ 75 years, 2; Diabetes mellitus, 1 point; Stroke/transient ischaemic attack, 2; Vascular disease, 1 point; Age 65–74 years, 1 point; Sex category for 1) score. Bleeding risk was assessed by the HAS-BLED (Hypertension, 1; Abnormal renal and liver function, 1 point each; Stroke/thromboembolism, 1 point; Bleeding history, 1 point; Labile INR [international normalised ratio], 1 point; Elderly [age > 65 years], 1 point; Drug consumption and alcohol abuse, 1 point each) score. All procedures were performed according to the rules of the Ethical Committee on human clinical trials and according to the Helsinki Declaration revised in 2008. Informed written consent was obtained from all participants. The name of the registry was "Prospective randomized controlled study of anti-platelet therapy in atrial fibrillation patients undergoing percutaneous coronary intervention".

Definitions

AF was defined as paroxysmal, persistent, permanent, or unknown according to guidelines [4]. Stroke was defined as the sudden loss of neurologic function, which was classified into ischaemic or haemorrhagic and verified by brain computed tomography or magnetic resonance imaging [5]. Systemic embolism was diagnosed as acute vascular obstruction of the limbs or any organ and was verified by angiography. Acute myocardial infarction (AMI) was defined according to the universal definition of the ESC/ACCF/AHA/WHF [6]. Stent thrombosis (ST) was defined according to the Academic Research

Consortium standard [7]. Thrombolysis in myocardial infarction (TIMI) major bleeding included intracranial or clinically significant haemorrhage with a haemoglobin decrease > 50 g/L according to the TIMI criteria [8]. Minor bleeding was also defined according to the TIMI criteria [8].

PCI

PCI was performed in accordance with international guidelines, using a standard technique, through the radial or femoral route [9]. A drug-eluting stent (DES) was used based on the angiography outcome. An intravenous bolus of unfractionated heparin (100 IU/kg) was administered immediately before the procedure. The administration of glycoprotein IIb/IIIa inhibitors was decided on by the attending cardiologists.

Antithrombotic therapy and clopidogrel modification

Warfarin was stopped 3 days before PCI and patients were treated with low-molecular-weight heparin until 12 h before PCI. A combined loading dose of 300 mg aspirin and 600 mg clopidogrel was used before PCI. After PCI, a combined administration of 100 mg aspirin, 75 mg clopidogrel, and INR-monitored warfarin was continued for 3 months according to guidelines [9]. The clopidogrel MD (Plevix, 75 mg per tablet, SANOFI, France, and clopidogrel bisulfate tablets, 25 mg per tablet, SALUBRIS, China) fluctuated between 75 and 225 mg for at least 1 year. All patients were treated with TT for 3 months, followed by clopidogrel plus warfarin for 9 months. VASP-adjusted clopidogrel MD commenced at the beginning of 3 months and was modified according to the VASP index in order to keep the platelet reaction index (PRI) below 50%. VASP was monitored at 3, 6, 9, and 12 months after PCI. The stepwise increase of clopidogrel dosage was adopted. After the first PRI monitoring, 100 mg clopidogrel was administered if PRI > 50%. The second PRI monitoring was undertaken 6 months after PCI, and 125 mg clopidogrel was administered if PRI was still > 50%. Subsequent additional doses were similar to the previous doses. Another 25 mg clopidogrel was given if PRI > 50% after every 3 months. The maximum clopidogrel MD at the end of 1 year was 175 mg. If PRI < 25%, clopidogrel MD was decreased to 75 mg. If PRI > 25% and was < 50%, the dose was not changed and the determined dose was maintained.

Blood samples

Three months after PCI, blood samples were drawn from the antecubital vein once every 3 months. The initial blood was removed to avoid platelet activation induced by the puncture action. Blood was transferred into a tube with 3.8% trisodium citrate. The tube was gently inverted up and down 3 to 5 times and was immediately sent to the monitoring laboratory.

VASP phosphorylation test

The VASP phosphorylation test was performed more than 1 h after blood collection by an experienced technician using Platelet VASP kits (Becton Dickinson, USA) according to the instruction manual [10]. Briefly, blood samples were mixed in vitro with adenosine diphosphate (ADP) and/or prostaglandin E1 (PGE1). Each blood sample was incubated with a 16C2FITC antibody, followed by a goat anti-mouse fluorescence staining in isothiocyanate polyclonal reagent. Flow cytometric monitoring was conducted with a Coulter EPICS XL cytometer (CA, U.S.A). The platelet group was identified on its side scatter and forward distributions. Every 3000 platelet events were gated and analysed for mean fluorescence intensity (MFI) using flow cytometry. The MFI corresponding to each experimental situation (ADP and ADP + PGE1) was determined to calculate a ratio directly related to the VASP phosphorylation value. The ratio, $[(MFI_{PGE1}-MFI_{ADP+PGE1})/MFI_{PGE1}] \times 100\%$, which indicates a percentage of platelet reactivity, is expressed as a PRI corresponding to a ratio of activated platelets versus resting platelets.

INR monitoring

For all patients who received warfarin, the predicted INR was set between 2.0 and 2.5 according to guidelines [2]. INR was regularly monitored after discharge. In the beginning, INR evaluations were performed every week after discharge. If the INR achieved the target range after monitoring three consecutive times, the measurement was then taken monthly.

Clinical endpoint

For the clinical follow-up, the primary endpoint was designated as the occurrence of MACCE, involving cardiovascular death, myocardial infarction (MI), target vessel revascularisation (TVR), ST, systemic embolism, and stroke. Secondary endpoints were defined as TIMI major and minor bleeding.

Follow-up

The clinical follow-up involved a clinic visit or telephone interview at 3, 6, 9, and 12 months after PCI. If a dose adjustment was made at 9 months, the patients were followed up for another 1 year from then on. The MD modification was as before. All patients with symptoms during the visit and interview were evaluated by at least two cardiologists. Death or MI events were recorded by hospital admission staff or community service.

Statistics

Continuous variables are described as mean ± SD and categorical variables as numbers and percentages. Differences between treatment groups were tested with one-way or two-way repeated-measures ANOVA, followed by Bonferroni correction for intergroup comparisons. Comparison between categorical variables was performed with the Chi-square test or Fisher exact test if frequencies were no more than 5. Event-free survival rates in different groups were calculated by Kaplan-Meier survival analysis and compared by the log-rank test. A two-sided P-value of < 0.05 was considered statistically significant. Data statistics were performed using Prism 5.0 (GraphPad Software, CA, USA).

Results

We prospectively recruited 503 patients with AF requiring anticoagulation and who underwent PCI between July 2014 and July 2017; 481 patients (VASP-guided, $n = 241$; control, $n = 240$) completed the 1-year follow-up (Fig. 1). In the VASP-guided and control groups, 89.7 and 89.9% of patients, respectively, had paroxysmal or persistent/permanent AF. The clinical and procedural characteristics and other medical histories were comparable between both groups. In the VASP-guided and control groups, the CHA_2DS_2-VASc score was 3.7 ± 0.6 and 3.8 ± 0.9, respectively, whereas, the HAS-BLED score was 3.1 ± 0.4 and 3.3 ± 0.5, respectively, indicating high thrombotic and bleeding risk profiles in both groups. The average INR on the day of the procedure was 1.2 ± 0.6 and 1.3 ± 0.7, respectively, indicating unsatisfactory warfarin therapy in both groups (Table 1).

Antithrombotic mediation after discharge

For patients prescribed antithrombotic therapy after discharge, there was high compliance in both groups. The median duration of TT and clopidogrel plus warfarin

was 3.2 and 9.5 months, respectively. There was no difference in duration between CHA_2DS_2-VASc 1 or ≥ 2 and HASBLED ≤ 2 or ≥ 3 (Table 2).

PRI

We analysed PRI at a mean time of 3, 6, 9, and 12 months after the PCI procedure. The baseline PRI showed no significant difference between both groups ($73.5 \pm 12.7\%$ [VASP] vs $68.4 \pm 17.2\%$ [control], $P = 0.4$). PRI in the VASP-guided group decreased significantly ($73.5 \pm 12.7\%$, $32.3 \pm 4.9\%$, $35.5 \pm 6.7\%$, and $29.8 \pm 7.3\%$ at 3, 6, 9, and 12 months after randomisation, respectively; $P = 0.001$); PRI in the control group also decreased, but not significantly ($68.4 \pm 17.2\%$, $48.5 \pm 13.2\%$, $51.6 \pm 19.8\%$, and $65.3 \pm 17.2\%$, respectively; $P > 0.5$). Compared to the control group, PRI in the VASP-guided group was significantly lower ($P = 0.04$, 0.03, and < 0.001 at 6, 9, and 12 months after randomisation, respectively) (Table 3).

Clopidogrel dose modification

Clopidogrel MD in the VASP-guided group was modified according to PRI. The number of patients that required clopidogrel MD individualisation was 162 (67.3%), 181 (75.4%), 197 (81.9%), and 208 (86.3%) at 3, 6, 9, and 12 months, respectively (Fig. 2). Regarding MD according to PRI at 3, 6, 9, and 12 months, 132 (81.5%), 100 (55.2%), 70 (35.5%), and 40 (19.4%) patients, respectively, had increased MD, 22 (13.6%), 41 (22.6%), 93 (47.2%), and 130 (63.1%) patients, respectively, had unchanged MD, while 8 (4.9%), 40 (22.1%), 34 (17.3%), and 36 (17.5%) patients, respectively had decreased MD (Fig. 3). At the study's completion, 33 of 241 (13.7%) patients in the VASP-guided group still had HTPR> 50% (data not shown).

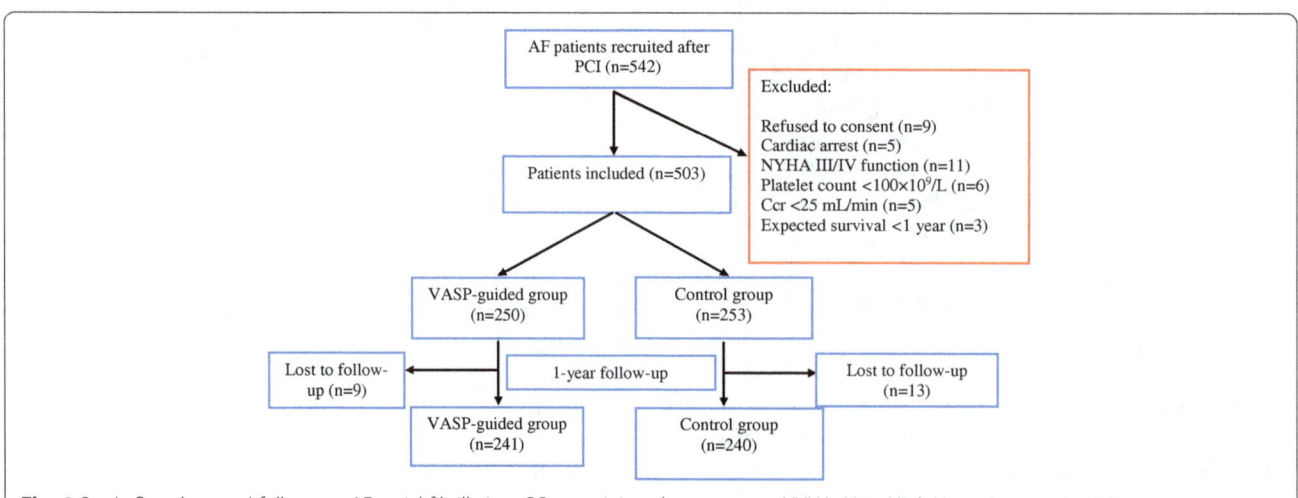

Fig. 1 Study flowchart and follow-up. AF: atrial fibrillation; CCr: creatinine clearance rate; NYHA: New York Heart Association; PCI: percutaneous coronary intervention; VASP: vasodilator-stimulated phosphoprotein

Table 1 Clinical, medical, and procedural characteristics

Characteristics	VASP-guided group	Control group	P-value
	($n = 241$)	($n = 240$)	
Age (y)	64.4 ± 3.2	62.8 ± 4.3	0.58
Age $\geq$ 75 years	61(25.3)	64(26.7)	0.72
Men	128(53.4)	122(50.8)	0.62
BMI (kg/m^2)	26.7 ± 4.2	25.3 ± 2.1	0.88
Current Smoker	87(36.2)	96(40.1)	0.55
AF category			
Paroxysmal	92(38.4)	96(40.2)	0.7
Persistent/permanent	123(51.3)	119(49.7)	0.84
Unknown	26(10.3)	25(10.1)	0.98
Medical history			
Diabetes	68(28.4)	75(31.3)	0.43
Hypertension	141(58.8)	144(60.3)	0.57
Previous heart failure	41(17.1)	52(21.9)	0.19
Previous stroke or thromboembolism	25(10.3)	28(11.6)	0.65
Previous bleeding	16(6.7)	13(5.5)	0.53
CHA2DS2 -VASc Score	3.7 ± 0.6	3.8 ± 0.9	0.87
CHA2DS2 -VASc Score $\geq$ 2	174(72.4)	168(70.3)	0.35
HAS-BLED Score	3.1 ± 0.4	3.3 ± 0.5	0.76
HAS-BLED Score $\geq$ 3	61(25.3)	59(24.8)	0.64
LVEF	52.3 ± 4.4	51.0 ± 3.9	0.59
Treatment on admission			
Previous aspirin	31(12.8)	33(14.0)	0.21
Previous clopidogrel	13(5.4)	14(7.3)	0.48
Previous oral anticoagulation	131(54.3)	119(49.7)	0.65
Indication for the catheterisation procedure			
Stable angina	188(78.5)	168(70.2)	0.74
Silent myocardial ischaemia	52(21.5)	71(29.8)	0.17
Platelet (×109/L)	202 ± 23	183 ± 17	0.28
Cr (µmmol/L)	98.3	89.4	0.13
Mean INR on day of procedure	1.2 ± 0.6	1.3 ± 0.7	0.72
Pharmacotherapy			
RAS inhibitors	212(88.2)	200(83.5)	0.61
Statins	237(98.3)	237(98.7)	0.98
β-Blockers	123(51.4)	132(55.3)	0.76
Digoxin	32(13.4)	41(17.2)	0.25
Amiodarone	62(25.9)	46(19.4)	0.09
Procedural characteristics			
No. of lesions treated per patient	1.4	1.5	0.88
No. of stents per patient	1.3	1.2	0.64
Patients receiving DES	241(100)	240(100)	1
GP IIb/IIIa inhibitors	61(25.4)	67(28.1)	0.38

Values are presented as mean ± SD or n (%)

AF atrial fibrillation, *BMI* body mass index, *Cr* creatinine, *GP* glycoprotein, *INR* international normalised ratio, *LVEF* left ventricular ejection fraction, *RAS* renin-angiotensin system

Table 2 Antithrombotic drug regimen at discharge

Medication	Median duration (months)				
	CHA_2DS_2-VASc = 1	CHA_2DS_2-VASc≥2	HASBLED≤2	HASBLED ≥3	P-value
Aspirin	2.3 ± 0.7	3.2 ± 1.1	3.8 ± 0.9	3.3 ± 0.9	>0.05
Clopidogrel	11.2 ± 2.8	12.9 ± 1.4	12.6 ± 2.5	10.3 ± 1.6	>0.05
Warfarin	10.5 ± 2.8	12.4 ± 1.3	11.8 ± 2.1	10.8 ± 2.7	>0.05

INR monitoring

During the 1-year follow-up, INR was measured at least every month. The representative value at 1, 3, 6, 9 and 12 months are listed in Table 4. INR increased at 12 months compared to baseline only in patients with CHA_2DS_2-VASc score ≥ 2 (from 1.9 ± 0.3 to 2.5 ± 0.8, $P < 0.05$).

Clinical outcomes during follow-up

Complete follow-up (median 365 days; range 300 to 395 days) was recorded in 95.6% of the whole cohort. The clinical events recorded in the two groups are shown in Table 5. The incidences of TVR and all MACCE were higher in the control group than in the VASP-guided group, whereas the occurrence of cardiovascular death, MI, ST, systemic embolism, and stroke was not significantly different between both groups. Regarding the secondary endpoints, major bleeding incidence was comparable between both groups, whereas the rate of minor bleeding was significantly higher in the VASP-guided group (15.3% vs 9.7%, $P = 0.032$). Kaplan-Meier survival analysis demonstrated that there was no statistical difference between the VASP-guided and control groups during the 1-year follow-up (log-rank test $P = 0.68$) (Fig. 4).

Discussion

To our knowledge, this is the first prospective study to show that individualised clopidogrel MD according to platelet function reduced the incidence of MACCE in AF patients requiring anticoagulation and scheduled for PCI. However, an increase in minor bleeding was noted. The study shows that our patients had a high risk of stroke and bleeding. Our clinical data demonstrate the protective effect of individualised clopidogrel MD in patients with AF undergoing PCI by decreasing the

incidence of adverse clinical events, without increasing major bleeding.

Owing to lack of well-founded evidence to date, there has been no consensus on the optimal therapy regarding the antithrombotic strategy for AF patients requiring chronic anticoagulation and coronary stent implantation. Most previous studies evaluating TT have either been small-scale retrospective or case-control clinical trials focusing on bleeding risk. Thus, there is a lack of evidence to support optimal medical therapy regarding the cardiovascular efficacy of different antithrombotic regimens. In the largest observational study of AF patients with stable coronary artery disease in Denmark, the addition of antiplatelet therapy (either aspirin or clopidogrel) to vitamin K antagonist therapy decreased recurrent cardiovascular events or thromboembolism but increased bleeding significantly [11]. In that study and in the present study, the high CHA_2DS_2-VASc score indicated a high thrombotic risk in both cohorts. The greater number of bleeding events in the previous study might be attributed to racial differences or the fixed TT strategy.

In the Karjalainen et al. [12] case-control study, warfarin plus aspirin failed to prevent more cardiovascular events. However, this combination increased the risk for stent thrombosis. In the study by Ruiz-Nodar et al. [13] regarding combined therapy with coumarins, aspirin, and clopidogrel, the incidence of adverse events in TT was low, with no increase in minor and major bleeding compared to dual antiplatelet therapy (DAPT). The prospective multicentre registry study, STENTICO, demonstrated an increase in severe and moderate GUSTO bleeding in TT compared to DAPT [14]. In addition, the AVIATOR Registry study [15], involving patients that received TT or DAPT, showed similar MACE rates, with a higher BARC ≥2 bleeding when discharged. In a prospective multicentre

Table 3 Platelet Reactivity Index (PRI) in the two groups during the 1-year study

	PRI (mean ± SD, %)				
	3 months after randomisation	6 months	9 months	12 months	P-value*
Control group	68.4 ± 17.2	48.5 ± 13.2	51.6 ± 19.8	65.3 ± 17.2	>0.05
VASP-guided group	73.5 ± 12.7	32.3 ± 4.9	35.5 ± 6.7	29.8 ± 7.3	0.001
P-value#	0.4	0.04	<0.001	0.03	<0.001

VASP vasodilator-stimulated phosphoprotein

*comparison between 3, 6, 9, and 12 months

#comparison between the control group and VASP-guided group

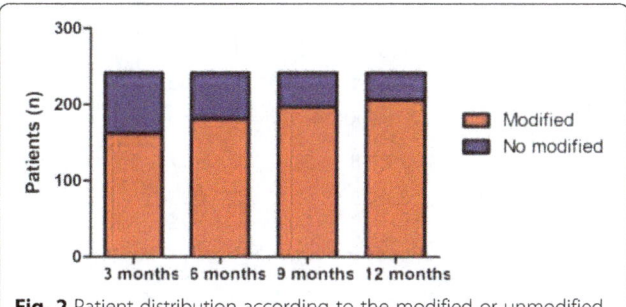

Fig. 2 Patient distribution according to the modified or unmodified clopidogrel maintenance dose in the VASP-guided group. VASP: vasodilator-stimulated phosphoprotein

study [16], TT was compared to DAPT in patients with AF undergoing PCI. The results showed that patients with a low CHA_2DS_2-VASc score had a high risk of bleeding without any benefit in reducing thromboembolic events. It also demonstrated that TT decreased the thromboembolism rate at the expense of an increase in major bleeding in patients with high CHA_2DS_2-VASc scores. These studies show the variability of antithrombotic agents in this kind of patients. There is no one-size-fits-all strategy for balancing thrombotic and bleeding risk.

In the present study, TT was used for an average of 3 months in all patients, which might be one reason major bleeding risk did not increase during the 1-year follow-up. Recently, the ISAR-TRIPLE trial [17] evaluated the effect of clopidogrel in addition to concomitant aspirin and warfarin following DES implantation. The study showed no significant difference in MACCE between 6 months and 6 weeks of TT. Furthermore, a longer duration of TT did not increase the bleeding risk in this study. This added evidence supports limiting the duration of DAPT and individualising therapy based on the patient's risk profile. In a recent study [18], 568 patients receiving TT were prospectively investigated according to a 1-month or > 1-month regimen. The endpoints of primary safety and secondary bleeding were not significantly different between both groups. The study suggested that 30-day TT had similar clinical

outcomes compared to longer TT durations. Because of the involvement of high-thrombotic-risk patients in the present study and guideline recommendations [2], we administered TT for 3 months.

Few trials have focused on antithrombotic therapy in Asian patients, particularly Chinese patients, who have undergone PCI and require oral anticoagulation. A prospective study involving 142 Chinese patients discharged with TT demonstrated a notable decrease in stroke and MACCE and its major bleeding risk might have fallen within acceptable ranges if the INR was strictly monitored [19]. In that study, the overall major adverse events in the TT group was 8.8%, and major and minor bleeding were 2.9 and 8.8%, respectively. In our present study, the major adverse events were 2.5% in the VASP-guided group and 5.0% in the control group, and major and minor bleeding were 2.8 to 3% and 9.7 to 15.3%, respectively. The difference between our study and theirs might be explained by the thrombotic risk of patients; the present study had a high-thrombotic-risk cohort (CHA_2DS_2-VAScScore ≥2, 71.5%). Another study with a small cohort of 37 patients requiring TT was conducted in South Korea [20]. The authors concluded that warfarin therapy reduced major adverse events without increasing bleeding risk. In that study, the percentage of $CHADS_2$ score ≥ 2 was 56.8%, whereas, all major adverse events and any bleeding were 0.97 and 1.94%, respectively. These differences may be attributed to the nationality and sample size, although this study was conducted in Asia.

Inter-individual variability of clopidogrel has been frequently reported and has been regarded as "clopidogrel resistance" and HTPR [21]. Hyporesponse to clopidogrel with a high risk of coronary ischaemia and hyper response to clopidogrel with a high risk of bleeding results in an increase in cardiovascular events. Clinical factors including diabetes, poor absorption, and drug-drug interactions may be one aspect of HTPR [21]. Genetic factors are another aspect to consider. The polymorphism of dominant genes such as *CYP2C19, ABCB1, P2Y12,* and *T2238C* result in

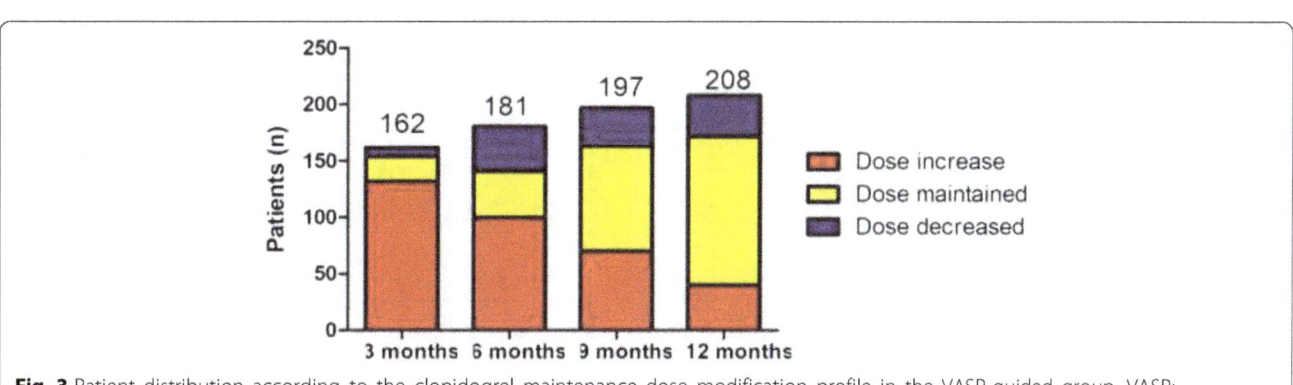

Fig. 3 Patient distribution according to the clopidogrel maintenance dose modification profile in the VASP-guided group. VASP: vasodilator-stimulated phosphoprotein

Table 4 INR monitoring during the 1-year follow-up

Categories	1 mo	3 mo	6 mo	9 mo	12 mo	P-value
VASP-guided group	1.8 ± 0.3	2.1 ± 0.5	1.9 ± 0.7	2.0 ± 0.2	2.2 ± 0.4	0.33
Control group	1.7 ± 0.9	2.0 ± 0.3	2.1 ± 0.5	1.9 ± 0.6	2.1 ± 0.2	0.48
CHA2DS2-VASc Score = 1	2.0 ± 0.2	1.7 ± 0.4	2.2 ± 0.9	2.0 ± 0.8	2.1 ± 0.7	0.56
CHA2DS2-VASc Score ≥ 2	1.9 ± 0.3	1.6 ± 0.6	2.3 ± 0.5	2.6 ± 0.9	2.5 ± 0.8	< 0.05
HAS-BLED Score < 2	1.6 ± 0.5	1.8 ± 0.4	2.0 ± 0.6	2.1 ± 0.4	2.2 ± 0.7	0.14
HAS-BLED Score ≥ 3	1.7 ± 0.2	1.9 ± 0.5	2.1 ± 0.6	2.2 ± 0.4	2.1 ± 0.8	0.35

P-value: 1 month vs. 12 months

HTPR, especially in Chinese patients [22–26]. Furthermore, the gene-based individualised clopidogrel strategy demonstrated no benefit from GRAVITAS [27], ARCTIC [28], Trigger-PCI [29], and ANTARCTIC [30].

In all patients in the present study, during the 1-year follow-up, INR was rigorously monitored and was within the therapeutic range. Our results from the present study demonstrate that the TT-induced bleeding risk will fall within acceptable ranges if INR is rigorously monitored. Likewise, the ACTIVE-W trial recorded a significant benefit from anticoagulation combined with DAPT in AF patients. The ACTIVE-W study also demonstrated that patients benefitted from anticoagulation therapy, with INR values within the therapeutic range [31].

Another problem is the use of the drug-eluting stent (DES) for AF patients, which is the predominant implantation scaffold for coronary intervention. DES use is also inevitably associated with delayed neointimal recovery and an increased risk of late ST, resulting in prolonged DAPT for up to 1 year. However, in patients requiring oral anticoagulation, prolonged DAPT may increase major bleeding risk [14]. Therefore, the use of bare metal stents (BMS) was suggested by some studies for such patients [32, 33] and DES should be implanted only in situations such as long lesions, small vessels, and

diabetes, in which the significant advantages of DES outweigh the disadvantages of BMS [34]. In our study, the scaffold used was exclusively DES. Individualised clopidogrel MD and close INR monitoring might overcome the disadvantages of DES in long-term antithrombotic therapy.

In the SPORTIF trial [35], the addition of aspirin to oral anticoagulants (INR 2.0–3.0) increased major bleeding risk without decreasing thromboembolism or AMI in AF patients. In addition, results from the WOEST trial [36] showed a significant increase in death and MI events in those who received vitamin K antagonist plus DAPT than in those treated with vitamin K antagonist plus clopidogrel. These results demonstrate that in patients whose bleeding risk surpasses stroke risk, combined warfarin and clopidogrel would be a reasonable treatment choice. In the present study, the average HAS-BLED score was 3.1, which indicated a relatively high-bleeding cohort. Consequently, we chose the close monitoring of warfarin and modified clopidogrel plus fixed aspirin for 3 months. The strategy was also in accordance with the consensus of antithrombotic therapy in AF patients with a combination of ACS and/or undergoing PCI [2].

The interaction of warfarin and clopidogrel was investigated in the Sibbing et al. study [37], in which they reported that both clopidogrel and phenprocoumon were metabolised synchronously through the hepatic cytochrome P450 system and there was an intra-drug interaction at this level. The result demonstrated that

Table 5 Outcomes during the follow-up

Outcomes	VASP-guided group n = 241	Control group n = 240	P-value
Cardiovascular death	1(0.4)	2(0.8)	0.34
MI	1(0.4)	2 (0.8)	0.34
TVR	1(0.4)	3(1.3)	0.03
Stent thrombosis	1(0.4)	1(0.4)	0.21
Systemic embolism	1(0.4)	2(0.8)	0.34
Stroke	1(0.4)	2(0.8)	0.34
All MACCE	6(2.5)	12(5.0)	0.02
TIMI major bleeding	7(3.0)	6(2.8)	0.72
TIMI minor bleeding	37(15.3)	23(9.7)	0.03

Values are presented as n(%)
MACCE major adverse cardiovascular and cerebral event, *MI* myocardial infarction, *TIMI* thrombolysis in myocardial infarction, *TVR* target vessel revascularisation

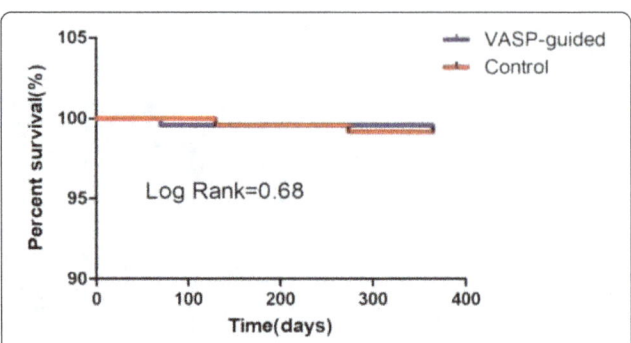

Fig. 4 Kaplan-Meier curves of survival during the 1-year follow-up. VASP: vasodilator-stimulated phosphoprotein

phenprocoumon notably attenuated the antiplatelet effect of clopidogrel. If this is true, the VASP-guided clopidogrel therapy compensated for the attenuation of warfarin on antiplatelet effects in the current study.

To date, only two studies have investigated the effect of prasugrel on TT strategy. In the Sarafoff et al. study [38], aspirin, prasugrel, and vitamin K antagonist were prescribed for 6 months. Compared to clopidogrel, prasugrel increased the bleeding risk in patients requiring TT. In the TRANSLATE-ACS study [39] of AMI patients treated with PCI, clopidogrel or prasugrel was administered in addition to aspirin and anticoagulant. The study concluded that among patients with TT, prasugrel administration was associated with a higher bleeding risk. Thus, prasugrel was not recommended in the consensus document.

Because of the high bleeding risk, a new oral anticoagulant therapy was evaluated. The RE-DUAL PCI study [40] compared TT with warfarin plus a P2Y12 antagonist (clopidogrel or ticagrelor) and aspirin (TT group) to dual therapy with dabigatran plus a P2Y12 antagonist (clopidogrel or ticagrelor) and no aspirin. The results demonstrated that among AF patients undergoing PCI, the bleeding risk was lower in patients who received the latter combination than in patients who received the former. Dual therapy was non-inferior to TT with respect to the risk of thromboembolism. In the PIONEER AF-PCI study [41], the combination of either low-dose rivaroxaban plus a P2Y12 antagonist or very-low-dose rivaroxaban plus DAPT significantly decreased the bleeding risk compared to standard therapy with a vitamin K antagonist plus DAPT for 1, 6, or 12 months. These two studies met the objective of decreasing bleeding risk; however, they exhibited no significant difference regarding thrombotic events. In addition, neither dabigatran nor rivaroxaban is used regularly in the real world, especially in China.

Limitations

There are some limitations to the present study. First, the study was conducted in the Chinese population, which demonstrates more "clopidogrel resistance" than the European and North American populations, so the conclusion should be cautiously extended to others. Second, the sample of patients recruited in the present study was relatively small. Third, the present study did not evaluate the effects of the new antiplatelet ticagrelor or new anticoagulants such as dabigatran or rivaroxaban. In the future, we will focus on the antithrombotic effect of these antagonists.

Conclusion

The present study verified that a modified clopidogrel maintenance strategy combined with aspirin and warfarin therapy decreased adverse cardiovascular events at the cost of increasing minor bleeding.

Abbreviations
ADP: adenosine diphosphate; AF: atrial fibrillation; AMI: Acute myocardial infarction; DAPT: dual antiplatelet therapy; DES: drug-eluting stent; HTPR: high on-treatment platelet reaction; INR: international normalised ratio; MACCE: major adverse cardiovascular and cerebral events; MD: maintenance dose; MFI: mean fluorescence intensity; PCI: percutaneous coronary intervention; PGE1: prostaglandin E1; PRI: platelet reactivity index; ST: stent thrombosis; TIMI: thrombolysis in myocardial infarction; TT: triple therapy; TVR: target vessel revascularisation; VASP: vasodilator-stimulated phosphoprotein

Funding
The present study was supported by the Science and Technology Commission of Shanghai Municipality (No. 17411968500) and the Key Disciplines Group Construction Project of Pudong Health Bureau of Shanghai (Grant No. PWZxq2017–05). The former helped fund the design of the study, collection, analysis, and interpretation of data. The latter helped fund the writing the manuscript.

Authors' contributions
CH collected all patients clinical and laboratory data, involving platelet activity index and anticoagulation function monitoring data and made major statistical analysis. XZ finished the follow-up during one-year follow-up and analyzed the relationship between triple/dual therapy and the clinical outcome. YG performed platelet activity examination in control group during one-year follow-up. XZ finished platelet activity examination in the VASP-guided group. YL1 performed coagulation examination in control group patients. HZ and YL2 performed the coagulation examination for every patient in the VASP-guided group. YL3 wrote the primary draft of this manuscript. XW put forward the conception of the study, conducted the proposal and revised the manuscript. All authors read and approved the final manuscript.

Competing interests
The authors declare that they have no competing interests.

Author details
[1]Key Laboratory of Arrhythmias of the Ministry of Education of China, Tongji University School of Medicine, Shanghai 200092, China. [2]Department of Cardiology, Shanghai East Hospital, Tongji University School of Medicine, 150 Jimo Road, Shanghai 200120, China. [3]Cardiovascular Medicine of Baoshan People's Hospital of Yunnan Province, Baoshan 678000, China. [4]Department of Anesthesiology, Renji Hospital, Shanghai Jiaotong University School of Medicine, 160 Pujian Road, Shanghai 200127, China.

References
1. Schömig A, Sarafoff N, Seyfarth M. Triple antithrombotic management after stent implantation: when and how? Heart. 2009;95:1280–5.
2. Lip GY, Windecker S, Huber K, Kirchhof P, Marin F, Ten Berg JM, et al. Management of antithrombotic therapy in atrial fibrillation patients presenting with acute coronary syndrome and/or undergoing percutaneous coronary or valve interventions: a joint consensus document of the European Society of Cardiology Working Group on Thrombosis, European Heart Rhythm Association (EHRA), European Association of Percutaneous Cardiovascular Interventions (EAPCI) and European Association of Acute Cardiac Care (ACCA) endorsed by the Heart Rhythm Society (HRS) and Asia-Pacific Heart Rhythm Society (APHRS). Eur Heart J. 2014;35:3155–79.
3. Wang XD, Zhang DF, Zhuang SW, Lai Y. Modifying clopidogrel maintenance doses according to vasodilator-stimulated phosphoprotein phosphorylation

index improves clinical outcome in patients with clopidogrel resistance. Clin Cardiol. 2011;34:332–8.

4. Kirchhof P, Benussi S, Kotecha D, Ahlsson A, Atar D, Casadei B, et al. 2016 ESC guidelines for the management of atrial fibrillation developed in collaboration with EACTS. Eur Heart J. 2016;37:2893–962.

5. Whiteley WN, Slot KB, Fernandes P, Sandercock P, Wardlaw J. Risk factors for intracranial hemorrhage in acute ischemic stroke patients treated with recombinant tissue plasminogen activator: a systematic review and meta-analysis of 55 studies. Stroke. 2012;43:2904–9.

6. Thygesen K, Alpert JS, Jaffe AS, Simoons ML, Chaitman BR, White HD. Third universal definition of myocardial infarction. Circulation. 2012;126:2020–35.

7. Cutlip DE, Windecker S, Mehran R, Boam A, Cohen DJ, van Es GA. Academic Research Consortium. Clinical end points in coronary stent trials: a case for standardized definitions. Circulation. 2007;115:2344–51.

8. Rao AK, Pratt C, Berke A, Jaffe A, Ockene I, Schreiber TL. Thrombolysis in myocardial infarction (TIMI) trial—phase I: hemorrhagic manifestations and changes in plasma fibrinogen and the fibrinolytic system in patients treated with recombinant tissue plasminogen activator and streptokinase. J Am Coll Cardiol. 1988;11:1–11.

9. Windecker S, Kolh P, Alfonso F, Collet JP, Cremer J, Falk V, et al. 2014 ESC/EACTS guidelines on myocardial revascularization: the task force on myocardial revascularization of the European Society of Cardiology (ESC) and the European Association for Cardio-Thoracic Surgery (EACTS) developed with the special contribution of the European Association of Percutaneous Cardiovascular Interventions (EAPCI). Eur Heart J. 2014;35:2541–619.

10. Bonello L, Paganelli F, Arpin-Bornet M, Auquier P, Sampol J, Dignat-George F, et al. Vasodilator-stimulated phosphoprotein phosphorylation analysis prior to percutaneous coronary intervention for exclusion of postprocedural major adverse cardiovascular events. J Thromb Haemost. 2007;5:1630–6.

11. Lamberts M, Gislason GH, Lip GY, Lassen JF, Olesen JB, Mikkelsen AP, et al. Antiplatelet therapy for stable coronary artery disease in atrial fibrillation patients taking an oral anticoagulant: a nationwide cohort study. Circulation. 2014;129:1577–85.

12. Karjalainen PP, Porela P, Ylitalo A, Vikman S, Nyman K, Vaittinen MA, et al. Safety and efficacy of combined antiplatelet-warfarin therapy after coronary stenting. Eur Heart J. 2007;28:726–32.

13. Ruiz-Nodar JM, Marín F, Hurtado JA, Valencia J, Pinar E, Pineda J, et al. Anticoagulant and antiplatelet therapy use in 426 patients with atrial fibrillation undergoing percutaneous coronary intervention and stent implantation implications for bleeding risk and prognosis. J Am Coll Cardiol. 2008;51:818–25.

14. Gilard M, Blanchard D, Helft G, Carrier D, Eltchaninoff H, Belle L, et al. Antiplatelet therapy in patients with anticoagulants undergoing percutaneous coronary intervention (from STENTing and oral antiCOagulants [STENTICO]). Am J Cardiol. 2009;104:338–42.

15. Mennuni MG, HalperinJL BS, Schoos MM, Theodoropoulos KN, Meelu OA, et al. Balancing the risk of bleeding and stroke in patients with atrial fibrillation after percutaneous coronary intervention (from the AVIATOR registry). Am J Cardiol. 2015;116:37–42.

16. Sambola A, Mutuberría M, García Del Blanco B, Alonso A, Barrabés JA, Alfonso F, et al. Effects of triple therapy in patients with non-valvular atrial fibrillation undergoing percutaneous coronary intervention regarding thromboembolic risk stratification. Circ J. 2016;80:354–62.

17. Fiedler KA, Maeng M, Mehilli J, Schulz-Schüpke S, Byrne RA, Sibbing D, et al. Duration of triple therapy in patients requiring oral anticoagulation after drug-eluting stent implantation: the ISAR-TRIPLE trial. J Am Coll Cardiol. 2015;65:1619–29.

18. Koskinas KC, Räber L, Zanchin T, Pilgrim T, Stortecky S, Hunziker L, et al. Duration of triple antithrombotic therapy and outcomes among patients undergoing percutaneous coronary intervention. JACC Cardiovasc Interv. 2016;9:1473–83.

19. Gao F, Zhou YJ, Wang ZJ, Shen H, Liu XL, Nie B, et al. Comparison of different antithrombotic regimens for patients with atrial fibrillation undergoing drug-eluting stent implantation. Circ J. 2010;74:701–8.

20. Suh SY, Kang WC, Oh PC, Choi H, Moon CI, Lee K, et al. Efficacy and safety of aspirin, clopidogrel, and warfarin after coronary artery stenting in Korean patients with atrial fibrillation. Heart Vessel. 2014;29:578–83.

21. Angiolillo DJ, Fernandez-Ortiz A, Bernardo E, Alfonso F, Macaya C, Bass TA, et al. Variability in individual responsiveness to clopidogrel: clinical

implications, management, and future perspectives. J Am Coll Cardiol. 2007;49:1505–16.

22. Mega JL, Close SL, Wiviott SD, Shen L, Hockett RD, Brandt JT, et al. Cytochrome p-450 polymorphisms and response to clopidogrel. N Engl J Med. 2009;360:354–62.

23. Wang XD, Zhang DF, Liu XB, Lai Y, Qi WG, Luo Y, et al. Modified clopidogrel loading dose according to platelet reactivity monitoring in patients carrying ABCB1 variant alleles in patients with clopidogrel resistance. Eur J Intern Med. 2012;23:48–53.

24. Fontana P, Dupont A, Gandrille S, Bachelot-Loza C, Reny JL, Aiach M, et al. Adenosine diphosphate-induced platelet aggregation is associated with P2Y12 gene sequence variations in healthy subjects. Circulation. 2003;108:989–95.

25. Strisciuglio T, Barbato E, De Biase C, Di Gioia G, Cotugno M, Stanzione R, et al. T2238C atrial natriuretic peptide gene variant and the response to antiplatelet therapy in stable ischemic heart disease patients. J Cardiovasc Transl Res. 2018;11:36–41.

26. Zhang S, Zhu J, Li H, Wang L, Niu J, Zhu B, et al. Study of the association of PEAR1, P2Y12, and UGT2A1 polymorphisms with platelet reactivity in response to dual antiplatelet therapy in Chinese patients. Cardiology. 2018; 140:21–9.

27. Price MJ, Berger PB, Teirstein PS, Tanguay JF, Angiolillo DJ, Spriggs D, GRAVITAS Investigators, et al. Standard- vs high-dose clopidogrel based on platelet function testing after percutaneous coronary intervention: the GRAVITAS randomized trial. JAMA. 2011;305:1097–105.

28. Collet JP, Cuisset T, Rangé G, Cayla G, Elhadad S, Pouillot C, et al. ARCTIC investigators. Bedside monitoring to adjust antiplatelet therapy for coronary stenting. N Engl J Med. 2012;367:2100–9.

29. Trenk D, Stone GW, Gawaz M, Kastrati A, Angiolillo DJ, Müller U, et al. A randomized trial of prasugrel versus clopidogrel in patients with high platelet reactivity on clopidogrel after elective percutaneous coronary intervention with implantation of drug-eluting stents: results of the TRIGGER-PCI (testing platelet reactivity in patients undergoing elective stent placement on Clopidogrel to guide alternative therapy with Prasugrel) study. J Am Coll Cardiol. 2012;59:2159–64.

30. Cayla G, Cuisset T, Silvain J, Leclercq F, Manzo-Silberman S, Saint-Etienne C, et al. ANTARCTIC investigators. Platelet function monitoring to adjust antiplatelet therapy in elderly patients stented for an acute coronary syndrome (ANTARCTIC): an open-label, blinded-endpoint, randomised controlled superiority trial. Lancet. 2016;388:2015–22.

31. Connolly S, Pogue J, Hart R, Pfeffer M, Hohnloser S, Chrolavicius S, et al. Clopidogrel plus aspirin versus oral anticoagulation for atrial fibrillation in the atrial fibrillation Clopidogrel trial with Irbesartan for prevention of vascular events (ACTIVE W): a randomised controlled trial. Lancet. 2006;367:1903–12.

32. Zahger D, Ilia R. Coronary stenting in warfarin treated patients. Euro Intervention. 2009;5:277–81.

33. Holmes DR Jr, Kereiakes DJ, Kleiman NS, Moliterno DJ, Patti G, Grines CL. Combining antiplatelet and anticoagulant therapies. J Am Coll Cardiol. 2009;54:95–109.

34. Lip GY, Huber K, Andreotti F, Arnesen H, Airaksinen KJ, Cuisset T, et al. European Society of Cardiology Working Group on Thrombosis. Management of antithrombotic therapy in atrial fibrillation patients presenting with acute coronary syndrome and/or undergoing percutaneous coronary intervention/ stenting. Thromb Haemost. 2010;103:13–28.

35. Flaker GC, Gruber M, Connolly SJ, Goldman S, Chaparro S, Vahanian A, et al. Risks and benefits of combining aspirin with anticoagulant therapy in patients with atrial fibrillation: an exploratory analysis of stroke prevention using an oral thrombin inhibitor in atrial fibrillation (SPORTIF) trials. Am Heart J. 2006;152:967–73.

36. Dewilde WJ, Oirbans T, Verheugt FW, Kelder JC, De Smet BJ, Herrman JP, et al. Use of clopidogrel with or without aspirin in patients taking oral anticoagulant therapy and undergoing percutaneous coronary intervention: an open-label, randomised, controlled trial. Lancet. 2013;381:1107–15.

37. Sibbing D, von Beckerath N, Morath T, Stegherr J, Mehilli J, Sarafoff N, et al. Oral anticoagulation with coumarin derivatives and antiplatelet effects of clopidogrel. Eur Heart J. 2010;31:1205–11.

38. Sarafoff N, Martischnig A, Wealer J, Mayer K, Mehilli J, Sibbing D, et al. Triple therapy with aspirin, prasugrel, and vitamin K antagonists in patients with drug-eluting stent implantation and an indication for oral anticoagulation. J Am Coll Cardiol. 2013;61:2060–6.

39. Jackson LR 2nd, Ju C, Zettler M, Messenger JC, Cohen DJ, Stone GW, et al. Outcomes of patients with acute myocardial infarction undergoing percutaneous coronary intervention receiving an oral anticoagulant and dual antiplatelet therapy: a comparison of clopidogrel versus prasugrel from the TRANSLATE-ACS study. JACC Cardiovasc Interv. 2015;8:1880–9.

40. Cannon CP, Bhatt DL, Oldgren J, GYH L, Ellis SG, Kimura T, et al. RE-DUAL PCI Steering Committee and Investigators. Dual antithrombotic therapy with dabigatran after PCI in atrial fibrillation. N Engl J Med. 2017;377:1513–24.

41. Gibson CM, Mehran R, Bode C, Halperin J, Verheugt FW, Wildgoose P, et al. Prevention of bleeding in patients with atrial fibrillation undergoing PCI. N Engl J Med. 2016;375:2423–34.

Dietary intervention with a specific micronutrient combination for the treatment of patients with cardiac arrhythmias: the impact on insulin resistance and left ventricular function

Elke Parsi[1][*] [ID], Norman Bitterlich[2], Anne Winkelmann[1], Daniela Rösler[3] and Christine Metzner[3,4]

Abstract

Background: Cardiac arrhythmias (CA) are very common and may occur with or without heart disease. Causes of these disturbances can be components of the metabolic syndrome (MetS) or deficits of micronutrients especially magnesium, potassium, B vitamins and coenzyme Q10. Both causes may also influence each other. Insulin resistance (IR) is a risk factor for diastolic dysfunction. One exploratory outcome of the present pilot study was to assess the impact of a dietary intervention with specific micronutrients on the lowering of IR levels in patients with CA with the goal to improve the left ventricular (LV) function.

Methods: This was a post hoc analysis of the randomized double blind, placebo-controlled pilot study in patients with CA (VPBs, SVPBs, SV tachycardia), which were recruited using data from patients who were 18–75 years of age in an Outpatient Practice of Cardiology. These arrhythmias were assessed by Holter ECG and LV function by standard echocardiography. Glucose metabolism was measured by fasting glucose, fasting insulin level and the Homeostasis Model Assessment of IR (HOMA-IR) at baseline and after 6 weeks of dietary supplementation.

Results: A total of 54 randomized patients with CA received either a specific micronutrient combination or placebo. Dietary intervention led to a significant decrease in fasting insulin ≥58 pmol/l ($p = 0.020$), and HOMA-IR ($p = 0.053$) in the verum group after 6 weeks. At the same time, parameters of LV diastolic function were improved after intervention in the verum group: significant reduction of LV mass index ($p = 0.003$), and in tendency both a decrease of interventricular septal thickness ($p = 0.053$) as well as an increase of E/A ratio ($p = 0.051$). On the other hand, the premature beats (PBs) were unchanged under verum.

Conclusions: In this pilot study, dietary intervention with specific micronutrient combination as add-on to concomitant cardiovascular drug treatment seems to improve cardio metabolic health in patients with CA. Further studies are required.

Keywords: Diastolic LV function, LVMI, Dietary intervention, Glucose metabolism, Premature beats

* Correspondence: praxisparsi@t-online.de
[1]Outpatient Practice of Cardiology, Suermondtstr. 13, D-13053 Berlin, Germany
Full list of author information is available at the end of the article

Background

Supraventricular (SVPBs) and ventricular premature beats (VPBs) are very common arrhythmias in patients with cardiovascular disorders. The incidence of SVPBs in Electrocardiogram (ECG) at rest is present in 10–20% [1], VPBs in 5–10% [2]. The prevalence is increasing with age. Patients with components of MetS like arterial hypertension (AH), abdominal obesity, type 2 diabetes mellitus (T2DM), impaired glucose tolerance (IGT) or HOMA-IR also show in addition to CA in different degree disturbances in cardiac metabolism and LV function. Based on abdominal obesity, IGT driven by IR leads already at an early stage to changes of diastolic function in different degree [3, 4]. The diastolic dysfunction is described with different parameters [5, 6] but according to the current ESC Guidelines for the diagnosis and treatment of acute and chronic heart failure, one of important parameter to describe the diastolic function is the left ventricular mass index (LVMI) [7].

Numerous studies on therapeutic interventions with magnesium [8–12], potassium [13], B vitamins [14–19], and Coenzyme Q10 [20–24] for CA and cardiometabolic risk factors have been published. An insufficient supply of magnesium can be clinical relevant as a trigger of CA and can also be linked with different components of the MetS like T2DM, and insulin resistance as well as by therapy with proton-pump inhibitors [25] and diuretics [12]. It may be caused by poor oral intake, elevated renal loss, diarrhea or alcoholism. The hypomagnesemia is also often combined with hypokalemia [26].

One objective of this pilot study was to investigate, if daily dietary intervention with a specific micronutrient combination improved LV function of CA in patients with disturbances in glucose metabolism after 6 weeks.

Methods

Study population

This was a post hoc analysis of the randomized double blind, placebo-controlled pilot study in patients with CA, which were recruited from patients who were 18–75 years of age in an Outpatient Practice of Cardiology in Berlin, Germany. 74 Caucasian patients with cardiac arrhythmias (VPBs, SVPBs, SV tachycardia) were screened from April 2014 to July 2015. Overall, patients who completed the study participated in 5 visits in the Outpatient Practice of Cardiology. At the first visit the patients were informed about the study in detail and the necessary examinations for inclusion and exclusion criteria were carried out. If the criteria were met and the patient gave his written consent to participate in the study, the placebo tablets for the run-in phase were issued at the second visit. Visit 3 marked the time baseline, again the inclusion and exclusion criteria were examined and the patients randomized. A further visit

followed after a 3-week intervention phase, before 6 weeks follow-up.

Inclusion criteria were: ≥ 500 VPBs or ≥ 200 SVPBs or ≥ 10 SV tachycardia's in Holter ECG at least 18 h. The general exclusion criteria were age > 75 years, LVEF ≤40%, intake of spironolactone > 50 mg/d, torasemide > 20 mg/d, supplementation of vitamins and minerals, hypo- or hyperkalemia, hypo- or hypermagnesemia, impaired renal function, hyperthyreosis, cardiac pacemaker, acute or chronic diarrhoea. Fourteen screened patients don't meet the inclusion criteria: They have not had the amount of supraventricular or ventricular ectopic beats, and one patient had a hypomagnesemia.

Figure 1 shows the trial profile of the 74 screened patients. All included subjects received placebo administration (2 tablets 2 times a day) during a one-week run-in period. After evaluation of the Holter ECG at baseline and check of the inclusion criteria 60 patients were randomly assigned to the verum or placebo group. Duration of dietary intervention was 6 weeks. Over this period of the randomized double blind, placebo-controlled pilot study, participants were required to take 2 tablets 2 times a day of verum (5 kcal, 145.8 mg magnesium, 469.2 mg potassium, 3.0 μg Vitamin B12, 400.0 μg folic acid, 48.0 mg niacin and 60.0 mg coenzyme Q10) or placebo (microcrystalline cellulose) with 200 ml water.

Outcomes for glucose metabolism and LV function

The exploratory outcomes were the changes in HOMA-IR and LV function after 6 weeks of dietary intervention in patients with CA.

Clinical measurements of components of the metabolic syndrome

At baseline the waist circumference (WC) was determined with a flexible tape with a measuring deviation nearest to 0.5 cm. WC was measured at the level midway between the lower rib margin and the iliac crest after breathing out normally and in standing position. MetS was determined by using diagnostic criteria of the International Diabetes Federation (IDF) [27]. The IDF definition requires increased WC, namely ≥94 cm and ≥ 80 cm for European males and females respectively, and any two of the following four components: systolic blood pressure (BP) ≥ 130 mmHg or diastolic BP ≥ 85 mmHg or treatment of hypertension, triglycerides (TG) ≥ 1.7 mmol/l, HDL-cholesterol (HDL-C) < 1.29 mmol/l in females, and < 1.03 mmol/l in males or treatment for lipid abnormality, fasting glucose ≥5.6 mmol/l or previously diagnosed T2DM. WC and Waist-to-Height-Ratio (WHtR) > 0.5 are proxy measures of abdominal obesity [28, 29].

In addition, an echocardiography (GE Medical Systems, Vivid S6), as well as a standard 12-leads ECG at rest (EINTHOVEN, GOLDBERGER, WILSON leads)

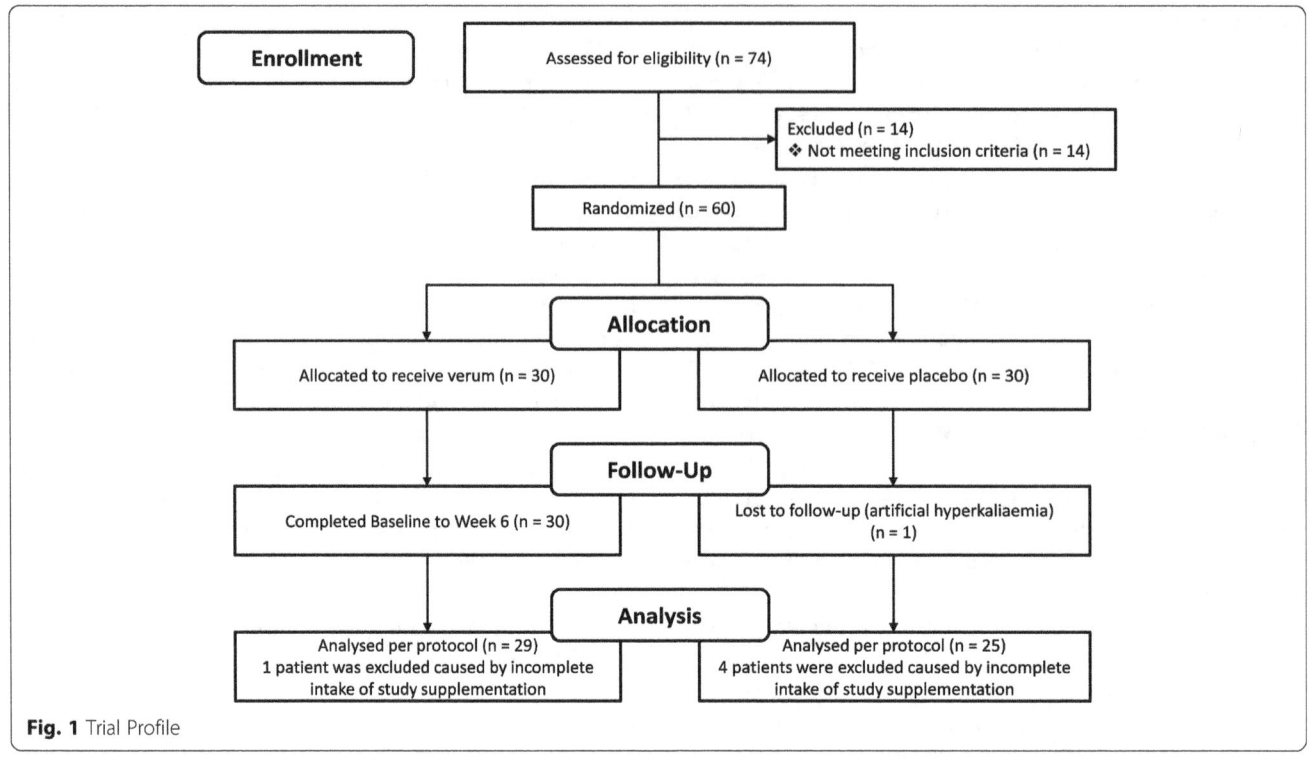

Fig. 1 Trial Profile

was performed and recorded on CUSTO CARD (custo med GmbH, Munich) as well as a Holter ECG (CUSTO FLASH 500 Multiday, custo med GmbH, Munich) for at least 18 h. ECG at rest and Holter ECG were analysed computer-assisted using Minnesota ECG Code Classification [30]. The SVPBs and VPBs were detected by software and confirmed by 2 cardiologists.

Echocardiographic studies were performed by 2 cardiologists in standard views [31]: parasternal long-axis view of the left ventricle in 2D, colour Doppler and M-mode, parasternal RV inflow- and outflow tract view in 2D and coulour Doppler, apical four- and five chamber view in 2D and colour Doppler, apical two-chamber view in 2D and colour Doppler, apical long-axis view in 2D and colour doppler, transmitral, transaortic and tricuspid velocities as well as tissue Doppler on mitral annulus (lateral velocities) in 4-chamber-view in accordence to the recommendations [32]. The upper cut off for LVMI in men is $\geq 115 \, g/m^2$ and women $\geq 95 \, g/m^2$ [7]. All echo parameters including LVMI were created by Vivid 6, GE Medical Systems, Ver. 11.2.0 b. 40.

Blood and urinary samples for biochemical assessment were collected at baseline, after 3 and after 6 weeks of dietary intervention (Fig. 2).

Laboratory tests

All laboratory analyses were conducted by Laboratory Schottdorf MVZ GmbH, Augsburg, Germany. The Analyses of serum glucose (hexokinase method),

gammaglutamyltransferase (IFCC method), glycated haemoglobin (HbA1c) (turbidimetric immunologic inhibition assay (TINIA)), insulin (ECLIA), total cholesterol (TC) (CHOD-PAP method), LDL-C and HDL-C (enzymatic colour test), TG (GPO-PAP method) and CRP sensitive (turbidimetry) were performed on a Roche analyser. 24 h urinary magnesium and potassium excretion was analysed by atomic absorption spectrometry. The HOMA is a measure for IR. HOMA-IR was calculated from insulin and glucose concentrations.

Statistical analysis

Statistical comparisons were made between groups using the nonparametric Mann-Whitney-U-test. The nonparametric Wilcoxon test was used for data comparison at different time points within groups. Differences in classified variables were tested by Fisher's exact test. The influence of covariates was analysed by analysis of variance (ANOVA). All statistical tests were based on per protocol population and two-sided. Differences were considered significant at $p < 0.05$. Data are reported as mean ± standard deviation (SD). Linear regression modelling was performed to detect the changes of different components of the cardiometabolic parameters as a function of LVMI and serum magnesium concentration. The effect size Cohen's d is defined as the difference between two means divided by a SD for the data. Effect size (ES) threshold: small 0.20, medium 0.50, large 0.80, very large 1.30 [33]. The first and third quartile (Q1 and Q3

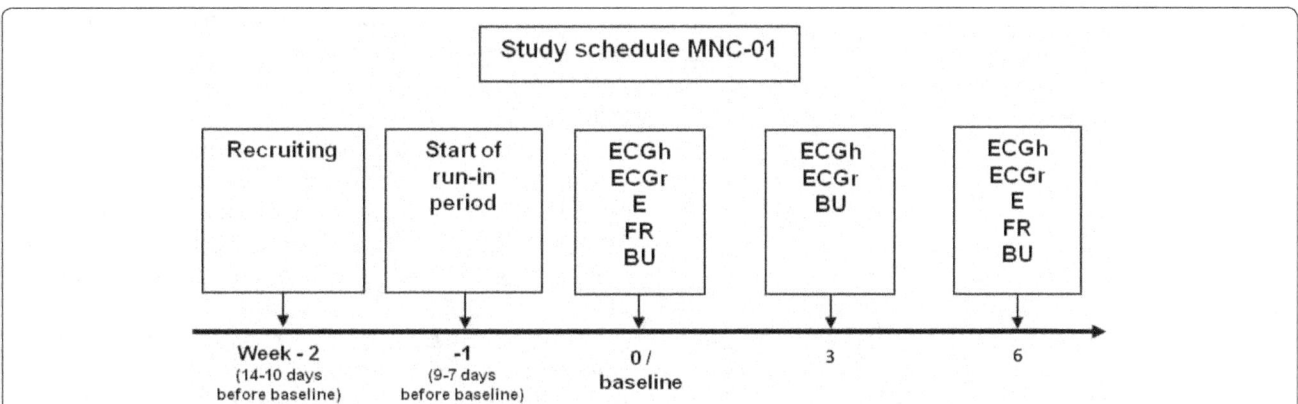

Fig. 2 Study schedule. Recruiting / Start of run-in period: At the first visit the patients were informed about the study in detail and the necessary examinations for inclusion and exclusion criteria were carried out. If the criteria were met and the patient gave his written consent to participate in the study, the placebo tablets for the run-in phase were issued at the second visit. Baseline: Inclusion and exclusion criteria were once again checked, then the patients were randomized. In addition anthropological parameters were collected at each visit. Abbreviations used: E, echocardiography; ECG, electrocardiogramm; ECGr, ECG at rest; ECGh, Holter ECG; FR, 3-day food record; BU, Blood and urinary samples

respectively) are shown. All analyses were conducted using SPSS® for Windows (version 22.0).

Results
Patients' characteristics
Fifty-four patients were evaluated per protocol, 29 in verum group, and 25 in placebo group (Fig. 1). Six patients did not finish the study per protocol: One patient in the placebo group has had an artificial hyperkalemia. 5 patients of the study population consumed less than 95% of study administration (8%), 4 of these patients were in placebo group.

No serious side effects were reported under dietary intervention. One patient in the verum group and one in the placebo group reported gastric pain. This could be caused by supplement intake. The supplementation has not been interrupted.

Pre-existing diseases und medications
Arterial hypertension (AH) was the most frequent pre-existing disease (65.5% verum group, 52.0% placebo group). Coronary artery disease (CAD) was present in 27.6% of patients in the verum group, and in 28.0% in the placebo group. A long-term medical treatment with beta blocking agents, ACE-inhibitors/AT II receptor antagonists, calcium channel blocker as well as spironolactone was given to 21 patients (72.4%) in the verum group and 16 patients (64.0%) in the placebo group. T2DM was found in 10.3% of patients in the verum group and 8.0% in the placebo group. At baseline 68.5% of patients had a dyslipidemia (verum 68.9%, placebo 68.0%). Treatment with statins was recorded in 34.5% in the verum group and 28.0% in the placebo group. Further baseline characteristics of both groups are shown in Table 1.

Metabolic syndrome and its components
Body mass index (BMI) $\geq 25 \, kg/m^2$ was recorded in 65.5% of the verum group and in 72.0% of the placebo group at baseline. An abdominal obesity with WHtR ≥ 0.5 was found in 72.4% of the verum group and in 80.0% of the placebo group (Table 1). The number of patients with criteria of MetS according to IDF compared to baseline to the study end decreased in the verum group of 16 to 15, and on the contrary in the placebo group increased from 8 to 12. At baseline 5 patients (17.2%) in the verum group and 4 (16.0%) in the placebo group had an atherogenic dyslipidemia and at study end 4 patients in the verum group (13.8%) and 3 (12.0%) in the placebo group.

LV function
In all patients at baseline the right ventricular end diastolic diameter (RVEDD), left atrium (LA), left ventricular end systolic diameter (LVESD), left ventricular end diastolic diameter (LVEDD), left ventricular ejection fraction (LVEF), intraventricular septum (IVS) and left ventricular posterior wall (LVPW) were in normal range. However, patients with LVEF 54–65% showed a significant increase of LVEF ($p = 0.020$, ES = 0.995, Q1;Q3: 0.5;15.0) in the verum group after intervention (Table 2).

After dietary intervention the LV mass index (LVMI) was significantly reduced in the verum group ($p = 0.003$, ES = 0.260, Q1;Q3: -26.5;-2.2). If a distinction is made between male and female this parameter is significantly reduced too, especially by reducing of this parameter in woman ($p = 0.035$). The LVEDD ($p = 0.050$, ES = 0.210, Q1/Q3: -5.0; 1.0) were reduced and E/A ratio ($p = 0.051$, ES = 0.401, Q1; Q3: -0.04; 0.27) in normal range was improved. In the placebo group these results were not

Table 1 Baseline characteristics

	Verum (n = 29)	Placebo (n = 25)	V vs. P
	x ± SD	x ± SD	p-value
Sex (n/%)			
female	14 (48.3%)	13 (52.0%)	1.000
male	15 (51.7%)	12 (48.0%)	
Age (years)	59.7 ± 10.2	59.8 ± 13.8	0.524
Height (cm)	171.9 ± 8.8	171.0 ± 9.1	0.740
Weight (kg)	82.0 ± 17.9	82.9 ± 14.7	0.561
BMI (kg/m^2)	27.6 ± 4.8	28.3 ± 4.2	0.535
< 25.0 kg/m^2 (n/%)	10 (34.5%)	7 (28.0%)	0.940
25.0–29.9 kg/m^2 (n/%)	11 (37.9%)	11 (44.0%)	
≥ 30.0 kg/m^2 (n/%)	8 (27.6%)	7 (28.0%)	
WC female (cm)	88.9 ± 13.1	87.6 ± 9.6	0.847
≥ 88 cm (n/%)	9 (31.0%)	5 (20.0%)	0.449
WC male (cm)	103.6 ± 14.6	106.6 ± 8.8	0.286
≥ 102 cm (n/%)	8 (27.6%)	9 (36.0%)	0.429
WHtR	0.558 ± 0.080	0.565 ± 0.064	0.602
≥ 0,5 (n/%)	21 (72.4%)	20 (80.0%)	0.545
BP systolic (mmHg)	142.2 ± 17.4	134.7 ± 12.5	0.077
≥ 130 mmHg (n/%)	23 (79.3%)	16 (64.0%)	0.239
BP diastolic (mmHg)	86.3 ± 9.7	82.2 ± 8.6	0.160
≥ 85 mmHg (n/%)	16 (55.2%)	9 (36.0%)	0.182
Heart rate/min	71.4 ± 12.5	72.9 ± 12.7	0.773

Abbreviations: BMI body mass index, WC waist circumference, WHtR waist to height ratio, BP blood pressure

found. But the differences between these both groups are statistical not significant.

The linear regression analysis showed that LVMI in the verum group depended on the initial value and the magnesium concentration in the serum during the course of the study. The change of LVMI is depending on the alteration in HDL-C and diastolic blood pressure. Only in the verum group the favourable changes of LVMI were found under this condition. In contrast, these results could not be shown in the placebo group (Table 3).

The interventricular septal thickness was reduced in tendency only in the verum group ($p = 0.053$, ES = 0.348, Q1; Q3: -2.0;0.5), while LVPW was unchanged in both groups. On the other hand, the LA parameters were significantly increased in the verum group after intervention but within the normal range ($p = 0.018$, ES = 0.314, Q1; Q3: -0.75; 3.75) (Table 2). Furthermore could be demonstrated a strong correlation between LVMI and LA in men ($p = 0.018$), but not in female ($p = 0.225$).

When looking at the results broken down by HOMA quartiles and parameters of LV function it can be noted, that in female diameter of LA increases age-adjusted significantly with the quartiles ($p = 0.001$) and in male the

LVEDD ($p = 0.055$) (Table 4). The influence of HOMA-quartiles was proofed by a regression model.

HOMA-IR

In the verum group abnormal fasting plasma glucose ≥5.6 mmol/l was distinctly reduced after 6 weeks of dietary intervention compared to baseline ($p = 0.055$, ES = 0.388, Q1;Q3: -1.30;-0.11), in the placebo group this difference was not found ($p = 0.328$, ES = 0.604, Q1;Q3: -0.94;0.28).

At baseline, elevated fasting insulin concentration (≥ 58 pmol/l) was recorded in 19 patients of the verum group and in 17 patients of the placebo group, a normal level (< 58 pmol/l) in 10 patients in the verum group vs. 8 patients in the placebo group. But only in the verum group it was in tendency reduced after intervention ($p = 0.053$, ES = 0.232, Q1;Q3: -35.1;9.4), and significantly in patients with fasting insulin ≥58 pmol/l ($p = 0.020$, ES = 0.340, Q1;Q3: -42.7; 1.4).

Elevated HOMA-IR > 2.5 was found in 14 patients in the verum group, and 11 patients in the placebo group. An euglycaemic IR (FPG < 5.6 mmol/l, HOMA-IR ≥ 2.5) showed at baseline 8 patients in the verum group and 4 patients in the placebo group. HOMA-IR was in tendency reduced in the verum group ($p = 0.053$, ES = 0.218, Q1;Q3: -1.25;0.25) at the end of study, particularly for patients with HOMA-IR > 2.5 in the verum group ($p = 0.068$, ES = 0.340, Q1;Q3: -2.90;-0.22) (Table 5). At the study end only 3 patients had a HOMA-IR ≥ 2.5 ($p = 0.063$), and in the placebo group 2 patients a HOMA-IR ≥ 2.5 ($p = 0.625$).

Other biochemistry cardiovascular risk factors

All relevant biochemical parameters are summarized in Table 5. In the blood cell count up to a significant reduction of leucocytes in normal range in the verum group ($p < 0.05$) all components were in normal range in the verum as well as the placebo group. Total cholesterol (TC) was unchanged in verum and placebo group after dietary intervention. LDL-cholesterol (LDL-C) was nearly unchanged in the verum group, and in the placebo group slightly reduced; HDL-C was unchanged in both groups. After dietary intervention TG were significantly increased in the verum group ($p = 0.011$, ES = 0.292, Q1;Q3: -0.01;0.30), but unchanged in the placebo group. TG concentrations ≥1.7 mmol/l were found at baseline in 27.6% of patients in the verum group and 28.0% in the placebo group. At study end this relation was 31.0 to 20.0%.

Renal function measured by creatinine and glomerular filtration rate (GFR) was normal in all patients. The changes in serum magnesium was significantly higher compared to the placebo group after intervention ($p = 0.005$, ES = 0.708, Q1;Q3: -0.02;0.05 vs. -0.06;0.01). The serum

Table 2 Changing of patient's characteristics: comparison of echocardiographic values before and after dietary intervention

	Verum (n = 29) x ± SD			Placebo (n = 25) x ± SD		
	Baseline	Week 6	Diff	Baseline	Week 6	Diff
LA (mm)	35.8 ± 5.9	37.1 ± 5.0	1.39 ± 2.92#	36.4 ± 6.4	35.8 ± 6.1	− 0.68 ± 4.26
RVEDD (mm)	26.8 ± 5.3	26.3 ± 3.4	− 0.52 ± 4.67	25.2 ± 4.1	25.1 ± 3.5	− 0.08 ± 4.29
LVEDD (mm)	49.0 ± 5.7	47.6 ± 7.1	− 1.34 ± 5.47#	47.9 ± 6.9	48.4 ± 7.5	0.52 ± 5.64
LVESD (mm)	30.4 ± 4.9	30.1 ± 5.5	− 0.31 ± 3.27	29.5 ± 5.2	30.2 ± 6.7	0.72 ± 4.20
LVEF (%)	68.6 ± 8.3	70.2 ± 9.0	1.66 ± 8.94	70.0 ± 9.3	70.3 ± 8.9	0.28 ± 10.81
< 65% (n/%)	10 (34.5%)	9 (31.0%)	–	6 (24.0%)	7 (28.0%)	–
< 65%	59.5 ± 4.2	66.8 ± 9.5	7.30 ± 8.22#	57.5 ± 5.4	64.5 ± 11.8	7.00 ± 7.75
≥ 65%	73.5 ± 5.5	72.5 ± 8.4	− 1.00 ± 8.07	74.0 ± 6.3	72.1 ± 7.3	− 1.84 ± 10.93
IVS (mm)	10.6 ± 1.6	9.9 ± 1.9	− 0.62 ± 1.78	10.6 ± 1.4	10.2 ± 1.5	− 0.44 ± 1.32
LVPW (mm)	10.7 ± 1.6	10.3 ± 1.6	− 0.41 ± 1.52	10.4 ± 1.5	10.2 ± 1.6	− 0.20 ± 1.12
E/E´ > 8 (n/%)	2 (25.0%)	3 (37.5%)	–	2 (33.3%)	0 (0.0%)	–
E wave	0.73 ± 0.19	0.71 ± 0.16	− 0.02 ± 0.18	0.73 ± 0.18	0.72 ± 0.15	− 0.01 ± 0.15
A wave	0.74 ± 0.24	0.68 ± 0.28	− 0.06 ± 0.19	0.71 ± 0.18	0.73 ± 0.15	0.01 ± 0.16
E/A ratio	1.05 ± 0.35	1.18 ± 0.49	0.13 ± 0.38#	1.45 ± 2.04	1.02 ± 0.21	− 0.42 ± 2.04
LVMI g/m2	98.2 ± 24.4	90.0 ± 37.0	−8.15 ± 35.48##	93.5 ± 26.5	90.9 ± 25.9	−2.61 ± 21.20
LVMI g/m² female[a]	87.2 ± 16.6	77.7 ± 20.9	−9.5 ± 15.6#	89.0 ± 26.2	80.2 ± 21.8	−8.7 ± 23.1
LVMI g/m² male[b]	108.4 ± 26.4	101.5 ± 45.1	−6.9 ± 47#	98.4 ± 27.1	102.4 ± 25.9	4.0 ± 17.5

Abbreviations: LA, left atrium; RVEDD, right ventricular end diastolic diameter; LVEDD, left ventricular end diastolic diameter; LVESD, left ventricular end systolic diameter; LVEF, left ventricular ejection fraction; IVS, interventricular septum; LVPW, left ventricular posterior wall; E/A ratio, ratio of the early (E) to late (A) ventricular filling velocities; LVMI, Left ventricular mass index
[a]n = 14 (verum)/n = 13 (placebo, [b] n = 15 (verum)/n = 12 (placebo)
# p < 0.05 within the group, ## p < 0.01 within the group

potassium level was significantly increased after intervention in the verum group ($p = 0.034$, ES = 0.512, Q1;Q3: 0.0;0.3 vs. -0.5;0.1), compared to the placebo group. However, the increase of both serum magnesium as well as potassium after intervention was in normal range.

In 24 h urinary collection potassium excretion ($p = 0.059$, ES = 0.326, Q1;Q3: -7.2;30.2) as well as magnesium excretion were elevated ($p = 0.018$, ES = 0.507, Q1;Q3: -0.18;1.66) in the verum group. The magnesium excretion was significant compared to the placebo group too ($p = 0.036$, ES = 0.377, Q1;Q3: -0.13;1.51 vs. -0.64;0.46). This result was an effect of compliance. The normal renal function could be shown in 24 h urinary collection: albumin excretion as well as the quotient albumin/creatinine/24 h was in normal

range. Only in the verum group this quotient was in tendency reduced after dietary intervention, while in the placebo group this quotient was increased. This difference in both groups was reduced ($p = 0.083$, ES = 0.521, Q1;Q3: -0.09;0.03 vs. -0.05;0.22).

Rhythm disturbances

In this pilot study a reduction of PBs could be observed in the verum group, but this result was not significant, probably due to the small number of patients and an enormous variance of the PBs. On the other hand, in the placebo group the reduction of VPBs was remarkable with the same enormous variance as in the verum group ($p = 0.005$, ES = 0.369, Q1;Q3: -935.0;5.0). The heart rate was

Table 3 Changing of LVMI depending on alteration in HDL-Cholesterol and diastolic blood pressure

	total P_ANOVA	Depending variable: Regression coefficient B (p-value)			
		LVMI Baseline	Serum-Mg Week 6	Changing of	
Verum (n = 29)	0,008	0,014	0,002	HDL-C	−0,567[1] (0,507)
	0,003	0,011	0,004	BP diastolic	1,623[2] (0,129)
Placebo (n = 25)	0,069	0,014	0,257	HDL-C	0,697 (0,283)
	0,109	0,020	0,421	BP diastolic	−0,164 (0,780)

Modell of linear regression, depending variable: changing of LVMI, age adjusted
Abbreviations: LVMI left ventricular mass index, Serum-Mg serum magnesium, HDL-C HDL cholesterol, BP blood pressure
[1]Increase of HDL-C correlates with decrease of LVMI
[2]Decrease of BP diastolic correlates with decrease of LVMI

Table 4 HOMA-quartiles for LVMI, LA, IVS, PW, and LVEDD in male and female

HOMA-quartile	1: 0.7 … 1.5	2: 1.6 … 2.4	3: 2.5 … 4.3	4: > 4.3	p-value
N (male/female)	7/7	5/8	5/9	10/3	
LVMI (male)	96.1 +/− 36.8	106.2 +/− 23.2	102.9 +/− 35.9	108.9 +/− 16.4	0.372
LVMI (female)	80.6 +/− 19.4	95.7 +/− 25.1	90.7 +/− 21.4	78.6 +/− 13.5	0.967
LA (male)	37.3 +/− 7.6	38.0 +/− 7.2	37.0 +/− 4.8	41.4 +/− 4.2	0.118
LA (female)	29.1 +/− 2.5	32.0 +/− 2.6	34.0 +/− 5.6	40.3 +/− 4.0	0.001
IVS (male)	11.6 +/− 1.8	11.2 +/− 1.3	10.8 +/− 1.8	11.0 +/− 1.3	0.533
IVS (female)	9.6 +/− 1.4	9.8 +/− 1.3	10.8 +/− 1.2	9.3 +/− 1.2	0.489
PW (male)	11.3 +/− 1.9	11.4 +/− 1.5	11.0 +/− 2.0	11.3 +/− 1.4	0.880
PW (female)	9.4 +/− 1.5	9.6 +/− 0.7	10.3 +/− 1.4	10.0 +/− 1.0	0.205
LVEDD (male)	47.0 +/− 8.5	50.0 +/− 7.1	51.4 +/− 6.7	53.5 +/− 4.1	0.055
LVEDD (female)	43.1 +/− 4.8	49.8 +/− 4.5	44.9 +/− 4.5	47.3 +/− 3.2	0.562

Abbreviations: HOMA Homeostasis Model Assessment, LVMI left ventricular mass index, LA left atrium, IVS interventricular septum, PW posterior wall, LVEDD left ventricular end diastolic diameter

decreased only in the verum group ($p = 0.027$, ES = 0.256, Q1;Q3: -7.8;0.8) (Table 6).

A change of awareness of symptoms measured by a visual analogue scale (VAS points) also could not be found.

Discussion

Metabolic syndrome and its components

The MetS is the burden of our century and in Germany could be found with prevalence depending on the region between 14 and 23% [34].

Precursors of MetS like disturbed glucose tolerance, triggered by elevated fasting insulin followed by IR, lead already at early stage to structural changes of the left ventricle and influence on diastolic function. These factors seem to be acting independently from CAD associated especially with diastolic dysfunction or heart failure [4, 5, 35]. Our knowledge based on experimental [36] and clinical studies concerning the MetS [4, 5, 37, 38] as well as meta-analyses [28].

The influence of micronutrients on these pathological processes in MetS is only partially known. There is evidence that magnesium plays an important role, especially in the glucose metabolism [10]. In addition, a positive effect on glucose metabolism is discussed for magnesium and for coenzyme Q10 [21, 24]. The effects of coenzyme Q10 on the glucose metabolism may be based on multifactorial mechanisms i.e. by reduction of oxidative stress [39, 40].

On average, the patients enrolled in this study were overweight, with abdominal obesity measured by WC and also by WHtR. These basic components of MetS as well as fasting plasma glucose were unchanged after intervention. The reduction of systolic blood pressure in the verum group at study end has not influenced this result. Therefore we did not found a reduction of the components of MetS in verum group. The results of this post hoc analysis seem to suggest that this specific combination of micronutrients improves the cardiometabolic profile in patients with CA.

LV function

The MetS and its components – IR/T2DM, AH and abdominal obesity – are associated with impaired mitochondrial function and increased oxidative stress. These pathophysiological mechanisms contribute to the development of diastolic dysfunction [4, 35, 37, 38]. Ikee et al. [41] found that diastolic dysfunction at first is an asymptomatic disorder of relaxation and/or compliance associated with normal systolic pump function. It depends on preload, end diastolic pressure and structure of the LV wall.

We found signs of preclinical LV diastolic dysfunction parallel to metabolic changes. This is consistent with the results of this pilot study in comparison of the verum and placebo group. At baseline the E/A ratio was in tendency lower in the verum group than in the placebo group. After intervention E/A ratio was significantly improved in the verum group, but not in the placebo group. Diastolic dysfunction assessed with the use of E/A worsened with the number of components of MetS [42]. The changes in diastolic function are age related [32, 42, 43] and furthermore depending on components of MetS like overweight, T2DM, AH, and CAD [4, 35]. Furthermore, the present study showed that the LVEF could only be improved if it was within the lower normal range (54–65%). Magnesium leads to an economization of cardiac pump function [44]. In a review it could be shown that also CoQ10 improves parameters of heart function like ejection fraction in heart failure [45]. This could be confirmed with this study: the results demonstrate a significant improvement of EF ≤ 65% in the verum group, but this effect was not significant between the both study groups (Table 2).

Table 5 Changing of patient's characteristics: comparison of biochemical values before and after dietary intervention

	Verum ($n = 29$) x ± SD			Placebo ($n = 25$) x ± SD		
	Baseline	Week 6	Diff	Baseline	Week 6	Diff
CrP (nmol/l)	26.0 ± 28.7	24.8 ± 22.6	−1.22 ± 23.37	20.8 ± 19.8	29.8 ± 42.1	9.07 ± 39.52
< 10 nmol/l (n/%)	9 (31.0%)	9 (31.0%)	–	10 (40.0%)	12 (48.0%)	–
10–30 nmol/l (n/%)	13 (44.8%)	13 (44.8%)		10 (40.0%)	6 (24.0%)	
> 30 nmol/l (n/%)	7 (24.1%)	7 (24.1%)		5 (20.0%)	7 (28.0%)	
FPG (mmol/l)	5.49 ± 1.58	5.30 ± 1.28	− 0.20 ± 0.75	5.35 ± 0.65	5.15 ± 0.77	−0.20 ± 0.63[#]
< 5.6 mmol/l	4.76 ± 0.54	4.79 ± 0.62	0.03 ± 0.39	5.04 ± 0.27	4.91 ± 0.70	− 0.13 ± 0.58
≥ 5.6 mmol/l	7.12 ± 1.94	6.42 ± 1.67	−0.70 ± 1.10	6.15 ± 0.65	5.79 ± 0.56	−0.36 ± 0.75
HbA1c (%)	5.77 ± 0.68	5.76 ± 0.63	−0.01 ± 0.35	5.64 ± 0.39	5.66 ± 0.33	0.02 ± 0.39
F Insulin (pmol/l)[a]	113.9 ± 127.5	89.5 ± 75.8	− 24.4 ± 73.4	83.6 ± 44.9	71.3 ± 51.3	−12.3 ± 54.0
< 58 pmol/l (n/%)	10 (34.5%)	11 (37.9%)	–	8 (32.0%)	10 (40.0%)	–
< 58 pmol/l	39.2 ± 9.9	44.7 ± 18.4	5.2 ± 19.5	41.3 ± 13.5	40.4 ± 13.3	− 0.9 ± 16.0
≥ 58 pmol/l	153.1 ± 143.2	113.1 ± 84.0	−39.9 ± 86.3[#]	103.5 ± 40.0	85.9 ± 56.3	− 17.7 ± 64.6
HOMA-IR[a]	4.93 ± 9.18	3.39 ± 4.00	− 1.54 ± 5.69[#]	2.97 ± 1.86	2.50 ± 2.17	−0.47 ± 2.26
≤ 2.5 (n/%)	15 (51.7%)	20 (69.0%)	–	14 (56.0%)	18 (72.0%)	–
≤ 2.5	1.55 ± 0.52	1.57 ± 0.59	0.03 ± 0.56	1.66 ± 0.52	1.95 ± 2.19	0.29 ± 2.02
> 2.5	8.56 ± 12.40	5.34 ± 5.12	− 3.22 ± 7.97	4.64 ± 1.60	3.20 ± 2.03	− 1.44 ± 2.28
Na (mmol/l)	143.0 ± 4.5	142.2 ± 2.7	−0.76 ± 4.25	141.9 ± 2.5	141.6 ± 2.8	−0.28 ± 2.51
< 140 mmol/l	138.0 ± 1.2	139.0 ± 3.5	1.00 ± 2.83	138.4 ± 0.9	138.8 ± 4.4	0.40 ± 4.22
≥ 140 mmol/l	143.8 ± 4.3	142.8 ± 2.2	− 1.04 ± 4.41	142.8 ± 2.0	142.4 ± 1.7	− 0.45 ± 2.01
K (mmol/l)	4.44 ± 0.53	4.55 ± 0.43	0.11 ± 0.44	4.59 ± 0.37	4.50 ± 0.31	−0.09 ± 0.33*
< 4.0 mmol/l	3.72 ± 0.17	4.08 ± 0.34	0.35 ± 0.26	3.70	4.10	0.40
≥ 4.0 mmol/l	4.56 ± 0.47	4.62 ± 0.40	0.07 ± 0.45	4.63 ± 0.33	4.52 ± 0.31	− 0.11 ± 0.32
Mg (mmol/l)	0.845 ± 0.069	0.858 ± 0.068	0.013 ± 0.047	0.874 ± 0.084	0.851 ± 0.068	−0.024 ± 0.056[#]**
< 0.75 mmol/l	0.727 ± 0.023	0.773 ± 0.021	0.048 ± 0.035	0.72	0.77	0.05
≥ 0.75 mmol/l	0.859 ± 0.058	0.867 ± 0.068	0.009 ± 0.047	0.881 ± 0.079	0.854 ± 0.068	− 0.027 ± 0.055[##]**
Cl (mmol/l)	102.0 ± 3.4	100.9 ± 2.6	−1.03 ± 3.80	101.4 ± 2.6	101.4 ± 3.2	0.00 ± 3.20
< 100 mmol/l	98.0 ± 1.2	99.6 ± 2.4	1.57 ± 2.51	97.8 ± 1.0	100.2 ± 2.5	2.33 ± 2.88
≥ 100 mmol/l	103.2 ± 2.8	101.4 ± 2.5	−1.86 ± 3.81[#]	102.6 ± 1.8	101.8 ± 3.4	−0.74 ± 3.00
Creatinine (μmol/l)	77.4 ± 14.6	76.4 ± 14.9	−0.95 ± 6.98	76.6 ± 17.4	75.3 ± 16.4	−1.31 ± 7.02
GFR (ml/min)	83.6 ± 13.9	85.4 ± 14.9	1.79 ± 8.09	86.1 ± 16.0	86.8 ± 16.3	0.76 ± 6.48
TC (mmo/l)	4.97 ± 1.00	5.12 ± 1.09	0.15 ± 0.66	5.25 ± 0.94	5.10 ± 1.04	−0.15 ± 0.69
≥ 5.2 mmol/l	5.74 ± 0.63	6.08 ± 0.79	0.34 ± 0.85	5.86 ± 0.75	5.89 ± 0.67	0.03 ± 0.37
LDL-C (mmol/l)	3.14 ± 0.97	3.10 ± 0.83	− 0.04 ± 0.44	3.39 ± 0.92	3.30 ± 0.97	−0.09 ± 0.45
< 2.6 mmol/l	2.02 ± 0.27	2.27 ± 0.48	0.25 ± 0.45	2.11 ± 0.56	2.33 ± 0.32	0.22 ± 0.25
≥ 2.6 mmol/l	3.59 ± 0.76	3.43 ± 0.70	−0.15 ± 0.40	3.64 ± 0.76	3.48 ± 0.94	−0.15 ± 0.46
< 3.3 mmol/l	2.43 ± 0.48	2.59 ± 0.51	0.16 ± 0.36	2.72 ± 0.57*	2.67 ± 0.40	− 0.05 ± 0.33
≥ 3.3 mmol/l	4.08 ± 0.55	3.78 ± 0.68	− 0.30 ± 0.41[#]	4.01 ± 0.71	3.88 ± 0.99	− 0.14 ± 0.54
HDL-C (mmol/l)	1.40 ± 0.41	1.39 ± 0.43	−0.01 ± 0.17	1.45 ± 0.47	1.40 ± 0.42	−0.05 ± 0.17
TG (mmol/l)	1.56 ± 0.77	1.97 ± 1.86	0.42 ± 1.30[#]	1.34 ± 0.53	1.36 ± 0.50	0.02 ± 0.58
≥ 1.7 mmol/l	2.63 ± 0.57	3.71 ± 2.95	1.08 ± 2.41	2.08 ± 0.28*	1.71 ± 0.61	−0.37 ± 0.76
Uric acid (μmol/l)	338 ± 90	331 ± 80	− 7.2 ± 42.1	315 ± 100	308 ± 91	− 6.9 ± 39.9
Gamma-GT (μkat/l)	0.64 ± 0.83	0.63 ± 0.72	−0.01 ± 0.17	0.53 ± 0.29	0.52 ± 0.26	−0.01 ± 0.17
ASAT (μkat/l)	0.42 ± 0.20	0.42 ± 0.11	0.00 ± 0.14	0.40 ± 0.11	0.40 ± 0.13	0.00 ± 0.09

Table 5 Changing of patient's characteristics: comparison of biochemical values before and after dietary intervention *(Continued)*

	Verum (n = 29) x ± SD			Placebo (n = 25) x ± SD		
	Baseline	Week 6	Diff	Baseline	Week 6	Diff
ALAT (µkat/l)	0.47 ± 0.24	0.46 ± 0.21	− 0.02 ± 0.16	0.43 ± 0.26	0.45 ± 0.28	0.02 ± 0.11
TSH (µIU/ml)	2.15 ± 1.17	1.96 ± 1.06	−0.19 ± 0.52#	2.19 ± 1.20	1.92 ± 1.00	−0.28 ± 0.57#
24 h urinary collection						
Na (mmol/24 h)	193.7 ± 73.6	186.7 ± 76.0	−7.0 ± 79.7	167.9 ± 53.5	177.4 ± 64.1	9.5 ± 46.8
K (mmol/24 h)	68.2 ± 25.3	76.6 ± 26.2	8.4 ± 28.0	67.3 ± 19.3	71.6 ± 22.5	4.2 ± 18.0
K i.S./K (24 h)	0.072 ± 0.023	0.067 ± 0.027	− 0.005 ± 0.028	0.076 ± 0.034	0.069 ± 0.021	−0.008 ± 0.030
Mg (mmol/24 h)	4.03 ± 1.14	4.79 ± 1.79	0.76 ± 1.85#	3.78 ± 1.45	3.86 ± 1.88	0.08 ± 1.75*
Mg i.S./Mg (24 h)	0.227 ± 0.070	0.221 ± 0.162	−0.006 ± 0.180	0.260 ± 0.095	0.268 ± 0.121	0.008 ± 0.093
Cl (mmol/24 h)	175.6 ± 70.2	174.9 ± 76.9	−0.72 ± 74.63	153.5 ± 54.9	161.2 ± 70.7	7.72 ± 43.40
Albumin (mg/24 h)	10.8 ± 19.2	12.0 ± 26.4	1.17 ± 15.42	9.5 ± 17.2	11.7 ± 18.8	2.24 ± 5.88
Albumin/crea (24 h)	0.82 ± 1.40	0.80 ± 1.36	−0.02 ± 0.36	0.77 ± 1.31	0.96 ± 1.55	0.20 ± 0.48

Abbreviations: HK haematocrit, *MCHC* mean corpuscular/cellular haemoglobin concentration, *MCV* mean corpuscular/cell volume, *CrP* C reactive protein, *FPG* fasting plasma glucose, *HbA1c* glycated haemoglobin A1c, *F Insulin* fasting insulin, *HOMA-IR* homeostasis model assessment-insulin resistance, *Na* natrium, *K* potassium, *MG* magnesium, *Cl* chloride, *GFR* glomerular filtration rate, *TC* total cholesterol, *LDL-C* LDL-cholesterol, *HDL-C* HDL-cholesterol, *TG* triglycerides, *ASAT* aspartate-aminotranferase, *ALAT* alanin-aminotranferase, *TSH* thyroid stimulating hormone, # $p < 0.05$ within the group, ## $p < 0.01$ within the group, * $p < 0.05$ between the groups, ** $p < 0.01$ between the groups, ªLarge variation coefficients indicate statistical outliers. By sensitivity analyses the influence of these statistical outliers was checked. The results in the full analysis set were confirmed

Different authors described that the prevalence of LV diastolic dysfunction measured by diameters of the LA, left ventricle, and LVMI is significantly increased the more components of MetS exist [4, 5, 7].

In the verum group of the present study the diameter of LA was increased and especially related to the HOMA quartiles, but no more than in upper limit of normal. In male but not in female a strong positive correlation between LVMI and LA at baseline as a sign of diastolic dysfunction was demonstrable. In contrary in the placebo group this diameter was reduced. To what extent the SVPBs are relevant in this process is yet unknown. Measured by effect size functional parameters are more improved in the verum group within 6 weeks than structural parameters like LVMI. Overall in literature the findings in disturbances in glucose metabolism and transthoracic echocardiographic evaluated structural and functional parameters are not consistent. This may be based on exclusion of older and patients with higher BMI [46]. In accordance with Rutter et al. [46] and

Hwang et al. [47] we found these relations to different parameters of LV diastolic dysfunction by transthoracic echocardiography. Similar results on LV function in patients with insulin resistance and glycaemic abnormalities were described by Velagaleti et al. [48] by means of MR imaging. These associations were more frequently significant in males. Overall is the reduction of LVMI due to intervention within 6 weeks an interesting finding. The mechanisms of modification of LVMI are not yet fully understood. It is accepted that arterial hypertension is contributing to the development of LV hypertrophy. But the changes in 24-h blood pressure measuring contribute only 25 to 30% of variation of LV mass [49]. Sundström et al. [50] described in 2000 that different parameters of MetS stronger related to the LV wall thickness and concentric remodelling than to LV hypertrophy.

Later could be shown, that the changes in LVMI are closely related to the insulin resistance in animals as well as humans. In an animal experiment comparable could

Table 6 Changing of patient's characteristics: comparison of Holter ECG before and after dietary intervention

	Verum (n = 29) x ± SD			Placebo (n = 25) x ± SD		
	Baseline	Week 6	Diff	Baseline	Week 6	Diff
VPBs > 500/24 h	2486 ± 2133	2316 ± 3232	− 170 ± 2469	5717 ± 7662	2649 ± 3287	− 3068 ± 5259##
SV tachycardia (hr > 100/min)	37.3 ± 66.1	23.7 ± 46.0	− 13.6 ± 67.4	52.2 ± 67.3	39.9 ± 103.8	− 12.4 ± 96.9
SVPBs > 200/24 h	2000 ± 1874	2204 ± 1474	204 ± 1541	1025 ± 406	585 ± 786	− 440 ± 427
SVPBs < 200/24 h with symptoms	20.5 ± 32.9	21.3 ± 46.9	0.85 ± 55.83	39.2 ± 36.4*	107.7 ± 298.0	68.6 ± 269.7
Heart rate (bpm)	71.4 ± 12.5	68.4 ± 10.8	− 3.0 ± 7.9#	72.9 ± 12.7	70.3 ± 13.2	−2.6 ± 9.3

Abbreviations: VPBs ventricular premature beats, *SV* supraventricular, *SVPBs* supraventricular premature beats
#$p < 0.05$ within the group, ##$p < 0.01$ within the group, *$p < 0.05$ between the groups

be found the development of structural changes due to insulin resistance in mice within 3 weeks [51]. Verma et al. [52] investigated in 2016 in a subgroup 10 patients with T2DM and performed echo studies at begin and 3 months later. They found a significant reduction in LV mass and an improvement of diastolic function. The mechanism is at all not fully known and needs further elucidation and is not finally to declare at time.

Influence on insulin resistance

Different compounds and durations of dietary interventions are not comparable in its effects. For this reason the results are not consistent [14, 22].

In this study 27.6% in the verum group and 16.0% in the placebo group showed an euglycaemic IR measured by HOMA-IR at baseline. That suggests that these changes in glucose metabolism could be found in overweight patients much longer before manifestation of T2DM. At study end we found in verum group a reduction in euglycaemic IR to 10.3% and in the placebo group to 8.0%. Only in the verum group these parameters of glucose metabolism were reduced after intervention ($p = 0.063$). The significantly increased serum magnesium concentrations in the verum group compared to the placebo group after intervention were only connected with the significantly decrease of HOMA-IR in the verum group. Chutia and Lynrah [53] showed a positive correlation between fasting insulin level and HOMA level in patients with T2DM compared to non-diabetic controls. The correlation between serum magnesium level and fasting insulin level was inversely.

Low vitamin B12 levels have been found in obese adolescents with clinical features of IR [15]. The supplementation of vitamin B12, folate, and coenzyme Q10 in this study was helpful in two ways: on the one hand in general a great part of the population has a deficiency in these micronutrients, especially seniors [54], and on the other hand the substitution may improve the glucose metabolism with a significant decrease in fasting insulin and HOMA-IR. The BMI remained unchanged throughout the study duration of 6 weeks.

The described effects of coenzyme Q10 on glucose metabolism are differently. In an interventional supplementation of coenzyme Q10 in patients with MetS a positive effect on serum insulin levels and HOMA-IR could be found [21]. In contrary Moazen et al. [20] and Azevedo et al. [5] did not verify an effect of coenzyme Q10 on fasting blood glucose and HbA1C level compared to the placebo group. Other investigators [24] found a significant reduction in fasting plasma glucose and HbA1C level but not in serum insulin and HOMA-IR. The effect on lipid profile was not favourable.

Influence on other biochemical parameters

The most frequently investigated substance is the coenzyme Q10. Supplementations like vitamin C, E, coenzyme Q10 and selenium only in a combination also improved the glucose and lipid metabolism [22]. Folic acid supplementation in patients with T2DM effects a reduction in homocysteine on the other hand it increases glutathione levels with an inverse effect on HbA1C, TG and HDL-C [14].

In accordance with other authors [21, 24] this study did not show a positive influence on lipids (TC, TG, LDL-C) by CoQ10, which was also given in higher dosages.

CrP was low grade elevated in 20 patients of the verum group and in 16 patients of the placebo group. Even with CrP serum concentrations of> 0.7 mg/l, there is a slightly increased risk [55]. The elevation of CrP indicates in patients with overweight and obesity as well as with metabolic disorders a higher risk for cardiovascular events. In our study was CrP was slightly reduced after dietary supplementation, and elevated in the placebo group. This effect may be due to magnesium intake by dietary supplementation [11]. After administration of coenzyme Q10, h-CrP was also reduced, according to the findings of Raygan et al. [21], and Shargorodski et al. [22] after intake of 60 mg Q10 combined with other antioxidants like vitamin C, E and selenium.

Influence on cardiac arrhythmias

Magnesium and potassium play an important role in management of CA [9, 12]. CA are often associated with hypomagnesemia but the pathomechanism of this process is not fully understand because of interaction with other electrolyte disturbances [44]. The hypomagnesemia and hypokalemia are closely linked together by triggering of CA [10]. In this pilot study an effect of the dietary supplementation on VPBs, SVPBs and VAS points could not be shown. The reduction of VPBs in the placebo group may be based on a placebo effect. In the verum group we found a significant reduction in heart rate. This may be caused on slowing of sinus node rate by oral magnesium administration [12]. In this pilot study a correlation between changes in LV function and CA could not be found.

Strength and limitations

The strength of this study includes a sample of patients with cardiovascular disorders like AH, CAD, and frequent PBs, and an averaged overweight, which were treated in an Outpatient Practice for Cardiology. Therefore, all were investigated in one centre and all procedures were under same standardized conditions. Limitations were the relative small number of patients and a post-hoc-analysis. In this echocardiographic study we have not measured routinely all parameters of diastolic function. Since outliers of several parameters are detected on different patients, a general clean-up of the data appears inappropriate, favouring the use of all available data. The tested parameters must be evaluated with other patient's condition too.

Conclusion

In this pilot study, dietary intervention with a specific micronutrient combination as add-on to concomitant cardiovascular drug treatment seems to improve cardio-metabolic health in patients with CA. The dietary intervention led to a significant decrease in fasting insulin ≥ 58 pmol/l ($p = 0.020$), and HOMA-IR was reduced in the verum group after 6 weeks ($p = 0.053$). At the same time, parameters of LV diastolic function were improved after intervention in the verum group: significant reduction of LV mass index ($p = 0.003$), and in tendency a decrease of interventricular septal thickness ($p = 0.053$) as well as an increase E/A ratio ($p = 0.051$). The heart rate was significantly decreased ($p = 0.027$), but the effect on reduction of rhythm disturbances like PBs was less pronounced. In both groups serious side effects were not observed. The results of this pilot study give indications for sign of further studies.

Abbreviations

AH: Arterial hypertension; ALAT: Alanin-aminotransferase; ASAT: Aspartate-aminotransferase; BMI: Body-Mass-Index; BP: Blood Pressure; CA: Cardiac arrhythmias; CAD: Coronary artery disease; Cl: Chloride; CrP: C reactive protein; E/A ratio: Ratio of the early (E) to late (A) ventricular filling velocities; ECG: Electrocardiogram; ES: Effect size; F Insulin: Fasting insulin; FPG: Fasting plasma glucose; GFR: Glomerular filtration rate; HbA1c: Glycated haemoglobin A1c; HDL-C: HDL-cholesterol; Hk: Haematocrit; HOMA-IR: Homeostasis Model Assessment- insulin resistance; IDF: International Diabetes Federation; IGT: Impaired glucose tolerance; IR: Insulin resistance; IVS: Interventricular septum; K: Potassium; LA: Left atrium; LDL-C: LDL-cholesterol; LV: Left ventricular; LVEDD: Left ventricular end diastolic diameter; LVEF: Left ventricular ejection fraction; LVESD: Left ventricular end systolic diameter; LVMI: Left ventricular mass index; LVPW: Left ventricular posterior wall; MCHC: Mean corpuscular/cellular haemoglobin concentration; MCV: Mean corpuscular/cell volume; MetS: Metabolic syndrome; Mg: Magnesium; Na: Natrium; PBs: Premature beats; Q1: First Quartile; Q3: Third Quartile; RVEDD: Right ventricular end diastolic diameter; SV: Supraventricular; SVPBs: Supraventricular premature beats; T2DM: Type 2 diabetes mellitus; TC: Total cholesterol; TG: Triglycerides; VPBs: Ventricular premature beats; WC: Waist Circumference; WHtR: Waist-to-Height-Ratio

Acknowledgements

We would like to acknowledge the team of the Outpatient Practice of Cardiology for their efforts on the conduct of the study.

Funding

This study was funded by a research contract from Trommsdorff GmbH & Co. KG, Alsdorf, Germany. The company had no influence on study design, data collection, analysis and interpretation of the results as well as the creation of this paper.

Authors' contributions

CM designed research, EP conducted the study and prepared the paper, NB conducted the statistical analysis, AW conducted the study, DR monitored the study. EP, CM, NB, AW and DR contributed to the interpretation of the data and the results. CM and DR supported the preparation of the paper. All authors read and approved the final manuscript.

Competing interests

The authors declare that they have no competing interests. EP received grants as consultant and as speaker for Trommsdorff.

Author details

[1]Outpatient Practice of Cardiology, Suermondtstr. 13, D-13053 Berlin, Germany. [2]Medicine and Service Ltd, Department of Biostatistics, Boettcherstr. 10, D-09117 Chemnitz, Germany. [3]Bonn Education Association for Dietetics r. A, Fuerst-Pueckler-Str. 44, D-50935 Cologne, Germany. [4]Department of Internal Medicine III, Uniklinik RWTH Aachen, Pauwelsstraße 44, D-52074 Aachen, Germany.

References

1. Conen D, Adam M, Roche F, Barthelemy J-C, Felber Dietrich D, Imboden M, et al. Premature atrial contractions in the general population: frequency and risk factors. Circulation. 2012;126:2302–8. https://doi.org/10.1161/CIRCULATIONAHA.112.112300.
2. Massing MW, Simpson RJ Jr, Rautaharju PM, Schreiner PJ, Crow R, Heiss G. Usefulness of ventricular premature complexes to predict coronary heart disease events and mortality (from the atherosclerosis risk in communities cohort). Am J Cardiol. 2006;98:1609–12. https://doi.org/10.1016/j.amjcard.2006.06.061.
3. Ryden L, Grant PJ, Anker SD, Berne C, Cosentino F, Danchin N, et al. ESC guidelines on diabetes, pre-diabetes, and cardiovascular diseases developed in collaboration with the EASD: the task force on diabetes, pre-diabetes, and cardiovascular diseases of the European Society of Cardiology (ESC) and developed in collaboration with the European Association for the Study of diabetes (EASD). Eur Heart J. 2013;34:3035–87. https://doi.org/10.1093/eurheartj/eht108.
4. Ayalon N, Gopal DM, Mooney DM, Simonetti JS, Grossman JR, Dwivedi A, et al. Preclinical left ventricular diastolic dysfunction in metabolic syndrome. Am J Cardiol. 2014;114:838–42. https://doi.org/10.1016/j.amjcard.2014.06.013.
5. Azevedo A, Bettencourt P, Almeida PB, Santos AC, Abreu-Lima C, Hense H-W, Barros H. Increasing number of components of the metabolic syndrome and cardiac structural and functional abnormalities—cross-sectional study of the general population. BMC Cardiovasc Disord. 2007;7:17. https://doi.org/10.1186/1471-2261-7-17.
6. Galderisi M. Diastolic dysfunction and diabetic cardiomyopathy: evaluation by Doppler echocardiography. J Am Coll Cardiol. 2006;48:1548–51. https://doi.org/10.1016/j.jacc.2006.07.033.
7. Ponikowski P, Voors AA, Anker SD, Bueno H, Cleland JGF, Coats AJS, et al. ESC guidelines for the diagnosis and treatment of acute and chronic heart failure: the task force for the diagnosis and treatment of acute and chronic heart failure of the European Society of Cardiology (ESC). Developed with the special contribution of the heart failure association (HFA) of the ESC. Eur J heart fail. 2016. https://doi.org/10.1002/ejhf.592.
8. Bashir Y, Sneddon JF, Staunton HA, Haywood GA, Simpson IA, McKenna WJ, Camm AJ. Effects of long-term oral magnesium chloride replacement in congestive heart failure secondary to coronary artery disease. Am J Cardiol. 1993;72:1156–62.
9. Falco CN, Grupi C, Sosa E, Scanavacca M, Hachul D, Lara S, et al. Successful improvement of frequency and symptoms of premature complexes after oral magnesium administration. Arq Bras Cardiol. 2012;98:480–7.
10. Geiger H, Wanner C. Magnesium in disease. Clin Kidney J. 2012;5:i25–38. https://doi.org/10.1093/ndtplus/sfr165.
11. Song Y, Ridker PM, Manson JE, Cook NR, Buring JE, Liu S. Magnesium intake, C-reactive protein, and the prevalence of metabolic syndrome in middle-aged and older U.S. women. Diabetes Care. 2005;28:1438–44.

12. Stühlinger HG. Die Bedeutung von Magnesium bei kardiovaskulären Erkrankungen. J Kardiol. 2002;9:389–95.

13. Aburto NJ, Hanson S, Gutierrez H, Hooper L, Elliott P, Cappuccio FP. Effect of increased potassium intake on cardiovascular risk factors and disease: systematic review and meta-analyses. BMJ. 2013;346:f1378. https://doi.org/10.1136/bmj.f1378.

14. Child DF, Hudson PR, Jones H, Davies GK, De P, Mukherjee S, et al. The effect of oral folic acid on glutathione, glycaemia and lipids in type 2 diabetes. Diabetes Nutr Metab. 2004;17:95–102.

15. Ho M, Halim JH, Gow ML, El-Haddad N, Marzulli T, Baur LA, et al. Vitamin B12 in obese adolescents with clinical features of insulin resistance. Nutrients. 2014;6:5611–8. https://doi.org/10.3390/nu6125611.

16. Knight BA, Shields BM, Brook A, Hill A, Bhat DS, Hattersley AT, Yajnik CS. Lower circulating B12 is associated with higher obesity and insulin resistance during pregnancy in a non-diabetic white British population. PLoS One. 2015;10:e0135268. https://doi.org/10.1371/journal.pone.0135268.

17. Sazonov V, Maccubbin D, Sisk CM, Canner PL. Effects of niacin on the incidence of new onset diabetes and cardiovascular events in patients with normoglycaemia and impaired fasting glucose. Int J Clin Pract. 2013;67:297–302. https://doi.org/10.1111/ijcp.12089.

18. Schwab S, Zierer A, Heier M, Fischer B, Huth C, Baumert J, et al. Intake of vitamin and mineral supplements and longitudinal association with HbA1c levels in the general non-diabetic population—results from the MONICA/KORA S3/F3 study. PLoS One. 2015;10:e0139244. https://doi.org/10.1371/journal.pone.0139244.

19. Sudchada P, Saokaew S, Sridetch S, Incampa S, Jaiyen S, Khaithong W. Effect of folic acid supplementation on plasma total homocysteine levels and glycemic control in patients with type 2 diabetes: a systematic review and meta-analysis. Diabetes Res Clin Pract. 2012;98:151–8. https://doi.org/10.1016/j.diabres.2012.05.027.

20. Moazen M, Mazloom Z, Ahmadi A, Dabbaghmanesh MH, Roosta S. Effect of coenzyme Q10 on glycaemic control, oxidative stress and adiponectin in type 2 diabetes. J Pak Med Assoc. 2015;65:404–8.

21. Raygan F, Rezavandi Z, Dadkhah Tehrani S, Farrokhian A, Asemi Z. The effects of coenzyme Q10 administration on glucose homeostasis parameters, lipid profiles, biomarkers of inflammation and oxidative stress in patients with metabolic syndrome. Eur J Nutr. 2015. https://doi.org/10.1007/s00394-015-1042-7.

22. Shargorodsky M, Debby O, Matas Z, Zimlichman R. Effect of long-term treatment with antioxidants (vitamin C, vitamin E, coenzyme Q10 and selenium) on arterial compliance, humoral factors and inflammatory markers in patients with multiple cardiovascular risk factors. Nutr Metab (Lond). 2010;7:55. https://doi.org/10.1186/1743-7075-7-55.

23. Turk S, Baki A, Solak Y, Kayrak M, Atalay H, Gaipov A, et al. Coenzyme Q10 supplementation and diastolic heart functions in hemodialysis patients: a randomized double-blind placebo-controlled trial. Hemodial Int. 2013;17:374–81. https://doi.org/10.1111/hdi.12022.

24. Zahedi H, Eghtesadi S, Seifirad S, Rezaee N, Shidfar F, Heydari I, et al. Effects of CoQ10 supplementation on lipid profiles and glycemic control in patients with type 2 diabetes: a randomized, double blind, placebo-controlled trial. J Diabetes Metab Disord. 2014;13:81. https://doi.org/10.1186/s40200-014-0081-6.

25. Classen HG, Grober U, Kisters K. Drug-induced magnesium deficiency. Med Monatsschr Pharm. 2012;35:274–80.

26. Kaye P. The role of magnesium in the emergency department. Emerg Med J. 2002;19:288–91. https://doi.org/10.1136/emj.19.4.288.

27. Alberti KGM, Zimmet P, Shaw J. The metabolic syndrome—a new worldwide definition. Lancet. 2005;366:1059–62. https://doi.org/10.1016/S0140-6736(05)67402-8.

28. Schneider HJ, Friedrich N, Klotsche J, Pieper L, Nauck M, John U, et al. The predictive value of different measures of obesity for incident cardiovascular events and mortality. J Clin Endocrinol Metab. 2010;95:1777–85. https://doi.org/10.1210/jc.2009-1584.

29. Browning LM, Hsieh SD, Ashwell M. A systematic review of waist-to-height ratio as a screening tool for the prediction of cardiovascular disease and diabetes: 0.5 could be a suitable global boundary value. Nutr Res Rev. 2010;23:247–69. https://doi.org/10.1017/S0954422410000144.

30. Prineas RJ, Crow RS, Blackburn HW. The Minnesota code manual of electrocardiographic findings: Standards and procedures for measurement and classification. Boston, Mass.: J. Wright; 1982.

31. Lang RM, Badano LP, Mor-Avi V, Afilalo J, Armstrong A, Ernande L, et al. Recommendations for cardiac chamber quantification by echocardiography in adults: an update from the American Society of Echocardiography and the European Association of Cardiovascular Imaging. Eur Heart J Cardiovasc Imaging. 2015;16:233–70. https://doi.org/10.1093/ehjci/jev014.

32. Nagueh SF, Appleton CP, Gillebert TC, Marino PN, Oh JK, Smiseth OA, et al. Recommendations for the evaluation of left ventricular diastolic function by echocardiography. J Am Soc Echocardiogr. 2009;22:107–33. https://doi.org/10.1016/j.echo.2008.11.023.

33. Cohen J. Statistical power analysis for the behavioral sciences. 2nd ed. Hillsdale: L. Erlbaum Associates; 1988.

34. Moebus S, Hanisch J, Bramlage P, Losch C, Hauner H, Wasem J, Jockel K-H. Regional differences in the prevalence of the metabolic syndrome in primary care practices in Germany. Dtsch Arztebl Int. 2008;105:207–13. https://doi.org/10.3238/arztebl.2008.0207.

35. von Bibra H, Paulus WJ, St John Sutton M, Leclerque C, Schuster T, Schumm-Draeger P-M. Quantification of diastolic dysfunction via the age dependence of diastolic function - impact of insulin resistance with and without type 2 diabetes. Int J Cardiol. 2015;182:368–74. https://doi.org/10.1016/j.ijcard.2014.12.005.

36. Koliaki C, Roden M. Alterations of mitochondrial function and insulin sensitivity in human obesity and diabetes mellitus. Annu Rev Nutr. 2016;36:337–67. https://doi.org/10.1146/annurev-nutr-071715-050656.

37. von Bibra H, Paulus W. Diastolische Dysfunktion. Kardiologe. 2016;10:47–55. https://doi.org/10.1007/s12181-015-0035-3.

38. Fontes-Carvalho R, Ladeiras-Lopes R, Bettencourt P, Leite-Moreira A, Azevedo A. Diastolic dysfunction in the diabetic continuum: association with insulin resistance, metabolic syndrome and type 2 diabetes. Cardiovasc Diabetol. 2015;14:4. https://doi.org/10.1186/s12933-014-0168-x.

39. Littarru GP, Tiano L. Clinical aspects of coenzyme Q10: an update. Nutrition. 2010;26:250–4. https://doi.org/10.1016/j.nut.2009.08.008.

40. Quiles JL, Ochoa JJ, Battino M, Gutierrez-Rios P, Nepomuceno EA, Frias ML, et al. Life-long supplementation with a low dosage of coenzyme Q10 in the rat: effects on antioxidant status and DNA damage. Biofactors. 2005;25:73–86.

41. Ikee R, Hamasaki Y, Oka M, Maesato K, Mano T, Moriya H, et al. High-density lipoprotein cholesterol and left ventricular mass index in peritoneal dialysis. Perit Dial Int. 2008;28:611–6.

42. Ahn M-S, Kim J-Y, Youn YJ, Kim S-Y, Koh S-B, Lee K, et al. Cardiovascular parameters correlated with metabolic syndrome in a rural community cohort of Korea: the ARIRANG study. J Korean Med Sci. 2010;25:1045–52. https://doi.org/10.3346/jkms.2010.25.7.1045.

43. Ochi A, Ishimura E, Tsujimoto Y, Kakiya R, Tabata T, Mori K, et al. Hair magnesium, but not serum magnesium, is associated with left ventricular wall thickness in hemodialysis patients. Circ J. 2013;77:3029–36.

44. Grober U, Schmidt J, Kisters K. Magnesium in prevention and therapy. Nutrients. 2015;7:8199–226. https://doi.org/10.3390/nu7095388.

45. DiNicolantonio JJ, Bhutani J, McCarty MF, O'Keefe JH. Coenzyme Q10 for the treatment of heart failure: a review of the literature. Open Heart. 2015;2:e000326. https://doi.org/10.1136/openhrt-2015-000326.

46. Rutter MK, Parise H, Benjamin EJ, Levy D, Larson MG, Meigs JB, et al. Impact of glucose intolerance and insulin resistance on cardiac structure and function: sex-related differences in the Framingham heart study. Circulation. 2003;107:448–54.

47. Hwang Y-C, Jee JH, Kang M, Rhee E-J, Sung J, Lee M-K. Metabolic syndrome and insulin resistance are associated with abnormal left ventricular diastolic function and structure independent of blood pressure and fasting plasma glucose level. Int J Cardiol. 2012;159:107–11. https://doi.org/10.1016/j.ijcard.2011.02.039.

48. Velagaleti RS, Gona P, Chuang ML, Salton CJ, Fox CS, Blease SJ, et al. Relations of insulin resistance and glycemic abnormalities to cardiovascular magnetic resonance measures of cardiac structure and function: the Framingham heart study. Circ Cardiovasc Imaging. 2010;3:257–63. https://doi.org/10.1161/CIRCIMAGING.109.911438.

49. Majahalme S, Turjanmaa V, Weder A, Lu H, Tuomisto M, Virjo A, Uusitalo A. Blood pressure levels and variability, smoking, and left ventricular structure in normotension and in borderline and mild hypertension. Am J Hypertens. 1996;9:1110–8.

50. Sundström J, Lind L, Nyström N, Zethelius B, Andrén B, Hales CN, Lithell HO. Left ventricular concentric remodeling rather than left ventricular hypertrophy is related to the insulin resistance syndrome in elderly men. Circulation. 2000;101:2595–600.

51. Zhang L, Jaswal JS, Ussher JR, Sankaralingam S, Wagg C, Zaugg M, Lopaschuk GD. Cardiac insulin-resistance and decreased mitochondrial energy production precede the development of systolic heart failure after pressure-overload hypertrophy. Circ Heart Fail. 2013;6:1039–48. https://doi.org/10.1161/CIRCHEARTFAILURE.112.000228.

52. Verma S, Garg A, Yan AT, Gupta AK, Al-Omran M, Sabongui A, et al. Effect of Empagliflozin on left ventricular mass and diastolic function in individuals with diabetes: an important clue to the EMPA-REG OUTCOME trial? Diabetes Care. 2016;39:e212–3. https://doi.org/10.2337/dc16-1312.

53. Chutia H, Lynrah KG. Association of Serum Magnesium Deficiency with insulin resistance in type 2 diabetes mellitus. J Lab Physicians. 2015;7:75–8. https://doi.org/10.4103/0974-2727.163131.

54. DGE. Referenzwerte für die Nährstoffzufuhr. 2nd ed. Neustadt an der Weinstrasse: Neuer Umschau Buchverlag; 2015.

55. Ridker PM. High-sensitivity C-reactive protein: potential adjunct for global risk assessment in the primary prevention of cardiovascular disease. Circulation. 2001;103:1813–8.

Better clinical outcome with direct oral anticoagulants in hospitalized heart failure patients with atrial fibrillation

Akiomi Yoshihisa* ⬥, Yu Sato, Takamasa Sato, Satoshi Suzuki, Masayoshi Oikawa and Yasuchika Takeishi

Abstract

Background: Atrial fibrillation (AF) is common in patients with heart failure and is associated with higher mortality. Although previous studies have reported that direct oral anticoagulants (DOACs) reduce the risk of cardiovascular events in out-patients with AF, it remains unclear whether DOACs reduce mortality in hospitalized heart failure (HHF) patients with AF. Therefore, we examined the impact of DOACs on mortality in this group of patients.

Methods: Consecutive 497 HHF patients with AF were retrospectively registered and divided into three groups on the basis of the presence of anticoagulant therapy: non-anticoagulant group (Non, $n = 90$), Vit K antagonists (VKAs) group ($n = 257$) and DOACs group ($n = 150$). We followed up all the patients for mortality.

Results: In the Kaplan-Meier analysis (mean follow-up of 1093 days), all-cause mortality was significantly lower in the VKAs and DOACs groups than in the Non group (31.1% and 15.3% vs. 43.3%, log-rank $P < 0.001$). In the multivariable Cox proportional hazard analysis after adjusting for other potential confounding factors, usage of DOACs and VKAs were independently associated with lower mortality in HHF patients AF (DOACs, HR 0.356, $P = 0.001$; VKAs, HR 0.472, $P = 0.002$). Furthermore, the propensity-matched 1:1 cohort was assessed based on the propensity score (DOACs, $n = 114$ and VKAs, n = 114). All-cause mortality was significantly lower in the DOACs group than in the VKAs group in the post-matched cohort (12.3% vs. 35.1%, log-rank $P = 0.038$). In the Cox proportional hazard analysis, the use of DOACs was associated with lower mortality in the post-matched cohort (HR 0.526, $P = 0.041$).

Conclusion: Appropriate use of anticoagulants in HHF patients with AF is important, and DOACs potentially improve all-cause mortality in such patients.

Keywords: Heart failure, Atrial fibrillation, Anticoagulant therapy, Direct oral anticoagulants, Vitamin K antagonists, Mortality

Background

Heart failure (HF) is a systemic disease with a devastating prognosis, which affects many organ systems, including the cardiovascular system. In HF patients, atrial fibrillation (AF) is a frequent co-morbidity and its prevalence is related to the severity of the clinical status of patients [1]. HF and AF share common risk factors and clinical backgrounds (e.g. inflammation and fibrosis), and the occurrence of either of them may induce the onset of a vicious circle which, in turn, facilitates the manifestation of the other [2–4]. AF subsequently causes stroke and/or HF [5]. On the other hand, the incidence of AF increases with severity of HF [4], and AF in HF patients is strongly associated with all-cause mortality including sudden cardiac death [6] and bleeding, rather than stroke or embolism [7–9]. Hence, all-cause mortality is the most meaningful endpoint in such patients.

Anticoagulant therapy is prescribed in consideration of balance of efficacy for embolic risk (e.g. CHADS score, CHA_2DS_2-VASc score) and safety for bleeding risk (e.g. HAS-BLED score) in AF patients [10]. Direct oral anticoagulants (DOACs) have the potential to reduce the burden of stroke as effective, safe, and more convenient alternatives to vitamin K antagonists (VKAs), such as warfarin [11–13]. A recent meta-analysis of randomized controlled studies revealed that DOACs significantly reduce the risk of stroke or systemic embolic events by

* Correspondence: yoshihis@fmu.ac.jp
Department of Cardiovascular Medicine, Fukushima Medical University, 1 Hikarigaoka, Fukushima 960-1295, Japan

19% and hemorrhagic stroke by 51% compared with VKAs, but increased the risk of gastrointestinal hemorrhage by 25% in out-patients with AF [12]. On the other hand, a few post-hoc analyses limited to AF out-patients with HF revealed that 1) DOACs were similarly effective or safer (less intracranial hemorrhage) compared to VKA in AF out-patients with HF compared with those without HF, and that 2) DOACs have not yet improved all-cause mortality of AF out-patients with HF [7–9, 14]. However, there were several problems in the previous studies [7–9, 14]: 1) out-patients with reduced left ventricular ejection fraction and no symptoms of HF were included in previous studies, [7–9, 14] and hospitalized heart failure (HHF) patients had higher accurate diagnosis of HF and risk of mortality than out-patients [15–17], 2) important factors for HF, such as Framingham criteria, etiology, presence of anemia and hyponatremia, natriuretic peptide, medications of HF, were partly absent or were not considered in these post-hoc analyses [7–9, 14], 3) anticoagulant therapy could not be used in all the patients with HF and AF in a real world setting [18] because of certain contraindications for anticoagulants (higher HAS-BLED score and presence of anemia) [18]. Additionally, studies on symptomatic HHF patient coexistence with AF have not been previously reported. The association between DOACs and all-cause mortality in HHF patients with AF is still unclear and controversial. Therefore, we examined the impact of anticoagulant therapy on all-cause mortality in symptomatic HHF patients with AF based on a retrospective study, using propensity score (PS) analyses to reduce selection bias, and taking into consideration the patients' clinical backgrounds,

including CHA_2DS_2-Vasc and HAS-BLED scores, other co-morbidities and pharmacotherapies.

Methods

Subjects and study protocol

This was a observational study analyzed using PS methods in which we enrolled consecutive HHF patients with AF, who were hospitalized with decompensated HF defined based on the Framingham criteria [19]., and discharged from Fukushima Medical University Hospital between 2011 and 2015. AF was identified by an electrocardiogram performed during hospitalization and/or medical records including past history. The patient flow chart is shown in Fig. 1. In HHF patients with AF ($n = 627$), patients with severe valvular etiology and/or post-operative state ($n = 75$), dialysis and/or creatinine clearance less than 30 ml/min ($n = 43$), acute coronary syndrome ($n = 6$), and documented advanced cancer ($n = 6$) were excluded, and 497 HHF patients with AF were finally enrolled. Patients were divided into three groups on the basis of the use of VKAs and DOACs at hospital discharge: non-anticoagulant group (Non, $n = 90$), VKAs group (warfarin, $n = 257$) and DOACs group ($n = 150$). The DOACs used in this study were as follows: apixaban ($n = 52$, 34.7%), rivaroxaban ($n = 35$, 23.3%), edoxaban ($n = 33$, 22.0%) and dabigatran ($n = 30$, 20.0%). We compared the clinical features and laboratory data that were recorded at hospital discharge. The CHADS score, CHA_2DS_2-VASc score, HAS-BLED score, and time in therapeutic range (TTR) of VKAs were measured as previously reported [10]. The left ventricular ejection fraction (LVEF) was calculated using Simpson's

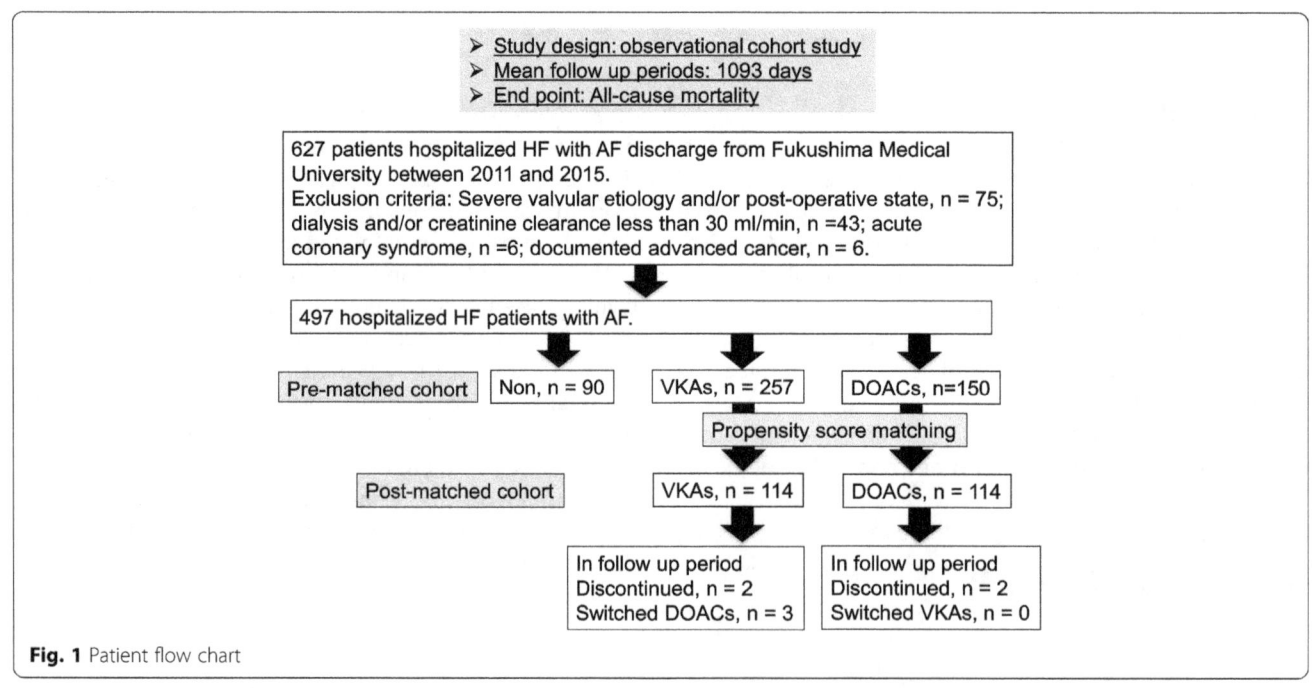

Fig. 1 Patient flow chart

method, and recordings were performed on ultrasound systems (ACUSON Sequoia, Siemens Medical Solutions USA, Inc., Mountain View, CA, USA). Preserved LVEF was defined as more than LVEF 50%. All patients were followed up until 2017 for all-cause mortality. Cardiac death was defined by experienced cardiologists as death due to worsening HF in accordance with the Framingham criteria [19], due to ventricular fibrillation determined by electrocardiogram or implantable devices, and acute myocardial infarction. Survival time was calculated from the day of discharge to the date of death or last follow-up. Status and dates of deaths were checked from medical recoreds of the patients. If these data were unavailable, status was examined by a telephone call to the patient's referring hospital physicians. The end-point classification committee, comprising two experienced cardiologists who were not study investigators, reviewed the data. We could follow up all the patients.

Written informed consent was obtained from each subject, and the study protocol was approved by the ethics committee of Fukushima Medical University (No. 823). The investigation conforms with the principles outlined in the Declaration of Helsinki. Reporting of the study conforms to STROBE along with references to STROBE and the broader EQUATOR guidelines [20].

Statistical analysis

Categorical variables are expressed as numbers and percentages, and the chi-square test was used for their comparisons. Normally distributed data are presented as mean ± SD, and non-normally distributed data are presented as median and interquartile range, or log-transformed. Data among the three groups were compared using analysis of variance followed by Tukey's post-hoc test. The Kaplan-Meier method was used for presenting the mortality, and the log-rank test was performed.

To eliminate imbalances in the measurement of baseline characteristics because of selection bias, we used multiple approaches, including multiple Cox regression analysis in the pre-matched cohort ($n = 497$) and PS matching in the post-matched cohort ($n = 228$). To prepare for potential confounding in the Cox regression analyses, we considered the following clinical factors, which are known to affect the mortality in HF patients: age, sex, B-type natriuretic peptide (BNP), presence of New York Heart Association functional class III or IV, ischemic etiology, preserved LVEF, hypertension, diabetes, CKD, anemia, hyponatremia (as sodium less than 135 mEq/l), and oral administration of renin-angiotensin-aldosterone system inhibitors, β-blockers, diuretics, inotropic agents, and anticoagulants. These factors, which predicting

mortality with value of $P < 0.05$, were selected in the final adjusted model.

Furthermore, the PS for treatment with DOAC was estimated for each patient by logistic regression with the following variables, which are important considerable factors to prescribe DOACs: age, body weight, CHA_2DS_2-Vasc score, HAS-BLED score and creatinine clearance. The PS is the propensity from 0 to 1 to receive treatment, and is used to adjust potential selection bias and confounding factors between the groups with or without treatment in the observational studies [21]. We used the PS to match patients who were administered DOAC and those who were administered VKA, using 1:1 nearest neighbor matching algorithm and a 0.2 caliper width of the standard deviation of the PS logit with caliper as of 0.03 [22]. The PS-matched datasets were compared using a pairwise analysis [23], and the post-matched cohort (DOACs, $n = 114$ and VKAs, $n = 114$) was defined. To assess potential heterogeneity of the effect of DOAC on mortality, we conducted subgroup analyses in the post-matched cohort ($n = 228$). We tested for first order interactions using multivariable Cox proportional hazard models by entering interaction terms between DOAC use and the subgroup variables. Missing values were handled by estimating one logistic regression model for each pattern of missing values. A P value of < 0.05 was considered significant for all comparisons. These analyses were performed using a statistical software package (SPSS ver. 24.0, IBM, Armonk, NY, USA).

Results

The clinical features of the study subjects are presented in Table 1. The Non group had the highest age, HAS-BLED score, prevalence of paroxysmal AF, female gender and anemia. It seems that this background is associated with abandonment of anticoagulants. The VKAs group had the highest prevalence of male gender and hypertension, and highest usage of β-blockers, diuretics, and inotropic agents. In addition, TTR was 70% in VKAs group (data not shown in Table 1). The DOACs group had the lowest prevalence of anemia. In contrast, $CHADS_2$ and CHA_2DS_2-Vasc scores, prevalence of NYHA class III or IV, preserved LVEF, other co-morbidities, BNP, C-reactive protein and sodium did not significantly differ among the three groups.

In the follow-up period (mean of 1093 days), 70 cardiac deaths (worsened HF $n = 42$, ventricular fibrillation $n = 22$ and acute coronary syndrome $n = 6$) and 72 non-cardiac deaths (stroke $n = 10$, gastrointestinal hemorrhage $n = 7$, aneurysms $n = 5$, trauma $n = 4$, pneumonia/respiratory failure/hemorrhage $n = 18$, cancer $n = 12$, infection/disseminated intravascular

Table 1 Comparisons of clinical features ($n = 497$)

	Non ($n = 90$)	VKAs ($n = 257$)	DOACs ($n = 150$)	P value
Age (years)	74.4 ± 12.0	69.9 ± 11.8**	70.4 ± 12.9*	0.010
CHADS$_2$ score	3.2 ± 1.3	3.1 ± 1.2	2.9 ± 1.3	0.286
CHA$_2$DS$_2$-Vasc score	4.8 ± 1.6	4.4 ± 1.7	4.3 ± 1.8	0.074
HAS-BLED score	3.4 ± 1.3	2.8 ± 1.2**	2.7 ± 1.4*	0.006
Paroxysmal af (n, %)	44 (48.9)	89 (34.6)	52 (34.7)	0.041
Male gender (n, %)	44 (48.9)	175 (68.1)	89 (59.3)	0.004
Body mass index (kg/cm^2)	22.7 ± 4.9	23.3 ± 4.0	23.5 ± 3.9	0.404
Systolic BP (mmHg)	130.8 ± 33.1	123.8 ± 28.8	132.3 ± 36.3	0.021
Diastolic BP (mmHg)	72.8 ± 19.2	72.6 ± 18.6	76.0 ± 24.3	0.265
Heart rate (bpm)	89.7 ± 35.0	84.1 ± 29.1	85.5 ± 35.8	0.371
NYHA class III or IV (n, %)	6 (6.7)	8 (3.1)	4 (2.7)	0.226
Preserved LVEF (n, %)	41 (45.6)	126 (49.0)	67 (44.7)	0.662
Etiology				0.130
Ischemic (n, %)	26 (28.9)	68 (26.5)	43 (28.7)	
Cardiomyopathy (n, %)	23 (25.6)	68 (26.5)	36 (24.0)	
Valvular (n, %)	19 (21.1)	70 (27.2)	25 (16.7)	
Others (n, %)	22 (24.4)	51 (19.8)	46 (30.7)	
Co-morbidity				
Hypertension (n, %)	67 (74.4)	202 (78.6)	98 (65.3)	0.013
Diabetes (n, %)	36 (40.0)	103 (40.1)	53 (35.3)	0.611
Dyslipidemia (n, %)	66 (73.3)	185 (72.0)	97 (64.7)	0.224
CKD (n, %)	49 (54.4)	163 (63.4)	85 (56.7)	0.213
Anemia (n, %)	58 (64.4)	144 (56.0)	70 (46.7)	0.023
Stroke (n, %)	23 (25.6)	65 (25.3)	32 (21.3)	0.628
Medications				
RAS inhibitors (n, %)	61 (67.8)	206 (80.2)	115 (76.7)	0.057
β-blockers (n, %)	63 (70.0)	219 (85.2)	116 (77.3)	0.005
Diuretics (n, %)	55 (61.1)	214 (83.3)	103 (68.7)	< 0.001
Inotropic agents (n, %)	9 (10.0)	52 (20.2)	7 (4.7)	< 0.001
Antiplatelet agents (n, %)	43 (47.8)	108 (42.0)	62 (41.3)	0.576
Laboratory data				
BNP (pg/ml) §	332.8 (140.3–656.1)	284.1 (157.4–625.9)	270.8 (101.8–552.2)	0.494
C-reactive protein (mg/dl) §	0.13 (0.05–0.53)	0.07 (0.03–0.18)	0.08 (0.04–0.25)	0.104
Sodium (mEq/l)	138.6 ± 5.1	138.7 ± 4.0	139.2 ± 4.3	0.561

Af atrial fibrillation, *BP* blood pressure, *NYHA* New York Heart Association, *LVEF* left ventricular ejection fraction, *CKD* chronic kidney disease, *RAS* rennin-angiotensin-aldosterone system; *BNP* B-type natriuretic peptide
*P < 0.05 and **P < 0.01 vs. Non group
§Data are presented as median (interquartile range)

coagulation $n = 5$, systemic embolism, $n = 3$, renal failure $n = 3$, others $n = 5$) occurred. As shown in Fig. 2, all-cause mortality was significantly lower in the DOACs and VKAs groups than in the Non group in the pre-matched cohort (Fig. 2; $P < 0.001$). In the Cox proportional hazard analysis after adjusting for potential confounding factors (Table 2), the usage of DOACs and

VKAs was independently associated with lower mortality in HHF patients with AF (DOACs, HR 0.356, $P = 0.001$; VKAs, HR 0.472, $P = 0.002$).

In addition, in the post-matched cohort, mortality was significantly lower in the DOACs group than in the VKAs group (Fig. 3; $P = 0.038$). The clinical features of DOACs group and VKAs group in the post-matched

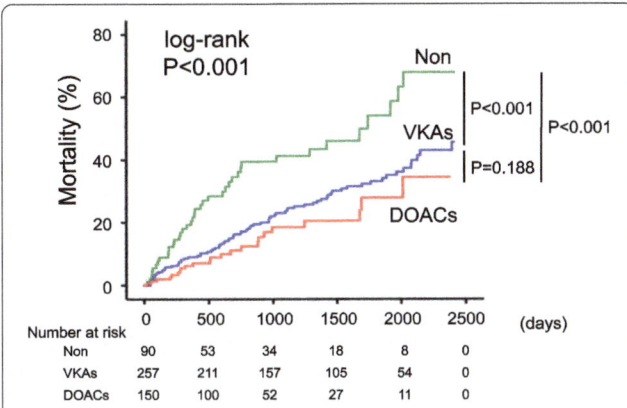

Fig. 2 All-cause mortality: pre-matched cohort. Kaplan-Meier analyses for all-cause mortality among the three groups (Non group, n = 90; VKAs group, n = 257; DOACs group, n = 150) in the pre-matched cohort (n = 497);

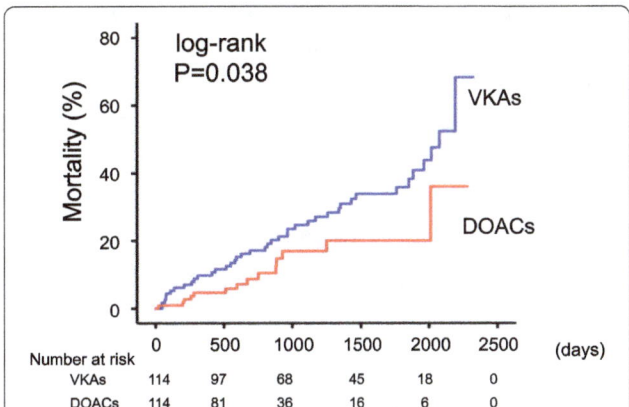

Fig. 3 All-cause mortality: post-matched cohort. Kaplan-Meier analyses for all-cause mortality between the groups (VKAs group, n = 114 and DOACs group, n = 114) in the post-matched cohort (n = 228)

cohort are summarized in Additional file 1: Table S1. Interactions between the DOACs group and clinically relevant variables were modeled with the Cox regression analysis, as shown in Table 3, for all-cause mortality in the post-matched cohort (n = 228). In the Cox proportional hazard analysis (Table 3), the usage of DOACs was associated with lower mortality in the post-matched cohort (HR 0.526, 95% CI 0.284–0.974, P = 0.041). There were no interactions between DOACs use and other important variables (e.g. CKD, anemia, LVEF, other pharmacotherapies) that affected mortality in all subgroups.

Discussion

To the best of our knowledge, the present study is the first to show the association between DOACs and lower all-cause mortality in HHF patients with AF based on a real world observational study using multiple Cox regression and PS analyses, considering clinical backgrounds, including CHA_2DS_2-Vasc and

Table 2 Cox proportional hazard model of all-cause mortality (event = 142/ n = 497)

Risk factor	Univariable			Multivariable		
	HR	95% CI	P value	HR	95% CI	P value
Age	1.045	1.028–1.063	< 0.001	1.025	1.007–1.044	0.007
Male sex	1.044	0.741–1.472	0.805			
NYHA class III or IV	4.662	2.718–7.995	< 0.001	1.561	0.826–2.949	0.170
Ischemic etiology	1.031	0.682–1.560	0.885			
Preserved LVEF	0.770	0.552–1.073	0.122			
Hypertension	1.089	0.719–1.651	0.687			
Diabetes	1.331	0.957–1.851	0.089			
Chronic kidney disease	1.842	1.274–2.664	0.001	1.352	0.899–2.032	0.147
Anemia	2.456	1.688–3.573	< 0.001	1.849	1.214–2.816	0.004
Hyponatremia	2.089	1.346–3.241	0.001	1.406	0.890–2.222	0.144
Log BNP	3.541	2.394–5.238	< 0.001	2.970	1.903–4.635	< 0.001
RAS inhibitors	0.632	0.433–0.921	0.017	0.750	0.492–1.141	0.179
β-blockers	0.636	0.437–0.927	0.018	0.657	0.426–1.014	0.058
Diuretics	2.290	1.379–3.802	0.001	2.008	1.137–3.546	0.016
Inotropic agents	2.026	1.377–2.982	< 0.001	2.126	1.366–2.308	0.001
Anticoagulants: Non	Ref			Ref		
VKAs	0.493	0.335–0.725	< 0.001	0.472	0.296–0.750	0.002
DOACs	0.352	0.210–0.590	< 0.001	0.356	0.199–0.638	0.001

NYHA New York Heart Association, *LVEF* left ventricular ejection fraction, *BNP* B-type natriuretic peptide, *RAS* renin-angiotensin-aldosterone system, *VKAs* vitamin K antagonists, *DOACs* direct oral anti-coagulants

Table 3 Subgroup analysis for all-cause mortality: DOACs vs. VKAs use in post matched cohort

Factor	Subgroup	n	HR	95% CI	P value	Interaction P value
DOACs vs. VKAs	Total	228	0.526	0.284–0.974	0.041	–
Age	≥ 70	126	0.604	0.299–1.219	0.159	0.537
	< 70	102	0.331	0.091–1.206	0.094	
Sex	Male	159	0.569	0.287–1.127	0.106	0.809
	Female	69	0.539	0.108–2.685	0.451	
NYHA class	I, II	222	0.561	0.301-1.044	0.068	0.978
	III, IV	6	0.024	0.000-397.4	0.540	
BNP	>median	114	0.341	0.115-1.012	0.053	0.168
	<median	114	0.690	0.319–1.489	0.344	
LVEF	Reduced	127	0.676	0.312–1.465	0.321	0.245
	Preserved	101	0.366	0.132–1.014	0.053	
Ischemic etiology	Present	63	0.926	0.319–2.002	0.466	0.269
	Absent	165	0.435	0.207–0.915	0.028	
Diabetes	Present	92	0.693	0.302–1.594	0.388	0.364
	Absent	136	0.401	0.159–1.011	0.053	
CKD	Present	131	0.598	0.302–1.185	0.141	0.994
	Absent	97	0.667	0.152–2.931	0.591	
Anemia	Present	106	0.474	0.215–1.044	0.064	0.498
	Absent	122	0.729	0.251–2.112	0.560	
RAS inhibitors	Present	188	0.664	0.336–1.313	0.239	0.171
	Absent	40	0.187	0.041–0.861	0.031	
β-blockers	Present	186	0.564	0.288–1.106	0.096	0.389
	Absent	42	0.293	0.061–1.394	0.123	
Diuretics	Present	166	0.630	0.333–1.191	0.155	0.475
	Absent	62	0.452	0.041–4.992	0.517	
Antiplatelet agents	Present	97	0.863	0.386–1.931	0.720	0.117
	Absent	131	0.295	0.109–0.796	0.016	

DOACs direct oral anticoagulants, *VKAs* Vit K antagonists, *NYHA* New York Heart Association, *BNP* B-type natriuretic peptide, *LVEF* left ventricular ejection fraction, *CKD* chronic kidney disease, *RAS* rennin-angiotensin-aldosterone system

HAS-BLED scores, other co-morbidities, and pharmacotherapies.

To improve the prognosis of HHF patients with AF, prevention of stroke and systemic embolism, as well as avoidance of major bleeding, may be the therapeutic target. To this point, appropriate use of DOACs is expected to be associated with better prognosis in HHF patients with AF. There are several randomized clinical trials in out-patients with AF regarding efficacy (prevention of stroke and/or systemic embolism) and safety (avoidance of intra cranial hemorrhage or gastrointestinal hemorrhage) of DOACs compared with VKAs. Firstly, dabigatran tended to lower all-cause mortality (RR 0.88, 95% CI 0.77–1.00) in the RE-LY trial, with enrolled 18,113 out-patients with AF (CHADS$_2$ score = 2.1, TTR = 67%, HF patients 32%) [24]. In the post-hoc analysis, the relative effects of dabigatran, compared to VKAs, on the occurrence of stroke or systemic

embolism and major bleeding were consistent among those with or without HF and those with reduced or preserved LVEF [7]. Secondly, rivaroxaban tended to lower all-cause mortality (RR 0.85, 95% CI 0.70–1.02) in the ROCKET-AF trial, with 14,264 enrolled out-patients with AF (CHADS$_2$ score = 3.5, TTR = 58%, HF patients 63.7%) [25]. In the post-hoc analyses, the efficacy of rivaroxaban was similar in AF out-patients with or without HF [9]. Among the AF patients with HF, the efficacy of rivaroxaban was similar, irrespective of NYHA class, CHADS$_2$ score, and LVEF [9]. Thirdly, apixaban significantly decreased all-cause mortality (RR 0.89, 95% CI 0.80–0.998) in the ARISTOTLE trial, with 18,201 enrolled out-patients with AF (CHADS$_2$ score = 2.1, TTR = 66%, HF patients 35%) [26]. In the post-hoc analyses, apixaban reduced the risk of stroke, systemic embolism or all-cause death, irrespective of the presence of HF and/or reduced LVEF [8]. Fourthly, edoxaban decreased cardiovascular mortality (RR 0.87, 95% CI 0.78–0.96) in the ENGAGE-AF TIMI 48, with 21,105 enrolled out-patients with AF (CHADS$_2$ score = 2.8, TTR = 68%, HF patients 58%) [27]. Although these previous post-hoc analyses [7–9] are partially concordant with our results, detailed data of HF, such as Framingham criteria, etiology of HF, natriuretic peptide and other co-morbidities, were unknown unlike in our results. Furthermore, there is no report regarding efficacy of DOACs on mortality in HHF patients with AF.

In previous studies regarding DOACs compared to VKAs in AF out-patients with HF, 57% took ACE inhibitors and 68% took β blockers in the RE-LY trial [7], and 60% took ACE inhibitors and 69% took β blockers in the ROCKET AF trial, in which rivaroxaban tended to decrease all-cause mortality (RR 0.93, 95% CI 0.82–1.07) [9]. In the ARISTOTLE trial, 71% took ACE inhibitors and 71% took β blockers; however, apixaban did not decrease mortality (reduced LVEF, RR 0.98, 95% CI 0.79–1.21; preserved LVEF, RR 0.89, 95% CI 0.69–1.13) [8]. Our study subjects were HHF, and had a relatively higher CHADS$_2$ score of 3.1, TTR of 70%, and higher usage of RAS inhibitors (76.9%) and β blockers (80.1%). In the present study, the use of DOACs was associated with lower all-cause mortality than VKAs and non-anticoagulant in HHF patient with AF. HF is reportedly associated with poor control of VKAs [28]. It has been recently reported that DOACs, compared with VKAs, is associated with lower prevalence of major bleeding [14] and avoidance of anemia, as well as lower occurrence of kidney injury [29], acute coronary syndrome [30] and HF [30]. These backgrounds may be associated with lower all-cause mortality in HHF patients with AF.

Study strengths and limitations

Our study has several strengths, and differs from previous studies [7–9, 14]. For instance, the present study is the first to show the effect of DOACs on reducing all-cause mortality in HHF patients with AF considering the clinical background, including CHA$_2$DS$_2$-Vasc and HAS-BLED scores, other co-morbidities, and pharmacotherapies. In addition, the diagnosis of HF and causes of death were accurately made by our experienced cardiologists, based on the Framingham criteria. Furthermore, there were no patients who dropped out.

There are some potential limitations. Firstly, our study was a observational study at a single institution, and thus the numbers of subjects were relatively small. Although the PS analyses are useful, they are inherently limited by the number and accuracy of the variables evaluated. Importantly, we cannot rule out residual confounding from unknown or unmeasured variables. There might be potential bias and although we analyzed present data using multivariate Cox proportional hazard regression analyses

and PS analyses to minimize selection bias under consideration of multiple confounding factors, the effects of the differences in clinical background between the groups might not be completely adjusted. Secondly, we have assessed this study using only variables on hospitalization, without consideration of changes in medical parameters and post-discharge treatment. There might be some cross over in medication during follow up. Thirdly, TTR of VKAs was insufficient; however, TTR in this study was higher than those of previous studies [7–9]. Finally, the differences of each DOAC were not considered in this study. For these reasons, the results of our study should be viewed as preliminary. Hence, further clinical trials for HHF patients with concomitant AF using DOACs are required with a larger population and/or randomization.

Conclusion

The appropriate use of anticoagulants in HHF patients with AF is important, and DOACs potentially improve all-cause mortality in such patients.

Abbreviations
AF: Atrial fibrillation; BNP: B-type natriuretic peptide; CI: Confidence interval; CKD: Chronic kidney disease; DOACs: Direct oral anticoagulants; HF: Heart failure; HHF: Hospitalized heart failure; HR: Hazard ratio; LVEF: Left ventricular ejection fraction; PS: Propensity score; RR: Relative risk; SR: Sinus rhythm; TTR: Time in therapeutic range; VKAs: Vit K antagonists

Acknowledgements
The authors acknowledge the efforts of Dr. Tetsuya Ohira (Department of Epidemiology) for his invaluable advice on medical statistics, as well as Ms. Kumiko Watanabe and Ms. Hitomi Kobayashi for their outstanding technical assistance, and Dr. Shunsuke Watanabe, Dr. Yuki Kanno, Dr. Akihiko Sato, Dr. Tetsuro Yokokawa, Dr. Shunsuke Miura, Dr. Satoshi Abe, Dr. Atsushi Kobayashi, Dr. Takayoshi Yamaki, Dr. Hiroyuki Kunii, Dr. Kazuhiko Nakazato, Dr. Hitoshi Suzuki and Dr. Shu-ichi Saitoh for their acquisition of data.

Funding
Not applicable

Authors' contributions
AY, SS and YT, making article, drafting the article and conception of this study; YS, TS analysis and interpretation of data; MO, and YT revising the article critically for important intellectual content. All authors read and approved the final manuscript.

Competing interests
The authors declare that they have no competing interests

References
1. Savelieva I, John Camm A. Atrial fibrillation and heart failure: natural history and pharmacological treatment. Europace. 2004;5(Suppl 1):S5–19.
2. Santhanakrishnan R, Wang N, Larson MG, Magnani JW, McManus DD, Lubitz SA, Ellinor PT, Cheng S, Vasan RS, Lee DS, et al. Atrial fibrillation begets heart failure and vice versa: temporal associations and differences in preserved versus reduced ejection fraction. Circulation. 2016;133(5):484–92.
3. Wang TJ, Larson MG, Levy D, Vasan RS, Leip EP, Wolf PA, D'Agostino RB, Murabito JM, Kannel WB, Benjamin EJ. Temporal relations of atrial fibrillation and congestive heart failure and their joint influence on mortality: the Framingham heart study. Circulation. 2003;107(23):2920–5.

4. Maisel WH, Stevenson LW. Atrial fibrillation in heart failure: epidemiology, pathophysiology, and rationale for therapy. Am J Cardiol. 2003;91(6A):2D–8D.

5. Lip GY, Laroche C, Ioachim PM, Rasmussen LH, Vitali-Serdoz L, Petrescu L, Darabantiu D, Crijns HJ, Kirchhof P, Vardas P, et al. Prognosis and treatment of atrial fibrillation patients by European cardiologists: one year follow-up of the EURObservational research Programme-Atrial fibrillation general registry pilot phase (EORP-AF pilot registry). Eur Heart J. 2014;35(47):3365–76.

6. Reinier K, Marijon E, Uy-Evanado A, Teodorescu C, Narayanan K, Chugh H, Gunson K, Jui J, Chugh SS. The association between atrial fibrillation and sudden cardiac death: the relevance of heart failure. JACC Heart failure. 2014;2(3):221–7.

7. Ferreira J, Ezekowitz MD, Connolly SJ, Brueckmann M, Fraessdorf M, Reilly PA, Yusuf S, Wallentin L, Investigators R-L. Dabigatran compared with warfarin in patients with atrial fibrillation and symptomatic heart failure: a subgroup analysis of the RE-LY trial. Eur J Heart Fail. 2013;15(9):1053–61.

8. McMurray JJ, Ezekowitz JA, Lewis BS, Gersh BJ, van Diepen S, Amerena J, Bartunek J, Commerford P, Oh BH, Harjola VP, et al. Left ventricular systolic dysfunction, heart failure, and the risk of stroke and systemic embolism in patients with atrial fibrillation: insights from the ARISTOTLE trial. Circ Heart Fail. 2013;6(3):451–60.

9. van Diepen S, Hellkamp AS, Patel MR, Becker RC, Breithardt G, Hacke W, Halperin JL, Hankey GJ, Nessel CC, Singer DE, et al. Efficacy and safety of rivaroxaban in patients with heart failure and nonvalvular atrial fibrillation: insights from ROCKET AF. Circ Heart Fail. 2013;6(4):740–7.

10. Camm AJ, Lip GY, De Caterina R, Savelieva I, Atar D, Hohnloser SH, Hindricks G, Kirchhof P, Guidelines ESCCfP. Focused update of the ESC guidelines for the management of atrial fibrillation: an update of the 2010 ESC guidelines for the management of atrial fibrillation. Developed with the special contribution of the European heart rhythm association. Eur Heart J 2012. 2012;33(21):2719–47.

11. Okumura K, Hori M, Tanahashi N, John Camm A. Special considerations for therapeutic choice of non-vitamin K antagonist oral anticoagulants for Japanese patients with nonvalvular atrial fibrillation. Clin Cardiol. 2017;40(2):126–31.

12. Ruff CT, Giugliano RP, Braunwald E, Hoffman EB, Deenadayalu N, Ezekowitz MD, Camm AJ, Weitz JI, Lewis BS, Parkhomenko A, et al. Comparison of the efficacy and safety of new oral anticoagulants with warfarin in patients with atrial fibrillation: a meta-analysis of randomised trials. Lancet. 2014;383(9921):955–62.

13. Albert NM. Use of novel oral anticoagulants for patients with atrial fibrillation: systematic review and clinical implications. Heart Lung. 2014;43(1):48–59.

14. Xiong Q, Lau YC, Senoo K, Lane DA, Hong K, Lip GY. Non-vitamin K antagonist oral anticoagulants (NOACs) in patients with concomitant atrial fibrillation and heart failure: a systemic review and meta-analysis of randomized trials. Eur J Heart Fail. 2015;17(11):1192–200.

15. Vaduganathan M, Butler J, Roessig L, Fonarow GC, Greene SJ, Metra M, Cotter G, Kupfer S, Zalewski A, Sato N, et al. Clinical trials in hospitalized heart failure patients: targeting interventions to optimal phenotypic subpopulations. Heart Fail Rev. 2015;20(4):393–400.

16. Ambrosy AP, Fonarow GC, Butler J, Chioncel O, Greene SJ, Vaduganathan M, Nodari S, Lam CS, Sato N, Shah AN, et al. The global health and economic burden of hospitalizations for heart failure: lessons learned from hospitalized heart failure registries. J Am Coll Cardiol. 2014;63(12):1123–33.

17. Fonarow GC, Albert NM, Curtis AB, Gheorghiade M, Heywood JT, Liu Y, Mehra MR, O'Connor CM, Reynolds D, Walsh MN, et al. Associations between outpatient heart failure process-of-care measures and mortality. Circulation. 2011;123(15):1601–10.

18. Camm AJ, Accetta G, Ambrosio G, Atar D, Bassand JP, Berge E, Cools F, Fitzmaurice DA, Goldhaber SZ, Goto S, et al. Evolving antithrombotic treatment patterns for patients with newly diagnosed atrial fibrillation. Heart. 2017;103(4):307–14.

19. McKee PA, Castelli WP, McNamara PM, Kannel WB. The natural history of congestive heart failure: the Framingham study. N Engl J Med. 1971;285(26):1441–6.

20. von Elm E, Altman DG, Egger M, Pocock SJ, Gotzsche PC, Vandenbroucke JP, Initiative S. Strengthening the reporting of observational studies in epidemiology (STROBE) statement: guidelines for reporting observational studies. BMJ. 2007;335(7624):806–8.

21. D'Agostino RB Jr. Propensity score methods for bias reduction in the comparison of a treatment to a non-randomized control group. Stat Med. 1998;17(19):2265 81.

22. Heinze G, Juni P. An overview of the objectives of and the approaches to propensity score analyses. Eur Heart J. 2011;32(14):1704–8.

23. Austin PC. A critical appraisal of propensity-score matching in the medical literature between 1996 and 2003. Stat Med. 2008;27(12):2037–49.

24. Connolly SJ, Ezekowitz MD, Yusuf S, Eikelboom J, Oldgren J, Parekh A, Pogue J, Reilly PA, Themeles E, Varrone J, et al. Dabigatran versus warfarin in patients with atrial fibrillation. N Engl J Med. 2009;361(12):1139–51.

25. Patel MR, Mahaffey KW, Garg J, Pan G, Singer DE, Hacke W, Breithardt G, Halperin JL, Hankey GJ, Piccini JP, et al. Rivaroxaban versus warfarin in nonvalvular atrial fibrillation. N Engl J Med. 2011;365(10):883–91.

26. Granger CB, Alexander JH, McMurray JJ, Lopes RD, Hylek EM, Hanna M, Al-Khalidi HR, Ansell J, Atar D, Avezum A, et al. Apixaban versus warfarin in patients with atrial fibrillation. N Engl J Med. 2011;365(11):981–92.

27. Giugliano RP, Ruff CT, Braunwald E, Murphy SA, Wiviott SD, Halperin JL, Waldo AL, Ezekowitz MD, Weitz JI, Spinar J, et al. Edoxaban versus warfarin in patients with atrial fibrillation. N Engl J Med. 2013;369(22):2093–104.

28. Nelson WW, Choi JC, Vanderpoel J, Damaraju CV, Wildgoose P, Fields LE, Schein JR. Impact of co-morbidities and patient characteristics on international normalized ratio control over time in patients with nonvalvular atrial fibrillation. Am J Cardiol. 2013;112(4):509–12.

29. Chan YH, Yeh YH, See LC, Wang CL, Chang SH, Lee HF, Wu LS, Tu HT, Kuo CT. Acute kidney injury in Asians with Atrial fibrillation treated with Dabigatran or Warfarin. J Am Coll Cardiol. 2016;68(21):2272–83.

30. Vaughan Sarrazin MS, Jones M, Mazur A, Cram P, Ayyagari P, Chrischilles E. Cost of hospital admissions in Medicare patients with Atrial fibrillation taking Warfarin, Dabigatran, or rivaroxaban. J Am Coll Cardiol. 2017;69(3):360–2.

Permissions

All chapters in this book were first published in CD, by BioMed Central; hereby published with permission under the Creative Commons Attribution License or equivalent. Every chapter published in this book has been scrutinized by our experts. Their significance has been extensively debated. The topics covered herein carry significant findings which will fuel the growth of the discipline. They may even be implemented as practical applications or may be referred to as a beginning point for another development.

The contributors of this book come from diverse backgrounds, making this book a truly international effort. This book will bring forth new frontiers with its revolutionizing research information and detailed analysis of the nascent developments around the world.

We would like to thank all the contributing authors for lending their expertise to make the book truly unique. They have played a crucial role in the development of this book. Without their invaluable contributions this book wouldn't have been possible. They have made vital efforts to compile up to date information on the varied aspects of this subject to make this book a valuable addition to the collection of many professionals and students.

This book was conceptualized with the vision of imparting up-to-date information and advanced data in this field. To ensure the same, a matchless editorial board was set up. Every individual on the board went through rigorous rounds of assessment to prove their worth. After which they invested a large part of their time researching and compiling the most relevant data for our readers.

The editorial board has been involved in producing this book since its inception. They have spent rigorous hours researching and exploring the diverse topics which have resulted in the successful publishing of this book. They have passed on their knowledge of decades through this book. To expedite this challenging task, the publisher supported the team at every step. A small team of assistant editors was also appointed to further simplify the editing procedure and attain best results for the readers.

Apart from the editorial board, the designing team has also invested a significant amount of their time in understanding the subject and creating the most relevant covers. They scrutinized every image to scout for the most suitable representation of the subject and create an appropriate cover for the book.

The publishing team has been an ardent support to the editorial, designing and production team. Their endless efforts to recruit the best for this project, has resulted in the accomplishment of this book. They are a veteran in the field of academics and their pool of knowledge is as vast as their experience in printing. Their expertise and guidance has proved useful at every step. Their uncompromising quality standards have made this book an exceptional effort. Their encouragement from time to time has been an inspiration for everyone.

The publisher and the editorial board hope that this book will prove to be a valuable piece of knowledge for researchers, students, practitioners and scholars across the globe.

List of Contributors

Fei Zhao, Shi Jiang Zhang, Yi Jiang Chen, Wei Dong Gu, Bu Qing Ni, Yong Feng Shao, Yan Hu Wu and Jian Wei Qin
Cardiothoracic Surgery Department, First Affiliated Hospital of Nanjing Medical University, 300 Guangzhou RoadJiangsu Province, Nanjing 210029, China

Yangjing Xue, Saroj Thapa, Jiaoni Wang, Zhiqiang Xu, Shaoze Wu, Luyuan Tao, Guoqiang Wang, Lu Qian and Kangting Ji
Department of Cardiology, the Second Affiliated Hospital and Yuying Children's Hospital of Wenzhou Medical University, Xueyuanxi Road, No 109, Wenzhou, Zhejiang 325000, China

Baohua Liu
Department of Rehabilitation, the Second Affiliated Hospital and Yuying Children's Hospital of Wenzhou Medical University, Xueyuanxi Road, No 109, Wenzhou, Zhejiang 325000, China

Xiaoning Wang
Department of Intensive Care Unit, Zhengzhou Central Hospital Affiliated to Zhengzhou University, Tongbaibei Road, No 195, Zhengzhou, Henan 450000, China

Luping Wang
Department of Endocrinology, the Fourth Affiliated Hospital, Zhejiang University School of Medicine, Shangcheng Road, No N1, Yiwu, Zhejiang 322000, China

Lianming Liao
Department of Oncology, Academy of Integrative Medicine, Fujian University of Traditional Chinese Medicine, Huatuo Road, No 1, Fuzhou, Fujian 350122, China

Hesheng Hu, Yongli Xuan, Mei Xue, Wenjuan Cheng, Ye Wang, Xinran Li, Jie Yin, Xiaolu Li, Na Yang, Yugen Shi and Suhua Yan
Department of Cardiology, Shandong Provincial Qianfoshan Hospital, Shandong University, 250014 Jinan, China

Oliver Königsbrügge, Ingrid Pabinger and Cihan Ay
Department of Medicine I, Clinical Division of Hematology & Hemostaseology, Medical University of Vienna, Währinger Gürtel 18-20, A-1090 Vienna, Austria

Alexander Simon and Hans Domanovits
Department of Emergency Medicine, Medical University of Vienna, Vienna, Austria

Cihan Ay
Department of Medicine, Thrombosis and Hemostasis Program, McAllister Heart Institute, University of North Carolina at Chapel Hill, Chapel Hill, NC, USA

Qingzhi Luo, Qi Jin, Ning Zhang, Yanxin Han, Yilong Wang, Shangwei Huang, Changjian Lin, Tianyou Ling, Kang Chen, Wenqi Pan and Liqun Wu
Department of Cardiology, Shanghai Ruijin Hospital, Shanghai Jiao Tong University School of Medicine, No. 197, Ruijin Er Road, Shanghai 200025, People's Republic of China

Jiangang Wang, Shiqiu Song, Jie Han, Yan Li, Meng Xin, Jun Wang, Tiange Luo and Xu Meng
Department of Cardiac Surgery, Beijing Anzhen Hospital, Capital Medical University, Beijing 100029, P. R. China

Changqing Xie
Department of Internal Medicine, Vidant Medical Center, Broody School of Medicine, East Carolina University, Greenville, North Carolina 27834, USA

Jiahai Shi
Department of Cardiothoracic Surgery, Affiliated Hospital of Nantong University, Nantong 226001, China

Bo Yang
University of Michigan Cardiovascular Center, University of Michigan, Ann Arbor, Michigan 48109, USA

A. Tsyganov, A. Shapieva, S. Fedulova and S. Mironovich
Cardiac Electrophysiology Department, Petrovsky National Research Centre of Surgery, Abrikosovsky per. 2, Moscow 119991, Russia

V. Sandrikov, S. Fedulova and A. Dzeranova
Department of Clinical Physiology, Radiology and Diagnostic Imaging, Petrovsky National Research Centre of Surgery, Abrikosovsky per. 2, Moscow, Russia

E. Lyan
Cardiac Electrophysiology Department, Mechnikov North-West State Medical University, Kirochnaya ul. 41, Saint Petersburg 191015, Russia

Jūratė Barysienė, Aistė Žebrauskaitė, Dovilė Petrikonytė, Germanas Marinskis, Sigita Aidietienė and Audrius Aidietis
Centre of Cardiology and Angiology, Vilnius University Hospital Santariskiu Clinics, 2 Santariškių St., LT -08661 Vilnius, Lithuania
Clinic of Cardiovascular Diseases, Faculty of Medicine, Vilnius University, 21 Čiurlionio St., LT-03101 Vilnius, Lithuania

Daniel Cortez, Maria Baturova, Jonas Carlson, Bertil Olsson and Pyotr G. Platonov
Department of Cardiology, Clinical Sciences, Lund University, Lund, Sweden

Daniel Cortez
Electrophysiology Department, Penn State Milton S. Hershey Medical Center, Hershey, USA

Maria Baturova
St. Petersburg University Clinic, St. Petersburg, Russia

Maria Baturova and Yuri V. Shubik
Cardiology Research, Clinical and Educational Center, St. Petersburg State University, St. Petersburg, Russia

Arne Lindgren
Department of Neurology and Rehabilitation Medicine, Skane University Hospital, Lund, Sweden
Department of Clinical Sciences Lund, Neurology, Lund University, Lund, Sweden

Pyotr G. Platonov
Arrhythmia Clinic, Skåne University Hospital, Lund, Sweden

Matthew D. Solomon, Jingrong Yang, Sue Hee Sung and Alan S. Go
Division of Research, Kaiser Permanente Northern California, Oakland, CA, USA

Matthew D. Solomon and Alan S. Go
Stanford University School of Medicine, Stanford, CA, USA

Martha L. Livingston and Judith C. Lenane
iRhythm Technologies, Inc, San Francisco, CA, USA

Alan S. Go
Departments of Epidemiology, Biostatistics and Medicine, University of California, San Francisco, CA, USA

Matthew D. Solomon
Department of Cardiology, Kaiser Permanente Oakland Medical Center, 3600 Broadway, Oakland, CA 94611, USA

Chuan Nan Zhai, Hong Liang Cong, Yu Jie Liu, Ying Zhang, Xian Feng Liu, Hao Zhang and Zhi Jing Ren
Department of Cardiology, Tianjin Chest Hospital, Taierzhuang South Road No. 291, Jinnan District, Tianjin, 300350, China

Chuan Nan Zhai, Xian Feng Liu, Hao Zhang and Zhi Jing Ren
Graduate School, Tianjin Medical University, Tianjin 300051, China

Chuan Nan Zhai
Department of Cardiology, Tianjin Gongan Hospital, Xinhua Road No. 162, Heping District, Tianjin, 300042, China

Ryan T. Borne, Paul D. Varosy, Lucas N. Marzec, Frederick A. Masoudi, Paul L. Hess and P. Michael Ho
Division of Cardiology – Campus Box B130, University of Colorado Anschutz Medical Campus, 12631 E. 17th Avenue, Aurora, CO 80045, USA

Colin O'Donnell, Paul D. Varosy, Paul L. Hess and P. Michael Ho
VA Eastern Colorado Health Care System, Denver, CO, USA

Mintu P. Turakhia
Veterans Affairs Palo Alto Health Care System, Palo Alto, CA, USA

Mintu P. Turakhia
Stanford University School of Medicine, Stanford, CA, USA

Cynthia A. Jackevicius
VA Greater Los Angeles Healthcare System, Institute for Clinical Evaluative Sciences, Western University of Health Sciences, Los Angeles, CA, USA

Thomas M. Maddox
Washington University School of Medicine, St. Louis, MO, USA

Vivian Wing-Yan Lee, Ronald Bing-Ching Tsai and Ines Hang-Iao Chow
School of Pharmacy, Faculty of Medicine, The Chinese University of Hong Kong, 8th Floor, Lo Kwee-Seong Integrated Biomedical Sciences Building, Area 39, Shatin, Hong Kong

Bryan Ping-Yen Yan and Yat-Yin Lam
Department of Medicine and Therapeutics, Faculty of Medicine, The Chinese University of Hong Kong, Prince of Wales Hospital, Shatin, Hong Kong

Mehmet Gungor Kaya
Department of Cardiology, Erciyes University School of Medicine, Kayseri, Turkey

Jai-Wun Park
Charité University Medicine Berlin, Klinikum Coburg, Coburg, Germany

Guo-Zhe Sun, Liang Guo, Jun Wang, Ning Ye and Ying-Xian Sun
Department of Cardiovascular Medicine, The First Hospital of China Medical University, 155 Nanjing Street, Heping, Shenyang, Liaoning 110001, China

Xun-Zhang Wang
Heart Institute, Cedars Sinai Medical Center, Los Angeles 90048, CA, USA

Zhiwei Zhang, Xiaowei Zhang, Mengqi Gong, Lei Meng, Guangping Li and Tong Liu
Tianjin Key Laboratory of Ionic-Molecular Function of Cardiovascular Disease, Department of Cardiology, Tianjin Institute of Cardiology, Second Hospital of Tianjin Medical University, No. 23 Pingjiang Road, Hexi District, Tianjin 300211, People's Republic of China

Panagiotis Korantzopoulos
First Department of Cardiology, University of Ioannina Medical School, Ioannina, Greece

Konstantinos P. Letsas
Second Department of Cardiology, Laboratory of Cardiac Electrophysiology, "Evangelismos" General Hospital of Athens, Athens, Greece

Gary Tse
Department of Medicine and Therapeutics, Faculty of Medicine, Chinese University of Hong Kong, Hong Kong, SAR, People's Republic of China Li KaShing Institute of Health Sciences, Faculty of Medicine, Chinese University of Hong Kong, Hong Kong, SAR, People's Republic of China

Rami Riziq-Yousef Abumuaileq, Emad Abu-Assi, Andrea López-López, Sergio Raposeiras-Roubin, Moisés Rodríguez-Mañero, Luis Martínez-Sande, Javier García-Seara, Xesús Alberte Fernandez-López, Carlos Peña-Gil and Jose Ramón González-Juanatey
Cardiology Department, University Clinical Hospital, A choupana s/n, 15706, Santiago de Compostela, Spain

Faye L. Norby, Pamela L. Lutsey, Richard F. MacLehose and Ian Rapson
Division of Epidemiology and Community Health, School of Public Health, University of Minnesota, 1300 S 2nd St, Suite 300, Minneapolis, MN 55454, USA

Lindsay G. S. Bengtson
Health Economics and Outcomes Research, Life Sciences, Optum, Eden Prairie, MN, USA

Lin Y. Chen
Cardiac Arrhythmia Center, Cardiovascular Division, Department of Medicine, University of Minnesota Medical School, Minneapolis, MN, USA

Alanna M. Chamberlain
Department of Health Sciences Research, Mayo Clinic, Rochester, MN, USA

Alvaro Alonso
Department of Epidemiology, Rollins School of Public Health, Emory University, Atlanta, GA, USA

Satoshi Higuchi, Yusuke Kabeya, Kenichi Matsushita and Hideaki Yoshino
Division of Cardiology, Department of Internal Medicine II, Kyorin University School of Medicine, Tokyo, Japan

Yusuke Kabeya
Division of General Internal Medicine, Department of Internal Medicine, Tokai University, Isehara, Kanagawa, Japan
Department of Home Care Medicine, Saiyu Clinic, Saitama, Japan

Keisei Tachibana and Hidefumi Takei
Department of General Thoracic Surgery, Kyorin University School of Medicine, Tokyo, Japan

Riken Kawachi
Department of General Thoracic Surgery, Nihon University School of Medicine, Tokyo, Japan

Yutaka Suzuki, Nobutsugu Abe and Masanori Sugiyama
Department of Surgery, Kyorin University School of Medicine, Tokyo, Japan

Yorihisa Imanishi
Department of Otorhinolaryngology, Head and Neck Surgery, Kawasaki Municipal Kawasaki Hospital, Kawasaki, Kanagawa, Japan

Kiyoshi Moriyama and Tomoko Yorozu
Department of Anesthesiology, Kyorin University School of Medicine, Tokyo, Japan

Koichiro Saito
Department of Otolaryngology-Head and Neck Surgery, Kyorin University School of Medicine, Tokyo, Japan

Satoshi Higuchi
Division of Cardiology, Department of Internal Medicine II, Kyorin University School of Medicine, 6-20-2 Shinkawa, Mitaka City, Tokyo 181-8611, Japan

Joerg Herold, Vasiliki Herold-Vlanti, Blerim Luani, Christin Breyer and Ruediger Braun-Dullaeus
Department of Internal Medicine/Cardiology and Angiology, Otto-von-Guericke University of Magdeburg, Leipziger Str. 44, 39120 Magdeburg, Germany

Mohammad Sherif
Department of Internal Medicine/Cardiology and Angiology, University of Rostock, Ernst-Heydemann-Straße 6, 18057 Rostock, Germany

Klaus Bonaventura
Department of Internal Medicine/Cardiology and Angiology, Ernst-von-Bergmannstrost Clinic, Charlottenstraße 72, 14467 Potsdam, Germany

Dong-Hyeok Kim, Jong-Il Choi, Kwang No Lee, Jinhee Ahn, Seung Young Roh, Dae In Lee, Jaemin Shim, Jin Seok Kim, Hong Euy Lim, Sang Weon Park and Young-Hoon Kim
Division of Cardiology, Department of Internal Medicine, Korea University College of Medicine and Korea University Medical Center, 73, Inchon-ro, Seongbuk-gu, Seoul 02841, Republic of Korea

Shirvan Salaminia
Department of Cardiac Surgery, Yasuj University of Medical Science, Yasuj, Iran

Fatemeh Sayehmiri
Proteomics Research Center, Shahid Beheshti University of Medical Sciences, Tehran, Iran

Parvin Angha
Social Determinants of Health Research Center, Yasuj University of Medical Sciences, Yasuj, Iran

Koroush Sayehmiri
Department of Social Medicine, School of Medicine, Ilam University of Medical Sciences, Ilam, Iran

Morteza Motedayen
Department of Cardiology, Faculty of Medicine, Zanjan University of Medical Sciences, Zanjan, Iran

Herbert J. A. Rolden
Council for Public Health and Society, The Hague, The Netherlands

Herbert J. A. Rolden, Gert Jan van der Wilt and Janneke P. C. Grutters
Department for Health Evidence, Radboud University Medical Center, Nijmegen, The Netherlands.

Angela H. E. M. Maas
Department of Cardiology, Radboud University Medical Center, Nijmegen, The Netherlands

Rungroj Krittayaphong, Arjbordin Winijkul, Pontawee Kaewcomdee and Ahthit Yindeengam
Division of Cardiology, Department of Medicine, Faculty of Medicine Siriraj Hospital, Mahidol University, 2 Wanglang Road, Bangkoknoi, Bangkok 10700, Thailand

Komsing Methavigul
Department of Cardiology, Central Chest Institute
of Thailand, Nonthaburi, Thailand

Wattana Wongtheptien
Chiangrai Prachanukroh Hospital, Chiang Rai,
Thailand

Chaiyasith Wongvipaporn
Srinakarind Hospital, Faculty of Medicine, Khon
Kaen University, Khon Kaen, Thailand

Treechada Wisaratapong
Faculty of Medicine, Prince of Songkla University,
Songkla, Thailand

Rapeephon Kunjara-Na-Ayudhya
Vichaiyut Hospital and Medical Center, Bangkok,
Thailand

Smonporn Boonyaratvej
Faculty of Medicine, Chulalongkorn University,
Bangkok, Thailand

Chulalak Komoltri
Department of Research Promotion, Faculty of
Medicine Siriraj Hospital, Mahidol University,
Bangkok, Thailand

Piyamitr Sritara
Faculty of Medicine Ramathibodi Hospital, Mahidol
University, Bangkok, Thailand

Chaoyue Hu
Key Laboratory of Arrhythmias of the Ministry of
Education of China, Tongji University School of
Medicine, Shanghai 200092, China

**Xumin Zhang, Yang Gao, Xiaohong Zhao, Hua
Zhou, Yu Luo and Xiaodong Wang**
Department of Cardiology, Shanghai East Hospital,
Tongji University School of Medicine, 150 Jimo
Road, Shanghai 200120, China

Yonghua Liu
Cardiovascular Medicine of Baoshan People's
Hospital of Yunnan Province, Baoshan 678000,
China

Yaling Liu
Department of Anesthesiology, Renji Hospital,
Shanghai Jiaotong University School of Medicine,
160 Pujian Road, Shanghai 200127, China

Elke Parsi and Anne Winkelmann
Outpatient Practice of Cardiology, Suermondtstr.
13, D-13053 Berlin, Germany

Norman Bitterlich
Medicine and Service Ltd, Department of
Biostatistics, Boettcherstr. 10, D-09117 Chemnitz,
Germany

Daniela Rösler and Christine Metzner
Bonn Education Association for Dietetics r. A,
Fuerst-Pueckler-Str. 44, D-50935 Cologne, Germany

Christine Metzner
Department of Internal Medicine III, Uniklinik
RWTH Aachen, Pauwelsstraße 44, D-52074 Aachen,
Germany

**Akiomi Yoshihisa, Yu Sato, Takamasa Sato,
Satoshi Suzuki, Masayoshi Oikawa and Yasuchika
Takeishi**
Department of Cardiovascular Medicine, Fukushima
Medical University, 1 Hikarigaoka, Fukushima 960-
1295, Japan

Index

P

P-wave Duration, 66-67, 70-72, 170

P-wave Vector Magnitude, 66-67, 69-71

Paired-like Homeodomain Transcription Factor 2, 87

Percutaneous Coronary Intervention, 121, 163, 182, 194, 199-200, 202, 207-209

Perioperative Atrial Fibrillation, 145-150

Pioglitazone, 118-121, 123-126

Pocket Hematoma, 171

Prasugrel, 200, 207-209

Pro-collagen I, 1, 5, 9-11

R

Randomized Controlled Trials, 30, 32, 90, 93, 119, 123, 174-175, 180, 183

Rivaroxaban, 29, 31-34, 36, 52-56, 59-60, 64, 90-95, 97-103, 105, 109-110, 133-144, 161, 164, 184-185, 188-192, 207, 224, 228-230

Rosiglitazone, 118-121, 123-126

S

Semaphorin 3a, 19, 27-28

Serum Creatinine, 30, 133, 147-148

Serum Magnesium Level, 174-175, 181-183, 219

Serum Uric Acid, 111, 113-116

Single-nucleotide Polymorphism, 81-82

Sinus Rhythm, 1-2, 4-5, 10-11, 31, 34-35, 47, 50, 54-55, 59, 64-65, 67, 73, 75, 125, 151, 163, 169, 196, 229

Sulfonylurea, 121

Supraventricular Arrhythmia, 59, 174, 177-178, 180

Symptomatic Aortic Valve Stenosis, 151, 157

T

T-allele, 81-82, 84-88

Tachycardia-bradycardia Syndrome, 172

Thiazolidinedione, 118, 125

Thrombi, 52, 55-56, 58-64

Thromboembolism, 29-30, 32-35, 52-53, 55-56, 58, 61, 64, 127, 131-133, 144, 150, 186, 191, 199-200, 203-207

Ticagrelor, 200, 207

Transcatheter Aortic Valve Replacement, 151, 163-165

Transesophageal Echocardiography, 52-53, 56-57, 64, 97, 103

Troglitazone, 119-121, 125

Tumor Necrosis Factor, 49, 124

V

Vasodilatorstimulated Phosphoprotein, 199

Ventricular Arrhythmia, 19, 21-22, 66-67, 73, 174-178

Ventricular Tachycardia, 21, 24, 28, 43, 74-77, 176-178

Vitamin-k-antagonist, 30, 32-35, 127

W

Warfarin, 2, 13-14, 30, 32-33, 36, 56-64, 90-93, 95, 97-103, 105, 108-110, 134-144, 168-169, 191-198, 200-202, 204-208, 223-224, 230

Z

Zinc Finger Homeobox 3, 81-82, 87, 89

www.ingramcontent.com/pod-product-compliance
Lightning Source LLC
Chambersburg PA
CBHW080409190526

45161CB00003B/177